Textbook of
Community
Health Nursing

SUNITA PATNEY

M.Sc. (Nursing), RN, RM

Faculty, RAK College of Nursing
Delhi University, Delhi

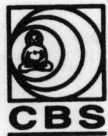

CBS

CBS Publishers & Distributors Pvt. Ltd.

New Delhi • Bengaluru • Chennai • Kochi • Kolkata • Mumbai
Hyderabad • Nagpur • Patna • Pune • Vijayawada

ISBN: 978-81-239-1557-9

First Edition: 2005
Reprint: 2008, 2011, 2013, 2017

Published by **Satish Kumar Jain** and produced by **Varun Jain** for
CBS Publishers & Distributors Pvt. Ltd.,
4819/XI Prahlad Street, 24 Ansari Road, Daryaganj, New Delhi - 110002
delhi@cbspd.com, cbspubs@airtelmail.in • www.cbspd.com
Ph.: 23289259, 23266861, 23266867 • Fax: 011-23243014

Corporate Office: 204 FIE, Industrial Area, Patparganj, Delhi - 110 092
Ph: 49344934 • Fax: 011-49344935
E-mail: publishing@cbspd.com • publicity@cbspd.com

Branches:
• *Bengaluru:* 2975, 17th Cross, K.R. Road, Bansankari 2nd Stage,
  Bengaluru - 70 • Ph: +91-80-26771678/79 • Fax: +91-80-26771680
  E-mail: cbsbng@gmail.com, bangalore@cbspd.com
• *Chennai:* No. 7, Subbaraya Street, Shenoy Nagar, Chennai - 600030
  Ph: +91-44-26681266, 26680620 • Fax: +91-44-42032115
  E-mail: chennai@cbspd.com
• *Kochi:* Ashana House, 39/1904, A.M. Thomas Road, Valanjambalam,
  Ernakulum, Kochi • Ph: +91-484-4059061-65
  Fax: +91-484-4059065 • E-mail: cochin@cbspd.com
• *Kolkata:* 6-B, Ground Floor, Rameshwar Shaw Road, Kolkata - 700014
  Ph: +91-33-22891126/7/8 • E-mail: kolkata@cbspd.com
• *Mumbai:* 83-C, Dr. E. Moses Road, Worli, Mumbai - 400018
  Ph: +91-9833017933, 022-24902340/41 • E-mail: mumbai@cbspd.com

Representatives:

• Hyderabad: 0-9885175004   • Nagpur: 0-9021734563
• Patna: 0-9334159340   • Pune: 0-9623451994
• Vijayawada: 0-9000660880

Printed at:
Neekunj Print Process, Delhi (India)

PREFACE

I take immense pleasure in presenting this book entitled **"Textbook of Community Health Nursing"**. During my over 25 years of teaching experience, I always felt the need of a book that is complete in all respects for students. I have written this book so as to fulfil the requirements of the students for better understanding and knowledge of the fundamentals of Community Health Nursing. Some special features of the book are :

- The language has been made as simple as possible with every effort to make it free of confusion, so that not only students learn better but they also develop an interest.

- Detailed theory has been supplemented with illustrations in the form of pictures, graphs, data, tables *etc.*, for better understanding.

- At the end of each chapter, subjective questions have been provided in two forms viz., Short Answer Type Questions and Long Answer Type Questions, so that students can test their knowledge of the chapter.

- Objective questions, with answers, based on all chapters have been provided for quick review of the syllabus.

- Previous years questions papers of the Delhi University have been provided.

- A special effort has also been made to minimise errors.

I do hope that the students will like the book and gain knowledge from it.

I take this opportunity to thank the MBD and their entire staff in general and *Mr. Brijesh Singh (Editor)* particularly for putting up his sincere efforts in compiling and publishing this book.

Inspite of our best efforts, some errors might have crept in. I will be very greateful to the teachers and students, if the same is brought to my notice. I also welcome constructive suggestions for improvement of the book.

—Sunita Patney

CONTENTS

UNIT – V

EPIDEMIOLOGY OF NON-COMMUNICABLE DISEASES   187–238

UNIT – VI

EPIDEMIOLOGY OF COMMUNICABLE DISEASES   239–390

=== UNIT – VII ===

HEALTH INFORMATION AND STATISTICS

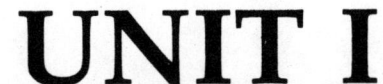

UNIT I

HISTORY OF COMMUNITY HEALTH AND COMMUNITY HEALTH CARE

- History of Community Health
- Changing Concept of Public Health and Primary Health Care
- Development of Community Health in India and Five-Year Plans

UNIT 1

HISTORY OF COMMUNITY HEALTH AND COMMUNITY HEALTH CARE

- History of Community Health
- Changing Concept of Public Health and Primary Health Care
- Development of Community Health in India and Five-Year Plans

History of Community Health

INTRODUCTION

The history of community health nursing can be traced to earliest record of civilization. Throughout its development there have been numerous programme **campaigns** often overshadowed by transient setbacks as health has been alternately given high priority and many of the advances in community health arose out of necessity. Epidemics and other devastating health conditions demanded resolutions that could not be postponed until a more propitious time.

Origin of Community Medicine

In ancient times, there was complete absence of scientific knowledge. Primitive medicine was based on trial and error basis. There was no definite diagnosis and treatment of various illnesses. History of medicine constituted errors, false theories and misinformations. In the stage of evolution, medicine has been drawn largely from traditional cultures and concepts of which it is a part and later from biological and natural sciences and then social and behavioural sciences. Medicine has evolved itself into a social system with social goals. Due to limited knowledge, the primitive man considered human sufferings as 'evil spirit' in the body and God's wish and influence of stars as well as planets and also due to individuals 'karma'. The concept of disease is said to be 'supernatural theory of disease'. They believed that disease can be treated by pleasing Gods by prayers, performing rituals, sacrificing animals and removing the evil spirits from the body.

Indian System of Medicine

The Indian system of medicine can be traced back to Vedic times, about 5000 B.C. During this period, the Ayurveda and the Siddha systems were in practice throughout the country, though Siddha was more common in southern part of India. Ayurveda had tremendous growth and development during Buddhist times. During the period 500 B.C. to A.D. 700, development in medicine took place to maximum. One of the principles of Buddhism was to help the sick. The king Ashoka (220-250 B.C.) was influenced by the Principles of Buddhism and worked towards the welfare of humanity—the common man, which is the main object of twentieth century. He established a large number of hospitals both for men and animals. The sick were treated at home and hospitals.

Ayurveda was practised throughout India in Vedic times around 5000 B.C. Atreya, Charaka, Sushuruta and Vaghbhatta were duly celebrated authorities in Ayurvedic medicines. **Atreya** (800 B.C.) was first known great Indian physician and teacher. Ayurveda had tremendous growth and development during Buddhist times. Buddhist kings established schools of medicine and public hospitals. **Charak** was the most popular name in Ayurvedic medicine. Charak mentioned the names of around 500 drugs. **'Sushuruta'** was the "Father of Indian surgery". His work is mainly devoted to surgery, e.g., treating fractures, performing amputations, excising tumours, cataract operations, plastic surgery and repairs of hernia. It is said that British surgeons learnt the surgery of Rhinoplasty from Indian surgeons. Though during Buddhist times, Indian surgeons suffered a setback due to Ahimsa.

Various other indigenous systems of medicine like **Unani** and **Homeopathy** were introduced by Muslim rulers in India. The Indian system of medicine is still practiced in India and has become a part of Indian culture. They are an important source of medical care among people.

In India, the diseases like leprosy, smallpox, etc. were believed as the punishment by the God and considered as presence of Goddess in the sick child. There were traditional healers, who were contacted to treat various illnesses by using some herbs and prayers. The similar beliefs and attitudes exist even today among some of the behavioural communities.

Chinese Medicine

The Chinese had complete faith in their traditional medicine. They were the first to name Public Health Workers as bare foot doctors. Acupuncture, which is famous worldwide even today was initiated by the Chinese system of medicine. The Chinese believed that the great doctor is *'one who treats not someone who is already ill, but someone who is not yet ill'*. Thus, they gave great importance to prevent diseases than to cure them. Their medical knowledge was based on two principles, that is the **Yang** and the **Yin**. The Yang is believed to be an active masculine principle and the Yin a passive feminine principle. The balance of these two forces was considered as a good health. Hygiene and good diet were also used to keep the health.

Egyptian Medicine

The medicine during Egyptian times (2000 B.C.) was integrated with religion. Egyptian doctors who were considered as equal to priests were trained in the temples. Sick people used to come to the temple for seeking the treatment. Egyptians worshipped many Gods. There were even specialists like eye doctors, head doctors and tooth doctors. They were officially paid by Government. They believed that disease was due to absorption of harmful substances in the intestine which gave rise to **petrification** of blood and pus formation. Diseases were treated by giving enema, catheterization and various drugs. Their God of health was **Horns**. Egyptian medicine was an important landmark in public health, since they believed in smallpox inoculation, under drainage system, prevention of mosquito bite and control of rats, etc.

Pre-Christian Era

They based health practices on magic and superstition rather than on facts about the cause of certain events on health. *Shamans* or medicine men cared for both health and religious needs and were highly esteemed. Two thousand years before the Christian era, securing an adequate supply of drinking water was a major concern. In Babylonia, the notion persisted that illness was caused by sins and displeasures of the God, that disease was caused due to punishment for sinning. Sick people were considered as unclean and in need of purification, and temples became place for medical care. Sick people were taken to the busy market where passerby could offer suggestions for treatment. In spite of primitive practices, both the Babylonians and Egyptians emphasised hygiene and possessed some medical skills.

Greek Medicine

Greek era was the year during 460 to 136 B.C. The early Greeks viewed people as part of nature and believed health results from harmonious relationship with nature.

The Greeks believed that people are a part of nature and health resulted from a harmonious relationship with nature. The Greeks also paid attention to the personal cleanliness, exercise, diet and sanitation.

Hippocrates was the greatest physician in Greek medicine who is popularly known as **Father of Medicine**. He studied and classified diseases based on observations and reasoning, and he initiated new approach to medicine, like applying the clinical methods in medicine, etc. Some of the sayings of Hippocrates became important aspects among physicians, *e.g.*, 'Where there is love for mankind there is love for the art of healing'. His famous oath 'The hippocrate oath' has become the keystone of medical ethics. This oath enables to set the high standards in medical education. Hippocrates will always be remembered as one of the masters of medical arts.

Hippocrates also studied the diseases which were epidemic and endemic in nature. His concept of health and disease stressed the relationship between man and environment. He also studied climate, water supply, clothing, nutrition, hygiene and their effects on health.

Greeks gave a new direction to medical thought. The first clear cut evidence of acute communicable disease is recorded in classical Greek literature. There are various references to severe sore throat, that often caused death. The Greek work mentioned about acute inflammatory processes of the throat, larynx, which is now recognised as diphtheria. Greek practitioners were going from place to place, knocking at the doors and providing the services to the sick and needy people. Big cities appointed the doctors and paid for their services through funds. They were the beginners of Community Health Physicians.

The Greek civilization fell into decay and was succeeded by Roman civilization.

Roman Medicine

The Romans followed the medicine from Greek. They were more towards practicing medicine and believed more in hygiene. Public health took birth in Rome with development of roads, sanitation, pure water supply, built sewer system and established hospitals for the sick.

Galen (130-205 A.D.) was a famous physician of that time. His important contribution was in the field of anatomy and physiology and his views on 'Health and Disease', health may be preserved and then how that may cure the disease. He also discovered three main factors of disease causation. These were predisposing, existing and environmental factors. His books were accepted as standard textbooks.

Romans were more of practical minded people than Greeks. They believed in cleanliness and sanitation, they developed bathrooms, sewers and aquaducts. They made fine roads and drinking water to all the people and established hospitals for the sick.

Middle Ages (Dark Era of Medicine)

The decline of Greeco-Roman era led to both decline in urban culture and disintegration of community health organisation and practice. This was the period between 500 to 1500 A.D.

During this period, there were **superstition** and **mysticism,** hence decline in the progress of medicine. People considered immoral to look at their own bodies, hence bathing was an infrequent practice and people often wore dirty clothes. Sanitation was inappropriate, refuse and body wastes were not removed from their places.

Dissections on human beings were prohibited. There was no progress in development of medicine and surgery. This age is also called as **Dark Era of medicine.**

During the dark ages, the Arabians took the Greek, Roman literature and translated into Arabic, and preserved the ancient literature. They also introduced many drugs, *e.g.*, benzoin, camphor, saffron, senna, etc, which turned out to be excellent remedies.

With the establishment of Christianity, various hospitals were established for poor and needy sick people. The rise of monasteries and convents as places for caring the sick. The monasteries admitted people from all ranks including kings and queens. They not only helped to preserve the ancient knowledge but also rendered active medical and nursing care to the sick.

FOUNDATION OF PREVENTIVE MEDICINE

The preventive medicine was isolated as a branch of public health after various studies on prevention of diseases. **Edward Jenney** (1749-1823) discovered vaccination against smallpox.

Pasteur (1883) founded the anti-rabies treatment and there was discovery of cholera vaccine (1892), anti-typhoid vaccine (1898) and diphtheria antitoxoid in 1894. With the bacteriological knowledge, it became possible to control the channel for disease transmission by specific measures, *e.g.*, quarantine, purification of water, pasteurisation of milk, preservation of food, disinfection and disposal of wastes, etc. There were laboratories for early detection of diseases which helped in control of infectious diseases. The three levels (primary, secondary, tertiary) of prevention of diseases were quite prominent during this period.

Development of Ayurveda and Siddha System in India

The Ayurveda is practiced throughout India and Siddha System was practiced only in Tamil speaking area of South India. Ayurveda is known as knowledge of life (Ayur– long veda– knowledge that means this is the knowledge to prolong life). The origin has been traced back to vedic times about 5000 B.C. Dhanvantri, the Hindu God of medicine is said to be as a result of churning of the sea during 'tug of war' between God and Demons. It is believed that medical knowledge in Atharveda (one of the four vedas) gradually developed into Science of Ayurveda.

THE RISE OF PUBLIC HEALTH

Public health developed in England in 1840. During that period, many cities and towns were without safe water supply, proper drainage and poor housing conditions. Due to rapid indus-trialization, the health problems were on increase in rural and urban communities. This led to high infant mortality rate, especially in industrial areas. **Edwin Chadwick** constituted the first Public Health Act in 1848, which stressed on environmental sanitation to remove the cause for spread of infection. By the beginning of 20th century, the broad foundation of public health was provision of clean water, clean surroundings, wholesome condition of houses, etc. were laid in all the countries of the civilized world.

PUBLIC HEALTH IN INDIA

Though public health in India is of recent development as compared to western countries, glimpses of public health practices and medicines, during the ancient period are found in Indian history. In early days the sick in the home was not treated by the nurses. The maternity and child health was mostly done by untrained *dais*. Care of the sick was considered as religious duty and prevention of disease was given first importance. Compulsory hygienic measures were adopted. **Midwives** were required to develop skills and maintain perfect cleanliness of self and the lying-in rooms (with cross-ventilation). Inocculation for smallpox was practised. Sick were cared in the institutions by old women and men.

In India, public health movement started only in 19th century, when in 1859 the British ruled over India. The high mortality in India arrested the attention of British Parliament. Florence Nightingale contributed a lot towards improvement of health and sanitary conditions for army men in India. She also suggested to improve health services for civil population.

A Royal Commission was sent in 1859 to find the reason for heavy mortality and morbidity among military and civil population in India. The Commission gave the report in 1863 and suggested the formation of Sanitary Commission of five persons in Bengal, Bombay and Madras. In 1864, such Commission was established to improve health mainly for military people and then civilians. In 1896, epidemic of plague broke out. Plague Commission was established to investigate the causes. The Commission submitted its report in 1904 and suggested the revival of the office of Sanitary Commissioner with the Government and establishment of Public Health Department. At present the Government of India has sufficient control over the Public Health Services.

●●●

2

Changing Concept of Public Health and Primary Health Care

INTRODUCTION

During 19th century emphasis was on physical environment and sanitation. The concept of public health by 20th century was that community has direct responsibility for the health of the individual. It was initiated with maternal and child health care, then school health services were developed. In the beginning, the health care was planned for poor only and not for the community as a whole. Gradually the idea grew that every healthy individual in the community is an asset, and sick person is a liability. Thus, the emphasis of primary health shifted to conservation of individual health, not only for the poor but for every citizen of the country. Industrial health services, accident prevention, and mental health services within the preview of public health also came into existence.

The public health may be stated in four stages:

(i) Disease Prevention Stage Phase (1880-1920).

(ii) Health Promotional Stage (1920-1960).

(iii) Social Engineering (1960-1980).

(iv) Health for All (1981-2000 A.D.).

Disease Prevention

During this period hygiene was given lot of importance. Public health was mainly stressed on sanitary conditions, i.e., control of physical environment like safe water supply and proper sewage disposal. Though main emphasis was to control the various diseases occurring due to poor environmental conditions, these measures were very useful to improve the health of the people by preventing various diseases and preventing deaths.

Health Promotion

The health of an individual was considered as the State responsibility for disease control measures and promotion of the health. The Public Health Departments started expanding various health programmes to promote the health of every individual. Special attention was paid to high-risk groups or special groups like maternal and child health, school health, industrial health, mental health and rehabilitation services, etc.

In 1920, **Winslow** defined public health as, "Science and Art of preventing disease, prolonging life and promoting health and efficiency through organised community efforts".

This definition is one of the landmarks in preventive medicine and which is largely true today. Various health units were opened all over, since the State has taken the direct responsibility for the health of an individual. The primary health centres and subcentres were started during this period to provide "Basic Health Services" for people. The first primary health centre was opened in 1920 by Lord Dawson in England. The establishment of health centres was important development in public health. The Bhore Committee in 1946 had also recommended establishment of health centres in India. The first primary health centre was established in 1952 at **Najafgarh, New Delhi**. Consequently, the primary health centres and subcentres were started in rural India.

Community Development Programmes were also started in 1952 to promote village development by active participation of the people by means of "People's health in people's hand," though this programme could not be successful due to inadequate resources.

Social Engineering

Many communicable and non-communicable diseases started emerging during this phase. Many acute illness problems were brought under control, but non-communicable problems began to emerge *e.g.*, cancer, diabetes, cardiovascular disease, drug abuse and alcoholism, etc. These problems could not be controlled by preventive measures like isolation, immunisation and disinfection, etc. The role of public health changed towards social and behavioural aspects, since these problems were considered as predisposing to social, economical and lifestyle of an individual. Hence, the name public health has also been called as community health, keeping in view that health of every individual on all **aspects of factor involved.**

Health for All

The explosion of knowledge during 20th century has made the medicine more advanced and complex and the treatment more costly, affecting the social groups and worldwide criticism as "social injustice". Current commitment of all the countries is to remove the inequalities in the distribution of health services and resources and attainment of "Health for all by 2000 AD". The goal of modern medicine is not merely treatment of diseases but prevention and promotion of health. Minimum health care must be accessible and affordable to each individual of the society, so as to maintain its optimum level of health. Majority of world's population, perhaps more than half, have no access to adequate health facilities. Either they adopt the home remedy or they go to traditional healers. The global awareness was stirred leading to fill the gap between health services and the people, especially in rural area.

In 1981, "WHO pledged a global strategy to an ambitious target to achieve the health for all by 2000 A.D., to attain the health of the people to lead a socially and economically productive life". Health resources will be made available to all the people at their own place of living and work.

'Health for all' means that health services are to be brought within the reach of everyone in the country, by removing various barriers like illiteracy barriers, like ignorance, provision of water supply, nutrition, housing in collaboration with other sectors indirectly related to health of public.

They defined HFA as : "attainment of a level of health that will enable every individual to lead a socially and economically productive life".

Health for all is a holistic concept which includes overall contribution to health like education, agriculture, communication, industry, medicine and housing, etc. The main aim of health for all is to provide an acceptable and accessible health services to all people of the country.

There is unequality of the health services provided to the people, the services are inaccessible to the people, like 70 per cent of population of our country lives in villages, whereas 70 per cent of health services, *e.g.*, big hospitals, specialised and superspecialised hospitals are opened in cities (with a population of 30%). The rural public had to travel a long distance to avail such services, which are expensive too and may be late for emergency.

World Health Assembly in 1977 at Geneva declared health for all by 2000 A.D. The main objectives of the movement is the equal distribution of health resources within the community, so as to maintain the equal health status of people.

Goals of Health for All

Long-term Goals

Mainly two types of goals are to be achieved under this perspective. Long-term goals means "attainment by all people of the highest possible level of health".

Short-term Goals

Which are to be achieved within defined period of time, are that minimum level of health of all the people must be maintained so that they are productive and are able to participate actively in the social life and can live a sound economical status.

The long-term goals are long awaited goals and can't be achieved or measured in a short period of time. To achieve long-term goals, they have to be splitted into short-term goals. Finally, all these short-term goals will enable to accomplish the long-term goals.

For example, if infant mortality and maternal mortality rate is to be reduced by 2020 A.D., it is important to set short-term goals, *e.g.,* provision of quality and quantity, antenatal care and facilities to pregnant women, so that at the end, she remains healthy and gives birth to a healthy child.

The main objectives of HFA is to provide health services at their doorstep, proper referral system and people's own participation for the health needs and achievement of health.

Alma Ata Conference held in 1978 stated that to achieve HFA, the best approach is by providing primary health care, especially to unreached rural population and urban slums. It was emphasised that essential health care should be accessible to all the people, which they can afford and accept by their own participation. All the countries were emphasised to formulate their national health policies and primary health care as an essential part of health care delivery system.

Global strategy was evolved in 1981, by WHO to adopt the HFA strategies by each country according to its conditions and requirements.

NATIONAL STRATEGY FOR HFA-2000 A.D.

As per Alma Ata Declaration in 1978, Government of India adopted the national strategy of HFA-2000. As per specific objectives laid down by WHO to be achieved, various attempts have been made to work towards these objectives. Based on this, National Health Policy was formulated in 1982, which commits the government and the people towards the achievement of HFA.

Specific Objectives

The main goals to be achieved by the year 2000 A.D. were :

- Reduction of IMR (Infant Mortality Rate) from 125/1000 (1978) to below 60/1000 for live births.

Table 2.1 : Current Status of Health Indicators

Indicators	Past Level	Current Level
Crude Birth Rate (per thousand population)	40.8 (1995)	25.0 (2002)*
Crude Death Rate (per thousand population)	25.1 (1995)	8.1 (2002)*
Infant Mortality Rate (per thousand live births)	146 (1951-61)	64 (2002)*
Maternal Mortality Rate (per 100000 live births)	437 (1992-93)	407 (1998)*
Total Fertility Rate (per woman)	6.0 (1951)	3.2 (1999)*
Couple Protection Rate	10.4 (1970-71)	52.0 (2002)
Life expectancy at Birth (in years)	1951	(2001-2006)
Male	37.1	63.87
Female	36.1	66.91
Immunization Status (% coverage)	1985-86	2003-2004
For pregnant women		
TT	40	82.9
For Infants		
BCG	29	102.5
Measles	44	91.8
DPT	41	96.6
Polio	36	97.0

Table 2.2 : Health Goals to be Achieved by 2000 A.D.

S. No.	Indicators	Level as quoted		Goals	
		1983	1985	1990	2000
1	2	3	4	5	6
1.	Infant mortality	Rural 136 (1978)	122		
		Urban 70 (1978)	60		
		Total 125 (1978)	106	87	Below 60
	Perinatal mortality	67 (1976)			30-35
2.	Crude death rate	Around 14	12	10.4	9.0
3.	Pre-school child (1–5 yrs) mortality	24 (1976-77)	20-24	15-20	10
4.	Maternal mortality rate	4-5 (1976)	3-4	2-3	Below 2
5.	Life-expectancy at birth (years)	Male 52.6	55.1	57.6	64
6.	Babies with birth weight below 2500 gm (percentage)	30	25	18	10
7.	Crude birth rate	Around 35	31	27.0	21.0
8.	Effective couple protection (percentage)	23.6 (mar.82)	37.0	42.0	60.0
9.	Net reproduction rate (NRR)	1.48 (1981)	1.34	1.17	1.00
10.	Growth rate (annual)	2.24 (1971-81)	1.90	1.66	1.20
11.	Family size	4.4 (1975)	3.8		2.3
12.	Pregnant mothers receiving antenatal care (%)		40-50	50-60	60-75
13.	Deliveries by trained birth attendants (%)	30-35	50	80	100
14.	Immunisation status (% coverage)				
	TT (for pregnant women)	20	60	100	100
	TT (for school children)				
	10 years		40	100	100
	16 years	20	60	100	100
	DPT (children below 3 years)	25	70	85	85
	Polio (infants)	5	50	70	85
	BCG (infants)	65	70	80	85
	DT (new school entrants 5-6 years)	20	80	85	85
	Typhoid (new school entrants 5-6 years)	2	70	85	85
15.	Leprosy-percentage of disease arrested cases out of those detected	20	40	60	80
16.	TB-percentage of disease arrested cases out of those detected	50	60	75	90
17.	Blindness-incidence of (%)	1.4	1	0.7	0.3

- To raise the life-expectancy at birth from 52 years to 64 years.
- To reduce crude birth rate from 33/1000 to 21 per thousand of population.
- To reduce the crude death rate from 14/1000 to 9 per thousand of population.
- To achieve net reproductive rate of 1 per cent. Which is 1.7 per cent at present.
- To provide safe drinking water to entire population by 1990.

The steps towards achievement of these goals have already been started by implementing various health programmes, strategies, sixth and seventh Five-Year Plans, 20-point programme and primary health care concept.

CHANGING CONCEPT OF HEALTH CARE

Despite the limited resources, there is disproportionate distribution of health services—dispensaries, hospitals, institutions for specialised treatment, majority of which are situated in urban areas of the country. The people from rural community have to travel very long distances to seek any medical relief due to unavailability of health services near their living place, which can readily and effectively be handled at the community level. Also, due to lack of proper referral system, it becomes difficult for people to approach to receive the medical care. To reduce such inconvenient, unsatisfactory situations, it was felt the need to restructure the health care delivery systems.

As stated in the Vedic prayer :

सर्वे भवन्तु सुखिनः सर्वेसन्तु निरामया ।
सर्वे भद्राणि पश्यन्ति माकश्चिद् दुःख भागभवेत् ॥

It states the health and happiness of the people as a whole, i.e., every living creature on this earth should be happy. In fact, in all ancient prayers we always prayed for the community as a whole. The way for achieving anything is from the individual himself, as the saying goes, "Charity begins at home". This states that individual has to be responsible for his own health. It is also said that "God helps those who help themselves".

In 1977, Government of India started, "Rural Health Scheme based on the principles of placing people health in people hands". Alma Ata Conference, 1978 set the goals for accessibility of health care through primary health care approach. Government of India committed to achieve this goal through the approach to provide universal comprehensive health care to the people which they can accept and afford.

PRIMARY HEALTH CARE

Historical Background

Primary health care in India dates back to the Vedic period with more evidence on environmental, sanitation, underground drainage, public baths in cities, etc. Health was given high priority in daily life, which included physical, mental, social and spiritual wellbeing. Lifestyle was conclusive to health promotion, e.g., health education, healthy personal hygiene habits, excercises, diet and spiritual values, treatment of minor ailments and injuries was stressed upon.

Due to various factors, e.g., British rule, economic constraints, the government did not lay much attention to primary health. Health services were mainly meant for Britishers and advocated medical components.

Comprehensive Health Care

After Independence, the government adopted several approaches and strategies to provide health care to public, which was mainly recommended by **Bhore Committee (1946)** with the concept of comprehensive health care.

- The Committee recommended that preventive, promotive, curative, rehabilitative services should be provided to the people from 'womb to tomb', from early days of individual's life.
- The services should be available to all citizens of the country.

There should be provision of consultants, laboratories and other special services, which may be necessary for diagnosis and treatment.

Objectives of comprehensive health care were :

- The services should make adequate provision for the medical care of a person, for curative and preventive field and active promotion of positive health.

- Services should be placed as close as possible to the people to ensure maximum utilization of health care.
- Health organisation should have the widest basis of co-ordination and co-operation between people, services and profession.
- Health care should be easily accessible irrespective of their economic status or inability to pay for it.
- Special target groups must be given priority, *e.g.*, maternal, child, handicapped, physically and mentally deficient, etc.
- Maintaining healthy environment around the people at home or workplace.

These recommendations formed the foundation of present health care system.

As per recommendation, the primary health centres with 75 beds were opened with a staffing pattern of :

- Medical officers—5
- Public health nurses—6
- Pharmacist—1
- Laboratory technician—1
- Auxillary nurse midwives—2
- Class IV employees—15
- Sanitary Inspector, etc.—1

Community Development Programme

India launched community development programme in 1952 for allround development of rural community. The country was divided into blocks and each block with a population of 1 lakh, health package was provided by primary health care.

Functions of PHC

The eight functions of Primary Health Centre were (Fig. 2.1, Table 2.2) :

- MCH,
- Control of communicable disease,
- School health,
- Medical care,
- Collection of vital statistics,
- Environmental sanitation,
- Health education and nutrition.

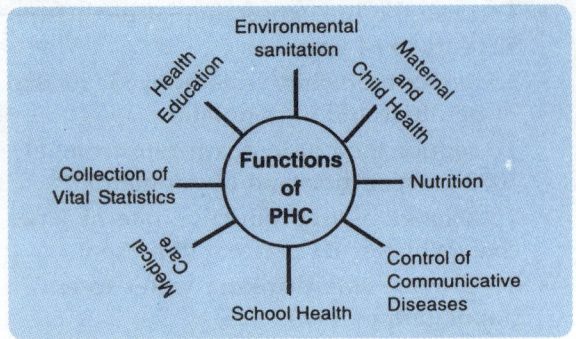

Fig. 2.1 : Functions of primary health centre

Each PHC was subdivided into subcentres to cover 10,000 of population.

Many other important committees like **Mudaliar Committee (1959); Mukharjee Committee (1966); Kartar Singh Committee (1975)** were appointed for recommendation on improving the health status of the country. Attempts were also made to expand and to re-orient the training for auxillary nurses, midwives and public health nurses and to strengthen the health and family planning services.

Basic Health Services

Basic health services were the organisation of functions essential to the health of an area and assuring the availability of competent professional and auxiliary personnel to perform their functions. The trained personnel were engaged in their specific field of work and were termed as basic health workers, in the areas of family planning, malaria control and immunization, etc. There was not much improvement in quality care, and there was lack of community participation and lack of inter-sectoral co-ordination.

NATIONAL HEALTH POLICY 1983

The Alma Ata (USSR) declaration in 1978, committed to attain the goal for health for all by 2000 A.D., through primary health care approach. Constant efforts were made to formulate and adopt National Health Policy, keeping in view the Health for All principles and targets. The National Health Policy was officially adopted for India by the Parliament in 1983.

Table 2.2 : Functions of PHC

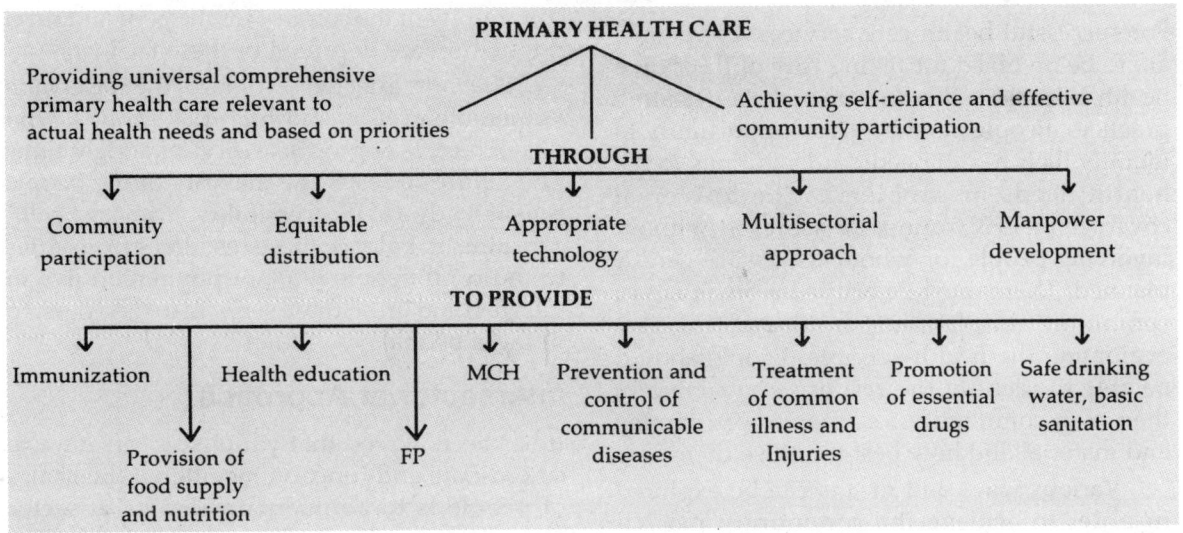

Primary Health Care

A new approach to health care came into force, which is known as "Primary Health Care". The old concept of primary health care was First Contact Care or primary level of health services. The Alma Ata defined primary health care with a different concept and meaning (Fig. 2.2).

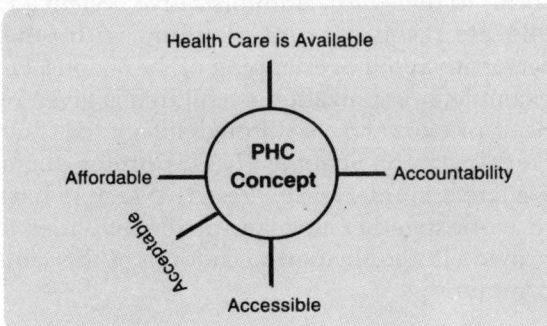

Fig. 2.2 : Concept of PHC

Definition

"Primary health care is the essential health care made universally accessible to individuals and acceptable to them, through their full participation and at a cost the community and country can afford".

PHC is based on practical, scientifically sound, socially acceptable, technologically accessible to individual, family and public, with their full participation and at a cost that individual and country can afford to maintain every stage of their development. It is the first level of health care that brings people and health system as close as possible.

PRINCIPLES OF PRIMARY HEALTH CARE

There are mainly five accepted principles of PHC (Fig. 2.3).

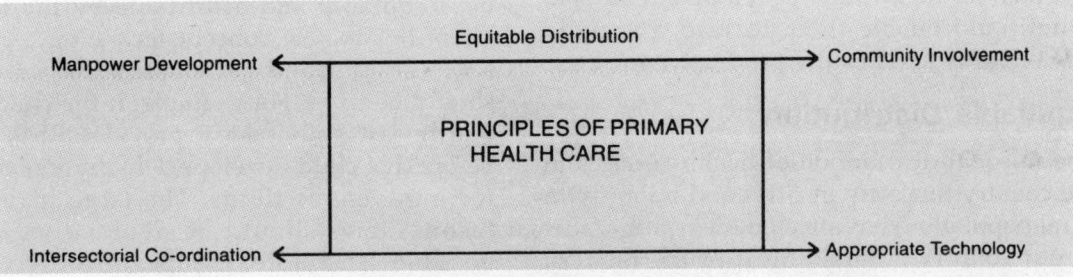

Fig. 2.3 : Principles of PHC

Community Participation

For successful health care services, the people are to be involved for taking care of their own health, by making them aware of certain healthy practices. People must be given opportunity to identify their health needs and solutions to the health needs or problems. The universal coverage of PHC cannot be achieved without involving people for whom the health care is planned. There must be active involvement of community in planning, implementing and evaluating the health services. People should be able to identify the resources available in their own community, *i.e.*, manpower, money and material and how best to utilise them.

Various ways and means can be explored in order to achieve the community participation, *i.e.*, through community leaders, voluntary health workers and trained *dais,* etc. These people are elected by the public themselves, therefore, they have more sense of belongingness and approaches.

Any type of health services can be reached through the influential people. The immediate services provided by these people should be comprehensive, scientific and adequate for the people. The health volunteers and traditional birth attendants (TBA) are the best approach to reach the general public.

"Participation is a way of living which needs to be inculcated in all the citizens of the world so as to enable and involve them actively, collectively and voluntarily to diagnose their problems and felt needs; find and implement socioculturally, economically and scientifically acceptable solutions in the community logistics, either with or without support so as to eliminate or minimise their problems; fulfil their felt needs and plan for their future development so as to benefit and enable them to lead a socially economically and healthy productive life".

Equitable Distribution

The unequal distribution of health services in the country (majority in cities and minority in rural population) has affected the health status of our country at large. Most of the modern technology hospitals, specialised and super-specialised are opening in big cities; urban community of the country for the poor and rural population are deprived of these facilities.

The most affected sections of the society are vulnerable groups and high-risk groups, who do not receive appropriate services at right time. The failure to reach the majority of the people is usually due to inaccessibility. Primary health care aims to balance these resources from cities to the rural people (70% of population live in villages) and bring these services to the doorstep of these people.

Intersectorial Approach

It has been agreed that various sectors have to co-ordinate and function together, if the health of people is to be maintained. Health sector alone may not be able to achieve the goal of health for all. For example, a person needs to have basic education, appropriate nutrition, housing and food to keep the health. All sectors must provide safe and healthy resources to the people. All these sectors like education, agriculture, housing, public works, food, industry, animal husbandry, communication and other sectors have to collaborate with health sector to review the administrative system and allocate resources and planning with other sectors to avoid overlapping of the actions. For example, immunization to children is given by health sectors and also through Integrated Child Development Scheme (ICDS) under social welfare sectors. Hence, these two sectors have to work together to plan for the activities to provide immunization to children of the same community.

Appropriate Technology

Technology which is applied for people must be acceptable and affordable by the users. According to PHC concept, technology, simple, scientifically sound and adaptable to local needs should be used. For example, if the child gets diarrhoea it is advisable to provide ORS to child, before that child develops dehydration and go for intravenous fluids. The large luxurious technologies should be avoided as far as possible. Therefore, cheaper, effective, safe, scientifically valid and acceptable procedures should be practised, than costly, sophisticated and complicated ones.

Manpower Development

The purpose of health care services is to improve the health status of the people. The goal of 'Health For All' have to be achieved through primary health care concept. Health manpower requirements are subject to change, both quantitatively and qualitatively as new programmes. Projects are introduced into health care system. For example, the new concept on primary health care to achieve 'Health For All', and emphasis on 'periphery health care' and 'community based care' needs trained workers to work at the root level. Therefore, many new categories of workers has been introduced since then. They include 'Village Health Guides' multipurpose health workers, technicians, TBAS, etc.

Health manpower accounts for both professionals and paraprofessionals to health care system. The health manpower requirements are based on health needs and demands of a country and desired results. Health needs are based on the health status of the country. Health manpower planning is an important object of community health planning. It is based on the accepted ratio of 1 village health guide is needed for 1000 of population which helps to identify the number of workers required for a community. These health personnel are specially trained for specific goals.

The total health manpower which have been trained till date :

Health Manpower	No. of Personnel
Village health guides	410904
Trained birth attendants	660996
Female health workers	124680
Male health workers	63875
Health assistants	22144

COMPONENTS OR ELEMENTS OF PRIMARY HEALTH CARE

According to Alma Ata Declaration, 'Primary Health Care' is essential health care made universally acceptable for individuals and families in the community by means acceptable to them through their full participation and at a cost community can afford. It forms an integral part both of the community health system of which it is the nucleus and of the overall social and economic development of the community. Alma Ata declaration further spelt out the minimum essential components of primary health care. These components are not merely independent but *Linked components*. Since primary health care is an integrated development approach to health; these components have an ongoing interface with education, health and development. These components are :

- Educating people about health and family welfare matters.
- Promotion of food supply and proper nutrition.
- Safe drinking water and basic sanitation measures.
- Maternal, infant care and family planning.
- Immunization.
- Prevention and control of locally endemic diseases.
- Appropriate treatment of common diseases and injuries.
- Provision of essential drugs.

Education Health Linkages

Education is an important factor responsible for individual as well as family's health. For example, in India, mothers are usually responsible for bringing up the children. So, the level of literacy and education of mothers assumes more significance in determining the health status of our children. This is more so where health care promotion is not always institutionalised.

Not only literacy and education give the chance and access to information and services but also it has inherent strength supported by knowledge for decision making towards conditions of health promotion. Education-Health linkages bring out a simple fact in this context for integrated planning is that 'An educated mother can ensure the optimal utilisation' of available resources for nutrition as also for better utilisation of the available health and medical services and bring accountability into them by demanding what she knows is her right.

Study of Kerela (1981) has shown that the high level of literacy and education among the females in Kerela is the 'one single' factor which has significantly contributed to the improvement of health status of infants and children. Lot of studies and statistics can be quoted to show the association, and differentials for high infant mortality, non-utilisation of health care, extent of low birth babies, 'non-coverage of immunisation', etc. with the educational status of females in India.

Education as factors determine political awareness and gives the indicative right to demand and use health and other welfare facilities. This itself is a function of awareness created by education.

Literature in India and other developing countries have brought out that among households (for any given income level), families were better fed where the mother education was higher. These differentials are known also for child survival.

Educating People About the Health and Family Welfare Matters

Educating People about the health and family welfare matters as follows :
- Promotion of proper nutrition.
- Basic sanitation measures.
- Maternal, infant care and family planning.
- Immunisation.

Integrated Child Development Services

Of many programmes and services, example may be given for one programme where linkage between health care services and educational efforts may be seen subtly forged.

Of many programmes, this countrywide programme of child development is known for its 'holistic approach' to improve health and educational environment of child. It has twin goals :

(*i*) to encourage school enrolment via early pre-school stimulation programme for children 3 to 6 years of old,

(*ii*) to improve the health and nutrition status of children 0 to 6 years via supplementary feeding to selected beneficiaries. But, it also brings mothers in picture and attempts to promote mothers education via 'Health and Nutrition Education Exposures'. A broad package of six integrated services are delivered through Integrated Child Development Services (ICDS) which could be further strengthened as an area for integrated planning :
- Health check-up
- Immunisation
- Referral service
- Supplementary nutrition
- Nonformal education
- Nutrition and health education to mothers.

Accessibility for Health Care Services and Educational Facilities

Physical accessibility to health services and also towards educational facilities have been enhancing over the period of time. However, there remain gaps for these 'social inputs' among some states, districts, rural and urban areas, terrains, within socio-economic strata organized vs unorganized groups, etc. These accessibility gaps are there not just in terms of general basic (elementary) services and facilities but also for type, frequency, qualitative aspects, etc. Besides these, observed 'locational biases' are also there.

Linkages between health care services and educational efforts must strive to brings mother in limelight and attempts to promote mother education through health and nutrition education exposures.

Promotion of Food Supply and Proper Nutrition

Measures should be taken to check and prevent the adulteration and contamination of food at the various stages of their production, processing, storage, transport and distribution. To ensure uniformity of approach, the existing law would require to be reviewed and effective legislation enacted by the centre, so that the food supplied to people should be adequate and of good quality.

Safe Drinking Water and Basic Sanitation

The provision of safe drinking water and the proper disposal of water, human and animal wastes, both in urban and rural areas must constitute an integrated package. The provision of safe drinking water and basic sanitation facilities should be accompanied by intensive health education campaign for improving the hygienic conditions and ultimately health. All water supply schemes must be fully integrated with efforts at proper water management, including drainage and disposal of water waste. To reduce expenditure and for achieving targets it is necessary to adopt appropriate technologies in planning and management of delivery system.

Immunization Against Major Infectious Diseases

It is essential to launch an organised, nationwide immunization programme arrived at cent per cent coverage of targeted population group with immunization for prevention and control of various communicable diseases. Such an approach will not only control the diseases and disabilities but also bring down the existing high infant and child mortality rate.

Maternal, Child Health and Family Planning

Mothers and children not only constitute a large group (60% of population), but they are also a 'vulnerable' or special risk group. The risk is connected with childbearing in the case of women; growth, development and survival in the case of infants and children. Mothers and children are always considered as an integrated unit, therefore, all the programmes are aimed at devoting efforts at launching special programmes for the improvement of maternal and child health, with a special focus on the less privileged section of the society. Such programmes need to be decentralised to the maximum possible extent, that their delivery being at the various national level and inter-national level health programmes have been initiated to reduce the MMR and IMR and encourage family planning services like CSSM programme initiated with a package for safe motherhood and better child survival chances and reproductive health, etc.

Primary level care are the health facilities nearest to the doorstep of the people. Emphasis must be given on training, retraining and orientation programme for TBAs who are responsible for 60 per cent of the deliveries conducted in rural areas. There must be adequate facilities for perinatal, natal and postnatal health care and prompt referral system for the complicated cases. It is essential to lower IMR for successful family planning measure.

Appropriate Treatment of Common Diseases and Injuries

Especially, the areas where there is inadequate health facilities available, there must be provision of treatment for ailments and injuries, etc. Such provision is emphasised by giving training of 6 months to community health volunteers and other community people who are capable of giving such services in the community.

Prevention and Control of Locally Endemic Diseases

Specific infectious diseases are common in certain places. Keeping in view preventive measures must be taken to control the recurrence and spread of such endemic diseases in the community by various methods, e.g., immunization, surveillance and chemopro-phylaxis etc.

Provision of Essential Drugs

The measures required to be taken to ensure against the manufacture and sale of substandard drugs. The essential drugs must be safe, cheap and available to the people so that they must not be deprived of these drugs.

Levels of Primary Health Care

(Flow Chart 2.1)

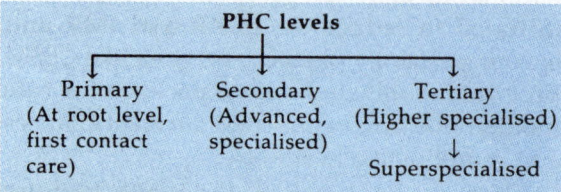

Primary Care Level

The first level is usually the point of contact between the individual and the health system, where the primary health care or essential health care is delivered.

Secondary Care Level

This is more specialised as obstetric, paediatric, psychiatry, medical and surgical, and is provided at the regional or central level. When the care is required more than the primary level of health care, patient is referred for specialised care.

Tertiary Care Level

This comprises superspecialised as mental, diabetic, heart problems and renal care at the regional or state level according to the health problem of the individual.

●●●

3

Development of Community Health in India and Five-Year Plans

INTRODUCTION—
BEFORE INDEPENDENCE

The history of public health during British rule is as follows :

1825 : Quarantine's Act for communicable diseases was passed.

1865 : Sanitary Commissioners were appointed at three main cities of Bombay, Madras and Calcutta to investigate the cause of poor sanitary and unsatisfactory conditions of health.

1869 : Public health commissioners were appointed.

1873 : Birth and Death Registration Act was started.

1880 : Vaccination Act was passed.

1881 : The first Indian Factory Act was passed, under the ESI scheme.

1896 : Major 'Epidemic of Plague' took place in India, which initiated government to take immediate measures to improve the health of public.

1897 : Epidemic Diseases Control Act was passed, ensuring the preparations before the epidemics during fairs and festivals and marriages, etc.

1909 : Central Malaria Bureau was established at Kasauli.

1911 : Indian Research Foundations Association (IRFA), renamed as Indian Council of Medical Research (ICMR) was established for research work in the field of health and public health in Delhi.

1918 : Lady Reading Health School was established in Delhi for training lady health visitors. This was to prepare the nursing workers for public health in the rural areas. The Nutrition Research Laboratory (NRL) was established in Coonoor, Madras.

1930 : All India Institute of Hygiene and Public Health (AIIHPH) was started in Calcutta, with the aid of Rockfeller Foundation. Various public health programmes were provided in this institution. Child Marriage Restraint Act (CMRA) came into force to stop the child marriage at young age and the age limit was fixed to minimum of 14 years for girls and 18 years for boys.

1931 : Maternal and Child Welfare Bureau (MCWB) was established by Indian Red Cross Society.

1935 : The Government of India Act was reinforced giving greater autonomy at Centre, State and periphery levels.

1937 : Central Advisory Board of Health (CABH) was started: Central Health Minister was designated as Chairman and State health ministers were the members of the Board to co-ordinate the public health activities.

1939 : Madras Public Health Act was passed. Rural Health Training Centre (RHTC) was started in Singur, Calcutta, with aid from Rockfeller Foundation.

Tuberculosis Association of India (TAI) started in Delhi.

1940 : Drug Act was promulgated, so as to keep the standards of drug under control.

1943 : Bhore Committee (Named as Health Survey and Development Committee–HSDC) under the Chairmanship of Dr. J. Bhore, who was appointed by Government of India to survey the existing situation regarding health conditions and make recommendations for future health prospects.

1946 : Bhore Committee submitted its report with various recommendations and suggestions which are important landmarks in health development even today. Committee recommended short-term and long-term objectives to be achieved for health sector development. The short-term plans suggested the establishment of primary health units to serve about 40,000 population. Long-term includes scheme of expansion of primary health units with primary and secondary health units.

PUBLIC HEALTH DEVELOPMENT AFTER INDEPENDENCE

India became independent in 1947, after a long British rule affecting the health and economy of the public. After independence, there have been a continuous expansion of national health activities in all aspects of community life to improve the health of people. The progress has been made in four main programmes of administration, training, health services and research. The important events in public health were as follows :

1947 : Ministry of Health was established at Centre and State level. The Director General of Health Services, Directorate of Health Services and Public Health were started at the Centre and State health ministries.

1948 : Indian Nursing Council Act was passed. India became a member of World Health Organisation (WHO).
Employees State Insurance (ESI) Act was passed.

1949 : The South East Asia Regional Office of WHO was established in New Delhi. Indian Research Fund Association was renamed as Indian Council of Medical Research (ICMR).

1950 : The Constitution of India came into force and India became a Republic in the Commonwealth. Planning Commission was setup by Government of India for overall development of all sectors, by drafting the Five-Year Plans. The Planning Commission consists of a Chairman, Deputy Chairman and five members.

The Five-Year Plans were conceived to improve rural health, industrial progress and overall development of all parts of the country, health being an important sector was given considerable importance to health programmes during Five-Year Plans.

First Five-Year Plan (1951–56)

1951

It was started with outlay of Rs. 2,356 crores and Rs. 140 crores (5.9%) for health sector.

- BCG vaccination programme was initiated in the country.

1952

- Primary Health Centre was setup at Najafgarh, Delhi. Community development programme started on 2nd October, 1952 for rural development.
- Central Council of Health was constituted with the Union health minister as Chairman and state health ministers as members to co-ordinate the health policies between central and state governments.
- Virus Research Centre (VRC) was setup at Poona (Maharashtra).

1953

- National Malaria Control Programme (NMCP) started.
- National Smallpox Eradication Programme (NSEP) launched.
- Family Planning Programmes (FPPs) were started.

1954

- National Water Supply and Sanitation Programme (NWSSP) initiated.
- National Leprosy Control Programme (NLCP) launched.
- Central Government Health Scheme (CGHS) started in Delhi.
- VDRL (Vinereal Disease Reference Laboratory) antigen production was setup in Calcutta.
- Prevention of Food Adulteration Act (PFAA) was passed by Parliament.

1955

- Hindu Marriage Act (MGA) fixed marriage age for boys 18 years and girls 15 years.
- Filaria Control Programme (FCP) started and Filaria Training Centre (FTC) was established in Kerala.
- Central Leprosy Research Institute (CLRI) started in Madras.
- T.B. sample survey started.

Second Five-Year Plan (1956–61)

- Second Five-Year Plan launched with an outlay of Rs. 4800 crore and 225 crore (5%) for health sector.

1956

- Central Health Education Bureau (CHEB) established under Ministry of Health.
- Family planning director appointed in Union Health Ministry.
- Trachoma Control Pilot Project (TCPP) initiated.
- Tuberculosis Chemotherapy Centre (TBCC) established.
- Demography Training and Research Centre (DTRC) was started in Bombay.

1957

- Demography Research Centre (DRC) started in Delhi, Calcutta and Thiruvananthapuram.

1958

- National Tuberculosis survey was completed.

- National Malaria Control Programme was changed to National Malaria Eradication Programme (NMEP).
- Leprosy Advisory Committee (LAC) was constituted.
- Three-tier structure was recommended as self-governing bodies at villages, districts and tehsils, etc.

1959

- **Mudaliar Committee (Health)** was appointed to survey the progress made after recommendations of **Bhore Committee** (1946) and suggestions for future development and extension of health programme.
- Central expert committee to study the measures for smallpox and cholera eradication.
- The First Panchayati Raj introduced in Rajasthan.
- National Tuberculosis Institute started in Bangalore.

1960

- National Nutritional Advisory Committee (NNAC) was constituted.
- School Health Committee (SHC) was formed.

Third Five-Year Plan (1961–69)

1961

- The Third Five-Year plan started with an outlay of Rs. 7,500 crores out of which Rs. 342 crores (4.3%) were provided to health sectors.
- **Mudaliar Committee** report was published.
- Central Bureau of Health Intelligence (CBHI) was established.

1962

- Central Family Planning Institute (CFPI) established in Delhi.
- National Smallpox Eradication Programme (NSEP) launched.
- School Health Programme was initiated.
- Goitre Control Programme (GCP) started.

1963

- Applied Nutrition Programme (ANP) started by Government of India with aid from WHO, UNICEF and FAO.
- National Institute of Communicable Diseases (NICD) was established in Delhi.
- **Chadha Committee** recommended a norm of one basic health worker for every 10,000 of population for multipurpose work.
- Safe Drinking Water Board (SDWB) was setup.
- Extended Family Planning Programme (EFPP) was launched.
- National Trachoma Control Programme (NTCP) initiated.

1964

- National Institute of Health Administration and Education (NIHAE) Munirka, Delhi was started.
- **Shantilal Shah Committee** was setup to study the legislation of abortions.

1965

- Reinforced Extended Family Planning (REFP) was launched.
- Direct house-to-house BCG vaccination was initiated.
- Director of ICMR introduced lippis loop as safe and effective method for family planning.

1966

- **Mukharjee Committee** was formulated to look into the minimum manpower required for Primary Health Centres.
- Minister for Family Planning was appointed under Ministry of Health and Family Planning, the department was created to co-ordinate family planning programmes at Centre and States for better results in controlling population.

1967

- **Madhoc Committee** was appointed to review the working of National Malaria Eradication Programme (NMEP) and to suggest further improvements.

- Small family norm was encouraged to provide suitable incentives to people who were willing for small family.

1968

- Birth and Death Registration Act (BDRA) was reinforced by Rajya Sabha for compulsory registration of birth within 15 days and death within 7 days.

Fourth Five-Year Plan (1969–74)

Fourth Five-Year Plan started with an outlay of Rs. 16,774 crores and Rs. 840 crores for health and Rs. 315 crores for family planning.

1969

- Central Birth and Death Registration Act was started.

1970

- Drug Control Policy (DCP) was initiated.
- All India Postpartum (Hospital) Family Planning Programme (AIPFPP) started.
- Population Council of India was formed.

1971

- Medical Termination of Pregnancy Bill (MTPB) (1969) was passed by Parliament.
- Expert Committee was appointed for control of air pollution.
- Family Pension Scheme (FPS) was initiated.

1972

- Medical Termination Act (MTA) came into force.
- National Institute of Nutrition (NIN) was setup in Hyderabad.

1973

- **Kartar Singh Committee** submitted its report with recommendations to form male and female multipurpose workers health scheme in subcentre in place of unipurpose worker.
- The committee proposed that Auxillary Nurses, Midwives should be replaced as female health workers and vaccinators, malaria workers, sanitary workers to be replaced as male health workers.

Fifth Five-Year Plan (1974–79)

Fifth Five-Year Plan was started with total outlay of Rs. 53,411 crores of which Rs. 796 crores for health and Rs. 516 crores for family planning.

1974

- Prevention and Control of Water Pollution (PCWP) Act was passed by Parliament.
- Reports of Evaluation Committee and Consultative Committee suggested Revised Strategy for National Malaria Eradication Programme.

1975

- India was declared smallpox free by WHO on 5th July.
- Government of India adopted revised strategy for Malaria Eradication Programme as suggested by N.M.E.P. Committee.
- E.S.I. Act was amended.
- Integrated Child Development Programme (ICDP) was started.
- **Srivastava Committee** submitted its report in regard to medical education and manpower support.
- Cigarette Regulation Act for production and distribution was passed by Parliament.

1976

- National Programme for Prevention of Blindness and Visual Impairment was initiated.
- Prevention of Food Adulteration Act (1975) was amended and passed.
- Indian Factory Act was formulated.

1977

- WHO adopted the goal of health for all by 2000 A.D.
- Eradication of smallpox declared in April by International Commission.
- Rural Health Scheme (RHS) initiated.
- Revised Modified Plan of Malaria Control was under operation.
- National Institute of Health and Family Planning formed in Munirka, New Delhi. Which was earlier named as National Institute of Health Administration and Education (NIHAE).

1978

- Alma Ata Declaration emphasing primary health care concept.
- Air Pollution Bill initiated in Lok Sabha.
- Child Marriage Restrain Act was approved by Parliament; with minimum age for boys 21 years and girls 18 years.
- Expanded programme on immunisation was launched by WHO against six killer diseases.

1979

- The offices of health and family planning were merged to formulate regional offices of health and family welfare.

Sixth Five-Year Plan (1980–85)

1980

- Total Plan investments were Rs. 97,500 crore
  Health : 1,821 crore
  Family welfare : 1,010 crore
- Smallpox was officially declare free for entire world by WHO.

1981

- Census were taken.
- Air Pollution Act was activated.
- International drinking water and sanitation decade started (1981-90).
- WHO and member countries adopted the strategy for health for all.

1982

- National health policy as health policy was adopted by Government of India.
- New 20-Point Programme was started to uplift the poor and rural sections of the country.

1983

- WHO Committee met in Geneva for special training of nurses and doctors on primary health care.
- National Leprosy Control Programme was converted as National Leprosy Eradication Programme.
- National Health Policy was approved by Parliament.

- Guinea Worm Eradication Programme (GWEP) was started.
- National Plan of Action against Avoidable Disablement known as **"IMPACT INDIA"** was initiated.

1984

- ESI Amendment Bill was passed by Parliament.
- Bhopal Gas Tragedy with major industrial accident in the history, taking at least 2,500 peoples lives and 50,000 seriously injured and more than this impairments.

Seventh Five-Year Plan (1985–90)

1985

- Seventh Five-Year plan was started with an outlay of Rs. 180,00 crores; Rs. 3392 crores for health and Rs. 3,256 crores for family welfare.
- Universal Immunization Programme was launched by WHO with the objective to immunize every child against six killer diseases.
- Lepers Act, 1898 was reinforced by Parliament.

1986

- Environmental Protection Act was started.

1987

- Indian Standard Institute renamed as Bureau of Indian Standard.
- Worldwide "Safe Motherhood" Programme was promulgated by World Bank.
- National Diabetes Control Programme (NDCP) and National AIDS Control Programme (NAIDCP) were initiated.
- High Power Committee was appointed by the Government of India for nursing standard and to assess the working condition of nurses, nursing education and related matters.

Eighth Five-Year Plan (1992–97)
1992

- The plan started with an outlay of Rs. 798,000 crores; Rs. 7,575 for health Rs. 6,500 crores for family welfare.

- The Health for All Paradigm should form on underprivileged and people of the country, within the vulnerable group like MCH has been done.
- Positive health approach with emphasis on disease prevention and health promotion including rehabilitation of physically and other handicapped.

1993

- CSSM (Child Survival and Safe Motherhood) Programme initiated.

1993

- Revised National T.B. Control Programme, with new strategy of DOTS (Direct Observation Therapy Scheme) was launched.

1994

- Panchayati Raj Act came into force completing the process of legislation in all states.
- Plague Epidemic in Rajasthan.

1995

- Pulse Polio immunization campaign took place on 9th December 1994 and 20th January 95.
- Department of Indian System of Medicine and Homeopathy established in Ministry of Health and Family Welfare.
- "Transplantation of Human Organ" Act was passed to regulate the removal, storage and transplantation of human organs for therapeutic purpose.
- Malaria control programme, expert committee submitted its reports on the guidelines for modified plan of action.

1996

- Pulse Polio Immunization. Second Phase on 7th December 1995 and 18th January 1996.

Ninth Five-Year Plan (1997–2002)
1997

- Introduction of Reproduction and Child Health Programme.

1998

- Annual Sentinel Surveillance for HIV infection started in the country.

1999

- A formal 9th plan document finally received all necessary clearance and was adopted on 19th February 1999.

2000

- Government adopted the National Population Policy for stabilizing population.

2001

- WHO declared India as Guinea worm free. Medical Care for remote and Marginalised Tribes and Nomadic Communities during IX Five-Year Plan. Glaucoma and Cornea Research Laboratories inaugurated.
- J.P. Narayan Trauma Centre inaugurated. National Programme for control and treatment of occupational disease.
- National technical committee on Child Health was constituted.

Origin of Public Health Nursing in India

Women's health during childbirth and desire to improve the health of children laid the foundation for public health nursing in India in the beginning of this century. Nursing care in military and civil hospitals had started much before the concept of public health nursing began. By this time, visiting nursing movement was firmly established in England. Trained nurses visited the sick in their homes. Ms. Nightingale called them Health Missionaries, since they donated health unlike others donated clothes and soap. She influenced Lord Dufferin to start services for women and children in India.

The birth of health visiting, midwifery, child care and public health nursing in India can be traced to the efforts of prominent British women like Lady Dufferin, Lady Chelmsford and Lady Reading. The National Association for Supplying Medical Aid by Women to the Women of India was established in 1885 under the leadership of Lady Dufferin. Hospitals were built for women and children in different parts of the country. Training of nurses and midwives started in several parts of India. Lady Chelmsford also gave impetus to maternal and child welfare in the early part of

the 20th century. The Baby Week Movement was launched and implemented successfully by Lady Reading. The Red Cross Society picked up the movement and started several maternal and child welfare centres in India.

Ms. Griffin and Ms. Graham started training *dais* near Kashmiri Gate in Delhi. In appreciation, Lady Reading gave them a building at Bara Hindu Rao which became the Lady Reading Health School, the first such school in the country. Ms. Griffin was its first Superintendent (Wilkinson, 1958). At first, getting Indian women to join the school was not easy, since visiting sick people in their homes was not a tradition in India.

At the time of the **Bhore Committee Survey**, there were health visitor training centres, midwifery training centres and nurses training centres, but, there were no training centres for public health nursing. The health visitor, according to the Committee, was inadequate to carryout the professional nursing, midwifery and general health roles required at the village level. While the health visitor originated from the district health nursing and health visitor of England, the foundations of the public health nurse were modelled along the lines prevalent in Canada and USA.

The **Bhore Committee** visualised the public health nurse as a highly qualified and efficient generalist professional. The Committee felt that such a person should be a fully qualified certified nurse and midwife (GOI, 1946, p. 395).

Public Health Nurses and Health Visitors

There are in India today about 750 or 800 health visitors, *i.e.*, 1 to 375,000 of the population in British India. Very few of these health visitors are registered nurses. Most of them are certified midwives and have had a 9 to 18 months training in the duties of health visitors. Their work has been almost entirely limited to maternity and child welfare. They function as maternity supervisors and train and supervise *dais* in order to provide for trained attendance on the mother at childbirth. They carry out much valuable work in their health centres and by home visiting, but the quantity of work to be done, the limited training of the health visitor and the widespread influence of superstition, ignorance and unhealthy habits, make effective health education of the public extremely difficult.

Public health nursing has proved to be more effective in operation and less expensive to administer than the provision of multiple specialised services such as maternity and child-welfare, school health and tuberculosis work.

Public health nursing includes all nursing services organised by a community or an agency to assist in carrying out any or all phases of the public health programme. Services may be rendered on an individual, family or community basis in home, school, clinic, or business establishment.

It is the responsibility of the public health nurse to assist in analysing health problems and related social problems of families and individuals; to help them with the aid of community resources, to formulate an acceptable plan for protection and promotion of their health, and to encourage them to carryout the plan – The Public Health Nurse.

Role of Community Health Nurse

If community health nurses are to be effective and be vital force for promoting the health of people, it is necessary to understand the history of community health nursing as well as current status of the health care system. Effective strategies for community health nurses must be designed so that they are consistent with the total mosaic of health care delivery. The Community Health Nurse (CHN) must understand the scope and nature of change and the future directions of the health care system.

SUMMARY

The history of community health nursing can be traced to the earliest recorded history of civilization. Throughout its development, there has been lot of progress. The work of **St. Vinent de Paul** and **Mademoiselle Lecras** established the first actual community health nursing programme. The life and work of Florence Nightingale influenced all nursing practices including education, hospital development and actual delivery of nursing care.

Primary health care starts at the root level of health services. It can be very successful by keeping all principles in collaboration towards achieving the optimum health of people. Hence, if people are involved in health care, services are available to all at cheaper rate and other sectors collaborate with health sectors the objectives can be achieved.

Nurse has a vital role to play in achieving the goal of health for all by 2000 A.D. through primary health care approach. Nursing profession, in broad sense, includes all nurses, auxillary nurses, midwives (female health workers). Nurses are one of the most crucial components and important health personnel in health care system. Nurses spend most of their time with people in the community and they are closest of all.

EXERCISE

1. Discuss the changing concepts of Public Health.
2. (a) Explain the concept of Primary Health Care.
   (b) Describe the principles and elements of Primary Health Care.
3. Enumerate the functions of Primary Health Centre.
4. Write Short notes on the following :
   (a) Chinese system of medicine
   (b) Dark era of medicine
   (c) Barefoot doctors
   (d) Indian System of Medicine
   (e) Health for all
   (f) Five-Year Plans

•••

UNIT II

INTRODUCTION TO COMMUNITY HEALTH NURSING

- Concept of Community Health Nursing
- Roles and Responsibilities of Community Health Nursing Personnel
- Community Health Nursing Specialised Roles
- Legal Aspects in Community Health Nursing

4

Concept of Community Health Nursing

INTRODUCTION

The new concept of health has made an impact on the role of Community Health Nursing because people want to seek quality health care. The country continues to face health crisis, how to provide access to all persons for quality health care at reasonable rates.

Educational preparations for health care providers have traditionally been conducted in illness setting. Learning about health must be from curative and restorative view rather than preventive or health promotion. This emphasis, however, is beginning to change. Schools/Colleges of Nursing in many areas are teaching students about the concept of preventive and promotive health and are providing clinical experiences in areas where student can apply the nursing process to a healthy population. In studying healthy community, student can begin to appreciate various lifestyle practices and seek knowledge about these practices that tend to maintain or promote healthy states. This will help them to change their behaviour and eradicate the unhealthy actions.

As community health nurses we should be advocating an approach of preventing, care and maintenance of healthy state.

Nurse working in the community with sound understanding and appreciation of the health concept will be able to provide realistic and attainable nursing care plans to the people with whom she works.

Concept

Due to the changes in health care delivery system, the need for community health nursing service is also changing. The government, private health institutions and consumers are supporting primary care, home care and health promotion so as to reduce the need for more expensive institutional based care. In the community, growing health consciousness is leading them to assume more responsibility for their own health and health care. Therefore, community health nurse has to work in collaboration with community to identify, their health needs and meet those needs.

Definition of Community

Different concepts and definitions of *'community'* have been given by experts.

It is defined as *a group of people living together in a defined geographical area, in the same locality, district and country, sharing the same resources, a social group; or class having common interest.*

Community is a group of inhabitants being in somewhat localized area under the same general regulations and having common norms, culture and organisations.

Community is made-up of many groups who serve as channels of communication audience and sounding boards.

Community includes a group of people who have common interest and needs which they can identify or be helped to identify.

The common thing in all the above definitions is a group of people, thus community cannot be without people. The community is also characterised by place and resources. The main focus is on specific community characteristics like geographical boundaries, educational status, environmental factors, demographical characteristics, culture, occupation, political structures and socio-economic status. All these factors affect the structure of a community. Individuals and families are likewise affected by community characteristics.

Community is also defined as *a group of people living together in the same geographical area sharing same interests, values, religious, political, economical and social factors.*

Geographical

Boundaries, landmarks, natural resources (water, soil, climate and season) are important factors to be considered about a place.

Demographical

Population, its agewise distribution, sexwise distribution, economic conditions, education and religion.

Social System

People in a community belong to different religions, castes, classes, which have variety of beliefs, customs, cultures and traditions. These factors help to determine the spread of disease, act as guidelines in delivering the health services and to determine the factors causing nonacceptability of health service.

Resources

The resources like men, money and materials available to run the health services. The funds may come from three levels :

- Government provides equipped hospitals.
- Medical colleges to provide health personnel.
- Health schemes to tackle with the health problems and private practitioners provide generalised and specialised health care.

COMMUNITY HEALTH

To ensure every individual a standard of living, maintaining the health, community health has a vital role to play. Public health as named earlier was defined by Wanglow in 1920 as : *Science and art of preventing disease, prolonging life and promoting health and efficiency through organised efforts for sanitation of environment, control of communicable diseases, health education, public health, medical care, nursing services for early diagnosis, treatment and maintenance of health.*

Public health deals in the health of public in general, while the preventive and social medicine has an academical field.

In early days of public health, the field extended up to prevention of communicable diseases, sanitation, chronic diseases, accidents, maternal and child health. Gradually, it included preventive measures of degenerative and hereditary diseases and geriatric problems. The recent problems of population growth is also dealt through family welfare programmes. Various communicable diseases are controlled through national programmes.

The discovery of synthetic insecticides like DDT, HCH, malathion and others, has brought drastic changes in the control of vector-borne diseases, *e.g.,* malaria, plague, rickettsial diseases, etc.

The availability of sulpha drugs, antimalarial, antibiotics, antitubercle and antileprosy drugs has enriched preventive medicine. Concept of disease eradication has been successful in eradicating smallpox and still few more like polio, leprosy and guinea worm will be eradicated. Emergence of preventive paediatric, geriatric and preventive cardiology reflects newer trends in the scope of public health.

Improving the living standard and health education will improve the overall health of public at large. Three levels of prevention as primary, secondary and tertiary have reduced the prevalence of chronic disability related to disease.

Objectives

Objectives of preventive health care have become prominent in the delivery of health services. Community health has four main objectives :

Prevention of Diseases

The first and foremost objective of community health is to prevent the disease from its occurrence, by blocking the modes of transmission from entering the agent into the host, or making the host resistant to a specific agent and protect against the disease by immunization, healthy practices, health education, etc.

Promotion of Health

Through various preventive ways health can be promoted by good nutrition, hygienic conditions (personal, food and environmental), health education and healthy ways of living, etc.

Curative Health

In case individuals fail to promote the health and prevent disease, illness might occur. In case of a person suffering from a disease which makes him unfit to perform daily activities, he is given all available treatment to cure the disease.

Rehabilitation Health

The person is rehabilitated by helping him to settle himself as an economic asset or himself dependent individual in the society, so that he does not feel unfit to work after his illness and not accepted in the family and society. Community health nursing practice is the field of nursing practice for which there exists a body of knowledge and related skills, applied in meeting the health needs of communities and of individuals and families in their normal environments such as the house, school and the place of work. It is an area of practice which lies primarily outside therapeutic and inturn reflects the areas of population parameters.

Community Health Nurse Practices

The community health nurse practices in a variety of settings and in different ways from the traditional nursing practiced to acute care facilities. Community health nursing is also carried out on an independent basis when the community nurse engages in an individual **contractual** type of practice. Community nursing is collaborative, interrelated and occasionally overlapping with other health disciplines, that is, role may become blurred depending upon the situation.

Community health nursing is a synthesis of public health science and nursing science (Fig. 4.1). The knowledge on which practice is based incorporates theory from both public

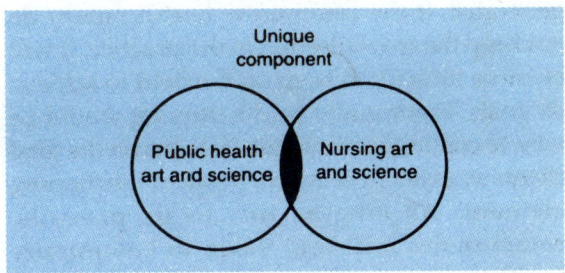

Fig. 4.1 : Public Health Nursing a synthesis of public health and nursing

health sciences and nursing science. Public health relates to control of communicable diseases, environmental sanitation, vital health statistics, laboratory services, maternal and child health, and health education. Within the nursing practices exist the means for providing the people with the knowledge and methods achieving their maximum human potentials through realisation of optimum health.

Thus, community health nursing is defined by American Nurses Association (ANA) and American Public Health Association (APHA) as :

Community health nursing is a synthesis of nursing practice and public health practice applied to promoting and preserving the health of population. The practice is general and comprehensive. It is not limited to a particular age, group diagnosis and is continuing not episodic. The dominant responsibility is on the population as a whole. Therefore, nursing directed to individuals, families or groups contribute to the health of total population. Health promotion, health maintenance, and health education, co-ordination and continuity of care are utilised in "holistic approach to the family, group and community. The nurse's actions, knowledge, the need for comprehensive health planning recognise the influences of social and ecological issues, give attention to populations at risk and utilize the dynamic forces which influence the change.

Scope of Community Health Nursing Practice

Majority of community health nurses are still practicing as generalised nurses. The ever increasing knowledge base and new technologies are making it difficult to work as generalist. If the community health nurses do not keep the specialisation in the practice, it will be more difficult to keep up the field to achieve its goals. Community health nursing would be wise to continue to maintain its focus on the total clients as a system of interdependent functioning element. As long as this focus prevails, communities will find value in community health nursing services.

The focus of community health nursing is on the prevention of illness and promotion and maintenance of health. Nursing activities to achieve these goals include client education, counselling, advocacy and management of care. The major emphasis in community health nursing is on primary care, which begins when clients enter the health care system and continues throughout the duration of the client's care. Secondary and tertiary care are accorded less emphasis. Primary care clients are considered to be active members of the health care team and the goal of care is to assist clients assume self responsibility of health care.

Community Health Nursing Training

Community health nursing training was started in 1952 at College of Nursing, New Delhi, to provide specialised training for community health nursing. Later, it was transferred to All India Institute of Hygiene and Public Health, Kolkata. Public health supervision training is also given at Lady Reading Health School, New Delhi and All India Institute of Hygiene and Public Health, Kolkata. Various colleges of nursing are providing specialised postgraduate degree in community health nursing.

ANM training schools are giving two years training to students to work in health centres.

The qualified community health nurse is one who has undergone :

- Basic general nursing.
- Midwifery training.
- Post basic education in community health nursing, where Community Health Nursing is considered as special training programme of Postgraduate Nursing in Community Health.

Until now, the rural health services were mainly provided by health visitors, midwives and trained *dais* whose activities were mainly concerned regarding MCH care. The ANM were replaced through primary health centres and subcentres. Training of ANM was inadequate to meet the changing needs of the people. In 1977, Indian Nursing Council revised the curriculum for ANM course in order to prepare candidates with high school certificate as Health Workers (female) under multipurpose worker's scheme. These workers are prepared to perform multiactivities like MCH, records and reports, prevention and control of communicable diseases and sanitation, etc. The female health worker is mainly accountable for MCH and field worker's services. Field health worker (FHW) is responsible for 5000 of population and works within an area of five kilometer.

Community Health Nursing Practices

New levels of specialisation are designated and areas of responsibility and independence are increased, new position, classification are seen. The commonly designated nursing practice in community health fields are :

- Public health nurses, now named as Community health nurses
- Visiting nurses
- School health nurses
- Occupational health nurses
- Clinic nurses
- Home care nurses.

The positions differ markedly from community health nurse generalists to highly specialised practitioners. Community health nursing consists of many interdependent parts, all working towards a common goal of community health promotion.

Professional Requirements for Community Health Nursing

Community health nurses primarily work outside the hospital setting. Their function is to provide preventive, promotive, curative and rehabilitative care to the defined population.

They may be professional group of nurses, who have specialised in this field of practice,

(PHN, DPHN, etc.) or they may be partially trained having semi-professional level in the field of practice, *e.g.*, Lady Health Visitors (LHV).

Voluntary Health Workers

They can also be short trained workers. They are prepared either on job or in brief training courses to function in a limited way, *e.g.*, Traditional birth attendants and village health workers (TBA and VHW).

Though the task is accomplished by all the levels of health workers, the level of health care varies from one in which most of the nursing services are completed by untrained traditional workers and other activities are to be performed by the most sophisticated professional specialist services in comprehensive care centres.

GOALS OF COMMUNITY HEALTH NURSING

The goals of CHN are as follow :

1. Contribute to improve the community health nursing practice and service to community by :
   - Continuing education and enhancing knowledge in the field of community health, must be an integral part of professional practice.
   - New entrants must be given adequate training and orientation to various programmes.
   - Research must be conducted in relation to community health needs, problems and solutions to the problems.
2. To increase the capabilities of individual, family and group or community to cope with health and illness problems :
   - By providing adequate information to family or group to serve as basis for making health decisions, that they are expected to make.
   - The community must have a positive and accepted attitude towards the services provided. They must get appropriate guidance to develop general problem solving ability to enable them to deal with health problems for self-reliance.

3. To support and supplement the efforts of health workers or agencies in controlling communicable diseases and in the restoration and preservation of health :
   - Reporting of occurrence of preventable diseases and presence of health threats and the response to the offered health services.
   - Nursing support should be given to other health team members for the care of families, group or community by providing required information about home condition and family problems of the patients and supporting sanitation workers by reinforcing instructions regarding environment.
4. To control physical and social environmental conditions that threatens health of people :
   - Community health nurse must ensure healthy and safe environment from health threats like accidents, communicable diseases, inadequate and unsafe water supply, etc.
   - Environment should be conducive to social behaviour, *e.g.*, self-respect and self-realisation, adequate affection between parents and children, child-bearing practices must be safe and healthy.

Community health nurse has to collaboratively accomplish all these goals. She cannot complete it single handedly and she cannot ignore any one of these. In these defined goals opportunity for creativity, independence, rewarding practice is limited only by personal inclination or by the failure to consistently and continuously expand one's professional competence.

The community health nursing goals must be supplemented by each nurse in her own situation and brought down to more measurable, observable and exact statements.

FUNCTIONS OF COMMUNITY HEALTH NURSING

The functions of community health nursing practice are independent, interdependent and dependent according to the role setting and legal aspects to practice nursing. For example, some places have a variety of legal aspects on practice of the independent nurse, midwife and the functions of community health nursing represents those broad areas of responsibility that is expected to assume functions of any professional group as generally defined by professional associations. Community health nursing functions are also defined by American Nurses Association (ANA) and American Public Health Association (APHA).

The functions and activities of the community health nurse influenced by preventing public health problems and the workload that she may carry.

The first expert committee of WHO on public health states that public health nursing is a combination of nursing skills and some phases of social assistance and functions as part of total public health programmes for the promotion of health, prevention of illness and disability and rehabilitation. Some of the important functions of community health nursing.

Community health nurse functions vary according to her designation and qualification. Some community health nurses work at staff levels, others may function as an administrator, supervisor or instructor in health organisations.

- Community health nurse provides comprehensive health care to individual, family and community as a whole. These health services may be preventive, promotive and therapeutic care to the unhospitalised sick and preventive tests and procedures that are within nursing competences, health guidance, support and counselling. To accomplish this function, she needs to :

  (i) Perform direct responsibility to provide direct care, supervise and guide others who provide nursing care to sick at home.

  Like, if the chronic diabetic patient has to get injectable insulin, she can give injection and demonstrate other family members to give injection. She must supervise the family members giving injections to the patient.

  (ii) Educating people and arranging the educational sessions and also supervision of others who give education regarding health care. Example, she may organize health education sessions based on needs of the people or of family members who have to look after the sick. She may arrange for educational sessions through other specialised organizations to conduct teaching for people regarding various health aspects, *e.g.*, first aid, home nursing and training for *Dais*, etc.

  (iii) Referrals to other health agencies is an important function of community health nursing, to get health services or for educational opportunities.

- Strengthening family life and promoting personal or family developmental and self-realisation.

  Helping the families in the adjustment of social and emotional conditions that affect health and development of favourable home environment.

- Nurse works in special setting with other health personnels, such as schools, industries, factories to plan, implement and execute the health programme.

  (i) Planning, executing and evaluation of programme in community, school, she develops goals to meet the health needs, evaluates the programmes and replans, if needed.

  (ii) Reviews and interprets the information such as absentees records, service reports, teacher-nurse conference relevant to health needs of special groups.

  (iii) Serving as committee member for health planning and action.

- Community health nurse participates in control of various communicable diseases by participating in national health programmes.

(i) Epidemiological investigations in the field of communicable diseases—malaria, T.B., leprosy, filaria and many others.

(ii) Preventive measures—early detection of disease, providing care and supervision to reduce the effects of the disease.

(iii) Using variety of channels to alert parents, teachers, patients, vulnerable groups and people regarding various preventable diseases.

• Community health nurse plans and evaluates the nursing services provided to the community by :

(i) Setting goals and clearly defining outcomes for nursing services and establishing a systematic method for checking progress.

(ii) Conferring and planning with other health workers for the care of family or group.

(iii) Working with nursing supervisor or administrator to evaluate nursing accomplishments and plan for improvements.

• Community health nurse contributes to the decision making and policy setting in the health agency and community by :

(i) Sending reports or suggestions by her own working experience.

(ii) Making recommendations in the community health meetings and planning the programmes and policies.

• Community health nurse actively participates to the extension of knowledge in nursing and health care by engaging in surveys, studies and research.

(i) Selecting the problem and using problem solving method to solve the problems.

(ii) Carrying out simple studies related to field experience to contribute to skillful nursing.

(iii) Participate in research done by others related to health and nursing fields.

• Co-ordinates her work with other members of the health team working in the community, e.g., sanitation engineering and schools, etc.

• Supervision and guidance of the work of midwives, TBAs and other nursing personnel.

PRINCIPLES OF COMMUNITY HEALTH NURSING

All health personnel involved in community health work follow certain principles in their daily activities. The following are some of the main principles which may be used as a guide for the nurse wherever she works.

An Effective Member of the Health Team

Community health nurse is an effective health team member. The basic health team consists of community health nurse, health assistants, sanitation workers, multipurpose health workers, TBAs and village health guides. The team will plan and execute the health programme. Community health nurse assists in planning, implementing and evaluating the various health programmes. She works with the family / community as a unit of services regard-ing nutrition, sanitation, MCH, family welfare and immunization. She co-operates and is co-operated by each health team member. She must be familiar with the duties and responsibilities of all the other workers in the health team for proper co-ordination of the work.

Community Health Nurse is Accountable to the Health Authority

Community health nurse, whether employed in government, private or local sector, she plans, organises and executes the work in consultation with the authority. She has to co-ordinate all the health programmes with the authority like officer incharge, district health officer or director of primary health, because she is again accountable to government for health services in her community.

Maintains the Professional Relationship and Ethics at the Workplace

Community health nurse has to develop relationship with other health organisers of the community like BDO, *Panchayat* members, TBAs and *Mahila Mandal*. She should work in collaboration with *Hakims, Vaidyas,* homeopathic and allopathic medical practitioners. She needs to explain her programme of work to get co-operation from all leaders, especially those people (*e.g., Dai*) on whom the people have more confidence. Local health practitioners may promote and support new health worker or they may hinder the progress. It is essential to take help from community for their own interest and work.

Involvement of Community to Carry-out Health Programmes

Community health nurse must involve community people who can contribute a great deal to the health programme. Village leaders can become highly interested and effective promoters to health activities. A village worker has excellent opportunity to teach nutrition, hygiene, environmental sanitation, antenatal care, immunization and family planning. The village *Dais* can also take the training to teach people. She can refer pregnant women to health centres for care; she can gather children for immunization and she can be useful in many ways.

Provides the Health Services to All, Irrespective of Age, Sex, Nationality, Social and Economic Conditions

Every individual has the right to health and environment conducive to health. So, community health nursing services must be available to all the people according to their health needs, for effective health programmes. Community health nurse must be neutral towards political and religious relationship with community.

She must respect their political and religious beliefs and must not interfere in their decisions, unless they are barriers to healthy living. Understanding their religious, social customs, attitudes and beliefs will help her for appropriate approach for acceptance of healthy practices. Community health nurse must not accept gifts and bribes.

She must work with the community irrespective of any expectations from them. If she has to collect some funds, financial contribution must be deposited with the concerned authority for proper accounts. She must not encourage the people to offer some sort of gifts etc., so as to develop her relationship. Health services must be based on health needs.

All health programmes should be based on a particular community needs and community health nurse must aim at meeting the needs of the people. The health services should not be rendered according to the goals and needs of the health agencies. The most appropriate way is to survey the community to assess the needs and resources and plan need based care within the resources available.

Plan the Health Services Which are Realistic According to the Resources Available (Manpower and Health Facilities)

Community health nurse must set the objectives for health services which are achievable and realistic according to availability of health workers and resources. Unrealistic planned services may lead to frustrations and failures in health system. Therefore, before planning, the money, men and material must be assured.

Family and Community are the Units of Community Health Nursing

Community health nursing is family and community centred care, where the family is the actual setting for health care. Health and illness of an individual affect the family and then community at large. Nurse can observe and assess the needs of the family. Ultimate goal of community health nurse is to help the family to solve the problems and provide health education regarding healthy practices. More emphasis is on promotion of health of all family members, through counselling, emotional support, teaching, demonstration and providing nursing care to the patients.

Health Teaching is an Integrated Part of Community Health Nursing

Health teaching is the backbone of community health nursing. Nurse plays an essential role in giving health education, planned to an individual, family and community on various aspects of health, *e.g.*, immunization, care of child, hygiene, nutrition, environmental sanitation, and family planning, etc. Teaching is usually based on individual's felt needs to make it more interesting and effective. Continuity of the service is an effective service.

Community health nurse must provide continuous services to the people by regular follow-up and keeping in touch with people's health problems, actions and progress, she can replan and implement due care to the patient. Health services should include continuous, repeated contact with individual family. With continuous contact, people can get to know and trust the community health nurse and will be more approachable to health system. Evaluation of care is an essential factor.

Evaluation Planning

No planning is complete unless evaluation is planned. Hence, for planning the health services, there must be wider scope for evaluation by setting the goals to be achieved. Evaluation is only possible when goals have been clearly established. Community health nurse should establish goals, formulate programme and review the progress in collaboration with her organisation. Evaluation helps to critically review programmes which help further planning of the programme.

Records and Reports are Essential in Community Health Nursing

Complete health records and reports are important tasks of community health nurse to ensure quality care, continuity of the care and evaluate the health services. Community health nurse must maintain accurate, complete factual, clear records for legal aspects. The community health records are of various types like family records, disease records, immunization records, health worker's daily activity records, home-visit records, MCH records, and family planning records. Community health nurse should be qualified in the field of community health nursing.

She must be a trained graduate nurse to work in community field. Undergraduate nurse who is not exposed to community health, may not be competent to work in the field, unless she had obtained a special training and skills.

COMMUNITY IDENTIFICATION

It is the systematic process of knowing and exploring a defined community for assessing the health status and determining the possible factors affecting the health of people. It is more than making a medical or nursing diagnosis relevant to the community. It implies to exploring the area, people in general, community leaders in particular, their lifestyle and resources, etc. All these informations can be obtained by:

1. Holding formal and informal meeting with community people, leaders and organising group which may include *Panchayat* members, School teachers, *Mahila Mandals*, Youth clubs/groups, young innovators.
2. Observation visit to community for observation of physical environment, biological environment and psychosocial environment.
3. Informal communication with people.
4. Records and reports.
5. Formal community/sample survey.
6. Discussion with health and health allied personnel working in community.

Community health nurse needs to prepare guidelines or proforma to collect relevant and complete information. After completion of information, a complete profile of community should be ready to plan for health care to community. Community identification will also help in making community diagnosis.

Community Diagnosis

The community diagnosis highlights the health problems and health needs of community to assess the health status of people. Community diagnosis include needs of population at large, agewise distribution of people, education level, mortality and morbidity indication, risk factors for communicable and noncommunicable diseases, traditional cultural practices, maternal and child health practices. Lack of knowledge and attitude towards healthy living, inadequate and inefficient facilities, etc. This diagnosis will help to plan, implement and evaluate the health services to that particular community.

ROLES OF COMMUNITY HEALTH NURSE

Since community health nurse functions in a variety of roles, the skills needed to function should be a part of the educational programme for nursing practice. These skills may be related to communication, teaching, learning interpersonal relationship, problem solving, critical thinking and decision making. *Learning how to learn and to continue learning is a skill in itself that does not become outdated as do facts and some concepts.* Continuously updating the content of nursing is necessary since our scientific base is expanding as explosively as any other field of knowledge.

Community health nurse plays a variety of roles as a care provider, promoter, teacher, advocate, organiser, manager, consultant, co-ordinator, evaluator, researcher and referrer.

Role of provider is most common role for community health nurse and it is usually the one at which she stands the largest percentage of time. The nurse working in health department can be a provider in different ways. The main functions may be as health educator, teacher, counsellor. She also performs various assessment activities.

Direct Care Provider

This role includes such activities as provision of direct nursing care, supervision of other care givers and management or co-ordination of care provided by a team of interdisciplinary workers. In all these functions, the community health nurse is performing the implementation phase of the care plan. Community health nurse involved in home care spends a great deal of time serving as provider, especially when there is no family member who can be taught to give the care or when the degree of difficulty of the care is such that professional skilled nursing is needed.

Nurses working in the clinics are providers, like occupational health and school settings. Whenever community health nurses are providers, they work towards relinquishing the role to someone else or to resolving goals so that the care is no longer needed.

Indirect Care Provider

Community health nurse also provides indirect care to the patient by supervising, guiding and teaching the family who is responsible to give the care to the patient. She evaluates whether care given by family is appropriate or not, otherwise she may have to guide them for appropriate care.

Advocate

An advocate is also a person who speaks for and on behalf of some other persons or group. Community health nurse is an advocate for her clients and speaks to support in all health aspects. She can be advocate in two ways, *e.g.,* by helping clients to obtain what they are entitled to by health system and by trying the health system to be responsive to the client needs. In most mediator situations, this role involves a great deal of interpretations to the people on both sides of the issue. As an advocate, community health nurse is concerned to explain the views of a particular client to others.

She is a kind of mediator and gives advices, who will explain to the doctor regarding problems in taking the treatment, talking to school authorities for prolonged absenteeism of students. She will also consult the sanitation workers for community sanitation. She is seen as one who can stands between family and health services.

Advocate as defined by Kohnke (1980), "is an act of informing and supporting a person so that he can make the best decisions possible for himself". Community health nursing is directed towards providing care which promotes and preserves health and wellbeing of communities. Therefore, it is necessary to examine ways in which community health nurse can implement this role when working in families or community.

Advocacy role is perhaps the easiest to understand in relation to work with individuals. She can provide the person with information about options available and allow them to make decisions. For example, to refer the patient to another health agency, she may provide three options and they have to select one, hence on deciding for one option she supports the family's decision.

Community advocacy involves working with the community people to determine solutions for identifying problems and supporting ultimate decisions.

Teacher

Community health nurse must be able to teach many kinds of people, many kinds of things, at many places even though it may not be formal. A community health nurse teaches subjects which are conducive to goal accomplishment. This may include growth and development, communicable diseases, environmental sanitations, self-help in promoting health and self-care in coping with disease states. Teaching involves imparting information and demonstrating the use of it in performing the desired behaviour. We must keep this information active and updated. To teach successfully, we must know some of the essential things about learner and teaching-learning process. The aim of learning is to change the behaviour, but such alterations are not always immediate or observable. In community nursing, we rarely get immediate feedback from the learner's behaviour. Yet, the teaching we do may be of great value as it is probably the only primary prevention for a number of chronic illnesses. Sometimes, changes in vital statistics in the community will indicate some effects of our teaching, although we must be aware that many other variables are existing in the situation.

Evaluator

Community health nurse is able to evaluate the need of health services and how to deliver the health care and the impact of health services on health of people. Community health nurse needs to develop the means to evaluate the health needs and impact of performance of health care.

Important considerations on whether entire system is actually achieving its purpose, meeting the ultimate goals and how efficiently its process is moving on those directions. As community health nursing, we have special awareness of the impact of health agencies on the lives of clients, which may thus place us in a position to evaluate that impact with particular acquity. The time to time evaluation helps community health nurse to know if she is going in right direction with desired goals to be achieved, or else she may have to change her goals if not achievable. The role of evaluator requires careful preparation of evaluation process to be used in selected situations. Preparations for the role of evaluator will include to know the purpose of evaluation, the person or content to be evaluated and communication skills needed to communicate effectively the finding of the evaluation.

Researcher/Data Collector

Data collection is a step in the process of nursing diagnosis. It is a role which requires continuous questioning approach. Data collection is a systematic curiosity about what is really going on in community health. Better health care interventions are based on organised information, which may be obtained by a variety of sources by a nurse who is developing a care plan, working with clients, to reach their own decisions; skills in collecting informations must be practiced and should become a regular nursing tool that we have many chances to use in work as community health nurse.

Manager

Community health nurse with some abilities to organise and mediate may find herself as a co-ordinator and manager in the performance of health professionals to achieve a desired unified task of care. The managerial role differs from the co-ordinator-facilitator role, which focuses, on care the client receives, which after he gets from unco-ordinated providers. In that, nurse manager works with providers so that they present a balanced programme of care.

She is accountable for keeping the clinics running smoothly, organise and supervise the auxiliary workers and organise home visits. She is expected to identify, maintain and interpret the link between the community and the hospitals. She is seen as one who keeps all the community health services under proper management.

Observer

An essential aspect in home-visiting is observation. A community health nurse's role as an observer has an important place. Community health nurse is expected to observe and report the environmental and home conditions. Many facts may not be told by people, but she comes to know by close observation by working with family and community. All health services to the community/family rely on observational skills of nurse.

Referrer

Making referrals of clients to other services has become nearly essential for community health nursing. This activity has a great deal of importance because we must work with many kinds of clients with variety of concerns related directly to health. Knowledge of resources available to deal with such a spectrum of problems is one hallmark of an experienced community health nurse. The people are dependent on health professional during crisis for referrals. Community health nurse must often take this task, by going directly to the health agencies to facilitate the use of their services.

Counsellor

Another dimension of nurse's role is counselling. It is a helping process between the nurse and the client of the family. This requires a friendly relationship, honesty openness, and respect between client or group and nurse. It is a method of assisting others to identify feelings and to clarify beliefs and values about a concern in order to make appropriate decisions. Health counselling is a valuable way of assisting the client or group in improving the health practices and self-care ability.

Adviser

Community health nurse is committed towards provision of good service and advices. Patients and families, are depending upon her advices

on practical and urgent matters. They always appreciate, when she listens to their problems willingly and accept whatever advice she gives. A good community health nurse will always help them to accept such offer. A family who has no faith in health services, community health nurse may gain their confidence by talking to them and listening them, advising on various household matters and tries to solve them. Hence, they will even start accepting the advices on all health aspects as given by her.

Facilitator

Facilitation is a process of listening, explaining, verifying and describing any situation with the result that client or group is involved in decision making process.

The nurse's knowledge of human behaviour and learning allows the client/group to make decisions regarding better health outcomes. This may be done in various areas like parent-child group, child abuse, drug abuse, teenage pregnancy and self-care discussions.

Planner

Commnunity health nurse may be involved for health planning process. This role could involve gathering data or participating in implementation. Community health nursing becomes more actively involved in the planning role, for initiating projects.

Preparation of community health nurse as planner, needs advanced education often at master level. Experimental practice greatly enhances academic learning. Whenever community health nurse gets opportunity, it must involve in planning activities to develop the capabilities.

Co-ordinator

The role of co-ordinator is commonly used by community health nurse. She is often responsible to co-ordinate the activities of other health agencies and at least for participating in the co-ordination. She has to co-ordinate the activities of health services and communities, family, or a patient. She has to co-ordinate with other sectors indirectly related to health. She is co-ordinator between medical care and nursing services, etc.

Community Health Nursing as Specialist

Some community health nurses specialize in a particular aspect of nursing care. A clinical specialist may be employed in a community health agency as well as in a hospital. Clinical specialists are prepared on the master's level with a speciality in a specific field.

The specialists include nurse practitioners educated in areas such as family health, paediatrics or midwifery. Other nurses specialize in mental health counselling and family therapy.

Preparation for the role of clinical specialist includes advanced education and advanced clinical practice. It is most helpful for the nurse who wishes to assume this role to practice in a clinical setting for several years, first to develop practice skills and to identify areas of particular interest. Then, the nurse can look into advanced educational programmes.

Community health nursing is a specialized area of nursing practice that serves individual families and aggregates of people in a variety of ways in many settings. Emphasis is on primary prevention and health promotion. Community health nurse functions in roles similar to other nurses but with an emphasis and focus unique to community health.

Expanded Role

There has been specialised training and educational programmes in the field of paediatric nurse practitioner, school nurse practitioner, gerontology, family planning, diagnostic disease specialities.

The expanded role is based on cost effectiveness, people's satisfaction and job satisfaction for professionals.

Nurse practitioners found different roles in institutional and non-institutional settings, *e.g.*, ambulatory care, healthy clinics and other health departments etc.

To accomplish this goal, community health nurses work with groups, families and communities as well as multidisciplinary teams and programmes. Identifying high-risk individuals, disabilities and premature deaths and directing resources towards these groups are the most effective approaches for accomplishing the goal.

Success in reducing the risk and improving the health of community depends upon involvement of people, especially high-risk group, and other community people in health planning and self-care activities.

BASIC SKILLS IN NURSING PRACTICE

Perceiving

Perceiving is the process of observing, organizing and interpreting sensations received from internal and external stimuli into a meaningful pattern that is usable in transaction with the environment. Perception is achieved by five steps :

- Noticing
- Organizing
- Analysing
- Synthesis
- Acknowledge as meaningful stimuli.

The process of perceiving is central to all nursing practices. The nurse who is perceptive demonstrates openness to experience and listens with awareness, hearing covert as well as overt messages in communication with others. Perceiving enables the nurse to observe the physical, emotional and mental states of clients, recognising common and recurrent health problems and potential illness and discrepancies between health needs and the care being provided.

Communicating

Communicating is the process of sharing personal meaning in order to influence behaviour. The goals of communicating is to achieve understanding or behavioural change in self or others. It is a process in which there is exchange of information between sender and receiver. Mainly four components are important for effective communication :

- Sender
- Receiver
- Message
- Media / channel and feedback.

Effective communications are essential to nursing practice. Those who have achieved the communication skills, will develop mutually satisfying working relationship with clients and colleagues. Effective communication contributes to learning by encouraging group discussions, in which reading, resources, clinical experiences, and insight are shared. Nurses who communicate effectively share their clinical work with colleagues in written as well as spoken, meet the professional standards for excellence. Through communication she can identify the health needs, implement and evaluate the health care to the people more effectively and efficiently.

Caring

Caring and communicating are interrelated to each other. She identifies the needs by communication and caring is based on health needs. While caring for the patient she needs to maintain working relationship by explaining.

Caring is the process being responsive to the needs of the others in relationship characterised by understanding, acceptance and empathy. Caring involves :

- Recognition of need
- Availability to respond to the need
- Availability of resources to alleviate the need, and
- Presence of mutuality of needs and response between client and nurse.

The caring nurse establishes a professional relationship that is supportive of mutual trust, communication and confidence and is able to communicate feeling of warmth, understanding and acceptance to the client. In addition to a concern for the psychosocial aspect of nursing care, the caring nurse is expert in providing the physical needs of the client as a caring process.

Knowing

Knowing has been described as comprehending, grasping the essential characteristics having knowledge or information and possessing a clear understanding or firm mental grasp. The process involves the incorporations of an idea to achieve logical integration and congruity and to change the existing organisation of knowledge.

Implementation

Using the chosen approach to achieve the established goals, community health nurse needs to take action towards right direction to achieve the goals.

Evaluation

Evaluation of the process and outcome to determine the effectiveness and need to employ the process repeatedly until the identified goals are achieved, revised or determined to be unattainable by available means.

The nurse uses problem solving approach intelligently in various fields of problem. Nurse who solves problems effectively employs the assessment, intervention and evaluating phases of the process.

CHANGING SKILLS IN NURSING PRACTICE

Inquiry

The ability to think critically, questioning and generate knowledge.

Helping

Involves purposeful, dynamic process within time limited relationship that is directed towards enabling a client to achieve a more satisfactory level of functioning in a variety of life situation. The purpose of helping is to enable a client to cope effectively. The focus is on the health needs of the client rather than needs of the helper.

Teaching

It is an ability to assist others to acquire the health related knowledge, skill and values that maintain cognitive interpersonal and psychomotor functioning.

The knowledgeable nursing practitioner is able to replicate and apply the factional and theory based knowledge upon which nursing judgements are based. A nurse is able to use the knowledge as intellectual competencies to facilitate cognitive functioning.

In teaching, the nurses assess the health related learning needs of individuals. They plans and implement the health education and guidance, focusing on ways to promote and maintain health and prevent illness and disability. As teacher, nurse evaluates the effectiveness of their teaching plans in terms of health related behaviour of the learner (expected to change).

Problem Solving

Problem solving is a goal oriented process of seeking solutions to dilemmas through the use of series of steps including simplest form of assessment, interventions and evaluation. The steps of problems solving are :

- *Problem identifications* : Include identification, clarifications and understanding of the problem. The problem should be stated clearly in such a way that it appears solvable.
- *Establishing priorities* : Which problem needs immediate attention and which to postpone according to severity of problem.
- *Establishing goals* : Requires describing a situation as a client would like it to be. Goals should be realistic and stated in a measurable and attainable way.
- *Generation of means* : Available for reaching each concrete goal. Enumerating the specific ways of strengthening the facilitating forces.
- *Selection of means* : It must be based on cost benefit analysis, which indicates the most positive results within less expenditure.

Collaboration

It is working together in an equilitarian spirit to achieve mutually defined and desired goal. Nurses who function collaboratively are able to demonstrate their professional competencies. Intradisciplinary work is prized for its opportunities for collaboration.

Consultation

It is an interactional process between professional in which the consultant shares specialised knowledge and expertise to assist the consultee to solve work related problem within the framework of the consultee's professional functioning. The nurse using consultation as an approach to creating change relies on the power of knowledge rather than on position or control within an organisation.

Administration

It is the process of policy determination and implementation to carryout the purposes and goals of an organisation. It is a skill concerned with the philosophy, purpose, policies, procedures and practices of complex organisation.

Supervision

It is the ability to assist people to function effectively by guiding their professional development and increasing their performance skills. The purpose of supervisory skills is to increase expertise of the staff members with the goals of their achieving professional autonomy. Nurses who employ the supervising process need to clarify their own philosophy of professional practice and supervision in order to assist others to accomplish the same goal. The focus should be on the growth of the staff by guidance about staff performance on the basis of agency policy and professional expectations. Supervisor needs to clarify the expectations of staff, reinforce the satisfactory aspect of staff performance and initiate supervisory regarding unsatisfactory aspect of performance.

Co-ordination

It is ability to bring together diverse approaches of health care in such a way as to deliver the quality health care. Quality health care requires the efforts of many health professionals, whose activities require co-ordination in order to provide the client with an organised system of care.

She must be a trained graduate nurse to work in community field. Undergraduate nurse who is not exposed to community health, may not be competent to work in the field, unless she had observed a special skills.

GUIDELINES FOR COMMUNITY IDENTIFICATION

Geographic Characteristics

This helps to know the area and climate and its impact on health.

- Name of the area
- Geographical boundaries
- Administrative boundaries
- Important roads, streets, buildings, institutions, maps, etc.
- Seasonal variations, etc.

Demographic Characteristics

This characteristics will help to know the type of people and number of people living in the area.

Population Characteristics

- Total population, total number of families, types and size of families
- Population density
- Population according to :
  - Age, sex.
  - Education, occupation, income.
  - Ethinic groups–caste, religion, language, etc.

Vital Health Statistics

Birth rate, death rate, life-expectancy, morbidity rate, procedure of collection and maintenance of data, etc.

Vulnerable or Special Risk Groups

Infants and toddlers, nursing and lactating mothers, multiproblem families, extensive poverty, etc.

Environmental Characteristics

Environment plays important role and its study will help to identify problems and their solutions.

Physical Environment

- Housing conditions : Number, type, living space facilities (bathroom, kitchen, laterine, electricity and water supply, etc.)

- Sources of water supply, water quality
- Removal and disposal of waste water
- Collection, removal and disposal of solid waste
- Vector control
- Environmental pollution
- Climate
- Structural organization and administration of environmental health services
- Educational opportunities.

Social Environment

These factors help to identify leaders who can help in giving community health care.

Community Organizations

- Kinship and caste organizations
- Value system in general and specific to health practices
- *Voluntary welfare organizations* : Caste organization, youth welfare association, youth clubs, ladies organizations, *Vikas Mandals*, occupational organization, volunteers, etc.
- *Trade unions* : Labour units, business organizations
- *Statutory body* : Gram panchayat, Nayay panchayat, Sadachar samities.

Leadership

- Local traditional.
  - *Biradari* leaders
  - Priests
  - Hereditary leaders
  - Teachers
  - Landlords and moneylenders.
- Informal leaders, influential persons
- Local corporators / MPs
- Leaders of political parties, trade unions, Mohalla welfare associations.
- Innovators.

Group Dynamics

- Major groups
  - Caste, occupational, religious and play groups

- Integrating factors
  — Common interests and security, etc.
- *Disintegrating factors* : Personal rivalries, caste rivalries.

Channels of Communication

- Existing channels
  — Kinship
  — Non-official
  — Traditional.
- Common meeting places
  — Reading room
  — Community hall
  — Community centre
  — *Chaupal*, etc.
- Important communications
  — Traditional like barbers, *numberdar*, teachers and retired people.
- Mechanism of communication of cultural heritage
  — *Katha, kirtan*, fair and festivals, religious and political gatherings, etc.
- Modern media of communication
  — Radio, T.V., cinema, etc.

Resources

Community Health Nurse needs to explore the resources available. Hence she must know the resources (men, money and material) available.

Economic Aspects

- Occupational characteristics
- Family income
- Per Capital Income
- Family members = 5

Institutional Resource

- Health and allied agencies
- Educational institution
- Social welfare agencies
- Health committees, etc.
- Transport and communication, marketing and industrial facilities, religious and recreational facilities.

Human Resources

- Professionals.
  — Doctors.
  — Teachers.
  — Lawyers etc.
  — Nurses etc.
- Para professionals.
  — Formal and informal.
  — Indigenous practitioners, traditional health workers, magic curers, etc.

Health Knowledge, Attitude and Practices

CHN must know about knowledge attitude and practices of health, so that she can remove the misconceptions and educate for healthy practices and gain more knowledge of people about health.

- Beliefs and knowledge on health and disease.
- Beliefs and knowledge on (outlook on) cause, spread, treatment and prevention of diseases.
- Existing health practices regarding prevention, treatment, cure, etc. of some of the specific diseases.
- Taboos during illness, epidemics, fevers, respiratory diseases, mental diseases, etc.
- *Promotional health practices* : Food, rest, relation and sleep, recreation, games, exercises, etc.
- *Attitude towards* : Health agencies, health programmes, social welfare programmes, community organizations, community leaders, etc.

Health Problems as Felt by the Community

- Major health problems and the needs
- Priority problems and the needs as felt by the people.

SOURCES OF DATA COLLECTION

1. Health and health allied records maintained by different agencies of the community
2. Officials working in these agencies
3. Community people in general
4. Community leaders
   — Formal/informal
   — Officials/non-officials
5. Census records.

METHODS OF DATA COLLECTION

- Interview
- Questionnaire
- Observations
- Study of records.

The study of these factors will give clear picture to a nurse to plan, implement and evaluate the health care services for people.

Roles and Responsibilities of Community Health Nursing Personnel

INTRODUCTION

Community Health Nursing Team and Nursing Personnel (Figs. 5.1 & 5.2)

A professional health team functions in home, hospital or other health agencies. Members of the team are the patient and his family, physician, graduate nurses, social worker and other allied professional worker.

Teamwork means "the smoothly co-ordinated synchronized activity that characterises a close knit group". It is based on :

(a) Team spirit in all members
(b) Of a small group
(c) Each of whom is able to make a practical contribution to the common goal
(d) Who have frequent and full two-way communication in face to face talk to plan and evaluate group activity
(e) Continued practice in supplementing each other as team member.

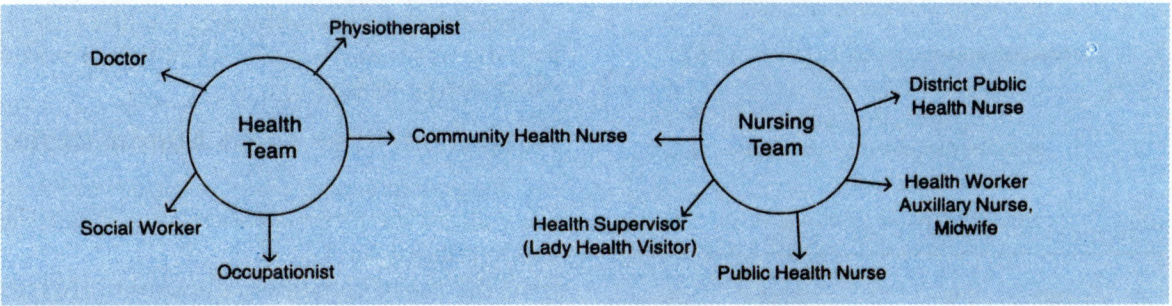

Fig. 5.1 : Community Health Nursing Team

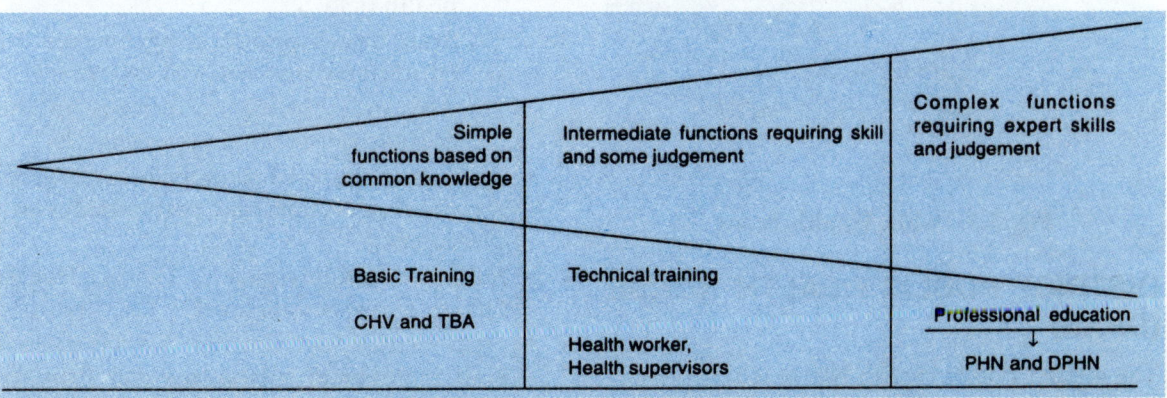

Fig. 5.2 : Levels of Community Health Nursing Personnel

FUNCTIONS OF NURSING TEAM

Nursing is unique, its uniqueness lying in the close and individualised service to the patient, the service may vary with his state of health from dependence in which the nurse performs for him, what he cannot do for himself through supportive and rehabilitative care, physical and emotional to self-direction of his own health.

The health care services in community health are based on **public health team** (Fig. 5.3). All members of the health teamwork together collaboratively, collectively and co-operatively to achieve the desired health outcome of people. As there have been changes in health care delivery system, the public health team has also been changing.

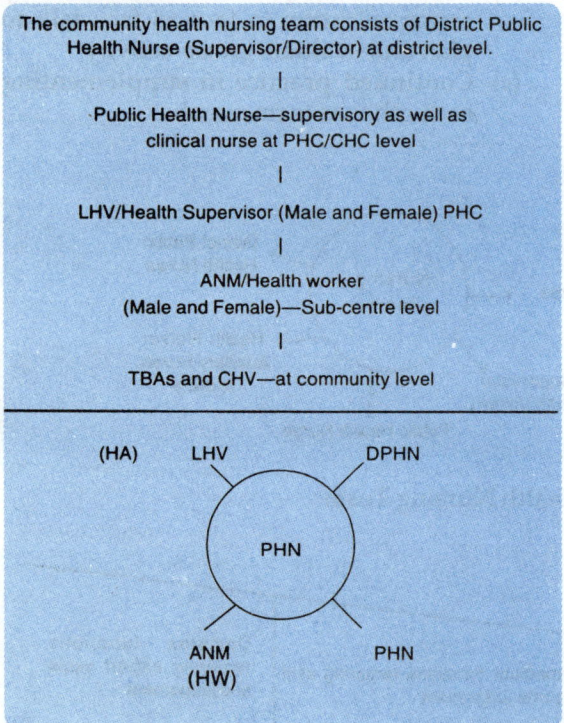

The community health nursing team consists of District Public Health Nurse (Supervisor/Director) at district level.

|

Public Health Nurse—supervisory as well as clinical nurse at PHC/CHC level

|

LHV/Health Supervisor (Male and Female) PHC

|

ANM/Health worker
(Male and Female)—Sub-centre level

|

TBAs and CHV—at community level

(HA)   LHV   DPHN

PHN

ANM   PHN
(HW)

Fig. 5.3: Public Health Team

DISTRICT PUBLIC HEALTH NURSE (DPHN)

The district Public Health Nurse is responsible for planning organising and directing the public health programme of jurisdiction where she is appointed.

- Participates in policy making activities in regard to health care.

She needs to learn and understand the organisation and administration of the state where she works. Public health nurse is affected by state administration and states public health programmes are affected by quantity and quality of public health nursing services available in urban and rural areas.

- Evaluation of nursing services is done by District public health nurse who plans for continuously improving the quality of client care.

The district public health nurse is attached to the district health office. She is directly responsible to the district health officer and delegates the responsibilities to all nursing personnel in the district community health field i.e., PHC, SC, family planning and all national health programmes. She is supervised by nursing officer at directorate level.

District public health nurse works in close co-ordination with community health nursing, nursing tutors and hospital administrators and other health workers.

Responsibilities as an Administrator

- Responsible for efficient implementation of policies and programmes relating to nursing in public health.
- Will make recommendations to district health officer on :
  (a) Requirements of nursing staff in public health field.
  (b) Staff development programmes for educational promotional awareness.
  (c) Any indiscipline occurrence in the community or nursing personnels.
- Determine the need for supply and equipment for her section, take part in budgetary planning.
- Submit monthly report to District Health Officer at directorate level.
- Field visits at least four times a day to each staff member in subcentres and Primary health centres and ensures the quality care, submit annual complete standard report for all Primary health centres and sub-centres

visits paid and recommendations for improvement of public health services.

Supervisory Responsibilities

- Conducting regular meetings and solving official as well as personal problems in best possible way.
- Encourage initiative and help in promoting professional growth of staff.
- Interpretations of policies, plans and rules to the staff so as to regulate and develop the services.
- Advice on organising and planning of work, helping the individual staff members to evaluate the needs of their particular areas and to select priority for her work.
- Help in improving the quality and quantity of health services by establishing good patterns of procedures and techniques.
- Guidance to staff regarding use of records, reports and the collection of statistical data and record keeping system.
- Ensure that public health nursing personnel have job descriptions, standing orders and understand their interpretations in the area of their work.

Educational Responsibilities

- Organise the inservice education programme for all nursing staff.
- Initiate and assist in planning and organising the orientation programme for new staff.
- Participate in community health field experience organised for nursing students of schools or colleges.
  - Suggest in selection of areas for practical experience.
  - Provide facilities and resources to students and staff.
  - Guide students during field experience.
- Help to supervise and guide the traditional birth attendants (TBAs).
- Keep her knowledge updated by reading, attending professional seminars and meetings, etc.

ROLES AND RESPONSIBILITIES OF COMMUNITY HEALTH NURSE

Community health nurse represents the most numerous of professional workers in the public health field and nursing services are employed to implement or support virtually all of the services offered to community.

- Community health nurse participates in planning, development and evaluation of the agency programme as a whole and advisement of other administrative staff in nursing matters. The special competencies and technical knowledge of nursing have a big contribution to make in relation to determining the care and content of public health programme.

  Application of nursing practice in public health field involves the use not only of technical and administrative skills with which the people are familiar but also the nursing skills of inter-personal and organisational in character. Nurse not only provides homely, comforting services, treatment provided for the care of the sick but also uses counselling and group work skills to teach and motivate families or groups toward better health care. She uses epidemiologic as well as physiologic bases in her observation of the health status of the family or community.

- She uses administrative as well as clinical skills in organising clinics and recruiting and training volunteers.
- Community health nurse considers the family as a service unit rather an individual, hence family health care is an important component of her functions.
- She plans her work and evaluates its effectiveness in terms of community as a whole.
- Provides nursing care to non-hospitalised sick, direct care or teaches the family member to give care to sick.
- **Medical supportive activities :** Assisting with medical procedures, identifying and reporting significant conditions or symptoms, providing inspectional services, *e.g.*, examination of school students, during high

incidence of communicable diseases, routine observation of industrial workers exposed to specific occupational hazards and interpreting home or community factors. She prefers diagnostic testing procedures that can be done safely without medical supervision, *e.g.*, collect specimens and blood slides.

- **Health counselling and teaching :** Family health counselling and teaching in all aspects of family care. Health counselling is the action taken to assist individual to make and carry-out his own plans to meet health problems. Teaching may be a part of counselling and involves provision of information in such a way that family or individual learns how to apply this information in his own situation and gains a desired health care.

  Control of environmental health hazard is an integral part of public health nursing, observation and teaching help to control the accidents, hazards at home, school and industries, prevent unnecessary exposure to injury or infection.

- Participation in development of the total public health programmes, the public health nurse plans with appropriate medical and administrative personnel within the agency or school regarding nursing participation in the health programmes and carries out the nursing activities.

- Participates in planning, conducting and evaluating instinct educational programmes for nursing personnel.

Responsibilities

General

- Responsible for organising and conducting the health clinics, *e.g.*, well baby clinic, antenatal clinic, family welfare and general clinics, etc.

- Supervising, organising and planning home visits for subordinate nurses and give suggestions for improvement.

- Organise and encourage the educational activities for improving quality care.

- Will interpret the need of the nursing and health services to medical officer.

Administrative

Responsibilities for the efficient implementation of policies and programmes.

- Outline the nursing requirements for nursing services and training programmes.

- Responsible for ascertaining the need for supplies and equipments in her section and arrange for adequate maintenance.

Supervisory

Promote harmony and efficiency within the team to improve the quality of work.

- Promote the professional growth of other staff and encourage initiative.

- Will interpret the staff policies, plans and rules laid down for developing and regulating the service.

- Review the use of records, reports and collection of statistical data and advise wherever necessary.

- Describe each staff member's **job description** and interpret in the area of her own work.

- Home visit as per schedule to supervise the staff.

- Arrange orientation programme of all new staff posted to training unit area to acquint them with the geography of the area, set-up, policies, duties of different staff and channels of communication.

Plan and carryout continuous and effective inservice training programme, arranging monthly meetings for all nursing staff.

Practical nurses are prepared to provide simple nursing care under the direction of a professional nurse or physician. They have been proved as useful in providing home care to the long-term illness and as assistants in clinics, where they relieve the professional staff for more existing work. In such cases community health nurse takes the responsibility of providing more complex services and delegates the task to practical nurse which they can do competently.

Nurse's Aids

They have been used in increased numbers in clinics. They are generally trained on jobs and work under close supervision of professional nurse. They assist in activities which do not require skills, *e.g.*, setting up clinics, equipments, carry-out for supply, assisting in doing procedures controlling the people gathering.

LADY HEALTH VISITORS/HEALTH ASSISTANT/SUPERVISOR (FEMALE)

They have been trained to provide specified health care in community health nursing. The multipurpose workers health scheme was designated LHVs as health supervisors (female). They have been given a special training of 6 months to promote as health supervisors and perform the activities to supervise the health worker's duty. The health supervisors are usually placed in primary health centre. Their job responsibilities have been listed as below.

Job Responsibilities of Health Assistant/Supervisor (Female)

Under the **Multipurpose Workers Scheme** a health assistant female is expected to cover a population of 30,000 (20,000 in tribal and hilly areas) in which there are six subcentres, each with one health worker female. The health assistant female will carryout the following duties :

- **Supervision and Guidance**
  - (*a*) Supervise and guide the health worker female, *Dais* and female health guides in the delivery of health care services to the community.
  - (*b*) Strengthen the knowledge and skills of the health worker female.
  - (*c*) Help the health worker female in improving her skills in working in the community.
  - (*d*) Help and guide the health worker female in planning and organising her programme of activities.
  - (*e*) Visit each subcentre at least once a week on a fixed day to observe and guide the health worker female in her day-to-day activities.

- (*f*) Assess fortnightly the progress of work of the health worker female and submit an assessment report to the medical officer of the primary health programme.
- (*g*) Carryout supervisory home visits in the area of the health worker female with respect to their duties under various National Health Programmes.
- (*h*) Supervise referral of all pregnant women for Venereal Disease Research Laboratory (VDRL) testing to Community Health Centre (CHC)/Sub-divisional hospital.

- **Team Work**
  - (*a*) Help the health workers to work as part of the health team.
  - (*b*) Co-ordinate her activities with those of the health assistant male and other health personnel including the *Dais* and health guides.
  - (*c*) Co-ordinate the health activities in her area with the activities of workers of other departments and agencies and attend meetings at primary health centre (PHC) level.
  - (*d*) Conduct regular staff meetings with the health workers in co-ordination with the health assistant male.
  - (*e*) Attend staff meetings at the primary health centre.
  - (*f*) Assist the medical officer of the primary health centre in the organisation of the different health services in the area.
  - (*g*) Participate as a member of the health team in mass camps and campaigns in health programmes.

- **Supplies, Equipment and Maintenance of Subcentres**
  - (*a*) In collaboration with the health assistant male, check at regular intervals the stores available at the subcentre and help in the procurement of supplies and equipments.
  - (*b*) Check that the drugs at the subcentre are properly stored and that the equipments is well-maintained.

(c) Ensure that the health worker female maintains her general kit and midwifery kit and *Dai* kit in the proper way.

(d) Ensure that the subcentre is kept clean and is properly maintained.

• **Records and Reports**

(a) Scrutinise the maintenance of records by the health worker female and guide her in their proper maintenance.

(b) Maintain the prescribed records and prepare the necessary reports.

(c) Review reports received from the health workers female, consolidate them and submit monthly reports to the medical officer of the primary health centre.

Additional duties where Kala-azar is endemic :

1. Supervise the work of health worker female during concurrent visit and will check whether the worker is performing her duties.

2. Visit minimum 10 per cent of the houses in a village to verify that the health worker female really visited those houses and carried her job properly. Her job of identifying suspected kala-azar cases and ensuring complete treatment has been done properly.

3. Carry with her the proper record forms, diary and guidelines for identifying suspected kala-azar cases.

4. Be responsible along with health assistant male for ensuring complete treatment of kala-azar patients in his area.

5. Be responsible alongwith health assistant male for ensuring complete coverage during the spray activities and search operations.

6. Also undertake health education activities particuly through interpersonnel communication, arranging group meetings with leaders and organizing and conducting training of community leaders with the assistance of health team.

Specific Duties where Japanese Encephalitis is Endemic—FHS will

1. Supervise the work of health worker female during concurrent visit and will check whether the worker is performing her duties.

2. Check along with minimum of 10 per cent of the houses in a village to verify that the health worker female really visited those houses and carried her job properly. Her job of identifying suspected kala-azar cases and ensuring complete treatment has been done properly.

3. Carry the proper record forms, diary and guidelines for identifying suspected kala-azar cases.

4. Be responsible for ensuring complete treatment of kala-azar patients in her area.

5. Be responsible for ensuring complete coverage during the spray activities and search operations.

• **Training**

(a) Organise and conduct training for *Dais* with the assistance of the health worker female.

(b) Assist the medical officer of the primary health centre in conducting training programmes for various categories of health personnel.

• **Maternal and Child Health**

(a) Conduct weekly MCH clinics at each subcentre with the assistance of the health worker female and *Dais*.

(b) Respond to calls from the health worker female, the health worker male, the health guides and the trained *Dais* and render the necessary help.

(c) Conduct deliveries when required at primary health centre level and provide domiciliary and midwifery services.

• **Family Planning and Medical Termination of Pregnancy—She will**

(a) Ensure through spot checking that health worker female maintains up-to-date eligible couple registers all the times.

(b) Conduct weekly family planning clinics (along with the MCH clinics) at each subcentre with the assistance of the health worker female.

(c) Personally motivate resistant case for family planning.

(d) Provide information on the availability of services for medical termination of pregnancy and for sterilisation. Refer suitable cases for MTP to the approved institutions.

(e) Guide the health worker female in establishing female depot holders for the distribution of conventional contraceptives and train the depot holders with the assistance of the health workers female.

(f) Provide IUD services and their follow-up.

(g) Assist medical officers at primary health centre (PHC) in organisation of family planning camps and drives.

- **Nutrition**

(a) Ensure that all cases of malnutrition among infants and young children (zero to five years) are given the necessary treatment and advice and refer serious cases to the primary health centre.

(b) Ensure that iron and folic acid and vitamin A are distributed to the beneficiaries as prescribed.

(c) Educate the expectant mother regarding breastfeeding.

- **Universal Immunisation Programme**

(a) Supervise the immunisation of all pregnant women and children (zero to five years).

(b) Guide the health worker (HW) (female) to procure supplies, organise immunisation camps, provide guidance for maintaining cold chain storage of vaccines. Health education and also in immunizations.

(c) Supervise the immunisation of all pregnant women and infants.

(d) Follow the directions given in Manual of Health Worker Female under National Immunisation Programme.

Acute Respiratory Infection (ARI)

1. Ensure early diagnosis of pneumonia cases.
2. Provide suitable treatment to mild/moderate cases of acute respiratory infection (ARI).
3. Ensure early referral in doubtful/severe cases.

School Health

1. Help the medical officers in school health services.

- **Primary Medical Care**

(a) Ensure treatment for minor ailments, provide oral rehydration solution (ORS) and first aid for accidents and emergencies and refer cases beyond her competence to the primary health centre or nearest hospital.

- **Health Education**

(a) Carry-out educational activities for MCH, family planning, nutrition and immunisation, control of blindness, dental care and other National Health Programmes like leprosy and tuberculosis with the assistance of the health worker female.

(b) Arrange group meetings with leaders and involve them in spreading the message for various health programmes.

(c) Organise and conduct training of women leaders with the assistance of the health worker female.

(d) Organise and utilize *Mahila Mandal*, teachers and other women in the community in the family welfare programmes, including International classifications of disease scheme (ICDS) personnel.

ROLES AND RESPONSIBILITIES OF ANM/HEALTH WORKER (F)

The auxiliary nurse midwives (ANMs) are designated as health worker (F), as per multipurpose workers scheme. They complete 2 years of training. They have been posted in subcentres to provide comprehensive health care services to community and assist the PHN and health supervisor in providing health care to defined area. Their main areas of jobs are :

Job Responsibilities of Health Worker (Female)

Under the multipurpose workers scheme, one health worker female and one health worker male are posted at each subcentre and are expected ultimately to cover a population of 5,000 (3,000 in tribal and hilly areas). She will carry-out the following duties :

Maternal and Child Health

(a) Register and provide care to pregnant women throughout the period of pregnancy.

(b) Test urine of pregnant women for albumen and sugar and estimate haemoglobin level during her home visits and at the clinic.

(c) Ensure that all pregnant women get VDRL test done.

(d) Refer cases of abnormal pregnancy and cases with medical and gynaecological problems to the health assistant female or the primary health centre.

(e) Conduct about 50 per cent of total deliveries in her area.

(f) Supervise deliveries conducted by Dais and assist them whenever called for.

(g) Refer cases of difficult labour and newborns with abnormalities, help them to get institutional care and provide follow-up to the patients referred to or discharged from hospital.

(h) Make at least three postnatal visits for each delivery conducted in her area and render advice regarding care of mother and care and feeding of the newborn.

(i) Assess the growth and development of the infant and take necessary action required to rectify the defect.

(j) Educate mothers individually and in groups in better family health including maternal and child health, family planning, nutrition, immunisation, control of communicable diseases, personal and environmental hygiene.

(k) Assist medical officer and health assistant female in conducting antenatal and postnatal clinics at the subcentre.

Family Planning

(a) Utilise the information from the eligible couple and child register for the family planning programme. She will be squarely responsibile for maintaining eligible couple registers and updating at all times.

(b) Spread the message of family planning to the couples and motivate them for family planning individually and in groups.

(c) Distribute conventional contraceptives and oral contraceptives to the couples, provide facilities and to help prospective acceptors in getting family planning services, if necessary, by accompanying them or arranging for the Dai to accompany them to hospital.

(d) Provide follow-up services to female family planning acceptors, identify side-effects, give treatment on the spot for side-effects and minor complaints and refer those cases that need attention by the physician to public health centre (PHC)/hospital.

(e) Establish female depot holders, help the health assistant female in training them, and provide a continuous supply of conventional contraceptives to the depot holders.

(f) Build rapport with acceptors, village leaders, health guides, Dais and others and utilise them for promoting Family Welfare Programme.

(g) Identify women leaders and help the health assistant female to train them.

(h) Participate in Mahila Mandal meetings and utilise such gatherings for educating women in Family Welfare Programme.

Medical Termination of Pregnancy

(a) Identify the women requiring help for medical termination of pregnancy and refer them to nearest approved institution.

(b) Educate community of the consequences of septic abortion and inform them about the availability of services for medical termination of pregnancy.

Nutrition

(a) Identify cases of malnutrition among infants and young children (zero to five years), give the necessary treatment and advice and refer serious cases to the primary health centre.

(b) Distribute iron and folic acid tablets as prescribed to pregnant and nursing mothers, infants and young children (zero to five years) and family planning acceptors.

(c) Administer vitamin A solution as prescribed to children from 1 to 5 years.

(d) Educate community about nutritious diet for mothers and children.

Universal Immunisation Programme

(a) Immunise pregnant women with tetanus toxoid.

(b) Administer DPT vaccine, oral polio-myelitis vaccine, measles vaccine and BCG vaccine to all infants and children.

(c) Maintain report of all eligibles those vaccinated and follow-up defaulters.

Diarrhoea Control Programme

(a) Educate mothers regarding home management of diarrhoea with ORT.

(b) Provide and indent ORS packets.

(c) Monitoring of cases of diarrhoea, if any increase, report to medical officer.

(d) Record deaths due to diarrhoea and give monthly report.

(e) Arrange for mothers' meeting and work closely with Anganwadi and other health workers.

Dais Training

(a) List *Dais* in her area and involve them in promoting family welfare.

(b) Help the health assistant female in the training Programme of *Dais*.

Communicable Diseases

(a) Notify the medical officer PHC immediately about any abnormal increase in cases of diarrhoea/dysentery. Polimyelitis, neonatal tetanus, fever with rigors, fever with rash, fever with jaundice or fever with unconsciousness, which she come across during her home visits, take the necessary measures to prevent their spread, and inform the health worker male to enable him to take further action.

(b) If she comes across a case of fever during her home visits, she will take blood smears, administer presumptive treatment and inform health worker for further action.

(c) Identify cases of skin patches, especially if accompanied by loss of sensation, which she comes across during her home visits and bring them to the notice of the health worker male for skin smears.

(d) Assist the health worker male in maintaining a record of cases in her area, who are under treatment for tuberculosis and leprosy and check whether they are taking regular treatment, motivate defaulters to take regular treatment and bring these cases to the notice of the health worker male or health assistant male.

(e) Give oral rehydration solution to all cases of diarrhoea/dysentery/vomiting.

(f) Identify and refer all cases of blindness including suspected cases of cataract to Medical Officer PHC.

(g) Where Kala-azar is endemic :
   — She will assist health worker male and identifying suspected kala-azar cases and guiding them to the nearest diagnostic and treatment centre.
   — She will ensure follow-up of all the kala-azar cases in her area for complete treatment.

(h) Where Japanese encephalitis (J.E.) is endemic :
   — She will assist the health worker male in identifying suspected encephalitis cases and guiding them to the nearest diagnostic and treatment centre.
   — She will ensure follow-up of all the J.E. cases in her area.

Vital Events

(a) Record births and deaths occurring in her area in the births and deaths registers and report them to the health worker male.

Record Keeping

(a) Register
   — Pregnant women from three months of pregnancy onward.
   — Infants day one to one year of age; and
   — Women aged 15 to 44 years.

(b) Maintain the prenatal and maternity records and child care records.

(c) Assist the health worker male in preparing the eligible couple and child register and maintaining it up-to-date.

(d) Maintain the records as regards contraceptive distribution, IUD insertion, couples sterilized, clinics held at the subcentre and supplies received and issued.

(e) Prepare and submit the prescribed monthly reports in time to the health assistant female.

Primary Medical Care

(a) Provide treatment for minor ailments, provide first aid for accidents and emergencies and refer cases beyond her competence to the primary health centre or nearest hospital.

Team Activities

(a) Attend and participate in stall meetings at primary health centre/community development block or both.

(b) Co-ordinate her activities with the health worker male and other health workers including the health guides and *Dais*.

(c) Meet the health assistant female each week and seek her advice and guidance whenever necessary.

(d) Maintain the cleanliness of the subcentre.

(e) Participate as a member of the team in camps and campaigns.

(f) Work as a team with *Anganwadi* workers in ICDS block/VHG/TBA.

Expanded Programme on Immunisation

- Follow the directions given in Manual of Health Worker (Female) under National Immunisation Programme.

Acute Respiratory Infection

- Ensure early diagnosis of pneumonia cases.
- Provide suitable treatment to mild/ moderate cases of ARI.
- Ensure early referral in doubtful/severe cases.

School Health

- Help the medical officers in school health services.

Non-Government Health Personnel

Due to inaccessibility of health services to the rural people, the need was felt to provide minimum health care to each individual at their own doorstep, so as to maintain the optimum level of health. The community health volunteers and traditional birth attendants are the community people who have been selected to provide simple training to provide health services at root level. There are the important ways and means of giving primary health care.

Village Health Guides or Community Health Workers

A village health guide is non-government personnel with an aptitude of social service. The VHG scheme was initiated in 1977 to encourage people's participation in the care of their own health and to make them self-reliant in health aspects. Mostly VHGs are women, who come from and are chosen by the community in which they work. They are the liason/link between government and community. They provide the first contact care to the people.

Criteria for Selection

A person preferably woman:
- Should belong to the same community, where he/she is going to provide care.
- Should be accepted and selected by the community people.
- Should be at least sixth standard and is able to read and write.
- Should be able to spare 2 to 3 hours everyday for community health work.
- Should be ready to work without financial gains and provide free health care.

Training

The village health guides (VHGs) undergo a three months training, which is being conducted in the primary health centres (PHCs) or subcentres (SCs) or any suitable place. During training they receive a stipend of Rs. 200 per month.

After training each village health guide receives a health manual and kit containing simple medicines. The duties assigned to health guides include treatment of minor ailments, first aid, maternal and child health, family planning, health education and sanitation. The health guide gives instructions of giving medication for minor ailments and what they can do, and what they cannot do and they are expected to do community health work in spare time for 2 to 3 hours daily in fixed regular period. They are paid an honorarium of Rs. 60 per month and drugs worth Rs. 600 per annum. Each village health guide (VHG) is expected to cover a population of 1000 per of a village. If population of village is more than one thousand another village health guide may be required. Since training involves expenditure by the government, hence she is expected to work for at least three years. At present more than 4 lakh village health guides are working in the country.

Traditional Birth Attendants/Local Dais

In rural areas, most of deliveries are conducted by untrained Dais, who are often the only people immediately available to the women during delivery. More than 70 per cent of the deliveries are conducted by traditional birth attendants (TBAs). They do not receive any training but they learn by virtue of their practice in the field or by elders or seniors who practice at home. Due to lack of scientific practice and knowledge, the maternal and infant mortality rate is very high especially in rural areas. Hence, the need was felt to train TBAs of all communities. An extensive programmes have been undertaken to train all categories of local Dais/traditional birth attendants to improve their knowledge in the basic concepts on maternal and child health and obstetric skills. They are provided training for 30 working days, twice a week and remaining four days they accompany the health worker to the villages preferably in dais own community.

During training each traditional birth attendant is expected to conduct at least two deliveries under the guidance and supervision of the health worker (female), auxillary nurse midwife (ANM) or health assistance (F). More emphasis is laid on aseptic technique during the process of delivery, which help in lowering the complications and reducing the maternal and infant mortality rate. They also learn to identify the high-risk cases and appropriate and timely referral and management of newborn emergencies and referrals.

After successful completion of training each Dai is provided with a delivery kit and a certificate to practice safe delivery. She is given Rs. 10 per delivery provided the mother is registered at health centre/primary health centre, etc. Each infant registered by her, will be given Rs. 3. These Dais are also expected to play important role in educating the people regarding family planning, nutrition, hygiene and immunization, etc. Each Dai is expected to cover population of 1000. At present there are more than 80 thousand trained Dais.

Anganwadi Workers : The Anganwadi workers are selected from the community they are expected to serve a population of 1000, under Integrated Child Development Scheme (ICDS) under Ministry of Social Welfare. There are about 100 Anganwadi workers in each Integrated Child Development Scheme project. At present 5320 integrated child development scheme blocks are functioning in the country. Each Anganwadi worker undergoes a training in various aspects of health, nutrition and child development for 4 months. She is a part time worker and is paid an honorarium of Rs. 250 per month for the services she gives to community, e.g., health check-up for mothers and children, immunization, supplementary nutrition, health education non-formal pre-school education and referral services, etc. These services are mainly rendered to mothers (15-45 years) and children below 6 years.

•••

6

Community Health Nursing Specialised Roles

INTRODUCTION

School Health Services were introduced early in 20th century in response to growing problems of communicable diseases among children. With increasing success in control of communicable diseases, the role of school health nursing shifted to health education. Earlier, community health nursing was interacting with parents, teachers, principals and school physicians. Today, she is expected to share responsibilities with guidance counsellor, psychologist, speech therapist, etc. She is even responsible for counselling children with health problems *e.g.*, drug abuse, teenage pregnancy, sexually transmitted diseases (STD), emergency care, etc.

Educational Preparation

For minimum preparation of professional practice, a school nurse must be a graduate from recognised college/school of nursing. Masters degree with specialisation is encouraged for professional commitment.

American Nurses' Association (ANA) in 1966 stated the philosophy of school nursing : "It is a highly specialised service contributing to the process of education—it must be deligently pursued through health and educational avenues".

Recent publication of American Nurses' Association (ANA), American School Health Association (ASHA, 1974) introduced as follow : School nursing as a professional entity is now in its eighth decade. School nurses have repeatedly attempted to define their role in the school and their responsibilities within the "**School Health Programme**". The primary focus of school nursing is enhancing the child's or youth's individual ability to utilize his intellectual potential and to make worthwhile decisions affecting present and future physical, social and emotional health.

Historical Perspective

In India, the school health services started in 1909 as medical examination for school children. In 1953, the secondary education committee felt the need for maintaining the health status of school children during their stay. In 1960, the Government of India constituted a school health committee to assess the standards of health and nutrition of children and to suggest the measures to improve the health of the children, the committee submitted its report with important recommendation. Many of the states government schools and private schools started providing health care *e.g.*, nutrition, medical examination, physical examination, immunization, first aid and health education to school children. In spite of services available most of the schools are still not getting proper health care due to lack of resources, manpower and facilities.

Common Problems to school children : Though health problems depend upon the geographical area and demographic aspects, but common health problems found in children are:
- Malnutrition
- Helminthic infestation
- Skin infection (scabrities)
- Communicable diseases
- Ear, nose, throat and dental problems
- Psychological problems, lack of concentration, stealing, nail biting, abusing, etc.
- Mental health problems.

OBJECTIVES OF SCHOOL HEALTH PROGRAMME

The main objective of school health care is to maintain the general physical and mental health of the children, so that they grow as healthy adults.

- To promote the health status.
- To prevent from communicable diseases and health hazards.
- Early detection and treatment of deficiencies.
- Health awareness among children.
- Provision of healthy environment (physical and psychosocial).

COMPONENTS OF SCHOOL HEALTH PROGRAMME

The types of health services to be provided can be as follows :

Healthful School Environment

The building site and equipment are part of the environment, where school children grow and develop. It is essential that school environment should be healthful in respect to physical, psychosocial and emotional development.

Location of School

The school must be located away from busy road traffic, factory, cinema halls, railway tracks and market places, etc. It should be centrally located with accessibility to community and roads. It should be properly fenced, placed on higher level, free from dampness and proper drainage. It has been recommended 10 acre land for senior secondary school and 5 acre for primary school, preferably single storied building.

Each classroom should not have more than 40 students, per capita space for children should not be less than 10 square feet. Furniture must be comfortable and appropriate to the age. It is suggested to provide single desk and chair to children. The classroom must be well-ventillated and cross-ventillation for air and sunlight. It should open towards varandah. The windows should be broad and at least two ventillators. The classroom should be white in colour and regular white washing should be done.

Classroom should have sufficient natural light (preferably from left and right, from front should be avoided.). The children should be encouraged healthy eating habits and provision of separate space for mid-day meal. The water supply must be safe and sufficient.

Lavatory

The urinals and laterines must be adequate, clean and separate for boys and girls. It has been suggested that one urinals for 60 students and one laterine for 100 children.

Regular Medical Examination (Health Appraisal)

The medical and physical examination of all school children and teachers must be done at least once a year. School Health Committee recommended medical examination for school children at the entrance to school and every four years or at least before leaving the school. The initial examination should be thorough e.g., physical examination, investigation, clinical examination for nutritional deficiencies, etc., special care to vision, hearing, speech and teething, etc.

Daily morning inspection must be done by class teachers and can detect changes in child's appearance, behaviour and guide for proper health care. Students showing any deviation than normal can be referred to school health clinic or nearby hospital. Children with communicable diseases should not be permitted to attend the school.

Teacher may notice the following symptoms for referral e.g., fever, injury, gestrointestinal problem, respiratory tract infection, neck rigidity, flushing face, convulsions, skin infection, bodyache, etc.

Treatment and Followup

Any deviation detected, school health nurse can educate children on :

1. Balanced diet rich in vitamin A. e.g., green leafy vegetables,
2. Rinsing/washing of eyes frequently to wash away dust at least 20 times a day,
3. Avoid any sharp instrument e.g., pencil, compass, pen, knife or scissors,

4. Be careful while playing and avoid injury to eyes,

5. Regular treatment in case of eye infections,

6. Avoid using others towel and handkerchief to clean the eyes,

7. Avoid putting *kajal* or *surmas*, etc. in the eyes,

8. Good reading habits, level of the book and light coming from left or back and not front.

School Health Records

These are important documents to assess the health of children, cumulative health records of each student should be maintained. These records should include personal history, family history and history of any illness, records of finding of medical check-up, etc. These records will help to find out the physical and mental status of school children. They are useful documents to evaluate the functioning of school health programme and are important link between school, home and community of the student.

Health Education

Todays children are tomorrows citizens. Healthy children will develop as healthy youth, and healthy citizen will be productive for the nation. Health education plays an important role in teaching healthy habits to school children, so that they can practice the same at home and teach others. The goal of health education should be to bring the desired change in healthy behaviour, attitude, practice and knowledge among childrens. Various aspects of health education can be included *e.g.*,

Personal Hygienes

Daily bath, care of nails, eyes, hair, clothes, teeth should be stressed upon, maintaining posture, and abnormal posture should be observed and corrected. Good health habits should be encouraged and bad habits, *e.g.*, smoking, drug use should be avoided.

Prevention of Diseases

School health nurse should be responsible to educate school children on all the three levels of prevention of disease.

Primary Level

Periodical examination
— Vaccination
— Healthful environment
— Prevent accident
— Good nutrition
— Healthy eating, sleeping and reading habits
— Regular exercise.

Secondary Level

Early diagnosis and treatment of communicable disease, dental problem, eye defect.

Tertiary Level

To help the child to rehabilitate to normal state of physical, mental and social dimension.

To prevent deformity and if occurred, then to help to correct any deformity, *e.g.*, eye defect; to wear glasses will help to correct the eye defect.

Environmental Health

To keep environment *e.g.*, house, school and surroundings clean to prevent various environmental problems and diseases. Various projects and programmes can be organised for people involvement, and students should be encouraged to participate actively.

Family Life Education

Children should be aware about healthy family life. They must be given sex education so as to prevent various sexual problems and diseases *e.g.*, acquired immunodeficiency syndrome (AIDS), and sexually transmitted diseases (STDs), etc., girls must be given special attention to avoid unwanted pregnancies, abortions and infections, etc. They need to learn about menstrual hygiene. They must learn reproductive system, which help them to know physiology of sex organs. They also need to know about healthy family life.

Nutritional Care

The diet is an essential component of physical health. If child is physically weak he will be mentally weak as well and cannot concentrate on studies. School children should be encouraged to take balanced diet for maintenance of optimum health and prevent from nutritional deficiencies, *e.g.*, xerophthalmia, rickets, anaemia, scurvy, malnutrition, etc.

To overcome these deficiencies mid-day meal can be encouraged in schools to supply half of daily protein and one-third calorie requirement. School Health Committee recommended at least one full meal everyday with all nutrients and bring lunch packed and have it in school.

Special nutrients can be provided to school children as per requirement to prevent nutrition deficiencies, *e.g.*, anaemia (iron), dental caries (calcium and vitamin C), endemic goitre (iodine), xerophthalmia (vitamin A), protein malnutrition (protein).

First Aid and Emergency

The most common problem among school children is falling and getting injured. It may be very serious emergency. The school teachers are the most approachable personnel to handle the emergency. Therefore, teachers must be trained adequately for first aid and emergency care. They should be able to judge, when and where to refer for emergency.

An Emergency Kit and First Aid Box should always be ready for students. The high school children should also be taught to provide first aid and emergency care.

Prevention of Communicable Diseases

Due to exposure among children in the school, the communicable disease spreads very fast. Hence communicable diseases are highly prevalent among children due to age and environmental factors. Immunization of all children should be encouraged to protect them from various diseases, *e.g.*,. tetanus, polio, tuberculosis, hepatitis B, etc. A record of all immunization should be maintained as a part of school health record. The record should be handed over, when child leaves the school.

Mental Health

School is most strategic place for keeping the mental health status of children. The mental health of the child affects his physical health and slows down the learning process and vice-versa. Mentally unhealthy child may develop less interest in studies and go for behavioural problems, *e.g.*, juvenile deliquency, maladjustment and drug addiction, etc. School teacher can have preventive role by helping the child to attain the mental health and help them to adjust by guidance and counselling. There should not be any discrepancy between sex, religion, age, race, caste, socio-economic status and intelligence level, etc. All children must be respected and treated equal. As per need, vocational counsellors and psychologists have been working in the schools to provide guidance and counselling which is today's need, due to industrialisation and urbanisation.

Dental Care

More than 80 per cent of school children suffer from dental diseases and defects. Dental caries and periodental diseases are two common dental problems in India. School health services should provide dental examination by dentist. Yearly school health nurse should assist in doing dental examination and health education on dental care. Health education should include :

1. Brushing the teeth twice a day (morning and before sleep), rinsing after every meal,
2. Balanced diet *e.g.*, Cheese, milk, vegetables and fruit consumption,
3. Avoid too hot, too cold and sweets especially chocolates,
4. Regular check-up,
5. Avoid chewing and eating too hard.

Eye Care

Eyes are precious organ of our body, it is important to take care especially for children, because they are essential for studies. School should be responsible for detection of any eye problem and treatment of eye infection. Administration of vitamin A to school children have shown gratifying results. Teacher should be able to identify if children find problem in reading or seeing the blackboard. School health nurse must ensure :

1. Regular eye check-up,
2. Health education,
3. Referral services, and
4. Health reading habits.

FUNCTIONS OF SCHOOL HEALTH NURSE

Assessment

Assessment is a systematic collection of information concerning the health needs of school children. Assessment includes description of students and their health statistics, description of community and an analysis of services available in the community.

Community Assessment

Student community consists of family, housing, socio-economic status, juvenile deliquency rate, drug and alcoholic usage, divorce rate, employment statistics. Information may be obtained by :

- Questionnaire,
- Interviewing through survey method,
- Direct observation of students, families and teachers in schools and community can be a rich sources of information concerning needs,
- Discussion with parents and students in parent-teacher association will provide comprehensive information.

Programme Planning

Planning begins when assessment is correctly interpreted and translated into goals and objectives. In planning, school health nursing needs :

- Determine the nursing health needs
- Establish priorities
- Identify strengths
- Form patterns of delivery services.

Screening Tests

Screening test includes procedures for :
- Testing vision and hearing
- Assessing growth and development
- Observation for scoliosis, dental and cardiac findings.

   The screening tests are selected according to their cost, availability, effectiveness and acceptability. Some tests might require parents permission for legal safeguard for most invasive procedure.

Vision

Usually annual examination help, detect signs for eye problem, *e.g.*, reading difficulty, eye irritation, excessive rubbing, forward head tilt.

Hearing

Good hearing is important to the learning process. Hearing loss may affect speech and personality of child. They are usually considered as disobedient, unco-operative and slow learner.

- Proficiency with an otoscope enables the nurse to detect ear infections that may affect hearing.
- Educating parents and children about potential for hearing loss resulting from infection is important.
- If hearing loss has already occurred, compensation may be made by preferential seating in classroom for better hearing.

Scoliosis Screening

- Spine curvature develops in early adolescence and may progress during rapid growth.
- Early detection and treatment may prevent costly major surgery.

RESPONSIBILITIES OF SCHOOL HEALTH NURSE

Responsibilities of school health nurse are :
- Organising and conducting school health clinic
- Assisting in periodical examination of school children and teachers
- Inspection of school health environment and mid-day meal programmes
- Instruction to teachers for regular inspection of school children
- Assisting in dental and eye check-up
- Counselling the parents and children with physical and mental problems
- Referral services
- Health education on good nutrition, healthy habits, reading habits, hygiene, and
- Performs comprehensive physical, cognitive and psychosocial evaluations
- Manages a variety of minor illness or injuries

- Place special emphasis on teaching students to be responsible for their own health promotion and maintenance
- Collaborates with physicians/other health care personnel and educators help in providing health care
- Uses advanced physical and health assessment skills to identify factors that may place the student at risk of acquiring learning disorders or other physical or emotional problems.

ROLES OF SCHOOL HEALTH NURSE

The school nurses role as a specialist can be effectively developed in a systematic manner. The school nurses have responded to changes in school health by assuming a wide variety of roles, often more than one at a time.

The school nurses have seven main roles to perform :

Nurse Practitioner

School nurse practitioners are concerned with identification of children and young at risk for specific health problem for management of certain chronic diseases (*e.g.*, children with diabetes) and acute health concerns (*e.g.*, teenage pregnancy) and for providing a comprehensive and continuous care programme to school children.

Nurse Teacher

School children are the future citizens and parents. The nurse teacher primary job is to teach health concepts and to identify ways of transmitting knowledge that supports change in health behaviour (teaching the relationship between nutrition and excercise) to school children.

Consultant

The nurse can be a consultant to students, parents and teachers to identify health problem and guide for good health practices.

Advocate

The nurse advocate represents the interest of individual student, special need group, or all children within the school in the community etc.

Functional Role

Nurses in the functional role may be responsible for a group of schools to fulfil the functions of screening, follow-up, control of communicable diseases (*e.g.*, outbreak of head lice), immunization, responding to call from different schools.

Primary Role

Usually generalised (primary) nurses are responsible for all direct health services like caring of sick children, control of communicable diseases and health education. They may also be advocates and consultants *e.g.*, working through others to get things done.

Team Member

Nurse is an active member of multidisciplinary team, consisting of school physician, counsellor, psychologist, social worker, teachers and parents. The school health team is problem oriented and is activated when the need arises. The nurse in the team may act as a co-ordinator or advocate, conveying information about problem areas to parents.

The nurse who elects the role of school nurse will have an opportunity for professional development and personal growth. Each nurse who makes the choice can help to clarify the school nurses role, define the domain of school nursing and participate in finding solutions to many dilemmas and issues facing those nurses who do work in schools. The qualified nurses in schools can care for school health services.

SCHOOL HEALTH SERVICES

It is an important and essential means of raising the health status of a community. It has been started as a narrower concept of health check-up of school children to the present concept of comprehensive care to the school children from age six years to 18 years.

The School Health Services have been divided into five parts :
- School health education
- Healthful school living
- Health supervision
- Health counselling
- School health services.

School health education is the process of providing learning experiences that favourably influence understanding, attitudes and conduct relating to individual and community health, which includes school health, safety instruction, general hygiene and prevention of accidents.

Healthful school living includes physical and social environment of the school and its effect on student health. School health services are concerned with the health conditions of the school children and can include observation, appraisal, screening tests following referral, care, control of communicable diseases and emergency care.

Health supervision includes such activities as health assessment, vision and hearing, screening, emergency care and indentification of health deficit.

Health counselling involves providing interpretation of health information, guidance and counselling regarding health behaviour and recommendations regarding individual and group health conditions.

School health services involve health education to school children and can be given on:

Personal hygiene, dental hygiene, prevention of accidents, prevention of worm infestation, balanced diet. Eye care and good reading habits, prevention of malnutrition, sex education, sexually transmitted disease/Acquired immuno-deficiency syndrome prevention, etc.

ADMINISTRATION OF SCHOOL HEALTH SERVICES

The school health services are provided through various organisations to provide adequate health care to children.

- Primary health centre at rural areas are covering all the schools, one medical officer and school health nurse visit every week to give regular care to children. The school health committee has recommended one medical officer for every 5000–6000 population. Though at present the services

in rural areas are not sufficient. The teachers refer the school children to private practitioners or primary health centre, etc.

- School health administration at urban schools are covered by school health clinic run by school health administration under local government. The schools have been equipped with one medical officer, a school health nurse, pharmacist and an attendant. These schools provide, medical check-up, vaccination, medication, health education and referral services.

After medical check-up children should be treated appropriately and follow-up. Special clinics should be conducted in rural schools, days and time should be intimated to students and their parents. The specialised care must be given in schools *e.g.*, eyes, ear, nose, throat, teeth, speech and mental health, etc. In urban areas each school should have health clinic and regular medical officer and school health nurse. There should be proper referral system for emergency cases.

OCCUPATIONAL HEALTH NURSING

Occupational health nursing is the synthesis of nursing principles and the public health services to observe the health of workers in all occupations. This speciality involves primary, secondary and tertiary prevention and requires skill and knowledge in health care, epidemiology, environmental sciences, toxicology and safety. The occupation health nurse employs process skills to meet the changing health care needs of increasing industrial workers.

The occupational health nurse retains the responsibility for direct nursing services to workers. She or he may also be involved in loss control management, environment surveillance, and programme development and evaluation.

Epidemiological Model in Occupational Health

Epidemiological model is useful to understand the relationship between work and health.

Host

Any susceptible man is a host. All employees and groups are potentials at risk of being exposed to occupational hazards. Certain host factors are associated with an increased risk of adverse response to hazardous exposure in the workplace. These factors include age, gender, chronic illness, work practices, immunological status and lifestyle habits. The population groups at greatest risk for experiencing a work-related accident with subsequent injury are young (30 years) men with less than six months experience in their current job.

Agent

Work related hazards or agents, represent potential and actual risks to the health and safety of workers. These agents may be classified as (Fig. 6.1):

- Biological.
- Chemical.
- Occupational.
- Mechanical.
- Physical.
- Psychosocial.

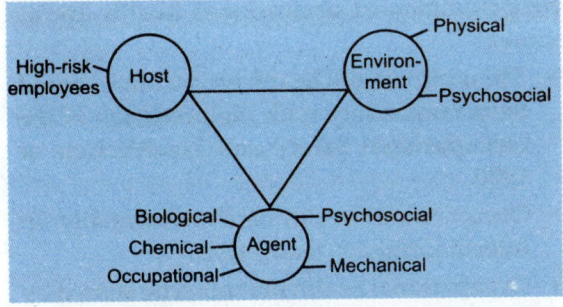

Fig. 6.1: Epidemiological agents in occupational health

Biological agents : These are living organisms whose excretions or parts are capable of causing human diseases usually by infectious process. Biological hazards are common in such places, *e.g.,* hospital and clinical laboratories. In these workplaces the workers are exposed to a wide variety of infectious agents including viruses and bacteria. For example, hepatitis B, AIDS, and tuberculosis are generally higher among hospital workers. Personnel in other occupations with exposures to biological agents include agriculture, *e.g.,* farmer's lung, worm infection.

Chemical agents : There are two million chemicals in existence and only 6000 have been tested for human effects. Of these, 1000 have carcinogen potentials and 400 are proven carcinogenic. As a result of environmental pollution with chemicals at work, home and community a variety of chemicals are found in the body tissues of general public.

Occupational agents : Exposure to chemicals has impact on reproductive health. Toxicity to both male and female reproductive systems have been demonstrated for common occupational agents *e.g.,* lead, mercury, cadium, nickle and zinc. High-risk or vulnerable workers should be screened carefully and monitored for optimal health protection.

Mechanical agents : The transfer of mechanical energy can produce adverse health effects, *e.g.,* vibrations, repetitive motions and lifting heavy loads. Localized effects are seen with hand-held power tools. Over work, faulty machines may cause accidents by machine.

Physical agents : Physical agents are those that produce effects on humans by the transfer of physical energy. Physical agents in the workplace include extremes of temperature, noise, radiations and lighting. The control of workers' exposure to these agents is frequently dependent on the workers' compliance with preventive actions such as wearing personal protection, equipment and safe work habits. These equipments include hearing protection, eye guards, protective clothes and devices for monitoring exposures to agents such as radiation.

Psychosocial agents : These are conditions that pose a threat to psychological and social well-being of individuals and group of people. Responses to poor interpersonal relationship particularly with authority in workplace are often cause of various health problems and an increased absenteeism rate.

Environmental Factors

The environmental factors influence the occurrence of host-agent interaction and outcome of these interactions. There may be aspect of physical environment (heat, odour, ventillation) that influence host-agent interaction.

The psychological environment includes characteristics of work itself, as well as inter-personal relationships required in work setting. Job characteristics like low autonomy, poor job satisfaction and limited control over the pace of work have been associated with increased risk of heart diseases among clerical workers. Interpersonal relationships are usually due to sources of conflicts and stress.

The physical environment includes the workplace, ventillation, hygienic condition, water supply, etc.

RESPONSIBILITIES OF OCCUPATIONAL HEALTH NURSING

Occupational health nursing is a new and rapidly growing area of specialisation within the nursing profession. Her primary role is the health care of the working population. Main concern areas are health maintenance, health promotion and health education. She has knowledge and skill to :

- Deal with minor laceration, broken bones, major trauma, *e.g.*, amputation, burns and multiple injuries.
- Deal with minor complaints *e.g.*, cold headache, splinters, respiratory diseases, myocardiac patients.
- Use skills learnt in psychiatric nursing to help individuals, recognise problems and seek appropriate counselling.
- Care of pregnant women.
- Skills in toxicology, epidemiology and environmental control.
- The focus of nursing care is mainly on primary prevention, since she is dealing with healthy people.
- Develop educational programmes for employees.
- Develop screening programmes to recognise major health problems, *e.g.*, hypertension, cardiovascular disease and diabetes. Preventive programmes for recognising

potential health hazards within the work setting that may result to respiratory diseases, dermatological problems, musculoskeletal disorders, mental health disorders.

- Actively participates in preplacement pro-gramme examination, periodical medical examination, treatment of occupational diseases or injuries, treatment of non-occupational diseases.
- Emergency interventions till further specialised care is available.
- Develop adequate record keeping system to find the potential health problem, and preventive and corrective measures.
- Evaluation of working conditions and measures to keep the healthy working situation, *e.g.*, hygiene, safety.

The criteria should be developed which includes information on physical set-up of the working place, physical hazards, chemical hazards, if present should be identified and notified.

PRINCIPLES OF OCCUPATIONAL HEALTH

The principles of occuptional health are as follows :

- The occupational health programme should be in conformity with the provision of the Occupational Safety and Health Acts of 1970.
- Occupational health care is essentially an interdisciplinary team effort.
- Occupational health unit must be staffed by qualified, professional personnel, must have administrative stability, and must have the understanding and support of management and labour.
- Quality of work environment is of vital importance and is centre to the prevention of disease.
- Workers themselves must participate to prevent injury in achieving a common goal and a high level of wellness as for quality of life.

- Occupational health professionals must understand the dynamics of work co-operatively.
- Occupational health is an essential component of community health, they are inter-related and independent.

OBJECTIVES OF OCCUPATIONAL HEALTH

These are as follows :

- Protect employee against any health hazards in the work environment.
- Facilitate placement and ensure the suitability of the individual according to the individuals ability and physical and emotional make-up.
- Ensure adequate medical care and reha-bilitation of the occupationally ill and injured.
- Encourage personal hygiene maintenance among all employees.

FUNCTIONS OF OCCUPATIONAL HEALTH

These are as follows :

- Occupational health nurse plans and develops nursing care that is consistent with overall objectives of the parent company health programme.
- Occupational health nurse plans and submits an annual budget proposal to support nursing services.
- Occupational health nurse participates in research designed to improve delivery of nursing services.

ROLE OF A NURSE

Nurse functions as an independent practitioner, manager, consultant, teacher and researcher. Close contact must be maintained with community agencies not only for the individual and family but also for community as a whole.

Nurses perform a variety of roles and functions in occupational setting. She offers the direct care to employee, as well as managerial skills such as programme evaluation and analysis of work related injuries and illnesses.

Nurses are often the first health care providers seen by an individual with a work related health problem. Nurses are in key positions to intervene in working population at all three levels of prevention.

MENTAL HEALTH NURSING

Mental Health

Persons with mental health problems and needs are clients of community health nursing. These problems are often complex and result from interaction of many factors including heredity, family relationships, living conditions, social and economic constraints.

Concept of Mental Health and Illness

The concept of mental health and illness is changing for last few centuries. The illness was considered to be due to introduction of bad evil in an individual. Recently efforts have been directed towards differentiating mental health from illness. Several characteristics to mental health have been accepted.

Mental health can be defined (**Taylor, 1982**) as : *"The state in the interrelationship of the individual and his environment in which the personality structure is relatively stable and the environmental stresses are within its absorptive capacity"*.

Like mental health, mental illness is usually determined in terms of an individual's relationship to the environment. The mental health is a system of care and significant change in the concept of mental health. Historically antecedents serve as determinants of many of today beliefs and forms of care in community mental health.

Mental illness and mentally retarded are among most critical health problems. They occur more frequently, affect more people, require more prolonged treatment, cause more suffering by the families of affected, waste more of our human resources, and constitute more financial drain upon both the public and personal finances of individual family than any other single condition.

Community mental health is an inter-disciplinary approach to meet the mental health needs of a group of people in the geographically defined area. It is concerned with promotion of mental health, prevention of mental illness and the care of the mentally ill.

COMMUNITY MENTAL HEALTH NURSING

Community mental health nursing is a vigorous and evolving field. Community mental health field deals with clients needs in the clients setting which can be home, school, business or any other location. Activities in community mental health nursing focus around the three levels of prevention. Primary prevention and health promotion focus on education and consultation. Secondary prevention is mainly concerned with early diagnosis and treatment. Tertiary prevention includes both the other two levels and concentrates on pre- and post-hospitalization services with the objective of helping clients establish, restore and maintain their optimum level of functioning.

NURSES' RESPONSIBILITY IN COMMUNITY MENTAL HEALTH

The community mental health nurse, with educational and clinical preparation provides comprehensive nursing services to meet community mental health needs at preventive, acute and rehabilitative levels.

A specialised area of nursing practice (preventive and corrective) employing theories of human behaviour as its science and purposeful use of self as its art.

It is a comprehensive approach to mental health services for individual, family, children, adolescents, elderly and groups in various community settings. While working in community health nursing must have certain attributes.

- Consistency
- Creativity
- Respect
- Independence
- Patience
- Warmth
- Self-criticism/self-evaluation.

Competencies

- Basic communication skills
- Community knowledge
- Teaching abilities on mental health concepts
- *Liaison work* : Liaison between doctor, patient, family friends, etc.
- Interviewing techniques
- Observation skills
- Crisis intervention technique.

She should have the knowledge of personality development, sociopsychological principles, family theory, group dynamism, mental health teaching, theories and methods of treatment for mental health care.

ROLE OF COMMUNITY MENTAL HEALTH NURSING

Direct nursing care provider to client by psychotherapy. Psychotherapy is a process of therapeutic work within the context of a relationship or as a member of a group.

SPECIALISED ROLE OF COMMUNITY MENTAL HEALTH NURSE

Techniques

Psychoanalytic psychotherapy is insight oriented treatment based on analytical understanding of human behaviour. The goal is to change the behaviour by clarification, interpretation and empathetic understanding.

Short Term Psychotherapy

Aimed at resolving an individual's difficulty within a given time-table. Therapeutic relationship can be defined as supportive or time limit. Supportive therapy focuses on the individual who usually is having an emotional crisis and needs professional help to decrease anxiety, increase coping ability and prevent further depression and psychopathology.

Group Psychotherapy

Therapeutic experience occurring in formally structured group members are often chosen, placed in a group and guided by a trained therapist for the purpose of helping each other.

The goal is to relieve psychic pain, bring about personality changes, provide corrective emotional experience for group members.

Family Therapy

A variety of techniques using different therapeutic approach aimed at bringing about change in the structure and process of a family. The basic need for family therapy is when problem does not exist within one individual but within the family system.

Play Therapy

Opportunity that is offered to the child to experience growth under most favourable conditions. Since play is his natural medium for self-expression. Child is given play to express his feelings, tension, frustration, insecurity, aggression, fear and confusion, etc. Play will help to face them, learn to control or abandon them.

GENERAL ROLES OF COMMUNITY MENTAL HEALTH NURSE

These roles are mentioned as follows :

- Community health nurse also provides indirect services as administrator, consultant and educator.
- She provides knowledge of general health matters physical as well as psychological aspect of illness.
- She can foster professional working relationship with family, psychiatrist, psychologist, and social worker.

Legal Considerations

Community health nurse must be registered and licensed to work in community health field. There is no additional licence given for experienced nurse in a specialised area.

Accountability

Community health nurse is accountable for her own nursing actions. She is responsible for competency and quality of nursing care provided.

Prevention of Mental Health Problem

Prevention of mental illnesses are of three levels. Community health nurse is responsible to prevent mental illness in the community of three levels.

Primary Prevention

The primary level constitutes the "improvement of social environment" and promotion of the social, emotional and physical well-being of all people. It includes working for better living conditions and improve welfare and health resources in the community.

- Education of the public on mental health concept,
- Prevention of mental health illness,
- Develop methods in increasing capacities to deal with problem.

Secondary Prevention

Early diagnosis and treatment of mental illness and of social and emotional disturbances through screening programmes in schools, industries, colleges and community, etc. Provision of treatment facilities and referral services. In the family, community health nurse must be able to identify emotional problems and early symptoms of mental illness, help family members to cope with overwhelming stress, treat problems of individual and social maladjustment when required and prepare each family member for psychiatric care. "Casework" or "counselling" is the most commonly method employed by community health nurse. The main responsibility of community health nurse is to provide counselling services and help the families with marital conflict, disturbed parent child relationship, and strained interpersonal relationship. Family counselling is one method of treatment intervention for mentally ill patients in the community.

- Focus on treatment of mental illness and prevention of associated complication by identifying the problem at early stage
- Intervention when in crisis
- Diagnosis and evaluation of mental health status
- Providing therapeutic care plan
- Liaison work with agency, professional to facilitate holistic approach.

Tertiary Prevention

Seeks to reduce the duration of mental illness and reduce the stresses they create for the family and the community. The goals are to prevent further breakdown and disruption.

- Health intervention focus on rehabilitative process
- Prevention of long-lasting mental illness
- Restoring their optimal level of health
- After care of individual in community.

Counselling

Community health nurse is key person in building mental health. The problems may often be related to family relationship and divorce is crisis that affects number of children.

Children of different ages may face different problems. Child abuse is most common among very young. At 5 to 6 years, separation anxiety, poor interaction and shyness are often found.

- New babies, death or illness in family can be source of mental problem.
- School environment is an additional factor in children's emotional health and needs special attention.

  Health Counselling will include :

- Pregnant teenagers, alcohol or drug abuse, chronic absenteeism, speech problem, recent death in family and overweight children.

Health Education

Nurse can be a valuable resource in assisting with selection of material and activities for health education.

Programme Evaluation

To find the extent to which service has had an effect on the health of group. Nurse must keep records and evaluate the programme periodically.

Prevention of Communicable and Non-Communicable Diseases

The control of disease is a dynamic process in the distribution of the disease, may change as social and economic conditions change. New methods of prevention and cure continue to be discovered at a rapid pace and incidence rates may fall precipitously over a very short period. Control programmes enhance efforts to define the nature and distribution of disease in the population, to constitute the preventive measures that are available and to secure prompt and adequate curative and rehabilitative care.

Define the Nature, Extent and Distribution of Diseases

Community health nurse must know the incidence and prevalence of specific disease entities in the population to judge the size of the problem with which health system must deal and help in programme planning.

Define Determinants of Diseases

A knowledge of determinants of disease is essential to control the disease. This is important to know not only the disease state of the population but also the pattern of states of disease associated conditions. For example, it may be useful to estimate the nutritional levels, immunization status, birth weight, smoking habits of people, which may suggest the relative vulnerability of specified population.

Knowledge of health and social consequences of disease is also essential for control of disease, since it provides an index of the urgency for the control measures and a means of determining the value of the programme to the community.

Primary and Secondary Preventive Measure

Preventive measures may be primary or secondary and have varying levels of specificity. Some measures, such as measles immunization are expected to prevent occurrence of the disease. Other measures, *e.g.*, early detection of disease or programme of rehabilitation that maximise functioning of the disabled, are expected to minimize the effects of the disease once occurred. Community health nurse must participate in control of various diseases of primary, secondary and tertiary level.

Prompt and Adequate Care

Prompt and adequate care means more than the provision of care facilities, requires that the condition be put under care as soon as the need arises and that the care encompasses secondary prevention and rehabilitation as well as curative care. It implies that the recipient is willing to accept the care provided and the cares provided by community health nurse are adequate and competent. It also implies that the facilities are both adequate to permit the community health nurse to work efficiently and accessible and acceptable to the users.

Prompt and adequate care includes provision of social, environmental and medical care.

Anticipatory Guidance

Community health nurse must provide anticipatory guidance when there is risk known to be high, *e.g.*, family member is suffering from diabetes or tuberculosis, a special anticipatory guidance will alert the family to early symptoms of the disease and to the value of periodic screening of the disease. This will help in early diagnosis and adequate care of the disease.

Implement the Regulations for Control

Community health nurse may be involved in the implementation of regulations for control of disease. The nurse may support the efforts of the disease control programme to secure adequate reporting of the disease. The school health nurse must be prepared to interpret and support regulations regarding exclusion from school for medical reason and requirements for hospitalisation for tuberculosis patients who have persistent positive sputum and lives in where they have small children. Community health nurse must have guide for such regulations and she may need to secure the information from the local or state health department.

COMMUNITY HEALTH NURSE AS A MEMBER OF EPIDEMIOLOGICAL TEAM

Community health nurse working with epidemiologist may participate in epidemiologic investigation through the following activities :

- Collects data essential to epidemiologic analysis. Community health nurse may collect data to be submitted to epidemiologist as a basis for her decision on the best way to evaluate the situation. It is important for her to have knowledge about disease and disease process.

- Participating in the design of epidemiologic investigation by identifying relevant area of information not already included or possible non-medical factors that might be significant in the analysis of data, *e.g.*, community health nurse must point out the absenteeism in industry which may not be due to worker's reason but due to supervisory styles, etc. Motivating and assisting in epidemiological investigations to co-operate in disease investigation and control. The patient may find it difficult to identify the probable source of infection or admit that he did not take perscribed medicine. The willingness of each patient to try to provide required medication and to level with the study personnel will influence the amount of knowledge that can be accummulated about disease and its treatment.

- Using the results of epidemiologic investigation for improving community health nursing practices. The findings of epidemiological studies may help to pinpoint the nursing needs of population group, to identify the crucial components of the care required, or to suggest areas of investigation in nursing practices.

Control of Communicable Diseases

The goal of communicable diséase control is "to reduce the incidences of the disease to a tolerable level as quickly as possible within the resources available". The "tolerable level" depends upon the degree to which the disease can be prevented and on the community's ability to take the required action. In many diseases, *e.g.*, malaria, tuberculosis, syphillis and leprosy, it is felt that complete eradication could be possible, though goal of eradication may be unrealistic in most of diseases.

Reporting Disease

In case of prevalence and incidence of disease, reporting is of prime importance. Reporting is carried out at all levels of government in order to maintain an epidemiologic intelligence system that facilitates control. The specific diseases to be reported are established by each government unit and internationally.

Community health nurse must be involved in several ways is ensuring adequate reporting. She may educate people concerning the importance of securing of care for what a communicable disease is. Nurse may assist family physician in reporting by seeing that he has necessary regulations and reminding him the need for reporting. She may report any suspicious symptoms, she herself observes, *e.g.*, gastrointestinal cases and she may consult epidemiologist for further confirmation.

Organisation of Immunization Sessions

Community health nursing contributes to the achievement of a safe level of immunization in the population. The need to intensify the immunization, effort has been recognised nationally and internationally. She must familiarise herself with the immunization measures that are available in the agency and can be given to the community. The sharp decline of the diseases is the indication of satisfactory immunization status of the community. She must be accountable to arrange the vaccination, organise immunization sessions and after care of immunization.

Control of Spread of Infection

Community health nursing contributes to control the spread of infection by :

- Monitoring the care provided for those who suffer from infectious disease and who are being cared for the non-hospital setting.
- Securing those regulations who have been exposed to communicable diseases, which might include exclusion from school or from job place and observing reasonable precautions in protecting others from infection.
- Inculcating personal health behaviour that prevents the spread of communicable diseases.

Isolation measure becomes less restrictive as more is known about the spread of infection and as treatment becomes more effective in controlling the infectivity, *e.g.*, effectiveness of chemotherapy in producing a negative sputum and the knowledge of the great importance of air-borne transmission of infection has made it possible to dispense with much of strict isolation.

Community health nurse must know the mode of transmission of diseases and their preventive measures. She must be aware about the group susceptible to infection and require special protection, *e.g.*, very young child or the elderly person.

She needs to participate in case finding by :

- Contact tracing and cluster identification
- Direct or delegated general case finding measures in vulnerable persons
- Participating population in mass or crash programme or screening measures.

●●●

7

Legal Aspects in Community Health Nursing

INTRODUCTION

Legal Applications in Clinical Areas

In each clinical care the community health nurses must know the standard of care applied to the situation. These standards may be found in institution policies, procedures, nursing and health care literature or other professional association standards, nursing curriculum, legislation such as Nurse Practice Act, accreditation and certification criteria. A community health nurse also reviews nursing documents to see if agency policy requirements were met. Self-evaluation assures that standards of care are met. Attention to daily practice to quality assurance, risk management and documentation will help to ensure that injuries to clients are minimized and adequate community health services are delivered.

Each community health nurse must consider legal implications of practice in each clinical area. Legal aspects of the roles and functions of general and specific areas, especially scope of practice and negligences, will prove to be useful information for nurses in community health. Community health nurses must consider the legal implications of their own practice in each clinical encounter.

Legislation and Regulation

Legislation is the type of law that comes from the legislative branches of government at different levels—central, state or local. Much legislation has an impact on community health nursing. In the past, situations dealing with the communicable diseases, the state exercised its power through legislation.

"**Regulations** are very specific statements of law that relate to individual piece of legislation."

Judicial Law

Judicial law is the law based on court or jurisdiction. The opinion of the court are judicial opinions and also referred to as case law. The court uses other types of laws to make its decisions.

Judicial law or common law is the last group of laws having an impact on community health nursing. The principles of judicial law are based on justice, fairness, respect for individual, autonomy, self-determination. These common law principles are part of our tradition and heritage as a society and play an important role in decisions made by courts.

Judicial opinions and common laws exist for a wide variety of legal disputes. The community health related laws are usually contract and criminal laws.

Contracts are the mutual agreements between two or more individuals, referred to as parties after contracts are written, but they can be made without writing them. A written contract is advisable if an agreement is complex or if it will make the parties agreement easy to prove. Verbal agreements are valid agreements if the elements of a contract are present. These agreements are commonly used in employment in community health nursing. Contracts can be created in other areas of employment situations. In community health nursing, agreements are made with clients almost everyday *e.g.*, nurses contract the clients to arrange a home visit. The nurse offers a visit and client accepts this offer.

Impact of Laws on Community Health Nursing Practices

The legal aspects are not only related to nursing practices but also community health nursing, since the community health nursing practice is the synthesis of nursing practice and community health practice. There are two legal aspects that apply to most of these practice situations.

1. Professional negligence
2. Scope of practice.

Professional Negligence

Professional negligence or malpractice is defined as an act or failure to act, when a duty is owned to another that was not reasonable and that leads to injuries compensable by law. For the client to succeed in persuading the judge or jury that a nurse was negligent, one has to prove the followings :

- The nurse owed a duty to the client
- The duty to act as a responsible nurse under circumstances is not fulfilled
- The failure to be responsible under circumstances caused harm to client
- The injuries claimed are injuries compensable through usual legal remedies.

Scope of Practice

This scope of practice involves the practices of physicians, nurses and other health care providers. This can be assessed by :

- Examining the usual practice of a profession.
- Taking into account how legislation defines the practice of a particular profession in a jurisdiction. This is an important issue for community health nurses who are practicing in a wide scope.

Every community health nurse should know and follow the proposed change in nursing, medicine and other related practices, acts. Nurse should always examine all related definitions to nursing practice, in relation to dependent and independent role.

SPECIAL COMMUNITY HEALTH NURSING PRACTICE AND THE LAW

The community health nursing field includes preparation of generalised and specialised community health nurses. The essential component includes the knowledge of community resources and other health professionals. The community health nurse delivers care to clients or groups at their residential areas, workplace, playground or school, etc. In addition, nurse encompasses further specialisation in clinical areas such as family health, school health, occupational health, or mental health.

Home Care and Hospital Services

The home care by community health nursing needs legislative, licensing and certification. In some countries, there is an impact on home care and hospice service through legislation related to rights to death with dignity, right of residents of long-term care facilities and use of living wills. The legal dimension in community health practices are important in this area of practice. Individual rights, *e.g.*, right to refuse treatment/services may lead to conflict in providing care to an individual. When rights and responsibilities are in conflict, appropriate decisions are needed to resolve the conflicts.

The laws and decisions related to the type and amount of services that must be given or made available to incarcerated individuals. For example, physical examination of each prisoner after they are sentenced are required. Prisoners must be provided minimum care especially when they are sick. If minimum services are not provided, it is a violation of a prisoner's right to be free of cruel and unusual punishment. Such decisions provide a framework that strongly influence the setting of nursing priority.

Legal Resources

One can find many resources in public libraries and law libraries that can help community health nurse find the law regarding their practices. One of the best ways to keep information is through daily newspaper. Some legislations can be identified under specific headlines of subjects *e.g.*, immunizations, family planning and types of clients being served *e.g.*, child, adolescents, minors or adults. Computer based laws are also available on looking for laws and regulations relevant to one's practice.

Functions of administrator, educationalists, researchers and consultants, legal aspects of community health nursing depends upon :

- Setting of delivering health services
- Clinical speciality
- Functions of community health nurse.

School and Family Health

School health legislation provides a framework for nursing functions. The legislation establishes a minimum of services that may be provided to children in school systems including public or private schools, *e.g.*, immunization to all children before entering school or in schools. Physical examination—every year. Legislation also suggests the type of health screening in schools regarding vision or hearing testing. Many jurisdictions carryout these activities specified by the legislature plus many other activities.

The important legislations that make an impact of community health nursing practice in schools and families of child abuse and neglect. The nurses are expected to report to police or social welfare agency any situation in which they suspect that child is being accused or neglected. The nurses may also witness a hearing, follow the investigation made by social welfare agency.

Many other community health nursing practices are also legislatively important *e.g.*, diagnostic screening tests, nutritional programmes, services for handicapped and health education. It is advisable that legislation becomes the part of agency's nursing policies and procedures, so that nurse can reform them on demand. Hence she must be oriented to the legislations.

Occupational health is another special area of practice that is greatly affected by law. Many occupational and industrial legislations have been introduced for health protection of all employees. A record keeping system required by agency gives the health record of a worker. Monitoring and inspections of industrial workers for safety, health services are provided by agency.

ETHICS IN COMMUNITY HEALTH NURSING

In order to practice community health nursing effectively, she must have an understanding and awareness of values and ethical belief. Community health nurse identifies potential ethical dilemmas that may be encountered and understands the process of ethical inquiries. This process involves clarification of issues, decision making, implementation and acceptance of the consequences.

Ethics is the study of general nature of morals and of the specific moral choices to be made by the individual in his/her relationship with others. Ethical dilemmas involve inter-relationships in which there are conflicts and tension (**Aroskar 1980**). Ethical standards may be different for different culture groups. For example, one group may believe that lying is acceptable behaviour; other may feel that it is very unethical.

Ethics is also defined as system of principles and rules of conduct. These are the basic principles of morally right action, therefore, professional ethics of nursing should follow these in practicing her profession. Professional ethics governing community health nursing practices are essentially the same as applied to nursing in other fields.

Some of the standards given in the code for nurses are stated in Nightingale pledge which has been universally accepted.

Nightingale Pledge

The Nightingale pledge is named after Florence Nightingale, the first founder nurse of modern nursing education.

As per her pledge, it is stated *"I solemnly pledge myself before God and in the presence of the assembly to pass my life in purity and to practice my profession faithfully. I will abstain from whatever is deleterious and mischievous and will not take or knowingly administer any harmful drug. I will do all in my power to maintain and elevate the standard of my profession and will hold in confidence all personal matters committed to my keeping and all family affairs coming to my knowledge in the practice of my calling with loyality, I will endeavour to aid the physician in his work and devote myself to the welfare of those committed to my care".*

This pledge holds the nurses their accountability for behaviour in professional capacity and includes her personal life.

Bioethical (health related ethics) issues centred around expected behaviour of health professionals, particularly nurses. There are few quotes from early texts regarding professional ethics.

In nearly all professions, there are various special moral obligations, due to hospital, due to patients and those they owe to each other (**Maxwell and Pope 1923**). The obligations due to patients are that she faithfully carries out the doctors order (**Maxwell and Pope 1925**), obligations due to hospital include conduct which maintains the good reputation of the institution.

Today, nurses are concerned with more complex ethical issues. They are more willing to become involved in ethical dilemmas and to help their clients who are confronted with decision making on ethical aspects.

The bioethical issues relate various conflicts in the field of practice, especially community health nursing, where most of the decisions are taken independently like should the wife of an AIDS patient be told about his disease ? Should she administer I.V. fluids to save the life of dehydrated child, when no time to refer and at long distance ? If there is opportunity to discuss with other member, it should be discussed. Community health nurse must involve family member in making the decisions. If you have any difficulty in making decision, you may have to identify a person who can help you in making decisions. In case physician has made initial ethical decisions, the job of community health nurse becomes easier.

In order to practice community health nursing effectively, the nurse must have an understanding and awareness of personal philosophy, values and ethical beliefs. The development of a philosophy helps the community health nurse clarify an orientation to life and to nursing practice. In turn, it clarifies the beliefs and values of the community health nursing for other people.

Every nurse encounters ethical dilemmas regardless of the area of practice.

MAJOR ETHICAL PRINCIPLES

Three general ethical principles for bioethics have been framed in respect of autonomy,

beneficence and justice. These three principles should not be construed as jointly forming a complete moral system or theory; but they are sufficiently comprehensive to provide an analytic framework through which we can begin to reason about problems in bioethics. Principles provide a starting point for moral judgement and policy evaluation. They are tested and reliable starting points, but they are rarely sufficient for moral thinking.

Respect for Autonomy

It is the principle rooted in the liberal importance of individual freedom and choice associated with several ideas, *e.g.*, privacy, voluntariness self-mastery, choosing freely, freedom to choose, choosing one's own moral position and accepting responsibility for one's choice.

The moral demands that we respect the autonomy of persons, can be formulated as a principle of respect for autonomy. Autonomy of action should not be subjected to controlling constrains by others.

The principle provides the justificatory basis for the right to make decisions, which in turn takes the form of specific autonomy related rights.

To respect the autonomy of self-determining agents is to recognize them as entitled to determine their own destiny, with due regards to their considered evaluations and views of the world. Medical and nursing codes have included the rules that are based on this principles. For example, the first principle of American Nurses Association code reads as follows :

"The fundamental principle of nursing practice is respect for the inherent dignity and worth of every client. Nurses are morally obligated to respect human existence and the individuality of the reasons who are the recipients of nursing actions, truth telling and the process of reaching informed choice underline the exercise of self-determination, which is basic to respect for persons. Clients should be as fully involved as possible in the planning and implementation of their own health care".

Many controversial questions about the conditions, under which a person's right to autonomy, demands action by others and also questions about restrictions, society might rightfully place on choices by patients or subjects when these choices conflict with other values. If the individual's choice endanger the public health, potentially harm another party, or involve a scarce resource for which a patient cannot pay, it may be justifiable to restrict exercises of autonomy. If restriction is in order the justification will rest on some competing moral principle such as beneficence or justice.

Principle of Beneficence

The welfare of patient is the goal of health care. Public health is based on prevention of disease, promotion of health and cure of illness. This value has long been treated as fundamental value in nursing ethics. Among the most quoted principles in the history of code of medical and nursing ethics is the maxim primum non-nocere : "above all, do not harm". It was present in nursing code as early as Nightingale's pledge for nurses. Many current ethics assert that health professional's "primary commitment" is to protect the patient from harm and promote the patient's welfare.

The 'term' 'beneficence' has a broad set of meanings, including the doing of good and the active promotion of good, kindness and charity.

Justice

Justice has been the subject of more treatises on the terms of social co-operation than any other principle. A person has been treated justly, if treated according to what is fair, due and owed. For example, any demands of a good service or piece of information to which a person has a right or entitlement based on justice is an injustice. It is also an injustice to place an undue burden on the exercises of a right, e.g., to make a piece of information owed to a person unreasonably difficult to obtain.

Thus, distributive justice refers to fair, equitable and appropriate distribution in society by justified norms of distribution that structure part of the terms of social co-operation.

Honesty should be an important issue for nursing ethics for public health nurse working independently in the field without supervision. They are usually considered as model citizens. There are some circumstances in which health professionals are probably exempted from society's general requirements of truthfulness. But not telling the truth is usually the same as telling a lie and a lie requires strong justification. Whether or not knowing the truth is essential to the patient's health, telling the truth is essential to the health of the nurse-patient relationship.

CONSUMER PROTECTION ACT

The Consumer rights have become an important issue in health care system. It was introduced in India in 1986, for the first time, providing consumers speedy redressal of their greivances against medical services. The active participation and dedication of health personnel is essential for quality care. Over the centuries the medical profession has been accorded respect by the society, since last few decades or so, increasing commercialisation of profession had eroded this faith.

Under the general law a profession is required to show a standard of care which a person is expected to possess. In developed countries e.g., USA, UK, patients do not encounter many difficulties, as the court has developed principles of law which give important rights to patients. In India, people were not going to Civil Courts freely because court fee is very heavy and there is long delay to get a final verdict. Parliament has provided an alternative, quick, efficacious and economic remedy for protection of patient's rights. According to Consumer Protection Act (CPA), 1986 the decision should be taken within 3 to 6 months and no court fee payment is done. The consumer can plead its own case.

COPRA is a piece of comprehensive legislation and recognises six rights of the consumer that is right to safety, right to be informed, right to choose, right to be heard, right to seek redressal and right to consumer education.

Consumer Protection Act committee consisting of medical professionals and senior advocates will hear the consumer and medical defaulters, make the judgement for situation. In case health personnels are held responsible for negligence, the panalty may be done to the organisation or an individual in person.

EXERCISE

1. Explain the concept and principles of community health nursing.
2. Discuss the functions and roles of community health nursing.
3. Define community identification. Discuss the factors to be studied for community identification.
4. Describe the purpose for community identification. Enumerate the methods and sources for data collection to explore the community.
5. Discuss the roles and responsibilities of district public health nurse (DPHN), public health nurse (PHN) and Health Supervisor (female).
6. Enumerate the responsibilities of health personnel at periphery level/grass root level.
7. Define community health nursing team. Discuss the functions of Community Health Nursing team. List the nursing team members.
8. (a) List the common problems among school children.
   (b) Discuss the role of nurse in providing school health care.
9. Discuss the occupational health problems and role of nurse in maintaining occupational health.
10. Define mental health. Describe the functions of Community Health nurse in prevention of mental health problems.
11. Write short notes on the following :
    (a) Scope of Community Health Nursing
    (b) Professional requirement for CHN
    (c) Changing skills of Community Health Nurse
    (d) Goals of Community Health Nursing
    (e) Role of traditional birth attendant (TBA) in reducing MMR
    (f) Role of *Anganwari* Worker
    (g) Administrative responsibility of district public health nurse (DPHN)
    (h) Educational responsibility of public heath nurse (PHN)
    (i) Legal aspects in community health nursing
    (j) Role of nurse in prevention of communicable disease
    (k) Levels of prevention of mental health
    (l) Administration of School Health Nursing
    (m) Components of School health services.

●●●

UNIT III

FAMILY HEALTH APPROACH

- Family Health Care Services
- Family Health Care
- Maternal and Child Health

8

Family Health Care Services

INTRODUCTION

The family is considered as natural and fundamental unit of society and occupies a unique position between individual family members and community. The family as society's most significant unit of social behaviour, has been undergoing considerable changes that have affected the family structure, functions and interactions, both within the family and in the community.

HISTORY

The concept of the family as a unit of community, health nursing care has been evolving overtime, especially during the twentieth century. The management of physical and emotional illness has been a responsibility assumed by the traditional family within the home environment. By 1850, families started to share the task of caring for ill family members with others such as physicians.

In 1880, visiting nursing associations began to develop and visiting nurses (initially called district nurses) started to provide short-term client care in homes. The nurse's home visits included instructions to families about how to care for the ill family members and in addition, emphasized a healthy lifestyle for all family members. Through contact with family and individual family members in the home setting, the visiting nurse became increasingly aware of the influence that the family had on the individuals health.

During 1990, there was a growing awareness of the relationship between the health of the family and health of the community. The identified interaction between the health of an individual, family and community led to the development of new ideas about the scope of practice of the community health nurse.

By middle of the same decade, the community health nurse was providing total nursing services for individuals and families.

Since 1920 numerous official publications and position papers have included statements addressing the concepts of the family as a unit of community health nursing services. One of the earliest statements was published in 1932 by the National Organisation for Public Health Nursing. Several decades later, WHO Expert Committee (1974, p.11) expressed concern over the diminishing importance of family health nursing in community health nursing and made following statements in a position paper.

"Family health nursing is based on the concept of family as a unit and is directed towards meeting the health needs and concerns of the family by encouraging it to use its own resources as well as available health services".

CONCEPT OF FAMILY

Family, a common word, is generalised as *"a structural unit composed of a man and woman who are married and have children"* (Fig. 8.1). Family is

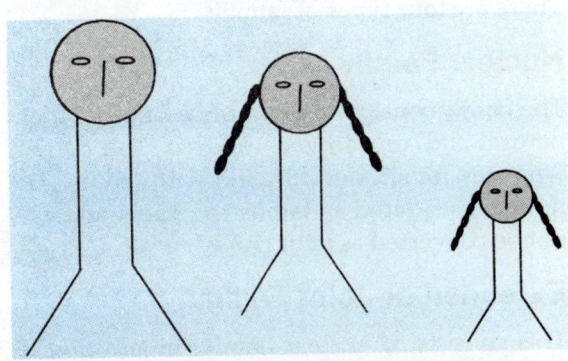

Fig. 8.1 : Family — A Biological Unit

also considered as *"a primary group with genetic characteristics in common with all small groups"*. These characteristics are mainly relationship of intimacy, extensive communication and common goal. The concept of family keeps changing due to developmental stages in the family.

DEFINITION OF FAMILY

The family forms the basic and strongest unit of a society. Therefore, society too defines family. Man is organized in different groups to live in it.

"Family is defined as a primary unit of society. The family members are biologically related individuals living together under the same roof, eating from same kitchen and sharing all the resources which can be money, material, manpower and having same culture, ways of living and religion".

Members have integrated relationship, by virtue of marriages and births and live as one group.

Family is defined as *"A group of two or more people, who are emotionally involved with each other and who choose to identify themselves, makes a family"*.

The definition clears that a family has minimum two members and they are attached to each other emotionally. They have sense of belongingness, and the comfort they get being a member of family.

TYPES OF FAMILY

There are four types of families :

Nuclear Family

The family consists of a husband, wife and their natural and/or adopted children. The people who stay for shorter duration with family will not be considered as family members and can not be converted as joint family.

Extended or Joint Family

This consists of nuclear family, in addition to others who are blood related or marriage related. They are grand parents, aunts, uncles and cousins (Fig. 8.2).

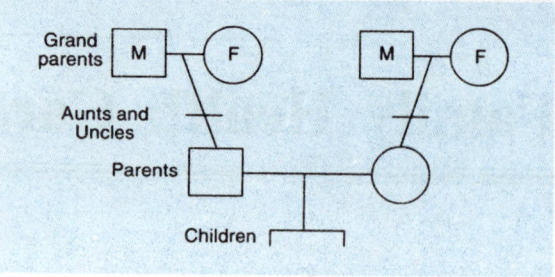

Fig. 8.2 : Blank genogram

Blended

This family includes a married couple, one or both of them have been married previously and have children from previous marriage, and couple have their own children as well (Fig. 8.3).

Single Parent

A single person either male or female, who lives alone with his or her child or children. That may be adopted child, foster child or naturally born child (with or without marriage).

FUNCTIONS OF A FAMILY

A function may be defined as *"an expected role or action given to someone"*. It is through the enactment of family role that family functions are fulfilled. Each family has certain functions to perform to maintain the integrity of the family unit and meet the needs.

The functions of the family assure major importance and responsibility because human personality is not born but must be made through the socialisation process. Children learn to perceive the world through the adult model in the environment.

Hill outlined basic requirements for family survival, continuity and growth. These include :

• **Reproduction :** Planning and controlling the family size. To reproduce the new members of the society, and to keep continuity of the family.

• **Socialisation :** Of the children into functioning adults, capable of assuming adult family roles of husband, father and wife, mother, to make them productive member of the society, as well as keeping the status of family members.

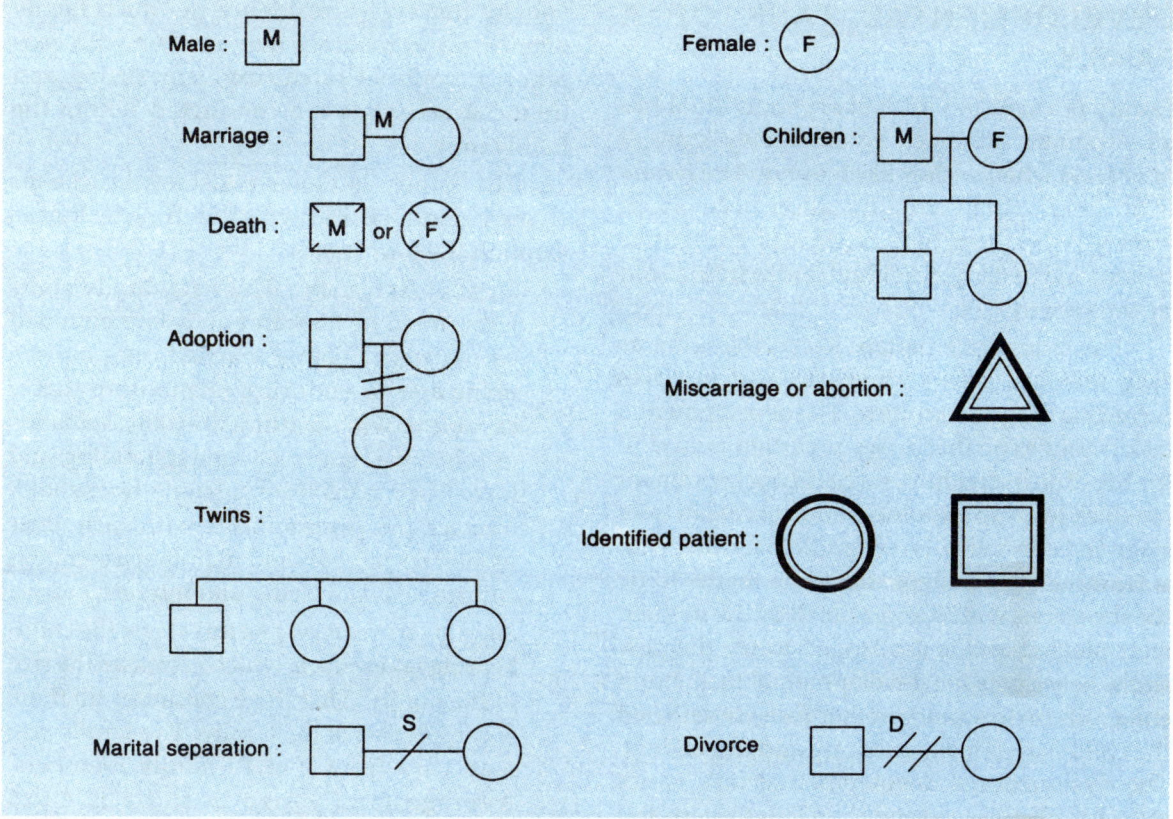

Fig. 8.3 : Symbols used in genograms

- **Economic Function** : To provide sufficient economic status by allocation of economic resources (income) and output.
- **Provision of Physical Necessities** : Physical necessities must be met for all family members, by providing food, clothing, shelter and medical care, which are basic needs for survival.
- **Family Coping Function** : Measures used for the maintenance of order within the family, providing a system of reward and punishment to keep members of family tasks, development of balancing and inspiring mechanisms for the upset or discouraged members.
- **Affective Function (Personality Development)** : To keep up the adult personalities, help children to develop healthy personality meeting the psychological needs of the family members.

- **Maintenance of Family Morale and Motivation** : To carry-out family tasks, keep up the family morale and encouragement.
- **Creating Emotionally Healthy Environment** : By meeting emotional needs of member's affectional ties with other members and channelising of sex drive, providing means of communication among all family members.

Other Functions of a Family

- To achieve economic survival
- To provide physical protection to individual member
- To pass on religious faith
- To educate its young
- To confer status.

Provide food, shelter, clothes, maintenance of health supporting psychosocial home environment.

DEVELOPMENTAL TASK OF A FAMILY

Family is a unit in which every individual has an important influence, whether they know it or not and whether they like it or not. The family is an interacting communication network in which every member influences the entire system and in turn individual is also influenced by the system.

The family role pattern keeps changing as each member grows, develops and matures according to age and culture. The developmental task is said to be that arises at certain period in the life of an individual, successful achievement of which leads to happiness and success in later stage and vice-versa. For example, a toddler who is learning to be independent and learns to tie the shoe laces, will be appreciated by the mother, feels pleased and is challenged to try the new skills, hence gets the developmental task. But if child fails to do so and mother feels dissatisfied the child may remain unhappy and dependent. The dysfunctional developmental task is not satisfactorily resolved and child fails to learn and appreciated. There are various listed developmental tasks :

- Development of conscience
- Learning biological and psychological sex role
- Achievement of appropriate dependent, independent lifestyle
- Learning to understand and control physical words
- Relating to changing social group
- Achieving an appropriate receiving-giving attitude
- Relating one's self to the others feeling (cosmos).

Cyclic Growth and Development of Family

Family involves people who are related in traditional and non-traditional senses by marriage, blood, adoption or friendship. It reflects tradition, rituals and customs. Family usually involves a residence in which family members and relatives may interact with each other. Emotional nurturing, supporting and financial activities are conducted within the family unit.

The family is never constant, but keeps changing and has its own growth cycle. It goes through the four stages.

- *Stage of Formation :* The new family starts with union of husband and wife bounded by marriage. Young married ones build a home and an enduring relationship that is capable of withstanding the daily demands of tolerance, maturity, understanding and love. They constitute a single household, interact and communicate with each other in their social roles and maintain a common culture, ways of living and interest, etc.

- *Stage of Development :* At this stage, the child-bearing takes place, which increases the size of the family. This stage continues till there is completion of the family. The family size may vary from 2 to 10 family members. Average family size in India is 4 to 5 (Parents + 2 to 3 children).

- *Stage of Retraction :* The children at this stage grow-up to get married, hence the children become independent and form a family. Married children may live with the parents or they may make the single family and parents are left alone. Couple re-adjust to the empty nest. This is difficult period after children have grown and moved away. They face retirement and possible re-settlement and try to cope with special problems and increasing dependence with old age.

- *Stage of Disintegration :* The parents start dying, so the number of older family members start ceasing to exist, hence leaving the children with their families.

There may be overlapping of one stage with another stage. There can also be two stages together. Like the parents may die before the children get married or there may be stage of formation of the family, birth of children and stage of disintegration, death of parents, etc.

CHARACTERISTICS OF A FAMILY

Family has specific characteristics :

Family Changes According to Time and Place

The way in which the family is organised and the societal tasks which are assigned will vary with time and place. The roles of father, mother and children are not likely to be clearly defined or rigidly fixed, increasing urbanization and industrialisation may encourage both parents to earn and consequently adjust in the family roles.

Family size also reflects the social and economic conditions. There may be rise and fall of socioeconomic condition in good and bad days. Subsequently, culture too influences the family.

Family Develops Its Own Lifestyle

Each family develops its own value system and behaviour style. In some families there is no or little communication between husband and wife and between parents and children. In other families there may be much communication and interaction. Still in other families there may be outward behaviours with depth of understanding and affection not quickly apparent to be observed.

Family also develops its own power system, which either be balanced, in that father, mother and children have their own area of decision and control, or there may be biasness among members by dominance of one over another.

In some cases, the power is distributed among members, like mother makes the decisions about home management, care of children and father decides regarding economical aspects of family.

Family Operates as a Group

Family develops its own way of operating and dealing with common problems. One family may face the problem as a group, deciding together, for example for decision on choosing the career for child. All family members give their own suggestions for the same and come to a conclusion, whereas in some families, it can be one man decision, *e.g.*, father may decide alone to choose the career for the child.

Family Accommodates to the Needs of the Individual

In the family each member is not only working as a group, but he is also considered as an individual human being. He must have some independence to grow and develop. Sometimes the family needs and individual's needs do not coincide which results into conflict among family members. Like, for adolescents, they make their own decision and may not be acceptable to parents resulting conflicts. There must be some adjustment between two different needs.

Family Relates to the Community

Family has interaction with the community, by utilizing the community institutions and contributes to whatever it can do for the community betterment. Some families have responsibility to the community development, whereas other families may feel a sense of isolation from the community. They keep their unsocial attitude towards community. They may accept all community benefits, but they do not contribute towards betterment of their own community.

UNIVERSAL CHARACTERISTICS OF A FAMILY

Every family is a small social system.
- Has its own cultural values of rules
- Has its own structure
- Performs certain basic functions
- Moves through stages of the life cycle.

FAMILY HEALTH

Concept

The concept of family health is based on the health of family as an integrated unit and is concerned with the health of all family members. The family as a social unit develops a system of values, beliefs and attitudes about health and illness that are imparted to and demonstrated through the health, illness, behaviour of family members. Through the family, the members learn the beliefs and practices concerning health of a large society. The WHO (1976, p. 17) defines family health *"as family health connotes the relative functioning of the family as a primary social agent in the promotion of health and well-being".*

The family and individual health should be viewed within the couple of interrelationships between family members' health. If the family is regarded as a unit in relation to health, with family pattern of illness, responses to symptoms, and use of health and illness facilities, it should be recognised that those behaviours are representatives of individual acting in the name of or through the influence of the family (WHO 1976, p. 20).

Family health is usually described as family's functioning, developmental task, interpersonal relationship, coping with strategies and family organisation and integration.

FACTORS AFFECTING HEALTH OF A FAMILY (Fig. 8.4)

- Sociodemographic factors,
- Family composition,
- Family functions,
- Health values, beliefs and attitudes,
- Health goals,
- Transmission of diseases, congenital defects, disability, long-term health, illness, health risk behaviour,
- Health care provider,
- Role of family in health, illness, and
- Health practices, attitudes and behaviour, coping behaviour and resources available.

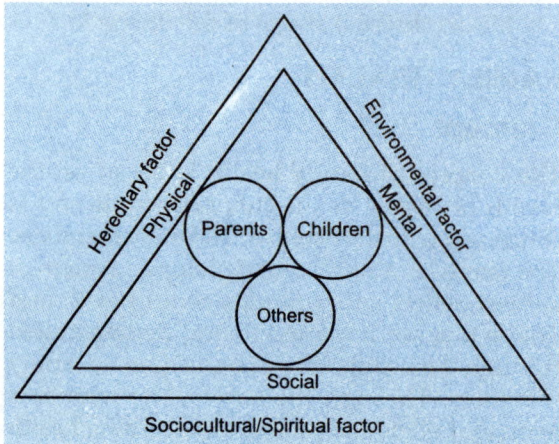

Fig. 8.4: Factors affecting family health

FUNCTIONS OF FAMILY HEALTH

- Provision of adequate food, shelter and clothings, maintenance of health supporting physical health environment.
- Provision of resources for maintenance of personal hygeine.
- Provision of meeting spiritual needs, health education. Health promotion (nutrition, excercise, etc.). Health and illness, decision making, recognition of developmental disruptions, recognition of health disruptions, seeking health care and illness care, seeking dental care and first aid, supervision of medications and illness care, rehabilitation care, and involvement with the community's wealth.

Family as a Unit of Health Services and Illness

The family is a basic unit of society and is also considered as a unit of health and disease. There are several factors which incorporate to justify the statement.

The Family is Natural and Fundamental Unit of Society

The family is based on the development of relationship by birth and marriage. The family originates after marriage and undergoes into various stages of childbirth, child rearing and their developmental tasks, etc. Hence, all functions of the family are carried-out within themselves. The qualities of family functions are the main concern for community health nurse. To understand the level of general family functioning, the degree to which the family can move as a unit to deal with its problems, can maximize the healthy situations and recognise the potentialities of the problems.

Family as a Unit, Generates, Prevents, Tolerates and Corrects Health Problems Within Its Members

Most of the health problems are generated from within the family due to lifestyle, family relationship and family behaviour and these problems can be prevented. Some diseases may be transmitted from mother to child and psychosocial problems may affect the emotional health of a child. Alcoholic father disturbs the home environment and child may develop certain psychogenic disturbances, etc. On the other side, emotionally healthy and stable family will contribute to social and emotional health. It is the family who is responsible to cause the illness and is responsible to prevent and correct the diseases.

Family Provides a Crucial Environmental Force

Each family interacts in its own way, with the physical and psychosocial environment created by the family, which affects the family. The continuous interaction influences the individual's attitude towards strengthening or weakening the cohesiveness of the family. The conducive family environment will bring up happy and healthy individuals (physical, mental and social health), whereas the poor environmental conditions, whether physical or mental may have negative influence on the individual's health leading to physical problems and mental ill-health like drug abuse, sexual assaults and juvenile deliquency, etc.

Health Problems of the Families are Interlocking

The health of one member of a family affects the health of other members in the family. The health of mother will affect the proper care of children and husband at home. A sick child will have to be looked after by all family members. The emotionally disturbed father reflects the emotional behaviour, affecting his wife and children. Though these problems may be acute, chronic or lifelong, but they keep appearing and disappearing within the family. Hence all family problems are inter-related to each other's health problems which affect the family as a whole. Whatever happens to one member of the family has some affect upon the whole family system.

The Family is the Most Frequent Locus or Position of Health Decisions and Actions in Personal Care

During illness of any one of the family members,

the family decides to seek the type of health facilities. Children of course merely depend upon parents, whereas the wife has to consult husband and vice versa. In joint family it is the grandparents who dominate in taking decisions for seeking the health care.

The dominant grandparents may encourage old remedies for sick members at home. The grandmother may insist on home delivery for pregnant daughter-in-law. But community health nurse needs to assess and evaluate the needs for going to hospital or clinic to prevent health crisis and advocate advice to family members.

The family is an important care provider in the home during illness. Care for minor illness, long-term illness or disability, pre-hospital and post-hospital cares are generally provided at home by family members. In many instances no care, other than home care is given to individual. The studies have shown that in low income group families, 97 per cent care for minor ailments, e.g., headache, fever, minor respiratory infection and gastroenteritis is given at home. Therefore, the family needs the abilities to provide appropriate care at home.

The Family is an Effective and Available Channel for Much of the Community Health Nursing Efforts

Family is most approachable and acceptable unit for providing health care to people. More numbers of individuals can be contacted at one time, and services can be provided effectively. Through the use of family approach, one is able to reach the total community. Community health nursing has opportunity to develop effective working relationship with members. This relationship helps to support and encourage the family and individual development to grow.

The community health nurse in family setting must focus primarily on the individual. Though there are some constraints in delivering family health care, but showing concern may remove these constraints and help in maintaining the relationship.

Hence, family health care as a unit is of advantage in most of the circumstances.

●●●

9

Family Health Care

INTRODUCTION

Family health care implies providing comprehensive health care for the purpose of preventing disease, promoting health, preserving and prolonging life and efficiency, through organised efforts by treating the minor ailment, control of communicable diseases, environmental sanitation, meternal and child health (MCH) and family planning.

Family health care is the component of a continuum of comprehensive health care, whereby health services are provided to individuals and families at their places of residence for the purpose of promoting, maintaining or restoring health or of maximizing the level of knowledge to be independent for minimizing the effects of disability and illness, including terminal illness. Services appropriate to the needs of the individuals and families are planned, co-ordinated and made available by the providers organised for the delivery of home health care through the use of employed staff.

OBJECTIVES OF FAMILY HEALTH CARE

The main characteristics of family health care are as follows :

- To identify the health problem by combined community health nursing efforts along with other professional workers, survey the family and community.
- To ensure family's understanding and acceptance of the problems. The family must be capable of recognising the problem and they must accept them.
- To provide need-based health care to each member of the family, which they cannot get themselves.

- To develop the competence of each family member to identify and solve their own health problems and be independent in tackling the health situation.
- To contribute to personal and social development of family.
- To promote the maximum utilization of health services for health promotion, medical care and prevention of diseases.
- To make the family aware of services available other than community health, which they can explore and avail for their health.

PRINCIPLES OF FAMILY HEALTH CARE

The principles of family healthcare are as under :

- Maintaining a good working relationship with the family is important to gain confidence and trust, so that they co-operate in assessing the health needs and implementing the care.
- Collecting adequate information regarding family composition, customs, traditions, incomes and health status, etc.
- Guidance to the family to make them independent for making decision and taking actions in health care.
- Identify health problems and set priorities.
- Provide need based support to the family to improve.

ADVANTAGES OF FAMILY HEALTH CARE

Community health nurse must plan the care which is family based because it has various advantages:

- Easy to understand health care needs of each family member since they are living together and can be easily approached.
- All members can be involved in planning and supporting the health care.
- It is economical and saves time, energy, materials and other resources etc.
- Overlapping and delay of the health care can be avoided.
- It helps the family to be self-reliant in meeting the needs of family member and improving health welfare and nutritional status of family.

FAMILY HEALTH NURSING PROCESS (Fig. 9.1 & Table 9.1)

Family health nursing process provides concrete problem-solving approach necessary to assist the family in its work to promote health, which requires a systematic approach provided by community health nursing, providing information about family.

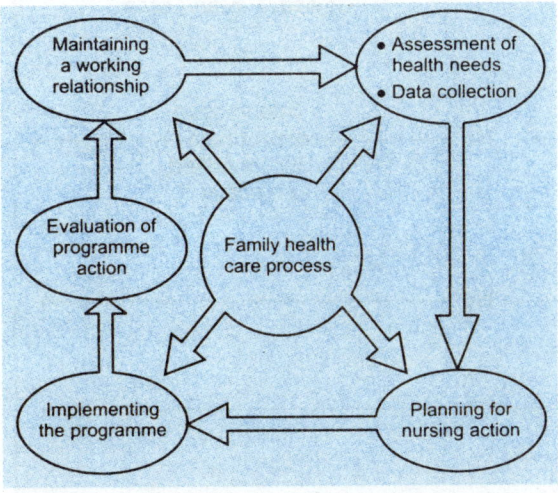

Fig. 9.1 : Family Health Nursing Process

DEFINITION OF HEALTH NURSING PROCESS

Nursing process is a scientific, systematic, continuous method of giving care to family or community by identifying health needs, planning the care, implementing the care and evaluating the effectiveness of care given.

It is defined as a systematic series of steps which if taken (to assess, plan and implement the care to a family) one expects to lead a desired results.

Nursing process is providing comprehensive care to each family member. There are organised series of steps that are carried out in providing health care. These are the steps to provide optimum care for making the family self-reliant.

Steps of Health Nursing Process

Family health care may be provided by five major steps :

1. Establishing a working relationship
2. Assessment of health needs
   - Data collection
   - Personal history
   - Family history
   - Home and environmental conditions.
3. Planning for nursing action
   - Goal setting
   - Resources available
   - Alternative plan of action.
4. Implementation of health care
5. Evaluation of the action taken
   - Formative
   - Summative.

The family health care is provided by visiting the families at their own living places by home visiting, an important aspect in family health care.

Table 9.1 : Family Composition

Sl. No.	Name of family members	Relationship with head of family	Age	Sex	Education	Occupation	Marital status	Immunization status	Health status	Remarks

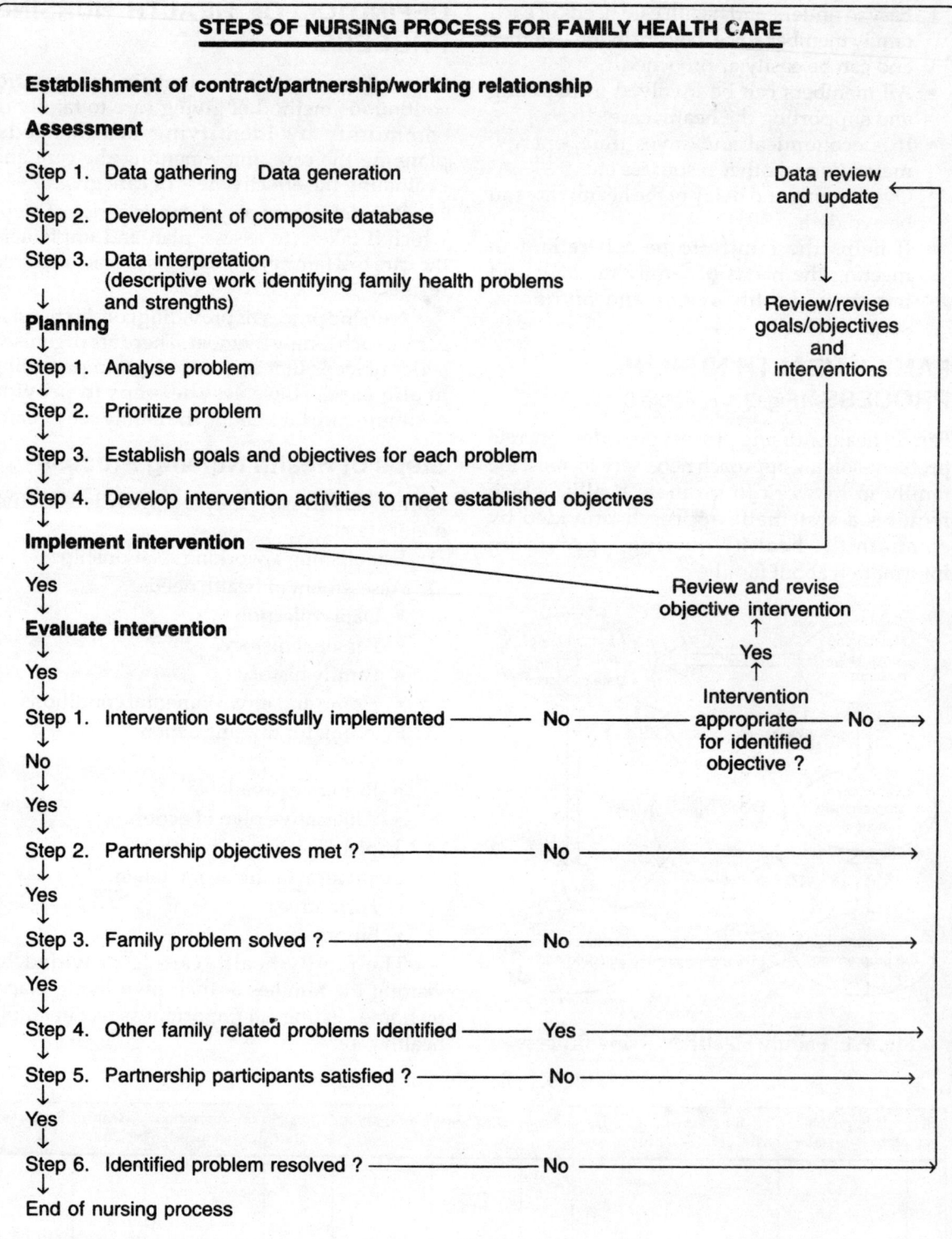

STEPS OF NURSING PROCESS FOR FAMILY HEALTH CARE

Establishment of contract/partnership/working relationship
↓
Assessment
↓
Step 1. Data gathering   Data generation
↓
Step 2. Development of composite database
↓
Step 3. Data interpretation
          (descriptive work identifying family health problems
↓   and strengths)
Planning
↓
Step 1. Analyse problem
↓
Step 2. Prioritize problem
↓
Step 3. Establish goals and objectives for each problem
↓
Step 4. Develop intervention activities to meet established objectives
↓
Implement intervention
↓
Yes
↓
Evaluate intervention
↓
Yes
↓
Step 1. Intervention successfully implemented ——— No ———
↓
No
↓
Yes
↓
Step 2. Partnership objectives met ? ——————— No ———————
↓
Yes
↓
Step 3. Family problem solved ? ———————— No ————————
↓
Yes
↓
Step 4. Other family related problems identified ——— Yes ———————
↓
Step 5. Partnership participants satisfied ? ———— No ————————
↓
Yes
↓
Step 6. Identified problem resolved ? ——————— No ———————
↓
End of nursing process

Data review
and update

Review/revise
goals/objectives
and
interventions

Review and revise
objective intervention
↑
Yes
↑
Intervention
appropriate——— No ——→
for identified
objective ?

Establishing a Working Relationship

The family and nurse maintain a working relationship. It is a relationship which is maintained while working together by developing trust, confidentiality and empathy. These are essential components or elements to find out the facts from families and making correct decisions. A working relationship must have scope of two-way communication. The family members must be given equal opportunity to give their views and ideas and express the feelings and vice versa. The nurse must have enough interactions with family members to guide and help them to solve the problem.

The development of such a working relationship becomes the foundation of all respective nurse interventions. To achieve the desired end, the nurse, family agency or community group must establish a relationship that permits them to work together in such a way that the best efforts of both can be fused into action for improving the situation.

HEALTH ASSESSMENT

Assessment is a continuous process which becomes more accurate as knowledge of people deepens. As defined by **Herpin** *"Nursing assessment is a continuous, systematic, critical, orderly analysing and interpreting information about physical, psychological and social needs of a person, the nature of self care deficient and other factors influencing condition and care".*

There are various means that community health nursing can do in family health assessment. She conducts family health assessment that is holistic in nature, which includes psychological, socioeconomic, physical and cultural factors. It also determines the conditions for nursing actions.

Purpose of Family Health Assessment

The purpose of family assessment are as follows :
- To identify the specific health deficits and guidance needed.
- To assume the probable effect of nursing intervention on these conditions and the

effectiveness of nursing efforts, while solving health problems.

Family health assessment consists of the following :

Data Collection

Collection of basic information—The information regarding family composition is collected about each family member's name, age, sex, educational level, marital status, occupation and health status.

In order to provide a family health service, the nurse must be alert to the health and welfare needs of the members. Care must be taken to deal with the family needs according to the priority, so that the problems with greater urgency are dealt first. Other needs can be recorded until such time that their resolution can be managed.

Methods of Data Collection

The information can be collected by various methods at home :
- Observation
- Interviewing
- Discussion
  1. *Observation :* The community health nurse must be good observer, during home visit. Collection of information by observation gives realistic situation of health practices. Observation of home environment (physical, psychological and economical) and living condition will help to assess the general condition. Interpretation of the data will help for nursing interventions.

  In community health nursing certain situations need direct observation. It is important to get acquainted with family/ environment along with patient and many things can be learnt by observation, *e.g.,* in a family how mother holds the infant, the feeding techniques and how safe the environment is for child to prevent from hazards and the cooking methods for food hygiene can only be done by home visiting and observation. Interpersonal relationship of husband-wife, mother-child can be observed and make interpretations to find different health problems.

2. *Interviewing :* "Interviewing is a face-to-face conversation with a purpose". Interview is a method of securing information, such as facts, opinion and personal history. When used on a professional level, interviewing as defined by **Abramovitz** is "a process of interaction and communication before people. Through this process an individuals can mutually clarify feelings, attitudes and meaningful information. In this way professional people can gain increased understanding of behaviour and personal reactions of individual they serve". Thus, interview process can help individuals to recognise and understand their own problems.

Any type of successful interview includes a satisfactory environment, privacy and assurance of confidentiality. The home is a suitable place for the community health nursing to interview the clients, especially when she has to interview for the first time, as the client will feel more comfortable, secure and relaxed in her own environment.

Interviews can also be conducted in the clinics, offices, health centres and the place of work.

Techniques of Data Collection

Community health nurse should have the knowledge of various techniques of data collection, which can be used to collect information on family health, family environment and other factors affecting health of families. The techniques / tools used can be :

- Questionnaire — Structured / Unstructured
- Observation checklist
- Rating scale
- Interview schedule — Structured / Unstructured

ASSESSMENT OF HEALTH PROBLEMS

Health problems can be identified into three categories :

Health Deficits

These are the instances of failure in health maintenance, *e.g.*, sudden or premature or untimely death, illness or disability and failures to adapt reality of life with emotional control and stability, which results into health problems.

The family fails to keep up the health of family members and leads to premature and sudden deaths, illness or disability and failure to accept the facts of life which leads to health breakdown.

Foreseable Crisis or Stresses

These are predicted time of unusual demands on the family or community. These demands may be pregnancy, retirement from work and adolescence. Though these conditions are expected but still lead to various types of crisis in family.

Health Threats Practices

These are conditions that are conducive to disease, accident, or failure to realise one's health potential. These situations are incomplete immunization among children, environmental hazards, poverty, family history of chronic illness, *e.g.*, diabetes, etc. may lead to threatening situations in family.

Community health nurse does the assessment of health problems and how effectively the family is able to deal with those problems, what barriers may have the family in solving the problems and the conditions require nurse's help in solving these problems.

ASSESSMENT OF FAMILIES

1. Assessment of environmental condition,
2. Health status assessment,
3. Family health practices, and
4. Family lifestyle.

Environmental Assessment

The environment of the family home should be examined carefully, the type of house, hygienic conditions, facilities available and safety factors (*e.g.*, not near a factory). When looking at family's physical and social environment, focus on the environment of the community as well as the type of community in which the family resides will give you clue about socioeconomic status, availability of resources, culture, living standards and safety, etc.

Health Status Assessment

The physical and emotional health status assessment must be done for all family members by using the available assessment tools.

Each family member should be evaluated even if she/he is not primary person whom you are seeing. Health of one affects the health of other members. Community health nursing may not provide the actual care to the each member but other measures, *e.g.*, referrals can be done for others. The basic informations which are helpful are as follows :

- Name, age, sex, height, weight;
- Immunization;
- Developmental stages;
- Health history; and
- Current health status.

Family Health Practices

Finding out their practices towards healthy living of nutritional status, sleeping pattern, exercises, rest and alcoholism, smoking, etc. use of health facilities. The type and ways in which a family uses health resources and providers give the information about health, will make community health nurse aware of their health practices about their strengths and weaknesses.

Family Lifestyle

Observe and describe family's interrelationship and communication pattern. Try to identify the role of each family member, patterns of decision making and family's attitude towards health care.

ASSESSMENT OF HEALTH RISK FAMILIES

Health risk families are those who experience a particular event or other events of any disease repeatedly, that make them more prone towards physical, psychological and environmental response.

The factors that cause a person or group of people to be vulnerable to unwanted, unpleasant or unhealthful agents, for example, home hazards, environmental pollution, smoking, drug abuse, overcrowding, alcoholism, genetic and broken homes, etc.

The presence of risk factors indicate that individual or family has higher probability of being affected by it than those who are not exposed to some risk factors. A child from low socioeconomic family is more likely to be malnurished than the one who belongs to high socioeconomic status.

The causation of a particular disease is not associated with one risk factor, but various attributed factors interact to cause the disease or conditions. A healthy person who comes in contact with any communicable disease, may fight against the infection under favourable conditions and may not get the disease. But if he is exposed to patient under unfavourable conditions like poor environmental sanitation, poor living condition, inadequate nutritional and hygienic state, he is more prone to infection.

People living in unhealthful conditions are more prone to diseases. Identification of risk factors and interventions to reduce or eliminate their impact on family are goals of improving the community health and family health.

IDENTIFICATION OF HEALTH RISK FAMILIES

The families which experience a particular event or several events that cause them to become more prone to the development of undesirable physical, psychological and environmental responses. Family members face stress and risk in their daily activities, in which coping mechanism is helpful. These events are without serious consequences. The extent of coping mechanism and stress situation will help to measure the risk factors for health and outcome of situation.

Identification of Health Risk Factor in Families (Fig. 9.2)

Assessment of health risk factor of the family will help community health nurse to plan and implement the care more effectively. These factors may be as follows :

- Developmental factors
- Situational factors
- Hereditary factors
- Lifestyle factors
- Economic factors.

Developmental Factors

Events that occur as a result of normal growth and development of an individual in the family. These are present throughout infancy, childhood, school age children, adolescence, adulthood and old age. Entering the schools, marriages, childbirth, menopause, retirement, anticipating death of self and others are typical developmental crisis.

A child is considered to be high-risk because of genetic factor, prenatal, natal, neonatal and environmental influences which may lead to subsequent development of a handicapped or developmental deviation.

Toddlers and adolescents are particularly prone to accidents that occur due to independency, developmental fact first time, will like to walk away and may meet road accident, or may try to climb stairs and they may fall from stairs without supervision of parents.

Adolescents like to be more independent with their peer group. They usually do not accept the advise of their parents. Such behaviour can lead to risk of accident while driving, use of drugs and alcohol with their friends, etc. which lead to health problems.

Situational Factors

These factors may appear in the family unexpectedly with no time for preparation. Although certain events may be anticipated and easily coped with, whereas some events are unpredictable and not subject to control risk factors, if such instances have not been identified or treated like natural, man-made disasters, illness, accident, assaults, etc.

Situation risk factor at community levels may be major calamities such as fire, flood and earthquake, etc. Death, rape, murder and automobile accident are events that may affect the individual, family or community. Sometimes it

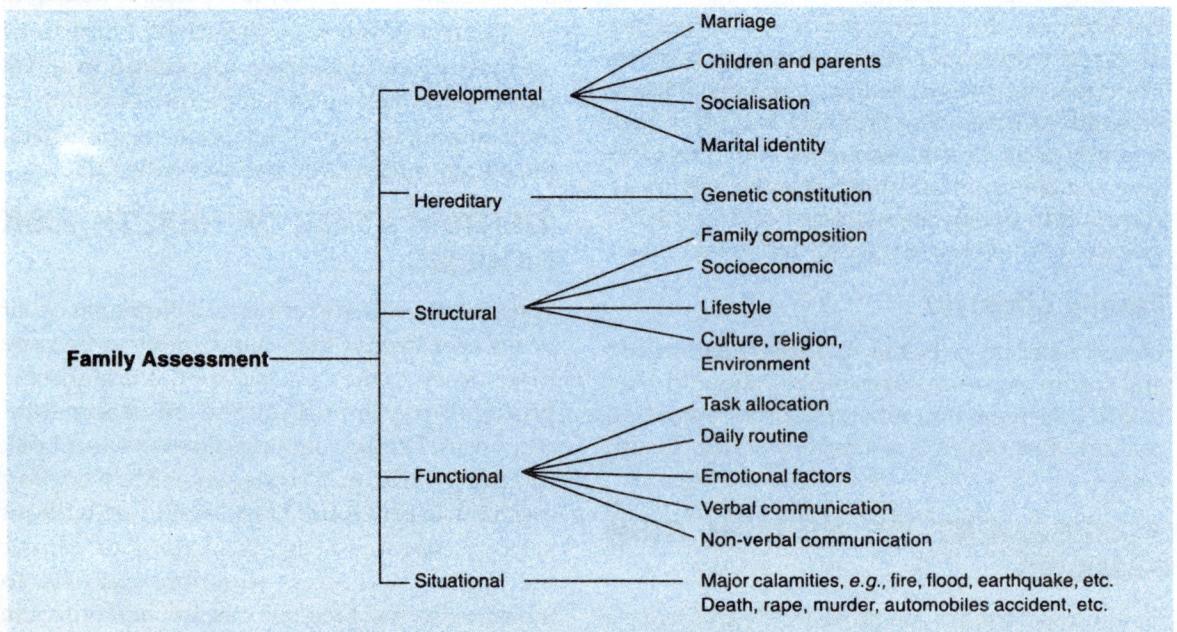

Fig. 9.2 : Identification of risk factor in families

is not possible to take the preventive measures, since they are unpredictable and sudden.

The families get separated and loose their possessions in natural disasters like earthquake and flood, etc. During this period, it is not possible to prevent it, but measures can be taken to prevent further destructions. The family affected by personal tragedy such as death, accident are likely to be vulnerable to health of individuals of family. Due to these potential risks, physiological and emotional trauma increase for all members of the family.

Hereditary Factors

The factor which affects the individual due to hereditary constitution of family. The genetic disease of parents may transfer the same to the offsprings leading to various congenital deformities like haemophilia is indicated. Genetic testing and premarital counselling will help a couple to prevent the birth of such children or undergo a treatment to avoid situations.

Lifestyle Factors

The way of living of a family like alcoholism, smoking, lack of exercise, ignorance and unhealthy practice can result into high-risk factor and affects all the family members. An alcoholic father may not be able to look after his family, that leads to poverty, inadequate nutrition of children and illness among children. The quarrel among husband-wife will lead to psychosocial problems like beating, abusing and even murder, etc. Hence, it affects the health of every family member.

Economic Factors

The factors related to source of income and other financial resources. Wages are the main source of income. When there is threat to job, it has impact on family's economic stability and coping ability of family. The lifestyle may change with economic conditions and physical as well as mental health may be disturbed. Previous coping patterns, reaction to stress and perception of economic conditions are the factors to be considered while working with family's economic issue.

The above factors may or may not precipitate the crisis situation in the family. *A family is in crisis when an event is perceived as being dangerous to normal functioning of family or fulfilling the needs of its members.* Though each family member will be affected and will try to cope with in its own way, but threat to the whole family as a unit still remains a major concern for community health nurse.

Functional Factors

These factors include the performance of family functions by each family member. The task allocated to them at a point of time and place within family by some other members of the family. These could be specific task allocation with reference to a particular time and place. It also involves the daily normal routine function for living, *e.g.*, bathing, clothing, cooking, eating and sleeping, etc. When a family member gets sick the task allocation of caring the sick is the functional factor for health assessment. It is important to assess these factors to solve the health problems.

The emotional factors, *e.g.*, feeling of sadness, anger, happiness which could be expressed verbally by direct communication within family members and non-verbal by body posture, eye contact and facial expressions, etc. It also deals with attitude, behaviour and expectations of the family.

IDENTIFICATION OF POTENTIAL HEALTH RISK FAMILY

Community health nurse needs to identify the health risk family, with potential problems, so that appropriate preventive measures can be taken. The families which have potential high-risk should be identified to prevent the actual risk factors. Assessment of the family functioning and risk factors provide the data for organising, implementing and evaluating the nursing actions.

Community health nurse can assess the health risk by working closely with the families and observations, taking history and physical examination, especially who has any complaint.

Identification can be done at three underlined categories.

CRITERIA FOR HEALTH RISK FAMILIES

The families can be mainly divided into three categories according to the factors present in the family. If any two of the factors are present, it can be categorised as high health risk, moderate, and low health risk family.

Criteria for High Health Risk Family

- Size of family is more than 6 members.
- Children below 6 years are more than three years and one or two may be malnurished and have incomplete immunizations.
- Mother is illiterate, cannot read and write, she is pregnant, lactating, malnurished and anaemic, etc.
- Number of school age children is two or more and suffering from malnutrition.
- Two or more old people with geriatric problems.
- Poor personal hygiene.
- Fatalistic (negative) attitude towards disease and death and not much interested in health.
- Dissatisfied with health services and not availing the services.

Criteria for Moderate Health Risk Families

- Size of family–six members.
- Children below six years are 2 to 3, slight degree of malnutrition, immunization may not be complete.
- Mother illiterate or primary school educated. School age children 1 to 2 with slight malnutrition or moderate nutrition.
- One old member with or without problem. One or two members sick and taking treatment.
- Personal hygeine maintained and environmental hygiene unsatisfactory.
- Neutral attitude towards health.
- Utilize health services when needed.

Criteria for Low Health Risk

- Family size—5 or below (parents and 2 to 3 children).
- Children below six years—one or two both healthy.

- Immunization complete or in process of completion.
- Mother literate—high school education or graduate.
- Mother pregnant but good health. Home and environmental sanitation satisfactory.
- Positive attitude towards health.
- Avail services as and when required.

ASSESSMENT THROUGH FAMILY HEALTH RECORDS

The family information can also be collected through family records. Family records are important sources of all family member's health information. Knowing cultural patterns that prevails in subgroups of population will also help in understanding the family, with which nurse works, thereby making it easier to collect relevant information to help the family in solving health problems.

The previous family records and reports are important means to gather information about family. The records provide important information about health situations of all family members. It gives brief description about family before we go into depth of family history. Documents available for each family members' health and illness which gives us evidence for the health risk situation. Knowing cultural patterns that prevails in subgroups of population will also help in understanding the families with which nurse works, thereby making it easier to collect relevant information to help family in solving health related problems.

Clinics

The family members coming to health centres to attend the clinics for medical care can also contribute to identify the health risk. Community health nurse can make observation and relate to the present health situation. Taking history of antenatal mother will help us to identify the potential health risk related to ANC mother and identify the needs and plan care. Community health nurse can not devote much of her time in clinic, hence she needs to go home to collect sufficient information and for close observations.

Observation

In community health nursing, certain situations need direct observation. It is important to get acquainted with family environment along with patient, and many things can be learnt by observation, e.g., in a family how mother holds the infant, the feeding techniques and how safe the environment is for child to prevent him from hazards, and the cooking methods for food hygiene can only be done by home visiting and observation. The interpersonal relationship of husband, wife, mother and children, etc. can be observed and make interpretation to find different health problems. Community health nurse needs to be a good observer.

Physical Health Assessment

Community health nurse may require to do physical examination of each family member to find individual's physical state of health. This may help her for early diagnosis and treatment and appropriate referral. If physical health is satisfactory, community health nurse may educate the family to promote health and prevent various illneses.

On assessment, she might find the health conditions with which family is unaware and could lead to serious problems, e.g., breast examination of mother above 40, may help in early stage of detecting breast cancer. If there is indication for primary breast cancer, she can save her life by treatment and prevent premature death and crisis.

PLANNING FOR NURSING ACTION

Constructing a Family Health Care Plan

It implies that a careful assessment leads to :
- Goal setting and selection of appropriate strategy
- Formulation of nursing diagnosis
- Resources available
- Choosing appropriate line of action.

GOAL SETTING AND SELECTION OF APPROPRIATE STRATEGY

A good assessment will make the selection of appropriate goals and strategies easier. Families determine the degree of change required. Often, people can easily identify their own goals. However, community health nurse has to assist in making a clear goal statement by achievable mens. Be sure that neither community health nurse nor family are too ambitious. Goal should be clear and concise statement. Clearly written goals give a sense of direction in how to proceed in the care of the family. This increases the self-confidence and trust and confidence of the family in you and your ability to provide care.

A goal must state a measurable outcome. This gives you the tool for determining whether or not your goal has been achieved. It is important to state one measurable outcome per goal. It helps you to keep the desired outcome separately and can be measured easily.

As a community health nurse, the goals which are written in care plan are preventive as well as rehabilitative goals, as well as crisis and more immediate goals. To facilitate the implementation, the goals can be broken down into three types :
(a) Immediate
(b) Shortterm
(c) Longterm.

Immediate Goals

The goals which require action within a short period of time as per need and crisis in the family. These may be derived from short or less term goals.

After assessment of data, establish the priorities for setting goals, you can determine the needs requiring immediate attention. You may set and achieve a goal during the visit in acute or crisis situation. For example, during assessment, the goals to be set for antenatal mother are providing antenatal care, postnatal care and MCH. It is also important to determine the family's attitude and expectations towards health agency. These attitudes may be a result of their previous experience or lack of know-ledge; hence nursing intervention is required.

If the antenatal mother starts antipartum haemorrhage, you have the immediate goal to care the mother with APH to save the life of mother and foetus.

One of the positive effect of setting and achieving an immediate goal is that the nurse and the client will both feel a degree of satisfaction and sense of accomplishment because it has been achieved. This also gives confidence to both nurse and the family, as they continue towards the achievement of their short- and long term goals.

Short Term Goals or Intermediate Goals

The goals that are to be achieved over a specific period of time. These are the steps towards achievement of long term goals. They have specific time limit to accomplish the goals, though in certain circumstances there may be some variation in time. The dates may be re-negotiated, to achieve the goals for correct course of action.

For mother, the long term goal is that she produces a healthy baby and she remains healthy till the end of the delivery and even after delivery. To achieve this goal various short term goals are established like to assess the general condition, to do the investigation, regular antenatal check-up and give health education, etc. These short term goals have specific time period to achieve them.

Long-term Goals

The goals that are oriented towards the future and state the ultimate level of health care can be achieved. It is important that goals are realistic in order to achieve them. Unrealistic goals can lead to frustration, discouragement, and abandonment (waste) of all efforts towards maximum health.

After assessment, the ultimate or long-term goals, must be set, as to what has to be achieved to keep the health status of the family.

The nursing needs which do not require immediate attention or action, the goals can be set as late priority than immediate or short term goals. For example, a child having diarrhoea requires immediate action to teach for oral rehydration solution (ORS) supplementation and control diarrhoea is an immediate goal and providing immunization and health status to child is long term action or can be taken later in long term, where community health nurse will find the results in later stage. Hence, community health nurse has to prioritise short and long term goals to provide efficient and effective health care to family.

The development of realistic, specific, relevant and acceptable goal is an essential requisite before planning for nursing actions to find the desired results. In community health nurse there are two types of goals which must reconcile the goals of professional care provider and the goals of the patient, family, community.

Two kinds of goals may be set for operation, the goals of the profession and the goals of the family. Sometimes these are in harmony, but in many instances there will not be complete agreement. Nursing goals must reconcile in three ways, with her professional preparation, with health agency and the patient.

The goals of community health nurse must reconcile with the goals of nursing profession, that means they must be consistent with ethical and expert characteristics that are expected from a professional. The set goal must reconcile with the health agency from where the health services are linked or provided. The goals must be acceptable to the recipient of the health cares. Community health nurse must set the goals which reconcile with her professional training, *e.g.*, if she is trained to provide preventive and promotive care, she should not set the goals for curative, which she is not prepared to do so.

The goals must be tested as realistic goals, unrealistic goals might exert a negative effect in the long-run, because if not achieved might lead to disappointment, frustration and loss of confidence.

DEVELOPMENT OF STRATEGY

In many instances there may be more than one possible course of action that appear suitable to the solution of the problem. Community health nurse must look for all possible ways of accomplishing a goal, make a selection. Along with the family select the strategy which you feel will best serve to achieve the goal. Once it has been selected, then review the reason for the choice made and record the rationale. Do not discard the other strategies which might be helpful further.

After selection of strategy, choose one or two alternatives, so that you can choose another one, if initial fails. Record the strategies together with the goals set. These strategies and alternatives must be discussed with family members.

A bedridden patient has to be given care at home. The different strategies may be that community health nurse gives the direct course, she supervises the daughter to give the care, nursing aid gives the care. One out of these alternatives can be selected and study all the possible actions. After selection, if one fails to give the care, other one should be ready to accomplish the work to achieve the goals.

These strategies become successful, when the family is encouraged to take the responsibility for selecting a given course of action, even though the action selected may be less productive than one the nurse would have choosen. But it enhances the ability of family to make decisions and solve their own problems in health matters.

FORMULATION OF NURSING DIAGNOSIS

Once assessment is complete, review all the data, compile the risk factors and formulate nursing diagnosis. Since assessment is an ongoing process, it should be periodically reviewed, deleted and revised as per need. It is important to look at assessment data in totality and compile as overall functioning and health of the family.

The final step of family assessment is formulation of nursing diagnosis. The nurse who practices in the community just like those practicing in other health care settings, formulates nursing diagnosis based on assessment data with complete data available. She can formulate more accurate and scientific diagnosis. This forms the foundation for development of a health care plan.

Resources Available

Availability of health related resources and financial resources used by family members. Sometimes families need help in identifying these resources; they may not define as broad as

community health nurse can do. Discussing the family's financial status may be difficult initially, and family may be reluctant to disclose their finances, to a stranger. The community health nurse must be sensitive to such possibilities. The primary reason to know financial resource is to know whether or not they are able to meet their basic needs and able to meet the needs during crisis. It is important to know how family pays for health care. Once family's health care resources are determined, it is important to know the significance of strengths and weaknesses related to resources. Sources of the family's income must be noted whenever possible.

FAMILY HEALTH CARE PLANNING

Advantages

The advantages of family health care planning are as follows :

- Provides systematic need based service.
- Provides scope for evaluation and replanning.
- Acts as a document for providing care.
- Prevents gapping and overlapping in providing family care.

Objectives of Family Care Plan

It helps to :

- recognise health needs of the family;
- make decisions to deal with these health needs;
- meet the health crisis effectively at its earliest possible time;
- provide comprehensive health care to all family members;
- carry-out medical recommendation;
- make environment conducive to health and personal development. Family care plan includes the following :

Choosing Appropriate Line of Action

In most instances there will be more than one possible actions which appear to be suitable to solve the problem. The selection of one course of action would depend upon many related factors like acceptability of the specific plan to family, level of judgement required in giving care, seriousness of the problem, expectation of family/community, sources of payment for nursing care.

In most actions there are negative and positive consequences. The positive outcomes anticipated must be seen against the possible negative responses. Selection among alternatives involves weighing the plus and minus values of each and identify the "best way". For example, to provide care to chronically ill-patient at home it can be done.

1. By the daughter of the family.
2. By qualified visiting nurse.
3. By nurse's aid and supervised by qualified nurse.
4. Combination of all the above while selecting the most appropriate action, it must be cost benefit, family must enhance ability of making own decisions and be independent as much as possible. Hence, community health nurse must try to teach the family member in improving their efficiency, so that they do not have to depend upon community health nurse all the time.

Selecting Appropriate Nursing Action

Supplemental

Intervention means providing or doing things for the family, individual or community; which they can not do themselves. The care may be therapeutic care to the side, making decisions during crisis in family or teaching healthy practices to family.

Facilitative

Intervention is to facilitate the situation by removing barriers to care, *e.g.*, economic, social cultural, ignorance, etc. so as to make the health care facilitative and feasible. For example, social, cultural barrier avoiding first breastfeed to newborn at home is a wrong practice. Community health nurse should facilitate the misconception and ignorance by teaching the importance of breast milk of first few days and should emphasize the mother to feed the baby immediately after birth, will facilitate healthy lifestyle for mother and child.

Developmental

Intervention is based on improving the capacity of the family or community to act themselves. Teaching families or group to make their own health decisions, guiding to deal with potential crisis and stresses.

The care planning involves all three types of interventions, though it depends which one of the intervention is suitable to the situation.

Family Care

Plan involves mobilization of all functional organisation of those involved in health care action. Various facilities and resources available within the family or community, like manpower who can facilitate in giving care. Money resources available and materials which can be used from within.

Planning

Several components of care plan for implementing nursing care needs to be drawn into organised schedule for action. This must involve establishment of priorities, the phasing and co-ordinating the activities.

Priorities are established by ordering the various aspects of care in terms of urgency or impact in order to define those who need earliest and most inclusive attention. A family in which a member has active tuberculosis, would definitely get the highest priority for regular treatment for curing illness and prevent the spread of infection than looking into health of other members.

Implementation of Health Care

Implementation of nursing process in family health care is foundation of nursing practice. Nurse uses family health care process to promote the health of families and differentiate from work with individual events. Implementing the health care requires home visits, working closely with families, community leaders, health workers, and other related agencies like social welfare and educational institution, etc. for comprehensive system to care.

Implementation is an ongoing process. Implementation of nursing care includes all activities that community health nurse undertake to carry-out the nursing care plan designed to improve the health of family and individual. In case of crisis situation in family, she should be prepared to crisis intervention by helping on appropriate resolution. The steps of crisis intervention which a nurse may follow are:

- Helping the family members to recognise the crisis and comprehend the reality of situation.
- Help the individual to tackle the situation in a manageable way.
- Help the family to solve their problems by exploring the alternative ways.
- Help them to recognise the strengths and encourage them to use their capabilities.
- Help family to accept assistance from others as needed and when available.

The presence of community health nurse will help family to explore their strength, use them and solve the problems by themselves, under her guidance and supervision.

Implementing a nursing care plan implies that a careful assessment and planning process has been accomplished. Activities for family are now available which will contribute to its well being and facilitate its coping behaviour as related to its specific health needs.

After goals and strategies have been set-up family is ready to implement the plan. At the beginning the family is ready to implement the plan and may be enthusiastic and eager to accomplish the goals. The role of nurse is to be supportive and advocating these positive behaviours.

As the implementation process goes on, it may be necessary to change or omit certain strategies according to situation. Nurse can also facilitate the growth of the well-planned programme. Family's satisfaction serves as the stimulus for adding further goal. Sometimes nurse observes the family's readiness and raises the possibility of care.

Many families are able to cope with and overcome most difficulties with a minimum of special help from outside beyond that provided by the society and government agencies. It is to strengthen the ties that bind the family and to help, keep the family safe from the ravages of sickness and disasters that community health guidance and service is provided. The guidance and help that community health nurse provides is based on individual needs.

MAINTAINING GOOD INTER-PERSONAL RELATIONSHIP TO PROVIDE HEALTH CARE

Nursing intervention must start with maintaining good professional relationship with family and helping them to do the work which they can not do on their own. Family should be made capable of meeting their own needs. Community health nurse needs to facilitate such action which makes the patients independent in actions. For example, a diabetic patient taking insulin at home. Community health nurse can teach to take (instead she gives it) the injection, so that he takes himself in future.

For successful implementation community health nurse must be fair in regard to caste, religion, economic status and age. She must know the family characteristics before nursing actions.

Evaluation

Evaluation of Action Taken Definition

"Evaluation is a process by which results are compared with the intended objectives or more simply the assessment of how well a programme is being performed". Evaluation should be always considered during planning and implementation of programme or activity. Planning and evaluation must be viewed as an interactive process leading to continuous modification both of objectives and plans.

Evaluation of the family problems resolution and nursing strategies for interventions occurs throughout the nurse's contact with families and at the point of terminating the relationship.

Evaluation is not an end to family health care programme, it is continuing process integrated in the other phases. The ultimate goal of community health nurse is for the family to be self-supporting and independent in identifying the presence or absence of preventive health behaviour and skills in determining strategies and using appropriate resources.

Evaluation of the health care requires careful appraisal of community health nurse's performance and behaviour as well as the family's response in regard to temporary and permanent change of behaviour. Evaluation involves measurement of behaviour and interpreting results in terms of the desired changes in behaviour.

The evaluation is based on the set objectives for family. For success in evaluation, it is better to involve family in setting the objectives to bring the desired changes in attitude.

Community health nurse should observe for change in attitude during and after the intervention of care. If she notices the failure brings to the desired change, then she needs to go back to reset the objective, replan and reimplement the programming.

Tools of Evaluation

These scales are used to elect the opinion, behaviour and attitude towards healthy practice.

Family is a basic unit of society, for all community health nursing services. The health of one members of family affects the welfare of all family member in a family. One family may find every member enjoying a good health, whereas another family may have an antenatal mother, two unimmunized toddlers, an hypertensive grandmother and grandfather with geriatric problems.

It is necessary to understand how family seeks and find ways of survival and how they live in a given environment. The nurse must recognise and understand the fundamental basis of family unity, love, protection and security.

Questionnaire

It is a tool in which the questions are formed in predetermined fashion, which are to be filled up by the respondents. Questionnaire can either be closed (Yes/No response) or open ended (response from people).

Interviewing Schedule

A tool for responses which are recorded simultaneously. It can be structured or unstructured. It is useful to get responses from illiterate people when written questionnaire is not possible.

Techniques

Questioning

The questionnaires are prepared to evaluate the programme. The questions are asked verbally for the programme participants who are illiterate and/or are unable to read and write and responses are recorded, tabulated, analysed and interpreted to find the impact of the programme.

Pen-pencil Technique

The questionnaires and opinionnaires are given to programme participants to get the responses and interpret the results to evaluate the effectiveness of the programme. The technique is limited to educate people only.

Observation Technique

(a) It is an effective tool in community health, because many things can be interpreted by observational skills, while tally which may not be interpreted by persons like housing condition and sanitation, breastfeeding practices and child care, etc. Observer must develop the skills of accurate and correct observation and timely recording. If good observation is made it gives an effective information regarding health, which can supplement to the interview or questionnaires. The opinionnaire is used to find the opinion of people regarding satisfaction level of health services available and helps to improve the health care facilities.

(b) The observation checklist is prepared on the items to be observed, e.g., housing conditions, child care, food hygiene and demonstration of ORT, etc.

Interviewing

It is a direct conversation between interviewer and interviewee. In interviewing the interviewer asks a set of questions to the interviewee and get responses on the interview schedule (prepared before hand) and the responses are recorded simultaneously.

Based on all methods, tools and techniques, a complete performa is prepared to observe and evaluate the community health activities.

COMMUNITY HEALTH NURSE'S RESPONSIBILITY IN FAMILY HEALTH CARE

The promotion of health care of families is a unique responsibility of community health nurse. Health care is an organising framework with a view to assist families to achieve the highest level of functioning.

Community health nurse applies the family health care process for family health promotion of strengths and weaknesses become apparent. Nurse helps them to identify the weaknesses.

- Community health nurse must be able to assess the family as a unit of health service of an integral part.
- In planning and implementing strategies, to promote family health, the nurse functions as a problem solver, resource link and health educator. She must not impose her own values and solutions to the problem.

Barriers to Family Health Care

- Multiproblem family and difficult to prioritise the needs. Community health nursing can help to set short-term goals to achieve.
- *Barrier to change:* The family may not understand to the concept of need. Community health nurse might remove anxiety by educating them.
  - **Language** may be a barrier, especially in rural population. They may not understand community health nurse's language. Community health nursing can involve informal or formal leaders from within the community and should be comprehensive in educating people.
  - **Sociocultural :** The culture of a family might interfere in providing family health care. Hence, community health nurse needs to study such cultural and social patterns and adjust to those and try to remove such barriers by assurance.

FAMILY VISITS/HOME VISITS

Community health nurse works in families in a variety of settings like clinic, schools, offices and homes etc. An important aspect of community health nurse's role in promoting health of people is by providing services to individual families in their homes.

Home visiting is one of the most important aspect of community health services. Besides the healthy and vulnerable people in the community, many of the sick people are there in houses. Health care at home requires knowledge and technical skills in providing comprehensive care to the healthy and the sick. Community health nurse must have teaching abilities, judgement, critical thinking, communication skills, problem solving abilities and skills in therapeutic measures.

Principles of Home Visiting

1. Plan the work for home visit, according to prioritised health needs and plan for regular visits to the homes in selected units at a time.
2. Keep the scientific base in mind while working at home.
3. Respect, understand and be sensitive to others feelings.
4. Use safe technical skills, *e.g.*, giving injection by safe technique and avoid giving harm to the person, use of handwashing technique and have good observation skills.
5. Gather relevant information regarding family, individual and the home environment and make an objective analysis of the facts as an initial step in visiting the home.

During home visit the community health nurse as well as family members should feel free to communicate about their own health problems. She can also observe various factors, *e.g.*, environmental sanitation, home condition, living standard and hygienic conditions, etc.

Working with families will help to know and record family in depth. This provides opportunities to assess the health risk by studying developmental situation, hereditary factors and lifestyle behaviours. The home visit is usually planning as per :

Objectives

- Need felt by the individual, families or community in case of health problems sickness, delivery and post-surgery.

- Planned visit by community health nurse for infants, toddlers and antenatal mother and follow-up of chronic illness, family planning, etc.
- To investigate the source of infectious diseases which may be spreading in the community.
- To identify the health problems and health status regarding immunization, nutrition, environment and give health education accordingly.
- To follow-up cases for treatment and care given by family members.
- To supervise and guide other health workers.

Purpose

- Opportunity to gain more accurate information of family structure and behaviour in the natural environment like certain information which people may not like to disclose in the interview, she can know the facts at home conditions, whether they are physical and psychosocial aspects.
- Provides opportunity to make observations of home environment and identifies both the barriers and supports for reaching family health promotion goal.
- Nurse can work with client first hand to adapt intervention to meet realistic resources.
- Home visit contributes to the family's sense of control and active participation in assessing their own health needs and meeting the health needs.
- Community health nurse gets opportunities to observe housing conditions and actual care given by family members.
- It provides an opportunity to look for new health problems.

PLAN FOR HOME VISIT

Initiation of Home Visit

Before going for home visit the nurse must have clear purpose of home visit. She must have basic knowledge about family in general. The initiation of visit starts with the needs of family and the nurse, through the health centres. The

family should also feel the need of home visiting to make the visits more successful.

Previsit Phase

If possible, prior information to the family for home visit must be given through either personal or telephonic message. The family should be aware of how community health nurse came in contact through records, school records, etc. The home visit must be scheduled in such a way that most family members should be available at the time of visit.

The family may possibly refuse to visit of the nurse to their home. Less experienced community health nurse may feel personal rejection when it is not. The nurse needs to explore the reason for such behaviours and try to resolve the situation by additional information of health services available to them.

In Home Phase

The nurse needs to provide her personal identification and professional affiliation. This is a part of introductory phase. Then there must be a social period, in which client needs to assess the nurse to establish rapport.

The important component of home visit is establishing the working relationship and implementing the nursing process. The nurse must be realistic about what can be accomplished in home visiting. Resources and needs of the family are to be explored. The nurse can assist in availing various health services available around the area and help in initiating the referrals. The frequency and intensity of home visit not only depends upon the needs of the family, but also with eligibility of services and agency's policies and priorities. It is realistic to expect at least the beginning of building a relationship and initiate assessment to occur on the first visit.

Termination Phase

When the purpose of the visit has been accomplished, the nurse reviews with the family what has occurred and has been accomplished. This provides opportunity for the client to recognise what has been done and provides a basis for planning any further home visits.

Ideally termination of the visit and ultimately, services begin at the first contact, with the goal or purpose being defined. Mostly community health nurse is not sure of the reason for the visit. Consequently the visits are aimless and end abruptly. If communication has been clear, the nurse can plan for future visits by setting goals and planning services for effective care.

Post-visit Phase and Follow-up

Even if nurse has terminated the visit and stopped the home visit, the community health nurse's responsibility is not yet over, the interaction still remains with family records and family. Record system and format may vary from agency to agency. The nurse needs to be familiar with the particular system used in her agency. All systems of records must include database, nursing specific goals, actual action and intervention and evaluation. These are the basic elements needed for legal and clinical purposes. It is important that all records must be accurate, complete, clean, neat, precise, current, dated and signed. The follow-up must be carried out and encourage the family to approach in need.

PUBLIC HEALTH BAG (Fig. 9.3)

The community health is designed to carry the essential equipment and materials needed during home visiting, visit to school or factory. These equipments are used to carry on various procedures for mothers and children and temperature taking, giving of medication, surgical dressing, eye care, cord care, postnatal care and newborn care. The public health bag is also used for providing domicillary care to the chronically ill patients.

Use of Public Health Bag

There are following uses of the public health bag :

- The bag is used during home visit to antenatal, natal, postnatal, infant care, pre-school and school children.
- To carry-out different procedures during home, school and industrial visit.
- Physical examination and regular check-up for all family members.

- To give the nursing care to the chronically ill-patients.

Equipment Inside the Bag

The public health bag consists of leather, with following articles.

Outer Pocket Contains

Hand washing articles specially, soap, hand towel, nail brush, and mackintosh. Inner pocket contains: dressing sets, cotton, bandages, scissors, medicines, syringe, needles, MP slide, solutions, lotions, foetoscope, thermometer, kidney tray, enamel bowl.

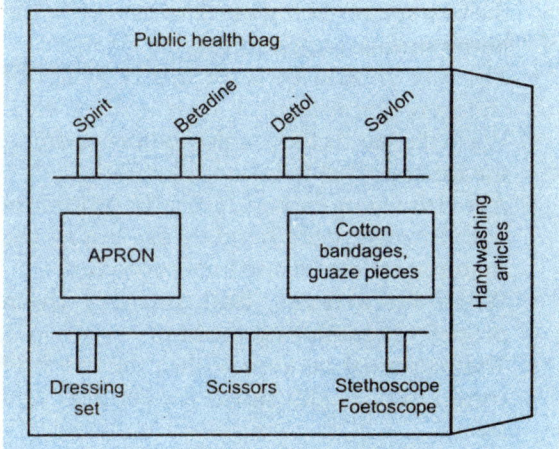

Fig. 9.3 : Public health bag

Indications

Public health bag is used to carryout emergency procedures in homes, factories or schools, etc. The important indications for utilizing the public health bags are :

- To provide maternal (antenatal, natal, postnatal and child health (newborn infant and toddler) care.
- To provide emergency and first aid services to the community people, in case of accident, minor ailments, at home or outside home.
- To provide nursing care to chronically ill-patient with communicable or non-communicable disease at home.
- To provide follow-up services to healthy as well as ill-patients.

- Identify the health needs and give nursing care to children, mothers, geriatric and sick, etc.
- To carry-out certain procedures *e.g.*, testing of haemoglobin, urine, antenatal check-up, newborn assessment, detection of high-risk cases, etc. and provide timely treatment and referral.

Principles of Using Bag

To carryout nursing procedures, certain points must be kept in mind while using public health bag.

- Keep the bag on higher level, clean area, and firm surface *e.g.*, table, cot or box, etc. Keep the newspaper lining or plastic sheet on the home surface to prevent contamination.
- The bag should be kept out of reach of children, domestic pets, such as dogs, etc.
- Wash the hands thoroughly before opening the inner pocket to take out articles.
- Avoid touching the bag during the procedure with contaminated hands. Take out all the required articles at one time procedure.
- Wash the articles, boil and dry them properly before using the bag.
- The bag must be kept within the reach of community health nurse for comfort and safety.
- Check the bag daily for cleaning, refilling and ensuring that all articles are in working conditions.
- Wash all used linen and dry it to keep it back in the proper pocket.

Care of the Public Health Bag

- Utmost care is required to keep the bag ready for handling the emergency and routine care. Clean the bag daily to preserve it in a good condition.
- Replace the used articles *e.g.*, drugs, dressing and linen, etc. daily in the bag.
- Wash the bag with soap and water if possible. At least once a week or more frequently as per need.

- Wash all the steel, enamel, rubber goods with soap and dry and replace them back.
- Check the gloves, lathers, thermometers and glass articles, etc.
- Place the bag in order after use for easy accessibility.

Steps for Using the Bag

During home visit it is essential to carry the public health bag, since it may be needed anytime.

- Community health nursing must follow certain techniques while using the bag.
- Select the safe workplace at home which protects the bag from contamination by children or domestic animals.
- Keep the bag on the newspaper lining or plastic sheet, make sure that outer pocket is placed towards the washing facilities.
- Take out the handwashing articles *e.g.*, soap, water, scrubber and hand towel.
- Wash the hands thoroughly either in running water or ask the family member to provide the water near by drain.
- Open the inner pocket after washing the hands and take out the required articles for the procedure you are doing at home.
- Do not mix the handwashing articles with inner pocket articles.
- Arrange the articles according to priority needs and carry-on the procedure.
- Do not mix the home articles with bag articles during the procedure.
- Remove all used articles, boil them, dry and keep them back in inner pocket after washing the hands.
- Dispose off the used things *e.g.*, paper bag, cotton bandage or guaze, etc.
- Wash the hands and put back the hand-washing articles.
- Record the procedure and care given to the families.
- Fold the newspaper so that surface touching the home area should be inside the fold.
- Place it properly in the health centre.

•••

Maternal and Child Health

10

INTRODUCTION

Maternal and children population constitute the major part of our country. They are also considered high priority on the health need, because of high-risk group. More than one lakh women die annually related to pregnancy and childbearing and many more suffer life-long disability, *e.g.*, chronic pelvic infection, infertility, dysfunctional uterine bleeding and fistula, etc.

Some complications during pregnancy also affect the child. These increase mortality due to increased foetal and perinatal death and morbidity *e.g.*, prematurity, low birth weight and infection among children.

Maternal and child must have integrated services and considered as one unit of health services, because the health status and health problems are interrelated to each other. The problems affecting the health of mother and child are multifactorial, hence there is a need for integrated approach in providing health care.

During antenatal period, the foetus is the part of the mother, therefore, child health is closely related to mother health, for example, if mother is anaemic, child will not be able to take sufficient blood from the mother and will be born anaemic, malnourished and weak because the foetus obtains all the building materials and oxygen from the mother's blood. A healthy mother will give birth to a healthy child, with less chances of maternal and neonatal complications and deaths. Even after the birth the child is dependent on the mother. His growth and overall development depends upon how she bring up her child. Mother is considered as the first teacher to child. If the mother is healthy she will take care in healthy way. Hence, child health depends upon mother health.

The existing health services are based on the principle of multifactorial approach, community participation and equal distribution of health services. Different health programmes have been integrated towards meternal and child health service.

    I. Family welfare programme

    II. Reproductive and child health

    III. Child survival and safe motherhood.

SAFE MOTHERHOOD INTERVENTION

The major causes of maternal death in India are haemorrhage (APH, PPH), sepsis, anaemia, obstructed labour and toxaemia, and most of them are preventable with good maternal care during pregnancy and delivery. Some complications during pregnancy affect the newborn, which increases the mortality and morbidity of both mother and child.

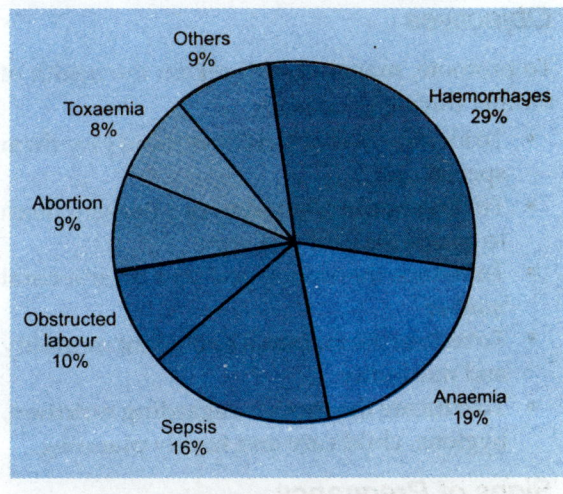

Fig. 10.1 : Composition of safe mortherhood

The aim of obstetric care is to ensure a maternal health throughout pregnancy and puerperium, and every pregnancy ensures healthy mother and a healthy baby.

Safe motherhood programme aims at reduction of maternal and child mortality and morbidity, spacing of pregnancies, prevention of communicable and non-communicable diseases, limitation of family size, improvement of nutrition to prevent malnutrition and anaemia, accessibility of health services to mother and child at periphery level of country. The period of safe motherhood extends from time of conception to 42 days after delivery. During this period the progress is not uniform. Hence the total pregnancy period is divided into three stages. Antenatal, natal and postnatal period. Each state has its own developmental changes, special features and specific risks.

Antenatal Care

The antenatal period is the period from conception to the onset of labour. The primary aim of antenatal care is to achieve healthy mother and baby at the end of pregnancy. The antenatal care should start soon after conception and continue throughout pregnancy. The mother should report to health agency as soon as she is pregnant.

Objectives

To promote, maintain, and regain the health of mother during pregnancy.
- To identify the high-risk cases and give them special care.
- To foresee complications and prevent them to ensure healthy delivery.
- To reduce the anxiety and fear of antenatal mother.
- To reduce the maternal and infant mortality and morbidity.
- To educate the mother regarding nutrition, hygiene, child care and family planning.

Signs of Pregnancy

Missing menstrual period, morning sickness, increased urination, breast changes, etc.

Antenatal Services

Registration

All pregnant women should be registered as soon as she becomes pregnant before five months. It is essential to provide routine care and timely screening to identify risk factors e.g., anaemia, pelvic disproportion, hypertension, diabetes, etc. Registration must include her personal history, family history, obstetrical history and health history.

Physical Examination

The physical examination includes height, weight, blood pressure, head to toe examination to detect any abnormality which might interfere with formal labour. Laboratory tests should include : Blood for haemoglobin. Sugar urine and tests for abnormal findings e.g., low haemoglobin, high sugar and albumin, etc. Measurement of fundal height and foetal heart sound to check the growth of child.

Radiological Examination

Ultrasounds can be done as per doctors prescription to identify any foetal abnormality and the exact condition of the foetus.

Obstetrical Examination

Complete obstetrical examination should include inspection, palpation and auscultation of abdomen.

Antenatal Visits

Ideally antenatal mother should visit the antinatal care clinic once a month during first seven months, twice a month during the next two months and once a week during last month, if everything is normal. During these visits she should undergo routine medical check-up e.g., measurement of height, weight, blood pressure and blood for haemoglobin, urine for sugar and albumin. It is difficult for most of the Indian women from lower socioeconomic status to attend antinatal care (ANC) clinic, which means loss of one day wages. At least three visits during the antinatal care entire pregnancy period, she should be aimed at the first visit to 20 weeks, second visit at 32 weeks, third visit at 36 weeks and at least one visit must be paid at home to assess the housing conditions conducive for delivery.

Care During Visit

(1) History—Personal, obstetrical (2) Lab Examination urine analysis, stool examination, blood group, count, Hb, RH, ELISA, VDRL, Chest X-Ray, Pap smear, (3) Obstetrical examination, (4) Health education, and (5) Identify high-risk mothers and referrals.

High-risk Group

The antenatal mothers who attend the clinic and has the following conditions, needs referral or special attention.

1. Too young mother below 15 years or elderly above 30 years.
2. Short statured primi (below 140 cm).
3. Elderly primi mother.
4. Elderly grand multipara.
5. Anaemia (below 10 g% Hb).
6. Malpresentation (breach, transverse lie, etc.).
7. Antepartum haemorrhage, history of threatened abortion.
8. Twin pregnancy, hydramnios.
9. Pre-eclampsia and eclampsia (complaint of hypertension, oedema and albuminuria).
10. Bad obstetrical history–previous stillbirth, intrauterine death, placenta previa, retention of placenta, manual removal of placenta.
11. History of previous caesarian or instrumental delivery.
12. Prolonged pregnancy (exceeding 14 days after expected date of delivery).
13. Medical problems associated with antenatal period e.g., cardiovascular diseases, renal diseases, diabetes, tuberculosis and liver diseases, etc.

The high-risk groups are identified to provide better services and special attention to those who need them most and maximum utilization of all resources e.g., involvement of community health workers, traditional birth attendants, etc. It helps to improve the quality care at all levels of health care especially at primary health care level.

Home Visit

Home visit is the essential component of meternal child health (MCH) care in community health nursing. Even if the antenatal mother is attending antenatal clinic regularly, she must be visited at home at least once during pregnancy by health worker, lady health visitor or public health nurse. More visits are required if she plans for home delivery. The mother feels more relaxed and comfortable at home and health worker also has enough time to spend for the mother. This will provide an opportunity for public health nurse to assess the general condition of mother and observe the home conditions (physical environment and psychosocial conditions) to advice for home delivery and give health education. The home visit will help to win her confidence, which is helpful for good working relationship. If the home conditions are not suitable, she may be advised for institution delivery. The public health nurse must warn the mother for danger signs: (1) Bleeding, (2) Loss of foetal movement, and (3) Swelling of feet and face or any other abnormal feeling must be reported to nearest health agency.

Antenatal Advice (Health Education)

The antenatal advices are the most important aspect of antenatal care, because she has to continue special care at home. Mother should be educated about herself and her baby.

Public health nurse must educate the mothers on the following aspects.

Nutrition

The women during pregnancy must take one extra meal everyday. The food should contain green leafy vegetables, pulses, fruits and milk, eggs, cheese, etc. She is expected to gain around 10 kg weight during pregnancy.

Reproduction Costs Energy

A pregnancy in total duration consumes about 60,000 kcal, extra than normal metabolic requirements. Lactation also requires more than 500 kcal/day. Further, child survival is correlated with birth survival and birth weight is correlated to the weight gain of the mother during pregnancy by consuming extra calorie and nutrients. If mother consumes less iron during pregnancy, leads to less storage, foetus may receive insufficient iron store. Such baby may show normal haemoglobin at birth, but may become severely anaemic later, due to lack of iron in breast milk and rapid growth and development, as well as exposure to diseases and infections. Balanced and adequate diet is essential during antenatal and postnatal period to meet the extra needs of the mother and prevent associated problems.

Hygiene

Personal hygiene is equally important during pregnancy. Mother must be advised to bathe daily and to wear clean and loose clothes. She must clean her hair, skin, teeth and feet with special attention to breast hygiene. She must take care to the cleanliness of the environment in which she lives, to prevent various infections and diseases.

Regular Exercises

Mother is advised to have regular walking exercises. She can perform light household work, though hard physical labour and lifting of heavy weight is not advised, which may affect the foetal growth.

Regular Bowel Movement

Avoid constipation, which may strain the mother and cause piles. She must have regular bowel movement, by regular intake of green leafy vegetables, milk, fruit and extra fruit. Purgatives should be avoided during pregnancy.

Rest and Sleep

At least eight hours sleep at night and two hour rest and relaxation after mid-day meal. In case of any deviation the mother is advised to take more rest and relax as and when she can. If mother has been adviced bedrest, she must follow the proper instruction to avoid complications, e.g., IUGR, preterm delivery, bleeding and abortions, etc.

Healthy Lifestyle

She must develop healthy lifestyle and avoid smoking or drinking alcohol, etc. Heavy smoking may lead to abnormality among foetus and placenta due to nicotine effect. Consumption of alcohol may lead to spontaneous abortion, intrauterine growth retardation, fertility problems among women and if children are born they may have various physical and mental problems.

Sexual Relationship

Sexual intercourse should be restricted during pregnancy especially during first and third trimester. If mother has the bad obstetrical history then avoid sexual intercourse during normal pregnancy.

Drugs

Certain drugs e.g., antibiotics, antipyretics, antitubercle, corticosteroids taken during pregnancy may, especially first trimester period, affect the foetal growth and cause foetal malformation. Streptomycin may cause eigth nerve damage and lead to deafness in the foetus. Corticosteroid may impair the foetal growth, tetracycline may affect the growth of bones and enamel formation of teeth. During breastfeeding, certain drugs taken may be excreted in breast milk and may affect the newborn. Hence the drugs must be taken with great caution and under medical supervision.

Radiation

The most common source of radiation is abdominal X-rays during pregnancy, which may lead to congenital malformation e.g., microcephaly, leukaemia and neoplastic anaemia. X-ray during pregnancy should be carried out under definite indication, otherwise it should be avoided as much as possible. Ultrasonic radiations appear to have no effect in pregnancy, this should also be restricted to once or twice during pregnancy.

Medication

The mother must be given vitamin supplementation, calcium and iron tablets regularly after first trimester; under safe motherhood programme every pregnant woman must take 100 iron tablets during her pregnancy.

Immunization

All antenatal mothers must get two tetanus toxoid immunization at the interval of at least one month period and if she is immunized during first pregnancy a year ago, then she can take one dose of tetanus toxoid at 5 months of pregnancy.

PREVENTION OF HEALTH PROBLEMS

Though pregnancy is a natural physiological phenomenon, complications do arise even with best antenatal care. It is, therefore, important to instruct the mother to recognise the danger sign and report immediately if :

1. Bleeding or discharge per vagina,
2. No foetal movement,
3. Swelling of the feet and face,
4. Blurring of vision,
5. Headache, and
6. Any other unusual symptom.

All women with danger sign must go to hospital for delivery. In case of bleeding, the women must be taken to hospital where blood transfusion facilities are available, otherwise loss of blood may cause death of women within two hours.

Prevention of health problems during pregnancy.

Toxaemia of Pregnancy

Hypertension and presence of albumin in the urine indicate toxaemia of pregnancy. It is important to diagnose at early stage and treat the patient. Efficient antenatal care minimize the risk of toxaemia and mortality due to toxaemia of pregnancy.

Anaemia

More than 60 per cent pregnant women in India are anaemic (Hb below 10 gm%) due to low sociogroup and lack of nutrition, more labour, multiple pregnancy, neglected female child, etc.

Anaemia may lead to premature delivery, antepartum haemorrhage, postpartum haemorrhage, puerperal sepsis, etc. Government of India has launched a programme that every pregnant woman must take at least 100 tablets (60 mg iron and 500 Mcq of folic acid) throughout pregnancy, which are available in antenatal clinics in primary health centres and subcentres.

Nutritional Deficiency

The nutritional demand is more than the normal requirement during pregnancy, which may be overlooked by mother due to various reasons. Hence she may develop other nutritional deficiencies of protein, vitamins and minerals. Mother must prevent these deficiencies by intakes of milk, vegetables, fruits and extra vitamin supplementation especially vitamins A and D.

Prevention of Infections and Communicable Diseases

STD

Syphilis is a common preventable infection during pregnancy. Syphilis may lead to spontaneous abortion, stillbirth, perinatal death or congenital syphilis to newborn and mental retardation VDRL (venereal disease research laboratory) is done regularly in antenatal clinics to detect any case of syphilis or gonorrhoea. Congenital syphilis can be prevented by providing injection procain penicilline 6 lac unit for 10 days.

Tetanus

Tetanus can be prevented by immunizing antenatal mother with tetanus toxoid at 5 months and 6 months, at one month interval between two doses. A woman who is immunized during early pregnancy, one booster dose is sufficient and not to give tetanus toxoid at every successive pregnancy to reduce the risk of hyperimmunization and side effect. The mother is advised not to have delivery by untrained hands and in unhygenic manner, which increases the risk of tetanus and other complications.

German Measles

The German measles can be prevented during pregnancy by preventing the disease in general public, and school children can be vaccinated against rubella vaccine. A mother with German measle infection may lead to foetal death or malformation like cataract, congenital heart diseases, deafness, etc. Therefore, it is important to prevent such infection.

Human Immunodeficiency Virus (HIV) Infection

Human immunodeficiency virus (HIV) infection may be transferred from human immuno-deficiency virus mother to her foetus, through placenta or to her newborn during delivery. One-third of children get HIV through placento-foetal route. Every pregnant woman during antenatal visit is adviced Enzyme-linked immunosorbent assay (ELISA) test to identify human immunodeficiency virus cases, to help infected women to choose therapeutic abortion or receive appropriate care.

Rhesus (Rh) Incompatibility

If the mother is Rh-negative and foetus is Rh-positive, it provokes an immune response to her which forms antibodies which can cross placenta and causes haemolysis (destroying foetal blood cells). These may lead to hydrops foetalis, congenital haemolytic anaemia and icterus gravis neonatorum (newborn patho-logical jaundice). The routine blood test for Rh factor is done during early pregnancy. If mother is Rh-negative and husband is Rh-positive, the blood is examined after 28 to 36 weeks for antibodies, Rh-anti-immunoglobulin should be given at 28 weeks of gestation, so that antibody production can be prevented during first pregnancy. If the child born is Rh-positive, then Rh-anti-immunoglobulin is given again within 72 hours of delivery.

Prenatal Genetic Screening

For early detection of chromosomal abnormali-ties associated with serious birth defects, congenital anomalies and haemolytic diseases, genetic screening is done for only recommended cases. In case of any defect therapeutic abortion is adviced.

Mental Health

The pregnant women needs to be prepared mentally to accept pregnancy as a normal and healthy phenomenon, especially the primi mothers. Mothers are advised to be mentally relaxed, without fear and anxiety. She must maintain good mental health along with physical health even after delivery to prevent puerperal psychosis.

Health Education

- Registration within three months of pregnancy.
- At least three visits during pregnancy.
- Rest and not to do heavy work.
- Take one extra meal everyday, the food should contain green leafy vegetables, pulses, fruits and milk.
- Tea should be avoided within one-hour of taking food. No fast should be observed during pregnancy.
- Take two tetanus toxoid vaccines at one month interval (5th and 6th month of pregnancy).
- Must take iron tablets for 100 days.
- Should be physically and mentally prepared for pregnancy changes and delivery procedure.
- Avoid smoking and alcohol.
- Avoid long journey and sexual intercourse, especially during first and last trimester.
- Motivation to adopt family planning measures.
- Must report the health agency for any danger sign.

Intranatal Care

The natal period starts from the onset of labour till the delivery is complete. Childbirth is a natural and normal physiological process but complications may arise, hence it is safest to have delivery in an institution with appropriate medical facility. Delivery in a hospital ensures newborn care and can reduce the incidence of infant mortality. In such institutions complications/emergencies e.g., bleeding, obstructed labour, can be promptly handled. In case delivery in the institution is not possible, at least it should be conducted by trained health personnel e.g., ANM, LHV or trained *Dai*. It is utmost important to maintain the aseptic technique, otherwise septicaemia and other complications might result from unskilled and septic manipulations and tetanus neonatorum from the use of unsterilized instrument. Need for effective intranatal care is indispensible, by emphasis on cleanliness which includes clean hands, clean finger nails, clean surface for delivery, clean cutting and care of the cord, keeping birth canal clean by avoiding harmful practices. Hospital and health centres should be well-equipped with all necessary instruments e.g., gloves, drapes, towel, midwifery kit, cleaning materials, soaps, antiseptic lotions, sterilized instruments and supplies.

Domicillary Care

During antenatal period, if the mother has normal obstetrical history, she can be advised to have confinement at home, provided home conditions are normal. Keeping in mind the risk to mother and child, home delivery is usually not recommended, especially the primipregnancies. Seventy per cent of deliveries in India are conducted by untrained *Dais* at home, resulting high infant and maternal mortality but if conditions are not feasible for institutional deliveries, at least trained health worker must conduct the delivery at home.

Advantages

The advantages of domicillar care are as under :
- Mother is relaxed in her own home, which removes her fear of being in a hospital.
- Less chances of cross infection.
- She can look after other children and household work and will feel more satisfied.

Disadvantages

These are mentioned below :
- Lack of medical and nursing care.
- Lack of rest due to resuming her work soon, may be on same day.

- Diet may be neglected due to superstitions and elders influence and workload.
- Home may not have sufficient space for her rest and sleep. Female health worker should be adequately trained to provide skilled care during intranatal care to produce healthy child and resume normal health of the mother and reduce the morbidity and mortality. Precaution for safe delivery when delivery is conducted at home following clean practices must be ensured during delivery.

The woman must lie on clean sheet. Hands must be washed thoroughly with soap and water. Nails must be cut (remove rings and bangles before washing hands). Use new blade to cut the cord. Tie the cord properly with clean string. These should be available in disposable delivery kit. Check the cord stamp for bleeding, if there is bleeding tie the cord again.

Avoid

Harmful practices during labour e.g., putting pressure on the abdomen to hasten delivery or putting finger or hand inside the cervix. They are dangerous and can cause rupture of uterus and infection endangering the life of mother and baby.

Care During Delivery

The care during delivery are as follows :
- Observation of progress of labour, i.e., intensity of pain, foetal heart sound, vital signs and general conditions of mother.
- Provide soft diet and plenty of water with glucose, as much as mother can take.
- Comfortable position to mother, e.g., sitting, lying, etc.

Psychological Support to Mother During Labour

- Preparation of mother how to bear down.
- Good perineal support to avoid tear.
- Observe for danger signs and refer.

During delivery some complications may arise. It is important to identify the danger sign to timely refer the mother to an appropriate health agency. These danger signs are :

1. Excessive bleeding,
2. Mother in labour for more than 12 hours,
3. Placenta not expelled,
4. Abnormal presentation breech, transverse, etc.
5. PPH,
6. Child did not cry at birth,
7. Yellow skin colour of child.

Institutional Delivery

Institutional care may start from antenatal period, if any deviation. Otherwise institutional care is recommended for all high-risk cases and all primi mothers even if they are normal and if home condition not conducive about one per cent deliveries are abnormal and four per cent difficult labour require skilled health care. The hospital stay depends upon the type of delivery. For normal labour she is advised one day rest and discharged on the next day. Instrumental delivery may stay for 2 to 3 days and caesarean case takes 7 to 10 days, if mother and child are healthy. They should be given health advices to continue at home after discharge *e.g.*, care of newborn, eye care, cord care, maintaining temperature, clothing, breastfeeding, hygiene care of mother, perineal care, nutrition, rest and family planning, etc.

Mother's Rooming-in

Keeping mother and baby very close to each other is rooming-in phenomena this gives psychological satisfaction to the mother because she gets an opportunity to care the child, feed the child and reduce the fear of misplacement.

POSTNATAL CARE

This period starts from delivery of placenta to 42 days. During this period the newborn and mother are vulnerable to new sets of risks. They are physically weak and need rest and proper nutrition to recover from labour and regain health.

Objectives

The main objectives of postnatal care are as follows :

• To provide nursing care for restoration of health of mother and child.

• To give health education on exclusive breastfeeding, family planning, hygiene, care of child and follow up, etc.
• To prevent the complications of mother and newborn due to postnatal period.
• Reduce morbidity and mortality of mother and child by giving quality care.

POSTNATAL CARE

The following care is necessary for complete restoration of health of the mother and proper care of newborn.

Physical Examination

Postnatal examination should be done immediately after delivery, which includes temperature, pulse, respiration, BP, head to toe examination of the mother, inspection for abdomen, cervix for any tear or bleeding, involution of uterus bladder and bowel movement, breast examination, etc. Community health nurse must observe for any deviation and examination should be carried out daily at least once, even if mother is discharged till cord is off. The follow up can be carried out by community health nurse at home till cord is off. The mother is advised for follow up after discharge. Further visits should be done once a month during first six months and once in 3 months till one year. Common problems observed during postnatal visits are subinvolution of uterus due to infections puerperal sepsis, retrovertal uterus, prolapse uterus and cervicitis due to mismanagement of second stage of labour. Identification of these complications are necessary during postnatal period.

Nutrition

Mother should eat more than her usual diet including milk, fruits, vegetables, etc., she needs additional nutrition like vitamins and minerals, she must take plenty of water so that she can regain her normal health and breastfeed her infant.

Hygiene

Mother and child must maintain proper hygiene to prevent infection and feel fresh. The mother must take bath with soap and water and put on clean and loose clothes.

Rest and Exercise

Postnatal mother should get enough rest and sleep. This helps to maintain breast milk production. It is necessary also to understand that rest is good for mother, prolonged bed rest may be harmful. It may cause mothers legs painful and swollen if she stays in bed for too long without moving about. Mother, with normal delivery should be made ambulatory within few hours. Mother must walk around and move her legs while in bed. She must start light excercise in a day or two. This will help in involution of the uterus and stop bleeding in normal cases. She must avoid straneous work for at least six weeks and follow abstinence during postnatal period.

Prevent Complications

A number of complications may arise after delivery. Some of them can be life-threatening *e.g.*, puerperal sepsis and postpartum haemorrhage. Follow-up is important to identify any danger sign and get appropriate treatment *e.g.*, fever, fowl smelling lochia, painful micturation, abdominal pain, swollen and painful legs, painful breast.

Breastfeeding

Postnatal care gives an excellent opportunity for the motherly touch to the child, physically as well as psychological by breastfeeding provides the main source of nourishment in first year of child's life. Timely and adequate breastfeeding is the best guaranteed aid of ensuring that the newborn is not malnurished, and it also ensures that the infant is not exposed to unnecessary and preventable infection. Breast milk is the best food available and is tailor-made to suit the child's needs.

An asset in Indian culture that breastfeeding is an accepted practice among most women in the country and breastfeeding rates are high. In spite of poor nutrition status, they have the ability to breastfeed her infant for prolonged period even for more than two years. The studies have shown that an Indian woman has the capacity to secret milk for 400 to 600 mL/day during first year of postnatal period. No other feed is required for 3 to 4 months.

Supplementary food is given after four months child's age *e.g.*, cow's milk, juice, soup, boiled water, etc. No water is required for breastfeeding up to 4 to 6 months of age. Water reduces milk intake and can also cause infection. Breast milk has enough quantity to meet the requirements of the child even in hot and dry conditions. Prelacteal feeds such as honey and glucose water must be avoided for the same reason.

Child should be given breastfeed within half an hour of delivery. Children delivered by caesarean, feeding should be put on the breast within 4 to 6 hours or as soon as the mother's condition is stabilised.

CHILD HEALTH

Care of children in the age group of 0 to 14 years is the most important factor in community, because infant and child mortality rates are important indicators which generally reflects the status of survival of children. Studies have shown that the health of women in reporductive age group and children below five years of age is of crucial importance for effective growth of population. If parents are assured of good health, they will have healthy children and be healthy citizens. Childhood period is also a vital period because this is also a period of socialisation process, where child learns the attitude, culture and social behaviour. Specific biological and psychosocial needs must be met to ensure the survival and healthy development of child and functional development components of child health.

(a) Neonatal period (0 to 28 days)

(b) Infancy (1 month to 1 year)

(c) Toddler/pre-school age (1 to 5 years)

(d) School age (6 to 18 years).

The child health starts from time of conception till child becomes independent. For normal healthy baby the antenatal care starts not only immediately after conceptions, but even before mother conceives and enters the maternal cycle, so as to prevent disorders like foetal and neonatal disorders including low birth weight (LBW) babies, neonatal asphyxia, infection inducing congenital anomalies. The antenatal care mainly includes genetic counselling, spacing at births and limitations of births to one or two. Delaying the young pregnancy till she is physically and socially mature to cope with pregnancy and baby care. Ensuring adequate maternal nutrition, protection of foetus from infection and other defects.

NEONATAL CARE

More than half of the deaths of infants occur during the neonatal period, the time after delivery till 25 days of life. The medical branch which deals with neonatal care is said to be neonatology. Care of newborn is the team work of paediatrician, obstetrician, gynaecologist, preventive medicine and community health care including nursing. Community health nurse plays the vital role in care of neonatology, though main role starts immediately after delivery, but consultation continues during antenatal, natal and postnatal period as well. The care of newborn can be divided as:

Immediate Care

The immediate care for neonates is as under :

- Clearing the airway to facilitate breathing
- Maintenance of temperature of newborn
- Assessment of APGAR, and appropriate action as per APGAR score including resuscitations
- Prevent complications
- Reduce the neonatal mortality and morbidity.

Clearing Airway

The newborn passes through stressful situation after procedure of delivery and child may aspirate the amniotic fluid in respiratory system.

ASSESSMENT OF NEWBORN

APGAR Score

After birth it requires immediate and careful observation of the heart rate, respiration, muscle tone, reflex action and colour of the skin. These can be done by APGAR score which includes all essential components. (Appearance, pulse, grimaces, activity and respiration). The APGAR score is taken at 1 minute and 5 minutes after birth. Each sign is given '0' for absence (zero), for mild 1, and 2 for good condition. It provides immediate assessment of general conditions of the newborn. The excellent general condition can be considered with 9 to 10 scores, 0 to 3 indicates the baby's poor general condition and 4 to 6 indicates fairly good general condition, 7 to 10 very good condition (Table 10.1). If the score is below 5 needs prompt action. Children with APGAR less than 4 remains for 5 minutes without progress, have higher chances of complications and death.

Maintenance of Body Temperature

A newborn delivered out of warm womb of the mother to an environment which may be as cold as 5 to 10°C or as warm as 40°C, whereas the

Table 10.1 : Condition of APGAR Score

Symptoms	(Absence) Score	(Good) Score	(Good) Score
Appearance/Colour	Blue, pale	Body pink extremities blue	Completely pink
Pulse/Heart rate	Absent	Less than 100	More than 100
Grimaces/Reflexes	No response	Grimaces slight	Grimaces present
Activity/Muscle tone	flacid	Some movement at extremities	Active movement
Respiration	absent	10 and irregular	20 regular
	0–3	4–6	7–10
Total 10 Conditions	Poor Condition	Fair Condition	Good Condition

normal body temperature of newborn is 36 to 37°C. They needs to adjust to this environment, if they are unable to adjust may cause complications *e.g.*, hypopyrexia, shock, etc. A newborn has less thermal centre and can loose body heat quickly after birth. Most of the heat loss occurs through evaporation of amniotic fluid from the body of wet baby and maximum (75%) of the heat loss through head. Therefore, it is important to cover and wipe the child to prevent heat loss with warm cloth and hand over to mother for skin to skin contact and breastfeeding the child soon after his vitals are stable. The sooner the child is given to mother, the more protection it is for mother and baby. Low birth weight babies and preterm are more vulnerable direct on to loose the heat through their skin because less developed subcutaneous fats. Avoid putting the child direct on surface of metallic tray, put rubber sheet to weighing scale, child should also be kept away from cold waves, from windows, doors, etc.

Neonatal Care

The neonatal period starts immediately after delivery as soon as the baby is born till 28 days. Out of these days the initial 24 to 48 hours are the most crucial period in the life of infant. This is because the newborn has to adapt or adjust rapidly to the external environment. The mortality during this period is very high. Fifty to sixty per cent of infant mortality is within one month of life and risk of death is greater within 24 to 48 hours after birth. The death rate is high in rural community than in urban due to lack of facilities and proper antenatal care for the mothers by expert obstetrician, also poor living condition for newborn, and poor referral system for emergencies.

As the child passes through vaginal canal during delivery he/she may aspirate/swollow the amonitic fluid or secretions, which may obstruct the airway. It is an important sign that child must cry immediately after birth. If child does not cry the lungs of the newborn do not expand and interfere with normal respiration. Establishing and maintaining cardio-respiratory function is the primary and life saving need of the newborn. To establish the breathing of the baby the airway should be cleared of secretions, fluids and mucus, etc., which can be helped by positioning the face towards one side and gentle suctioning to remove the amniotic fluid, secretions, etc. If, still child does not breath, within one minute resuscitation with the help of suction, oxygen administration, should be well-equipped, before labour and anticipated problems. If heart does not beat within five minutes child has very less chance of survival.

Resuscitation of Newborn Who Does Not Cry Soon After Birth

Most newborns cry soon after birth and suction of the mouth and throat is not needed. However, if baby does not cry immediately or till the time taken to wipe, dry and wrap him/her in clean linen (15–20 seconds after birth) resuscitation steps must be initiated immediately.

- Extend the neck of the baby at 30 degree by placing a folded towel under the shoulders.
- Clean the mouth and throat with a mucus extractor, most newborns who have not cried will cry after this procedure.
- Do not use a guaze or cloth to clean the secretions. It is not only infections but may cause injury and infection.
- If newborn does not cry or start breathing even after suction has been done, then stimulate the baby by pinching the sole with fingers two or three times. Do not slap the baby or hang it upside down.
- If still baby does not start breathing or is gasping, assisted ventilation will be required, hence the child should be referred immediately where facility is available.

Prevention of Hypothermia

The newborn is at risk of hypothermia, because of poor thermal centre development and inability to generate sufficient body heat to match heat loss. Hypothermia can be prevented in newborn by keeping the baby in close physical contact with the mother. The baby should be wrapped in several layers of cotton or woollen clothes depending upon environmental temperature. The room for baby should be kept warm enough that an adult feels uncomfortable and should be free from droughts.

Hypothermia can be fatal for the child. A child with hypothermia feels cold when the dorsum of the hand is placed on its body. The baby becomes lethargic and refuses feeds. Hypothermia is an emergency and must be treated promptly. The baby can be rewarmed rapidly by keeping the baby under a 200 watt bulb placed 45 cm above the baby. If baby does not improve within 30 to 45 minutes of initiating rewarming, refer the child quickly to health institute with facilities available. Mother must be advised to keep the baby wrapped and close to her body during transportation. Newborn should not be given bath immediately after delivery and for 24 hours of life. The child can be cleaned with soft moist cloth to remove vernix, meconium stains and blood clots. The first bath should be given by trained personnel, while bathing ensure that room is warm, free from exposure to cold. This is important to prevent the baby from hypothermia, and should be followed even during summer. The skin of the newborn should be clean throughout, even after passing meconium and urine, so as to prevent from infection, etc.

Eye Care

The eyelids should be cleaned with sterile wet swab during delivery procedure before the baby opens the eyes. One for each eye from inner to outer side (medial to lateral). Do not apply any eye drops or Kajal to the eyes. Any deviation or discharge from the eye of the baby should be reported immediately to paediatrician.

Ophthalmia Neonatorum

Foetus may get variety of organisms from mother during antenatal period, which may cause serious defects. Therefore, specific preventive measures should be taken and maternal genital tract infection should be treated effectively, prior to or during pregnancy to prevent such defects. The most serious cause of conjunctivitis of newborn is N.Gonococcus infection, since it can cause blindness. Trachomatis is another important cause of neonatal

conjunctivitis, which can be treated by silver nitrate (1%) or tetracycline (1%) ointment can be applied.

Cord Care

The cord of normal newborn should be tied with a clean cord tie 5 cm or less from umbilical cord and cut with new razor blade or autoclaved scissors. If the cords is cut after pulsation, the baby derives 10 mL of extra blood, inspect the stump for bleeding and apply any antiseptic preparation on the cord stump. Cord should be kept as dry as possible. It dries and shrinks and separates by necrosis within 7 to 8 days leaving an umbilical mark. Assessment of birth weight should be recorded soon after birth, so as to assess the low birth weight babies and more than normal weight. Newborn with less than 2 kg are low term weight babies and need special attention and if they show the sign of illness should be referred to an institution with newborn care facilities. Low birth weight child with illness can be fatal, hence specialised care is recommended. Children with more than 3.5 kg weight are also examined for blood sugar, etc.

Breastfeeding

All newborns who cry soon after birth and do not show any sign of illness must be kept with their mothers and put on the breast soon after birth. This will ensure warmth, initiation of breastfeeding and emotional bonding. Breastfeeding should be initiated within first hour after birth. This ensures establishment/stimulation of lactation and early involution of the uterus. No prelacteal feeds e.g., glucose water, honey, gur ghutti, etc. should be given. Malpractices of not giving first milk and keeping baby for longer period without milk should be avoided.

The first milk is called colostrum is most important and suitable for the baby, because it contains essential proteins and other nutrients which body requires. It is also easily digestable and contains anti-infective material, which prevents the child from respiratory and gestrointestinal infections. No need for any additional feed, not even water.

The regular milk starts coming on 3 to 4th day of delivery. The baby should be breastfed on demand, at least for 10 minutes on each breast.

Exclusive breastfeeding which keeps child healthy and saves life of many babies by preventing malnutrition and infection *e.g.*, ARI, pneumonia, diarrhoea, etc.

Newborn Infection

Newborn infection increases the infant mortality and morbidity, which is transmitted through transplacental. Early detection of newborn at risk of infection is important. These infections can be :

- **Hepatitis B :** If mother is hepatitis B may transmit the infection to babies at birth. The risk of transmission may be 20 to 30 per cent.
- If newborn gets infection, it will be a chronic carrier and gets hepatitis, cirrhosis of liver in later stage.
- It is important to prevent perinatal transmission by giving serum prophylaxis with hepatitis B vaccine 2 mL, intramuscular injection.

PHYSICAL EXAMINATION OF NEWBORN

The newborn should be immediately examined physically in the labour room to assess any injury, malformation and maturity. Head to toe examination should be done to identify any deviation on the head, eyes, ears, extremities, chest, abdomen, lower extremities anal region and back, etc. There may be haematoma, cynosis, breathing difficulty, cerebral irritation (convulsions, neck rigidity, bulging of anterior fontanel, etc.), persistent vomiting and temperature alteration. In case of any abnormality immediate action should be taken.

GENERAL EXAMINATION OF NEWBORN

Physical Assessment

Weight, height, head, chest and midarm circumference.

Weight

The baby weight should be taken soon after immediate care has been given. The weight should be taken preferably without clothes on a clean towel on a weighing scale. At home the weight is taken by placing the baby in a sling bag and using spring balance which is available in public health bag. The normal Indian weight is 2.5 kg to 3.5 kg.

Length

The length of the baby can be taken by measuring with measuring scale and infant lies supine with its legs fully extended and the feet flexed at right angles to lower legs. The normal length of newborn at birth is about 50 cm. The measuring scale should be capable of measuring to an accuracy of 0.1 cm; it is essential for accurate measurement of height. Errors in the measurement of a joining child may lead to significant errors in assessment of nutrition status.

Head and Chest Circumference

This measurement is taken with a measuring tape at the maximum circumference of the head at the occipitofrontal diameter to assess the baby head circumference and find if there is any congenital anomaly *e.g.*, macrocephaly.

Physical Assessment for Any Deviation

Weight

Low birth weight, excessive weight.

Body Temperature

Hypothermia, hyperpyrexia.

Skin

Observe for cynosis of lips and skin, jaundice, pallor, generalised erythemia.

Head and Face

Hydrocephalus, bulging fontennal.

Eye

Cataract, conjunctivitis.

Mouth and Lips

Harelips, cleft palate.

Cardiopulmonary Activities

Heart, murmur absence of femoral pulse, central cynosis, respiratory rate above 60/min.

Neurological Activity

Reflexes.

Limbs and Joints

Deformities of joints, congenital dislocation of the hips, extradigits.

Spinal

Neural tube defects.

Infected Newborns

The infections a newborn contain are as under :

Neonatal Infections

Neonatal infections are the main cause of high mortality, particularly in developing countries, due to unhealthy practices, poor environmental conditions. Transplacental contamination is one of the most important cause of infection in newborns. Early detection of newborns at risk of transplacental infection is important, by close monitoring and preventive measures may be undertaken.

Congenital Syphilis

Venereal Disease Research Laboratory (VDRL) test is a regular feature for antenatal mother for identification of syphilis. In case of doubt and risk of inadequate subsequent medical surveillance of baby, 2.4 to 4.8 million units of benzathine pencilline may be recommended.

Neonatal Tetanus

The neonatal tetanus is on rise in rural community, due to unsafe delivery by untrained *Dais*, and improper antenatal care. It can be prevented by giving tetanus toxoid vaccine to the mothers during pregnancy.

Newborn with Hepatitis B Positive Mothers

Newborn babies may be infected at birth when the mother is a HBV carrier. The risk of transmission is around 20 per cent when the mother has HBs antigen only, and 90 per cent when the mother has HBe antigen. Transmission of infection occurs through blood and genital secretions and affects during immediate perinatal period and throughout infancy. Breast milk is not contraindication. The infected newborn may become chronic carrier and develops hepatitis, cirrhosis and cancer of liver during adulthood. The perinatal transmission can be prevented by seroprophylaxis vaccine, 2 mL intra muscular (IM).

Newborn with HIV Positive Mother

Transmission of infection from HIV mothers occurs at the end of pregnancy; it is not influenced by the type of delivery. Thirty per cent of babies born to HIV positive mothers get infected. Virus has been isolated in breast milk. Although there is probability of transmission of infection through breast milk, prohibition of breastfeeding is doubtful. The risk of transmission depends upon the severity of infection.

Newborn Assessment

The newborns can be assessed by measuring height, weight, head circumference.

Height

The height should be recorded within three days of birth. It can be measured by infantometer with fixed head piece, on which infant lies with fully extended legs, flexed feet at right angles to the lower legs. The normal height measures around 60 to 70 cm at birth.

Weight

The birth weight should be taken within first few hours soon after the baby is stable. The baby should be placed on clean towel on weighing scale pan. At home delivery the weight is taken by wrapping the baby in thin cloth and weigh by spring balance. The normal weight should be 2.5 kg to 3.5 kg.

Head Circumference

The head circumference is taken with tape measure at the maximum circumference of the head in the occipitofrontal diameter, to assess the normal size against known standard. Large size may indicate hydrocephalus or caput formation. At birth the head circumference is 34 cm.

High-risk Newborns

It is necessary to identify high-risk newborns who need intensive care to reduce neonatal mortality and morbidity rates. These high-risks may be :

- Low birth weight (less than 2.5 kg),
- Twin newborns,
- Birth order 5 or more,
- Weight 70 per cent of expected weight, and
- Artificial feeding.

Child Health Services

Infant and child mortality rates are important indicators which generally reflect the status of survival of children. The experience gained within the country and outside has amply established that health of women in the reproductive age group and of small children below the age of five years is of crucial importance for effective tackling of the problem of growth of population. This is because if parents are assured of good health of their children they take initiative to keep the family small.

Child Health Problems

Major health problems encountered in children comprise of :

- Low birth weight,
- Infections and parasites,
- Malnutrition,
- Accidents and Poisoning, and
- Behavioural problems.

Low Birth Weight Child

LBW has been defined as a birth weight of less than 2.5 kg. There are two main types of LBWs, those born premature and those with foetal growth retardation. LBW is an infant with birth weight less than 2.5 kg regardless of gestational age.

Babies can also be classified as :

- *Preterm* : Babies born before 37 weeks of gestation and low birth weight.
- *Term* babies born at gestation period but low birth weight.
- *Post-term* born after 40 weeks of gestation, but weight less than 2.5 kg.

Malnutrition

Malnutrition is major health problem among children. Malnutrition makes the child more susceptible to infections, leading to high mortality. Malnutrition among children leads to growth retardation. Prevention and early treatment of infections, measles, diarrhoea are important to reduce malnutrition and related problems.

Infectious and Parasitic Diseases

Children are susceptible to diseases *e.g.*, diarrhoea, ARI, tuberculosis, diphtheria, measles, polio, pertussis and neonatal tetanus which are common because of poor environmental conditions and unsafe drinking water, poor socioeconomic status, etc. The preventation and control will reduce the morbidity and mortality due to these preventable diseases.

Accidents and Poisoning

Children are most vulnerable to accidents, especially burns and trauma, as a result of home accidents. Children and young adults are particularly vulnerable to home accidents *e.g.*, fall, drowning, burns and poisoning, etc.

Psychosocial Problems

The incidence of psychosocial problems are increasing in most countries, due to urbanisation and changing social system. These behavioural problems can be prevented by love, affection and security to young children.

FACTORS AFFECTING HEALTH OF CHILDREN

Many factors play important role in maintaining the health of children. These factors can be listed as :

Maternal Health

Mother's health is significant for child and family health because mother is centre of the family.

If mother is unhealthy, she is unable to care for the child. The mother health is important from time of conception, throughout pregency, delivery and postnatal and thereafter. A healthy mother brings a healthy baby, better chances of survival.

Family

Family composition, family environment and social environment have impact on child health in which the child is born and brought up. The healthy family provides conducive and happy environment, which influence the child personality and intellectual potentials. The child should be provided normal family relationship and family stability.

Socioeconomic Conditions

Physical and mental health is directly related to social and economic conditions, like educational status of parents, income, housing and lifestyle of the family. The difference in health between rich and poor children have been observed.

Environmental Conditions

Environment is an important determinant related to child mortality and morbidity. Healthy environment keep children healthy. The poor environmental conditions like poor housing conditions, unsafe drinking water, poor waste disposal, etc., may lead to infections like tetanus, diarrhoea, pneumonia and many others.

The psychosocial environment at home or school is an essential factor for health. Children exposed to happy and healthy homes, makes them physically and mentally healthy. Other factors affecting the health status of children include community and social support measures, etc.

CAUSES OF CHILD MORTALITY

A reliable indicator of the health status of children is infant mortality rate (IMR). The National Population Policy mandates the reduction of IMR to below 30 per thousand by the year 2010. Infant mortality rate has declined over the years. From 146 per thousand live births in 1951, the IMR declined to 66 per thousand in 2001. There are, however, interstate variations.

During 2000, the IMR ranged from 14/1000 in Kerala to 96/1000 in Orissa. Among larger states West Bengal (51), Karnataka (57), Maharashtra (48), Punjab (52) and Tamil Nadu (51), have achieved IMR below 60/1000 as per National Health Policy. However the states of Orissa (96), Madhya pradesh (85), Rajasthan (70), Uttar Pradesh (83) and Assam (75), continue to be above the National average of 66. Major cause of IMR include acute respiratory infection, diarrhoea and vaccine preventable diseases like measles, and tetanus (in areas where immunization coverage is not optimal). A high proportion of infant mortality (64%) is accounted by neonatal mortality. High incidence of low birth weight babies (birth weight less than 2.5 kg) and premature births continued to be high neonatal mortality.

Child Health Initiatives

Special attention is made to empower few states (where IMR is very high) to improve the child health care services like Immunization Strengthening Project– Three year project implemented with two components :
1. Support for pulse polio,
2. Support for routine immunization, including cold chain equipment, staffs, ensuring infection safety and strengthening of supervision and monitoring. Under immunization strengthening project, a study was conducted to assess the infection safety practices in India. Report has shown the unsafe injections are in use both in urban and rural areas.

Newborn Care

States were provided newborn care equipment to upgrade neonatal care facilities. The National Neonatology Forum (NNF) has imparted training to the medical staff, etc.

Anaemia Control Programme

Iron deficiency anaemia is widely prevalent in young children. The National family health survey revealed that 74.3 per cent of children under the age of 3 were anaemic. There is a marginal difference the prevalence of urban and rural areas. Under the National programme iron, folic acid tablets 20 mg of iron and 0.1 mg of folic acid are provided at subcentre level.

Hepatitis B Vaccine

Introduction of Hepatitis B vaccine in the National Immunization Programme was approved by the Government. Under this programme hepatitis B vaccine is being administered to infants along with, primary doses of deptheria-pertussis-tetanus (DPT) on sixth, tenth and fourteenth week. Overall coverage of infants in all the districts at present is 56.4 per cent of target infants.

Border District Cluster Strategy

It aims at providing interventions for reducing the infant mortality and maternal mortality rates by at least 50 per cent over the next two to three years in 49 districts in 16 states by :

1. Development and training of nutrition team,
2. Additional supply of equipment and drugs,
3. IEC for social mobilization,
4. Training of medical officers,
5. Upgrading of first referral unit.

Integrated Management of Neonatal and Childhood Illnesses (IMNCI)

IMNCI strategy has already been integrated in more than 100 countries all over the globe, with the objective to manage and prevent five major childhood illnesses *i.e.*, Acute respiratory infection, diarrhoea, measles, malaria and malnutrition. An integrated approach in India is an effective strategy to promote child health care. The activities undertaken are :

- Training of trainers or IMNCI physician package for key personnel.
- IMNCI training package for health workers.
- Piloting of IMNCI health worker package.
- Training at district level.

- Follow-up after training (training of master supervisors and supervisors).

UNDER SIX CHILD CARE

The care of children under six years is undertaken in well-baby clinics. These clinics combine the concept of prevention, promotion, treatment, rehabilitation, through supervision, nutritional surveillance and health education, within the resources available.

Objective of Under Six Clinic

The main objectives are as under :

1. Promotion of health and prevention of diseases.
2. Early diagnosis and treatment of acute and chronic illness.
3. Referral services.
4. Health education of child health care and family planning.

Components

Preventive Aspects

Immunization : Immunization against seven-killer infectious diseases is the goal for HFA. These diseases are tuberculosis, diphtheria, tetanus, measles, polio, pertussis and hepatitis B.

Nutrition surveillance : Nutritional surveillance is extremely significant for identifying nutritional disorders like PEM, anaemia, rickets, nutritional blindness. ICDS in India has taken up supplementary feeding of children below six years of age.

Oral Rehydration Therapy

Children living in a poor community in developing countries will suffer at least 2 to 6 times of diarrhoea episodes. Each episode is lowering the child's health status; and adds in high mortality rate. Timely introduction of oral rehydration therapy (ORT) to children with diarrhoea can reduce the mortality and morbidity among children.

Health Check-up

Physical examination and appropriate laboratory tests enable early diagnosis and timely treatment. These check-ups are provided every 3 months for infants and 6 months for toddlers. Health check-ups are useful to identify high-risk children, done at health centres.

Family Planning

The family planning measures will enable mother to adopt small family and spacing between children, which inturn will help the mother to take adequate care for the child.

Health Education (Fig. 10.2)

Health education is essential components of all child health areas. Educating mother regarding child nutrition, hygiene, immunization, growth and development, prevention of health hazards, etc. is necessary for child care.

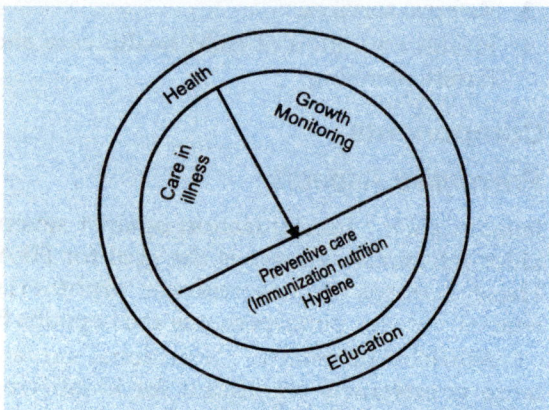

Fig. 10.2 : Health education to children

Care in Illness

Care and treatment of sick child is mother's 'felt need'. Majority (90%) of the sick children can be managed by trained nursing personnel. Basic philosophy of under six clinic is to give effective training to nurses on child health care. If proper training is given and timely help is provided to children can lower the child morbidity and mortality, which includes diagnosis and treatment of acute illness and growth disorders. Referral of unmanagable cases to the nearest health agency.

Growth Monitoring

The regular weight records of children enables health worker to detect growth failure at early stage and find the cause for growth retardation like inadequate or faulty nutrition, intestinal menifestation, poor breastfeeding and any other infection. The child should be weighed monthly or at least once in three months on the growth chart (Road to Health Card) which analyses the growth whether normal or any deviation in normal growth of child.

REPRODUCTIVE AND CHILD HEALTH

India launched National Family Planning Programme in 1952, with the objective to control the growing population. In the early beginning of the programme was modest with establishment of family planning clinics and distribution of educational materials, training and research. During Third Five-Year Plan (1961-66). Family planning was declared as the very centre of planned development. Emphasis was shifted from the purely "clinic approach" to more vigorous "extention education approach" to accept "small family norm". To assist couples in planning small families, the programme had made available both spacing and permanent methods of contraceptions. Programme was not successful, because people were not sure if children born would survive and be healthy. To ensure this Govt. of India launched various successful initiatives to reduce child mortality and ensure family health. Thus the Family Planning Programme was renamed as Family Welfare Programme in 1977.

High child mortality was mainly due to vaccine preventable diseases *e.g.*, diphtheria, whooping cough, polio, tetanus, tuberculosis, etc. Large scale immunization of children was carried out under Universal Immunization Programme. Diarrhoea was a major cause of deaths among children. The Oral Rehydration Therapy programme succeeded in reducing deaths due to diarrhoea.

Poor maternal health also had a profound impact on health of their children. High maternal mortality was due to bleeding during pregnancy and toxaemia. The Child Survival and Safe Motherhood (CSSM) Programme was started to improve the health and survival of mothers and children.

Concept of Reproductive and Child Health

The concept of RCH is to provide to the beneficiaries need based, client centred, demand driven, high quality and integrated RCH services. The RCH programme is composite programme incorporating the inputs of the government of India as well as funding support from donor agencies *e.g.*, World Bank and European Commission.

The RCH programme will provide relevant services for assuring reproductive and child health to all citizens. However, RCH is even more relevant for obtaining the objectives of stable population for the country. It is now well-established that parents keep the family size small, if they are assured of health and longevity of the children and there is no better assurance of good health and longevity of children than health care of mothers and for young children. Therefore, RCH programme by ensuring small families also ensures stable population in short-term and long-term.

Definition

People have the ability to reproduce and regulate their fertility, women are able to go through pregnancy and child birth safely, the outcome of pregnancies is successful in terms of maternal and infant survival and well-being, and couples are able to have sexual relations free of fear of pregnancy and of contracting disease.

Objectives

Improving the health status of young women and children through integration of family welfare programme, universal immunization programme, oral rehydration therapy, child-survival and safe motherhood programme and acute respiratory infection control programme.

Strategy

The overall strategy is to strive for obtaining RCH arrangements for the whole country's population and promote and make available contraceptives/terminal methods for desired couples. The objectives determined are as follows :

- Availability of adequate resources to all urban and rural communities in the country.
- Accountability of performance among health workers and efficiency of the health system. Provision of quality of health care and accessibility of services.
- Improvement of educational and economic status of families.
- Policy support expressed publicly by opinion leaders in different sectors–the national system and the community at large.

Highlights of the RCH Programme (Fig. 10.3)

RCH programme incorporates the components covered under the child survival and safe motherhood programme, includes additional components related to sexually transmitted diseases (STD) and reproductive tract infections (RTI).

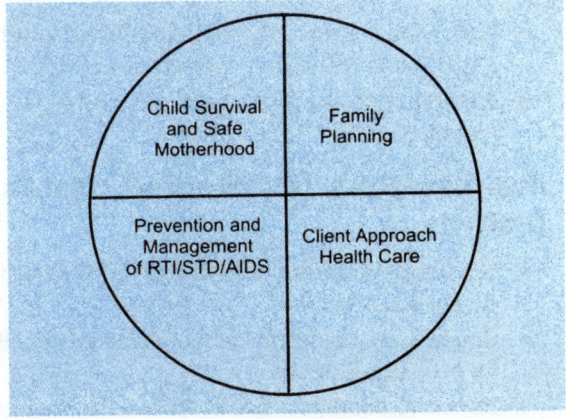

Fig. 10.3 : Highlights of RCH programme

The main highlights of the RCH programme are:

Programme Interventions

The RCH programme will be implemented based on different approach. Inputs in all the districts have not been kept uniform because efficient delivery will depend upon the capacity of the health system in the district. Basic facilities are proposed to be strengthened and streamlined specially in the weaker districts.

Interventions in All Districts

- Child survival interventions i.e. immunization, Vitamin A (to prevent blindness) oral rehydration therapy and prevention of deaths due to pneumonia.
- Safe motherhood interventions e.g. antenatal check up, immunization for tetanus, safe delivery, anaemia control programme.
- Implementation of Target Free Approach.
- High quality training at all levels.
- IEC activities.
- Specially designed RCH package for urban slums and tribal areas.
- District sub-projects under Local Capacity Enhancement.
- RTI/STD clinics at District Hospitals (where not available)
- Facility for safe abortions at PHCs by providing equipment, contractual doctors etc.
- Enhanced community participation through Panchayats, Women's Groups and NGOs.
- Adolescent health and reproductive hygiene.

Interventions in Selected States/Districts

- Screening and treatment of RTI/STD at sub-divisional level.
- Emergency obstetric care at selected FRUs by providing drugs.
- Essential obstetric care by providing drugs and PHN/Staff Nurse at PHCs.
- Additional ANM at sub-centres in the weak districts for ensuring MCH care.
- Improved delivery services and emergency care by providing equipment kits, IUD insertions and ANM kits at sub-centres.
- Facility of referral transport for pregnant women during emergency to the nearest referral centre through Panchayat in weak districts.

Components of RCH

Maternal and child health care was a part of family welfare programme from its inception.

In 1992 child survival and safe motherhood programme integrated all the schemes for better compliance. This programme has the following components:

Maternal Health

Obstetric care : The antenatal care includes registration, antenatal check-up, immunization, health education on rest, sleep and nutrition, detection of high-risk pregnancies and prompt referral, clean delivery by trained personnel. Birth spacing and promotion of institutional deliveries.

Essential obstetric care : Essential obstetrics care provide the basic maternity services to all pregnant women through :

(a) early registration of pregnancy (12-16 weeks).

(b) Provision of minimum three check-up by trained health worker or medical officer to monitor progress of pregnancy and detect any complication or high-risk.

(c) Provision of safe delivery at home and in an institution.

(d) Provision of three postnatal check-ups to monitor postnatal recovery and detect any postnatal complication like, puerpural sepsis or postpartum haemorrhage.

Emergency obstetrical Care : Emergency obstetrical intervention is essential component to reduce the maternal mortality. Under CSSM programme, 1748 referral units were identified and supported with maternity kits. *Dai* training was a uniform countrywide activity to ensure that mother delivers in safe hands.

Delivery services for 24 hours : Provision of round the clock delivery facilities at the primary health centres and the community health centres to promote institutional deliveries, by giving additional benefits to health personnel.

Control of STD/RTI/AIDS

The control of STD/RTI/AIDS in collaboration with National Aids Control Organisation (NACO) has been initiated under RCH programme. NACO will provide assistance for clinics at the district levels. The Central Government will facilitate the manpower training and drug kits including disposable equipment.

Medical Termination of Pregnancy

MTP enables a woman to terminate unwanted pregnancies under unavoidable circumstances without endangering her life, as per MTP Act. MTP act also aids in small family norm. The main aim is to reduce maternal mortality and morbidity, due to unsafe abortions. The Central Government is providing manpower training, equipment and engaging doctors involved in training.

Essential Newborn Care

The main objective of essential newborn care is to reduce the perinatal and neonatal mortality. The components are resuscitation, prevention of infection, exclusive breastfeeding and referral of sick newborn. The strategies are provision of necessary facilities, equipment and training of medical and other health personnel.

Oral Rehydration Therapy

Diarrhoea is one of the leading cause of child mortality. ORT programme started in 1986 is implemented to reduce the mortality due to diarrhoeal diseases. The programme emphasises on the rationale use of drugs for management of diarrhoea. Adequate nutritional care of the child with diarrhoea and proper education to mothers on breastfeeding.

Acute Respiratory Infection (ARI) Control

Prevention and control of ARI is an integral part of RCH programme. Health workers at root level are being trained to recognise and treat pneumonia. Cotrimoxazole is being supplied to the health workers through the CSSM drug kit.

Prevention and Control of Vitamin A Deficiency

Large number of children suffer subclinically from vitamin A deficiency. Under the programme vitamin A is given to all children under six years of age. First dose of 1 lakh I.U. is given at one year and subsequent other dose 2 lakh I.U. is repeated every six months till five years.

Immunization

The Universal Immunization Programme (UIP) became a part of CSSM programme in 1992; and RCH programme in 1997. Under this programme all the vaccines e.g., polio, tetanus, DPT, D.T., T.T, measles and BCG are made available. The cold chain is maintained to give immunization.

Reproductive Child Health (RCH)

Project II : This project has been implemented in the year 2005 with objectives of strengthening the manpower and training programmes for grassroot level workers and other health personnel who closely and collaboratory work together in lowering the IMR and MMR in most affected states and rural areas. This project also emphasises in providing adequate infrastructure to facilitate the RCH activities in various states of the country.

KANGAROO MOTHER CARE (KMC) FOR LOW BIRTH WEIGHT BABIES

It is estimated that approximately 20 million low birth weight babies are born each year mostly in less developed countries. Incubators are not sufficiently available to meet the need of LBW babies. Hypothermia, feeding problem, nosocomial infection are frequent among these children. Children in the incubators are deprived of mother touch. Only ray of hope is the initiation of Kangaroo Mother Care which is an effective way to meet the babies need for warmth, breastfeeding, protection from infection, safety and love, etc.

Definition

Direct skin to skin contact of the baby to the mother or any care given. The baby is placed between the mother's breasts. It is particularly useful in carrying the LBW babies below 2 kg.

Concept

The concept to Kangroo Mother Care is as under :
- Early continuous and prolonged skin to skin contact
- Exclusive breastfeeding

- Physical, emotional and educational support
- Early discharge and follow-up.

Advantages

The advantages of Kngaroo Mother Care are :
1. Effective thermoregulation.
2. Earlier bonding and improved lactation.
3. Decreased separation anxiety.
4. Self-satisfaction in the care of baby.
5. LBW babies recover faster with less complications.

Procedure

All mothers irrespective of age, parity, education can provide KMC. After preparation the mother, unit and baby, the baby should be placed between the mother's breasts in an upright position. The head should be turned to one side and slightly extended position. Slightly extended head position keeps the airway open and allows eye to eye contact between the mother and the baby. The hips should be flexed and baby's

abdomen should be at the level of mother's epigastrium. Mother's breathing stimulates the baby and reducing the occurrence of apnoea. The baby should be supported with the binder. The upper border of the binder will be below the level of ear. Then close the mother's gown in such a way that baby's head should be outside the gown like a baby Kangaroo.

Mother can provide KMC at sitting or recline in a bed or a chair. She can keep herself in slightly backward reclining position and support baby's body and neck using her own hands.

KMC can be started as soon as baby is stable and can be kept at least for one hour in each sitting. When mother needs to be away from her baby, other family member can continue this position. KMC can be done as long as possible day and night. Mother can sleep with the baby in Kangaroo position and recliner or semi-recumbent position. The KMC can be continued up to 40 weeks of post conceptional age or till the weight reaches at 2500 gm.

EXERCISE

1. (a) Define family and family health.
   (b) Describe the function of family health.
2. 'Family is considered as a unit of health and disease'. Justify the statement with examples.
3. (a) Explain the concept of family.
   (b) Discuss the cyclic growth, development and characteristics of a family.
4. Discuss the steps of providing family health care services.
5. Explain the objectives of family health care. Describe the process of family health interventions.
6. State the purposes of giving family health care. Describe the role of nurse in giving care to families.
7. State the importance of categorizing health risk families. Write the criteria for identifying high-risk families.
8. State the need for providing integrated maternal and child health care. Discuss the antenatal care for effective MCH care.
9. Discuss the components of providing maternal health care.
10. Discuss the components of child health care.
11. State the reasons of high maternal and infant mortality rate. Describe the role of nursing in reducing these indication.
12. Discuss some of the indicators to assess the maternal and child health status. Explain the recent National Programme to provide MCH care.
13. List the National Health Programmes related to MCH services. Explain any one in details.

14. Write short notes on :
   (a) Functions of a family
   (b) Development task of a family
   (c) Meaning of family
   (d) Public health bag
   (e) Home visiting
   (f) Role of nurse in evaluation of family care
   (g) Working relationship
   (h) Mobilizing resources
   (i) Health crisis and health deficits
   (j) Moderate health risk families
   (k) Maternal health care
   (l) Under six clinic
   (m) Role of nurse in RCH care
   (n) Role of nurse in family planning
   (o) Kangaroo mother care.

●●●

UNIT IV

INTRODUCTION TO HEALTH, DISEASE AND EPIDEMIOLOGY

- Concept of Health
- Concept of Disease
- Concept and Methods of Epidemiology of Diseases
- General Measures of Disease Control

11

Concept of Health

INTRODUCTION TO CONCEPT AND DEFINITION OF HEALTH

Health is a dynamic state and that is individually perceived. To understand health, illness requires careful study of both, self and people with whom one works. Modern medical science is often occurred for its preoccupation with the study of disease and neglect the study of health. More health facilities are available for care of sick but very few efforts are taken how to prevent the disease and promote health. Health is often taken for granted and its value is not appreciated, till health is lost.

Health is a topic of concern in every country. Either directly or indirectly, individually or collectively, consciously or unconsciously. Health is linked with all aspects of daily living, is a prerequisite for living a productive and satisfying life. The concept of health is related to the notion of well-being, health is not an end in itself, but represents ongoing efforts to enrich over level of well-being. Health is not just "feeling good" but is concerned with social, emotional, physical and mental aspects of life. It includes the cognitive, affective and action domains of human behaviour as it refers not only to individuals but also to the capabilities of families, communities, institutions and societies.

Basic Concept of Health

Health was usually considered as "absence of disease". An understanding of health is the basis of all health cares. Health is not perceived the same way by all members of the community which gives different concepts about health. In changing concepts of health, new concepts are emerging on new patterns of thoughts. The changing concepts of health has been identified as :

Biomedical Concept

In the past years, health was considered as merely absence of physical illness and scientists had been giving different views regarding health. They described human body and its functions, like machine. When machine fail functioning, needs repairs. Similarly, man, like machines, fails to function causing disease and doctors treat the disease to keep the body functioning. Though this concept was not sufficient hence many other views were expressed in relation to maintenance of health and causation of disease.

Ecological Concept

The impact of environment is another concept of health, because biomedical concept was not considered sufficient in maintaining health and causation of disease. According to ecological concept, the health is maintained in favourable environment and disease is caused when there is any deviation in the environment, which is unfavourable. It is determined as the "Dynamic equilibrium between man and his environment and disturbed equilibrium between environment and man may cause disease". Healthy environment will help the individual to lead a healthy and better quality of life.

Psychological Concept

Health has been viewed not only by absence of disease or environmental influences, but various psychosocial/economical and cultural factors contribute towards health. These negative factors play important role in causation of disease.

Holistic Concept

All the above concepts are important in causation of health and diseases. Health is considered as multidimensions and multi-determinants. To keep up the health, a person must be free from sickness in healthy environment and having positive psychological, social and economical factors. Health is multisectorial, *i.e.*, all sectors are responsible to keep the health, *e.g.*, education, animal husbandary, agriculture, food, industry and public works, communication, etc. Holistic health emphasises on promotion and protection of health and prevention of diseases.

DEFINITION OF HEALTH

There are many definitions of health and illness. It is important to consider that there is no one accepted definition of either term.

To the layman health implies a sound mind, in a sound body, in a sound family and in a sound environment.

Various definitions have been given by scientists from time to time. These can be given as :

- Health is a dynamic constantly varying attribute rather than a complete state of any kind including diseases—(Skrovan).
- Health is a state of physical, mental and social well-being and the ability to function and not merely the absence of illness or infirmity.
- The condition of being sound in body, mind or spirit, especially freedom from physical disease or pain (Webster).

- Soundness of body or mind, that condition in which its functions are duly and efficiently discharged (Oxford).
- A state of relative equilibrium of body form and function which results from its successful dynamic adjustment to forces tending to disturb it. It is not passive interplay between body substance and forces. Impinging upon it but an active response of body forces working towards readjustment (Perkins).

Definition of Health by WHO

WHO in 1948, had given definition of health, which has been widely accepted. It has been defined as health is *"a state of complete physical, mental and social well-being and not merely an absence of disease or infirmity"*.

This definition has not been completely accepted, because of various criticisms. Health is considered as a 'state', whereas this is not a state, because it keeps changing and is a process of continuous adjustments to the changing needs and demands in the life. Hence it is dynamic and not static. Healthy person may get unhealthy by the next moment. The WHO's definition is idealist to sound, but not realistic, because it may not be possible that individual will enjoy all physical, mental and social aspects of health at one time. One of these may be affected, but still appears to be healthy. Hence, according to this definition not any individual is healthy.

Dimensions of Health (Fig. 11.1)

Health is multidimensional *e.g.*, physical, mental and social. Many other dimensions can also be

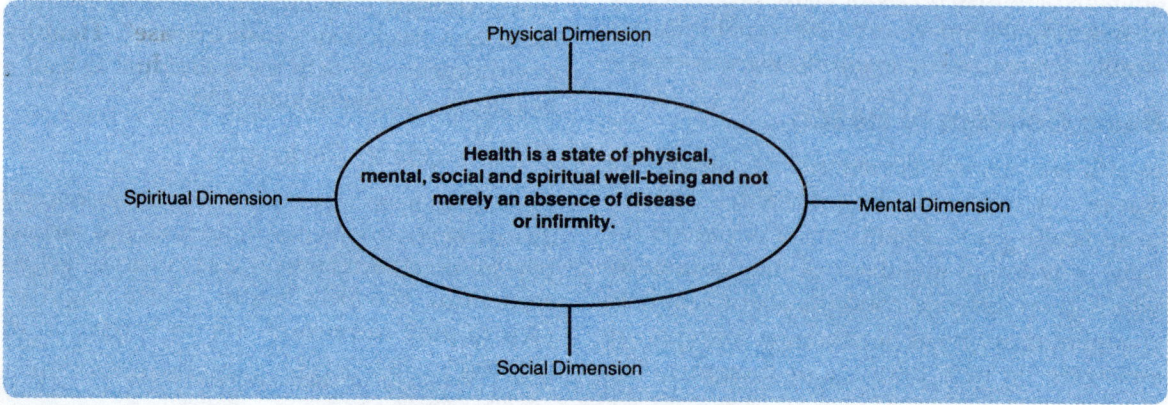

Fig. 11.1 : Dimension of health

considered. These dimensions are interrelated to each other.

Physical Dimension

It is important dimension of health. The physical health is easy to comprehend, since it implies the perfect functioning of the body. It is considered that all the cells, organs and systems of the body are functioning at optimum capacity and in perfect harmonious relationship with rest of the body. Physical health of an individual is good complexion, a clean skin, bright eyes, shiny hair, clean clothes, not too fat or thin, a sweet breath, good appetite, sound sleep, regular bowel and bladder movements co-ordinated body movements. All organs function normally, vital signs (temperature, pulse respiration and B.P.) are within normal range, according to age and sex. The physical health can be measured by anthropometry (height, weight), diet, physical examination, nutritional assessment and laboratory tests and investigations to maintain the physical health, all findings of the examination should be normal.

Mental Health

Mental health and physical health are interrelated. According to the ancient concept a sound mind in a sound body has been important to justify that poor mental health affects the physical health of individual and vice versa. If a person is physically sick will be worried about his health and upsets him mentally. And if a person is not mentally healthy he may stop eating and taking care of his physical needs and get sick. Psychological factors are considered to play major role in disorders such as essential hypertension, peptic ulcer and asthma, etc. Major mental illness e.g., depression and schizophrenia are caused due to biological factors.

Mental health is the ability to respond to the day-to-day life activities. Mental health is defined as a state of balance between the individual and the surrounding world, a state of harmony between onself and others. Though mental health is an essential component of health, but it is difficult to measure mental health. Psychologists have listed some of the characteristics for mentally healthy individual :

- A person is free from internal conflicts. He can make correct decision without having internal war with himself.
- He is well-adjusted i.e., he gets along with others and feels comfortable in any new situation. He accepts the criticism and does not get upset.
- He has self-respect, self-reliance and self-esteem. He respects his feeling and wants to be respected by others.
- He understands his needs, goals and problems.
- He is emotionally mature. He is able to control his emotions in a particular situation. He is able to balance his emotions.
- He has problem solving abilities. He is capable of facing problems and solving them intelligently and is able to cope with stress situation.

Mental health care should be assessed by various standardised psychological tools available to determine the mental disorders. One of the important key to good health is positive mental health, which can be assessed by determining the mental functioning, e.g., cognitive (knowledge) and affective (thinking) impairment.

Social Dimension

Social health is also an essential element of health which implies harmony and integration within the individual and society. Social health is defined as "quantity and quality of an individual interpersonal ties and the extent of involvement within the community". Social health includes the social skills, social functioning and ability to act as a member of society. A socially healthy individual is able to adjust in society and society accepts the individual. An individual participates in all social activities and is free from all unsocial behaviours which people usually do not accept.

It is not possible to raise the level of people's health without changing their social and cultural environment. Social health takes into account that every individual is part of a family and of wider community.

Spiritual Health

Spiritual health refers to that part of individual which reaches out and strives for meaning and purpose of life. It includes integrity, principles and ethics, commitments, belief in concepts. Spiritual health has been integrated in the concept of holistic health and is considered as an essential component of health. The evidences have shown that people's belief in spiritual concept has better health promotion and protection of life.

Emotional Health

Emotions have been separated from mental health, because they have different impact on health than mental health. Emotions can be negative, e.g., anger, fear, anxiety which affects the health and positive emotions, e.g., love, affection and have positive impact on health.

Vocational Health

Work often contributes towards promotion of physical and mental health. Physical work is usually associated with an improvement in physical capacity and goal achievement and self-realisation in work are the sources of satisfaction and improve self-esteem.

The negative impact occurs when there is loss of job at retirement or job frustration and stress. The acceptance of such situations is different among different people, hence affecting their health. Which may cause psychosocial or physical problem.

Socioeconomic Dimension

Socioeconomic conditions play important role in maintaining the health of an individual. Poverty is an important factor in causation of disease. High socioeconomic status community can afford better health services and standards of living. Adversely, poor community may find difficult to avail health facilities during sickness and may cause high mortality and morbidity. Though high socioeconomic people may get certain diseases due to lifestyle and stress which may not be common among low socioeconomic group.

Cultural Dimension

Culture contributes towards healthy lifestyle. Some cultural practices have healthy effects, whereas others may have adverse impact on health. Therefore, it is essential to study the cultural aspect in maintaining the health of an individual, e.g., performing culture during childbirth, antenatal care will affect the health of child and mother e.g., the rituals of not giving colostrum at birth may hinder the child from nutritious food.

Educational Dimension

Basic education helps in enhancing the knowledge of people regarding health aspects. Incidences show the educated people as practicing better health habits than illiterate people, e.g., Kerala state has 100 per cent literacy and has lowest mortality and morbidity, whereas U.P. has lowest literacy rate (25%) and highest morbidity and mortality rate.

Nutrition Dimension

An essential component of health is nutrition, balanced diet which prevents the deficiency diseases, as well as obesity problem, which leads to cardiovascular diseases, diabetes and hypertension, etc. Hence adequate nutritional status helps to maintain the health of an individual.

Preventive and Curative Dimension

Preventive measure, e.g., immunization and adequate treatment at an early stage will help in promoting and regaining the health.

All the above dimensions contribute towards healthy life, which might help an individual to attain optimum level of health, to lead socially and economically productive life.

POSITIVE HEALTH

WHO defines health in four dimensions e.g., physical, mental, social and spiritual well-being. A person who enjoys all the four dimensions of health is said to be in a state of positive health. The concept of perfect positive health can not become a reality, because a person can never be in the perfect state of all four dimensions.

Though the health has been described as the capability of an individual to adjust to the changing environment and keep the balance in environment and body. For example, in the changing climate the individual takes due care and prevents from extremes of climatic changes that will prevent him from any sickness, hence he remains healthy. Similarly, if person is able to adjust in a society of any situation, will help to keep mental and social health.

The state of positive health implies to the normal functioning of body and mind. Biologically it can be described as a state in which every cell and organ is functioning at normal capacity and in harmony with the rest of the body. Psychologically it is a state in which the individual feels a sense of perfect well-being and mastery over his environment. Socially it is a state in which individual capacity to participate in all social activities and considers himself a member of society and society accepts him.

ECOLOGY OF HEALTH (Fig. 11.2)

Ecology is defined as a mutual relationship between living organism and their environment. Ecology of the health is the study of relationship between variations in man's environment and his state of health. The basic theme of ecology is that everything is related to everything else. Health has been defined as a state of dynamic equilibrium or adjustment between man and his environment.

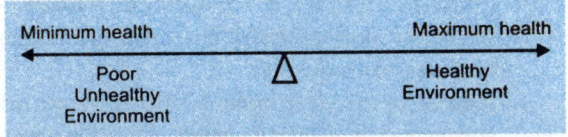

Fig. 11.2 : Ecology of health

Man is constantly altering his age, sex and other biological characteristics due to the operation of external or internal stimuli.

Health is a pendulum oscillating between a range or spectrum one end of which represents the minimum end and the other end maximum. There are degrees of well-being as there are degrees of severity of illness.

Ecological Model

Man is surrounded by his social, biological, physical environments, and change in any of these environments may initiate change in the others, affecting the relationship between man and agent and the environment. As long as a state of equilibrium exists between host, agent and environment, a state of health is maintained. For example, an increase in the host susceptibility resulting from lack of sleep, malnutrition excessive stress, ageing or many other factors also increase the risk of disease. Changes in environment, contribute to changes in most susceptibility as well as the conditions for viability of agent.

DETERMINANTS OF HEALTH

Health of a person is influenced by complex of genetic, environmental, social and economic factors related to each other (Fig. 11.3). These may be classified as :

1. Human biology
2. Lifestyle or ways of living
3. Socioeconomic status
4. Environmental conditions
5. Health and health-related services.

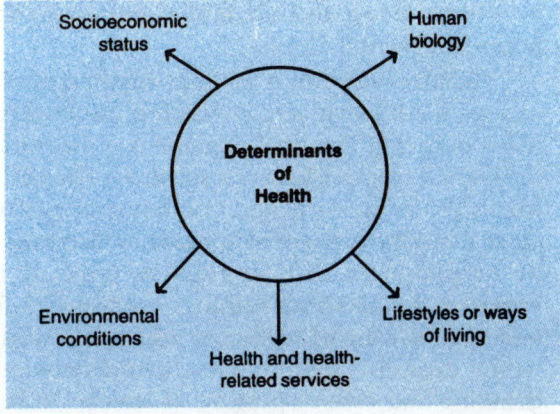

Fig. 11.3 : Determinants of health

Human Biology

Genetic constitution plays an important role in physical and mental traits of every human being. These genetic factors are unique and cannot be changed after conception. Many congenital diseases are known to be due to genetic origin, *e.g.*, haemophillia, congenital heart disease, mental retardation and some types of diabetes. The parents with genetic defects will transfer the same genes to their offspring causing the congenital illness. If a mother had cleft lip at birth there may be possibility of having the same in her child. These diseases occur due to faulty genetic constitutions during conception due to certain factors. The state of health, therefore, is also affected by genetic constitution of an individual.

The positive health defined by WHO implies that a person should be able to express as completely as possible the potentialities of genetic constitution, that is only possible when a person lives in a healthy environment, with healthy relationships that transform the healthy genetic potentialities.

Lifestyles or Ways of Living

The health of an individual has direct relationship to the lifestyle or ways of living. A person who has healthy practices of day-to-day living will remain healthy and vice versa. Major health problems emerging have significant relationship with the lifestyle and standard of living like cardiovascular diseases, road traffic accidents, drug and alcohol abuse, suicide, homicide, mental illness.

Health education is an important aspect to change the lifestyle and practicing the healthy ways of living. Personal hygiene is a matter of individual responsibility or self care. The child learns this at the early age, but they may not be clear about the concept of hygiene, which has to be emphasised during routine care. It is important to talk about bathing, washing of hair and clothes, care of teeth, ear and eyes, eating habits, excercise, sleep and rest, avoid smoking, drinking and care of posture. If anyone of the habits are neglected, it may lead to ill-health. The school children must be taught good health habits and include health topic in curriculum.

Socioeconomic Status

The health of a community is also related to the social and economical conditions. Many of the diseases are more prevalent among poor socio-economic status, because poverty leads to illiteracy, ignorance and lack of resources. It is said that poverty leads to sickness and sickness to poverty. Studies have shown that prevalence and distribution of disease is strongly influenced by economic factors. In fact, most of the infectious and nutritional deficiency diseases, *e.g.*, malnutrition diarrhoeal diseases, etc. which are common in developing countries, are due to poverty. Poverty also predisposes to high maternal mortality, infant mortality and child mortality rate, crime, violence, drug abuse, depression, alcoholism and many other behavioural problems, etc.

Many chronic diseases like cardiovascular, diabetes, hypertension are more prevalent among high socioeconomic status due to their way of living. Hence, it is clear that socioeconomic factors play a leading role in maintaining the health of people.

Environmental Conditions

Environmental factors that contribute to the health of an individual are : air, water and climate. *"Environment is the surrounding in which an individual lives"*—which can be classified into two that is, internal and the external environment. The internal environment relates the human body about each and every component of cells, tissues, organ systems and the body as a whole and their harmonious functioning. The external environment constitutes the things outside the human body to which man is exposed. This can be classified as :

1. *Physical environment :* Water, air, climate.
2. *Biological environment :* Plants, animals, virus, bacteria, rodents, etc.
3. *Psychosocial environment :* Socioeconomic status, caste, culture, stress, lifestyle, occupation, etc.

The environment has direct effect on the physical, mental and social health of an individual. Most of the diseases are caused due to unhealthy environment. There is increased evidence of chronic diseases, accidents and mental illnesses due to rural adjustment in the environment.

WHO emphasizes on achievement of highest level of health, is only possible in an environment which contributes towards healthful individual and family living. The people are exposed to various environmental hazards—air pollution, water pollution, noise pollution. United Nation Environmental Programme (UNEP) aims at promoting the quality of life and protecting the world against health hazards in the environment.

Health and Health Relaled Services

The accessibility, availability and quality of health services have impact on the health of a community. These services include medical care, preventive and promotive health services.

For example, if the vaccines are easily available for children, the mother can get them immunized on time, whereas if they have to go far away and there is more wastage of time, they will not be much careful in getting complete dose, which results in more evidences of illness. Provision of safe water supply prevents various water-borne diseases e.g., polio, cholera, typhoid. Adequate antenatal care will contribute to healthy mothers and children and reduction in maternal and infant mortality rate. These effective services too can add in healthy living.

The purpose of these health facilities are to improve the health status of people. To be effective, these services must reach at the periphery level, it should be equally distributed; in rural and urban areas, accessible at the cost that people and the country can afford and should be socially acceptable. The health services are essential for socioeconomic development of any community. The availability of adquate services will ensure good health of people and who inturn will be socially and economically productive for the country.

Not only the availability but also the quality of health care available, and the type of health professional providing care to the people also affect the health of a person.

INDICATORS OF HEALTH

Various measures are adopted to assess the health of an individual, but it is very difficult to assess the health of a community or country. Indicators are required to measure the health status of the community as a whole. Indicators are the indications of a given situation. WHO has defined them as variable, which help to measure change.

Purpose of Health Indicators

1. To assess the health care needs and planning the health care services
2. To allocate the scarce resources according to needs
3. To monitor and evaluate the health service activities and the programme in function and replanning them
4. To measure the extent to which the objectives and targets of the programme are being attained.

Characteristics of the Health Indicators

The indicators to measure the health must be :

Valid

Which actually measure what they are supposed to measure.

Reliable

Measurement should be stable if measured by different people in similar circumstances.

Sensitive

Indicators should be sensitive to the situation for application.

Specific

They should reflect changes only when situation is specific.

Objective

There must be objectivity in selecting classi-fication and measuring the indicators.

CLASSIFICATION

Types of Indicators

Measurement of health is not very simple. Since health is multidimensional, hence each dimension has to be measured. Health can not be in terms of single indicator. Hence the health has been framed in terms of illness (lack of health), consequences of illness (morbidity and mortality), economic, domestic and occupational factors that promote ill-health disease. Types of indicators are as follows :

1. Life-expectancy
2. Mortality indicators
3. Morbidity indicators
4. Disability indicators
5. Nutritional status indicator
6. Health care delivery indicators
7. Utilisation rate
8. Social and mental health indicators and utilisation rate
9. Environmental indicators
10. Socioeconomic indicators
11. Health policy indicators
12. Other indicators.

Life-Expectancy

Life expectancy at birth is *"the average number of years that will be lived by those born alive into a population if the current age-specific mortality rate persists"*. Life-expectancy at birth is highly influenced by the infant mortality rate; where this is high. Life-expectancy at the age of one year influences the infant mortality, and life-expectancy at the age of five years influences child mortality. It is estimated for both sexes separately. Increase in life-expectancy is related to improvement in health status of community.

Life-expectancy is an effective indicator to know the effectiveness of health services and socioeconomic development in general. This is considered as positive indicator which is mainly based on longer years of survival. It had been accepted as a global indicator for health goal to be achieved by 2000 AD as minimum life-expectancy at birth 64 years.

Mortality Indicators

The measurement of deaths for specific age group and general death rate, provides an effective tool to assess the overall health of a population. The deaths in specific community will also help to identify the causation of premature death and plan the health services as per health needs.

- *Crude death rate (CDR)* : This is an important indicator, to find the health of people. Crude death rate is defined as *"The number of deaths per 1000 mid-year population per year in a given community"*. The death rate provides rate at which people are dying. Although it is not the perfect measure of health status, but decrease in death rate provides a good tool for assessing the overall health improvement in a population. The decreased death rate indicates the advancement in the field of medicines and health care. The existing crude death rate in India is 9/1000.

- *Infant Mortality Rate* : Infant mortality rate is the most universally accepted indicator of health status not only for infants but of the whole population. It is a significant indicator to determine the availability, utilisation and effectiveness of health care, particularly peri-natal care. The national policy under global strategy of health for all has set a goal of infant mortality rate to be not more than 50/1000 live births. IMR is the number of deaths under one year of age in a given year to the total number of live births in the same year, usually expressed as a rate/1000 live births. It is 67/1000 in India.

- *Child Mortality Rate (CMR)* : The number of deaths of children of 1 to 4 years age are related to overall health status of the people. It is defined as *"The number of deaths at ages 1 to 4 years in a given year, per 1000 children in that age group at the mid-point of the year"*. The infant mortality is not included in it.

  Various causes of death can be related by child mortality, *e.g.*, malnutrition, poor immunization, environment hazards and inadequate MCH services.

- *Under-five proportionate mortality rate* : It is the proportion of total deaths occurring below five years of age. This mortality rate may vary according to health facilities and healthy living standards. High rate determines the high birth rate, high child mortality rate and shorter life-expectancy.

- *Maternal mortality rate (MMR)* : The number of deaths of women during reproductive age due to maternal cause (15-45 years) per live births. There are variations in mortality among women according to living standards to community and country. Average MMR is 3 to 4/1000 in India.

- *Disease-specific mortality (DSM)* : Mortality which occurs due to specific diseases, *e.g.*, communicable and noncommunicable, such as, cancer, cardiovascular, accidents, diabetes, etc. will help to know the emerging and re-emerging health problems and find the solution to those specific problems. Health services can be targeted towards control of such diseases with high mortality.

  Proportional mortality rate (PMR) : The proportional mortality rate from communicable diseases is useful indicator to assess the health status, which help to adopt various preventive measures. The proportional mortality rate helps to assess the deaths with proportion to various diseases.

Morbidity Indicators

Morbidity indicators are used to assess the mortality data, which help to describe the health status of the population. The morbidity rate is used for assessing morbidity among community.

1. Incidence and prevalence of diseases
2. Notification rate
3. Patients admission, readmission and discharge of the indoors and outdoors
4. Hospital stay of patients
5. Sickness spells and absenteeism from work or school, etc.

Disability Indicators

The period of disability of a patient during illness, limitation of morbidity and limitation of activity related to illness or injury indicates the mortality and morbidity of the community.

Nutritional Status Indicator

The nutritional status of the community also determines the general health status of people. This is a positive health indicator which can be measured by :

1. Anthropometric measurement of infants and preschool children by taking height, weight, mid-arm circumference.
2. Prevalence of low birth weight babies.

Health Care Delivery Indicators

These indicators reflect the equal distribution of health resources in different parts of the country and the provision of health care services. The commonly used indicators are :

Doctor Population Ratio	: 1 : 3500
Nurse Population Ratio	: 1 : 5000
Health workers Male/Female	: 1 : 5000 Population in plain and 1 : 3000 in tribal and hilly area.
Health assistants M/F	: 1 : 30000 population in plain areas and 1 : 20000 in hilly and tribal areas.
Pharmacist	: 1 : 10000 population
Laboratory technician	: 1 : 10000 population
Trained birth attendants (TBAs)	: 1 : 1000 (or one in each village).
Health Facilities →	
1 Subcentre	: 5000 population
1 PHC (Primary Health Centre)	: 30,000 population
1 CHC (Community Health Centre)	: 1 lakh population
1 DHC (District Health Centre)	: 1 million population.

Utilization Rate

The health of people is also affected by availability and accessibility of health facilities and their utilization by the people. The relationship exists between utilization of health services and health needs/status of the people. The health utilization rate can be measured by :

- Per cent of infants fully immunized
- Per cent of pregnant women received antenatal, natal, postnatal care by trained midwife, including per cent of immunization covered
- Per cent of Family Planning methods used by various eligible couples
- Bed occupancy rate is the rate at which average daily inpatients census are taken.
- Average length of stay *i.e.*, the days of health care received by patient from trained health personnel.
- Bed turnover ratio—frequencies of the discharge of patients from the hospital.

Social and Mental Health Indicators

These indicators measure the indirect measurements like indicators of social and mental pathology which includes accidents, suicides, violent act, crimes, juvenile deliquency, alcohol, drug abuse, smoking, obesity, etc. The other measure may be child abuse or battered babies, battered wives, family violence, neglected children and youths, etc. These indicators reflect the social and mental health status of particular community and guide for social action to improve the community.

Environmental Indicators

These indicators measure the quality of physical and biological environment in which people live in and is conducive to health or illness. It includes air pollution, water, noise radiation, solid wastes, exposure to toxic substances, food and drink adulteration. Most important indicator is measuring the proportion of population accessible to safe drinking water and sanitation facilities.

Socioeconomic Indicators

They are indirect indicators of health measurement. The socioeconomic status is not directly related to health of people, but is important in interpretation of health care indicator which includes: (1) Per capita Gross National Product (GNP), (2) Status of employment, (3) Education, (4) Family size, (5) Housing status, and (6) Per capita family income.

Health Policy Indicator

The important indicator of political commitment as allocation of adequate resources which includes: (1) Gross Net Production (GNP) spent for health care and health related activities *e.g.*, water supply, sanitation, housing, nutrition, etc., (2) The total health resources devoted to primary health care. Adequacy and accessibility of health care reflects the health utilization and improved health status of a community.

Indication of Quality of Life

Increased life expectancy does not reflect the quality of life, but the life enjoyed by an individual with positive health. An individual may live longer but has poor health status. Quality of life is difficult to define or explain to even measure. But some physical, mental and social measurements may help to measure quality of life.

Other Indicators

(1) *Health for all indicators :* For monitoring the goals for Health for All as per WHO guideline. These indicators will help to measure the extent of achievements for good health status of community.

(2) *Basic need indicators :* These includes the extent of basic needs being met for people to maintain the health of people which includes nutrition, water supply, housing, health facilities, etc.

(3) *Social indicators :* These indicators reflect the social health care like social security, social welfare services, culture and social stratification, etc.

All these indicators are important to give comprehensive view of overall health status. Each available indicator reflects an aspect of health. Use of multiple indicators arranged in profiles or patterns should make comparisons between areas, regions, and nation's health and measuring society's performance and quality of life.

Table 11.1 : Frequently used Rates and Ratios in Community Health Nursing Practices

Rate of Ratio	Formula	Commonly used Multiplier
Mortality Statistics		
Crude death rate	Number of deaths from all causes during a given year ÷ population estimated at mid-year	× 1000 population
Age-specific death rate	Number of deaths for a specified age group during a given year ÷ population estimated at mid-year for the specified age group	× 1000 population
Cause-specific death rate	Number of deaths from a specific condition during a given year ÷ population estimated at mid-year	× 1000 population

Maternal mortality rate	Number of deaths from puerperal complications during a given year ÷ number of live births during the same year	× 100,000 live births
Infant mortality rate	Number of death under 1 year of age during a given year ÷ number of live births during the same year	× 100,000 live births
Neonatal mortality rate	Number of deaths under 28 days of age during a given year ÷ number of live births during the same year	× 1000 live births
Foetal mortality rate	Number of foetal deaths 20-weeks gestation or more during a given year ÷ number of live births and foetal deaths during the same year	× 1000 live births and foetal deaths
Birth-death ratio	Number of live births in a specified population ÷ number of deaths in a specified population	× 100
Case fatality ratio	Number of deaths from specified disease or condition ÷ number of reported cases of the specified disease or condition	× 100
Mortality Statistics		
Incidence rate	Number of new cases of a specified disease or conditions occurring population during a given time period ÷ population at risk during the same time period	×100,000
Prevalence rate (ratio)	Number of old and new cases of specified disease or condition existing at a point ÷ total population at a point	× 100,000 population
Vital and Demographic Statistics other than Mortality		
Crude birth rate	Number of live births during a given year ÷ population estimated at mid-year	× 1000 population
General fertility rate	Number of live births during a given year ÷ population estimated at mid-year for females ages 15 during the same year	× 1000 female population (15 years old)
General marriage rate	Number of marriages during a given year ÷ number of persons 15 years of age and over in the population in the same year	× 1000 persons
General divorce rate	Number of divorces during a given year ÷ number of persons 15 years of age and over in the population in the same year	× 1000 persons
Dependency ratio	Persons under 20 years of age and persons 65 years and over ÷ total population ages 20-64	× 100
Life-expectancy	Average number of years expected to be lived by an individual	

Rates most frequently used as indexes of community health.

GENERAL MORTALITY

$$\text{Crude rate} = \frac{\text{No. of deaths during a year}}{\text{Average (mid-year) population}} \quad \text{Per 100,000 population}$$

$$\text{Cause-specific rate} = \frac{\text{No. of deaths from a stated cause in a year}}{\text{Average (mid-year) population}} \quad \text{Per 100,000 population}$$

$$\text{Age-specific rate} = \frac{\text{No. of deaths among persons in given age group in a year}}{\text{Average (mid-year) population in same age group}} \quad \text{Per 100,000 population}$$

$$\text{Proportional rate} = \frac{\text{No. of deaths from a specific cause in given time period}}{\text{Total deaths in same time period}} \quad \text{Per 100 population}$$

MORBIDITY

$$\text{Incidence} = \frac{\text{No. of new cases of disease in a place from time to time}}{\text{No. of persons in a place at mid-point of time period}} \quad \text{Per 100,000 population}$$

$$\text{Prevalence} = \frac{\text{No. of existing cases in a place at given time}}{\text{No. of persons in a place at same time}} \quad \text{Per 100,000 population}$$

●●●

12

Concept of Disease

INTRODUCTION TO BASIC CONCEPT OF DISEASE

The concept of disease in modern era has been changed from superstitions to the natural and multifactorial causation. There are people in many parts of the world who still consider disease as a supernatural and spiritual powers. These misconcepts have direct impact on the maintenance of health and prevention of disease.

The term disease has been described as uneasyness that means when an individual is not at ease and having some discomfort, pain due to body disfunctioning 'Illness' refers not only to the presence of specific disease, but also relates to individuals perception to disease and its behaviour in response to disease.

DEFINITION OF DISEASE

The WHO has defined health, but not disease because of its variations, *e.g.*, mild, moderate, severe and disease without clinical manifestations and some diseases manifest more than one signs and symptoms. The disease might appear acutely or chronically.

The disease might result in either recovery or disability or life-long illness or death of the patient.

Disease is a physiological and psychological dysfunctioning. Illness is described as a person not feeling well and is said to be subjective state.

It is possible to be victim of disease without feeling ill and to be ill without manifesting the signs and symptoms physical impairement etc.

Many attempts have been made to define disease. An adequate definition is yet to be found which should be accepted universally and is realistic.

Definitions given by Webster, it defines disease as *"A conditions in which body health is impaired, a departure from a state of health, an alteration of the human body interfering the performance of vital functions"*.

According to Oxford Dictionary, the disease is defined as *"A condition of the body or some part or organ of the body in which its functions are disrupted or deranged"*.

Ecologically, the disease occurs when there is imbalance in the environmental condition conducive to the health of man *e.g.*, the individual remains healthy in clean environment with adequate sunlight, healthy family and social environment; adversely when the environment changes to unclean and poor sunlight (slums, etc.), there may be family disturbance etc; will lead to diseased conditions. The diseases due to unhealthy environment may be physical, mental and social illness. Disease is defined as *"Maladjustment of the human organism to the environment"*.

Sociologically, disease is identified as a social phenomenon, which occurs in all the sections of society.

It can be defined as any deviation from normal functioning or state of complete physical, mental and social well-being. Though, none of the disease is considered as complete.

DISEASE—SICKNESS OF THE BODY AND MIND

Disease is an abnormal condition of an organism or part, especially as a consequences of infections, internal weakness or environmental stress that impairs normal physiological functioning.

Disease

A reaction to a stimuli which extends beyond the bounds of the individual reserve and adaptibility (Francis).

Disease is a maladjustment of the existing environment to the host.

Illness is a failure or disturbance in the growth development, function and adjustment of the organism as a whole or any of its system (Engel).

Disease is a state in which individual is no longer in a state of equilibrium with the forces in his external and internal environment (Beland).

Aetiological Factors in Causation of Disease

Various concepts have been explained in factors responsible in causation of disease.

Germ Theory of Disease

Various theories have been explaining the causation of disease. The disease was recognised scientifically by different bacteriologists. When **Louis Pasteur** (1822-1895) discovered the presence of bacteria in the air, **Robert Koch** (1843-1910) showed that anthrax was caused by bacteria. **Pasteur** and **Koch** confirmed the germ theory of disease, the disease is caused by bacteria.

Multiple Causation of Disease

Due to advancement in public health, chemo-therapy and vector control, the communicable diseases began to decline and arising of new type of diseases. The germ theory of diseases or "single cause factor" of diseases overshadowed the multiple causation of diseases. The non-communicable diseases which are emerging is not caused due to our single factor, but there are other risk factors in the aetiology of diseases like socioculture, economical, genetic and psychological factors, which e.g., contribute in disease prevalence. Like tuberculosis, is not only due to tubercle bacilli but other factors also contribute towards causation of disease e.g., environment, social factor, housing, living standards. Similarly, noncommunicable diseases e.g., diabetes mellitus and cancer are caused due to multiple factors e.g., poor dietary habits, smoking, lack of exercise, obesity, and human behaviour, etc. These all risk factors are to be controlled to control the disease. These multiple factors make a web around the person, hence they all contribute towards causation of single disease. This is also called as web of causations of diseases. This is important to understand all the factors in causations of diseases, so that diseases can be prevented and controlled by avoiding all risk factors and adopting healthy lifestyles.

Web of Causation

The web of causation is application in case of chronic noncommunicable diseases, where disease agent is not exactly known and disease is caused due to interaction of multiple factors. The web of causation is considered by all predisposing factors which contribute towards causation of disease. For example, web of causation in case of anaemia, has various factors e.g., poor diet, malnutrition, poverty, lack of knowledge, nonavailability of food, blood loss, etc. (Fig 12.1).

Epidemiological Triad

The germ theory explains the single causative organisms in causation of disease, but it was found that all persons exposed to infection do not show the signs and symptoms of the disease. Therefore, there are many other factors which contribute in causation of disease. These factors are related to the host factors (age, sex, culture, etc.) and environment (for bacteria to grow and cause the disease). Hence, disease is described as not only agent factors, but must have susceptible host and conducive environment (poor environmental condition, physical, social and psychological). These three factors have to interact to cause the disease (Fig 12.2).

Epidemiological Triad for Causation of Disease

The causation of any disease, whether communicable or noncommunicable, is determined by interaction between the agent, host and environment. They together constitute the epidemiological triad. The agent, host and environment of a particular disease have to interact to cause any disease. Before interaction

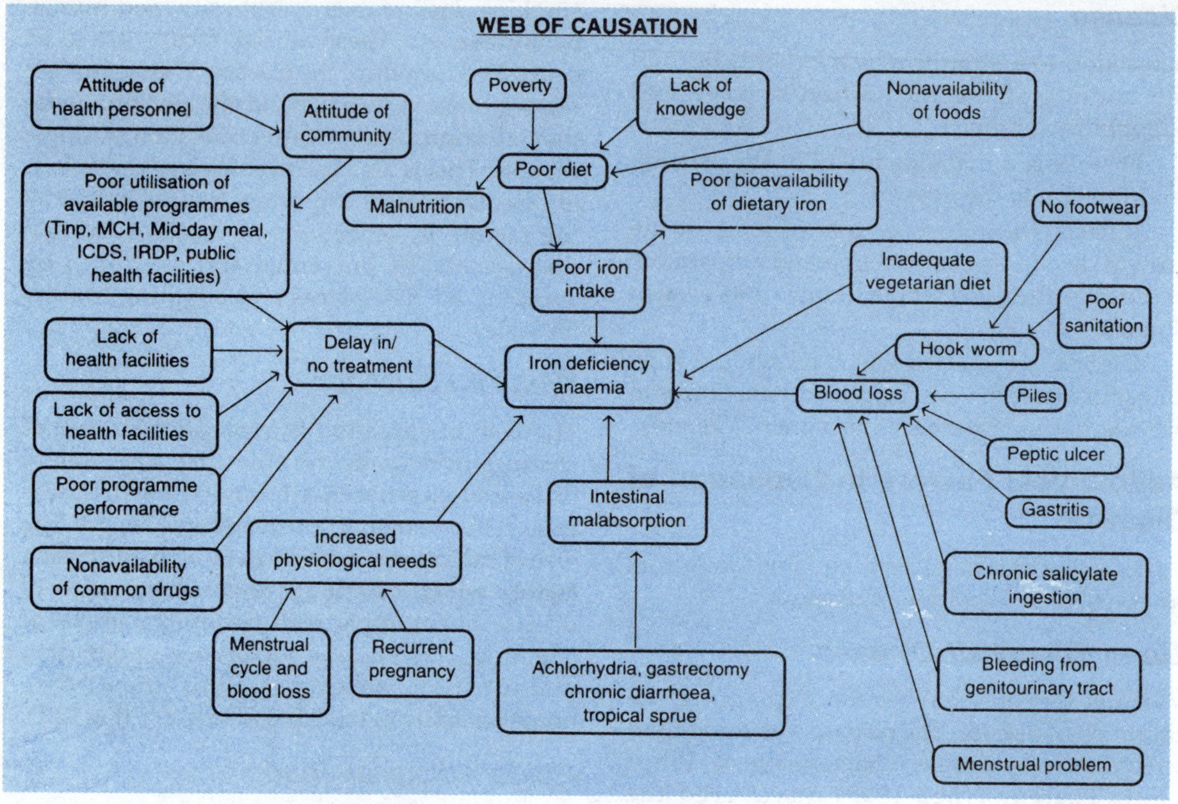

WEB OF CAUSATION

| Attitude of health personnel | → | Attitude of community | | Poverty | | Lack of knowledge | | Nonavailability of foods |

Poor utilisation of available programmes (Tinp, MCH, Mid-day meal, ICDS, IRDP, public health facilities)

Malnutrition

Poor diet

Poor bioavailability of dietary iron

No footwear

Inadequate vegetarian diet

Poor sanitation

Poor iron intake

Lack of health facilities

Delay in/ no treatment

Iron deficiency anaemia

Hook worm

Blood loss

Piles

Lack of access to health facilities

Peptic ulcer

Poor programme performance

Gastritis

Intestinal malabsorption

Nonavailability of common drugs

Increased physiological needs

Chronic salicylate ingestion

Menstrual cycle and blood loss

Recurrent pregnancy

Achlorhydria, gastrectomy chronic diarrhoea, tropical sprue

Bleeding from genitourinary tract

Menstrual problem

Fig. 12.1 : Biomedical pathophysiological factors

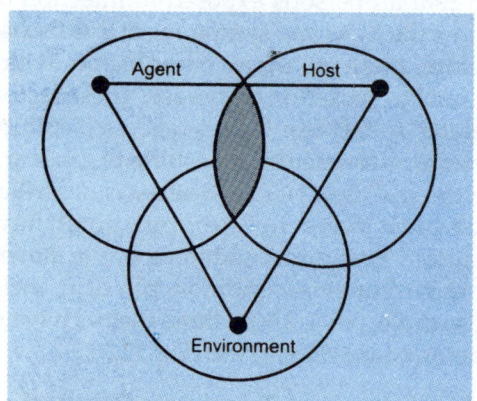

Fig. 12.2 : Epidemiological triad

these three are in isolation. There are specific agents, hosts and environmental conditions for specific diseases. When these three interact, the disease occurs. In the absence of any one of these three factors will not cause disease.

Isolation of agent, host and environment will not cause any disease.

Epidemiological Triad

Interaction of agent, host, environment for causation of disease.

Example : Tuberculosis is caused by specific tubercle bacilli–*Mycobacterium tuberculosis,* poor environmental conditions and susceptible host. If anyone of these three is not favourable, the disease will not occur. Everybody exposed to disease agent will not get the disease unless a person is malnourished, with low resistance and living in slum areas. That means, there are various factors related to host and environment which contribute to the causation of disease.

This model is known as epidemiological triad. This means the disease will only be caused when host is weak, agent is strong and enters the host through right mode of transmission, and the environmental conditions facilitate the interaction of host and agent.

This model is applicable to communicable and infectious diseases and not to noncommunicable diseases, where there is no agent for causation of disease, but various predisposive factors are involved. These diseases cannot be prevented by isolation, immunization and environmental sanitation. These diseases are multifactorial and are called **multifactorial causation of disease,** which interact to cause the disease. These factors can be lifestyle, hereditary human behaviour and environmental conditions, etc. This refers to web of causation of disease (MacMohan and Rugh). This model suggests clusters of causation and varieties of interventions for prevention and control of diseases.

Cardiovascular diseases are caused by overweight, smoking, lack of exercise, stress, etc. and can be prevented and controlled by suggestive interventions related to predisposive factors e.g., avoid smoking, diet control, reduce weight, regular exercise and health check-up.

EPIDEMIOLOGICAL FACTORS

Human Host

The host's contribution to disease is first through his characteristics. These characteristics determine how the man (human host) reacts to the agent in the environment. Various host factors are accountable in causation of a disease. They are :

Age

Certain diseases are more frequent in certain age groups than in others like chickenpox, measles in children, cancer in middle age, athrosclerosis, heart diseases, AIDS, hypertension, arthritis and cataract in old age.

Sex

The disease is also distributed according to sex like cancer cervix and breast-disorders are associated with pregnancy in female, diseases related to prostate, arthrosclerosis and coronary heart diseases in male; whereas rheumatoid arthritis are in female, though exact cause of these diseases is unknown.

Race

The effect of race for disease distribution is related to social customs and culture of the people, e.g., sickle cell anemia in Negroes.

Hereditary

This is an important factor in causation of various diseases like haemophilia.

Nutrition

Variation in balanced diet may aggregate various diseases.

Occupation

Many diseases are directly related to the occupation of an individual who is exposed to occupational hazards, e.g., silicosis, anthracosis, accidents (Machines) and health professionals exposed to various infections, e.g., AIDS, hepatitis B, etc.

Immunity Status

The resistance of human host to infection depends upon his immunity status. If the individual has high immunity status, by virtue of diet and vaccine, he is less susceptible to any infection, whereas if the status is poor then, he is more susceptible to get any infection.

Marital Status

Many diseases are associated with the marital status of a woman. Cervical cancer is more among married than unmarried, whereas breast cancer is more among unmarried women.

Lifestyle

The lifestyle of a person reflects the health status. The custom, culture and habits may favour the spread of diseases. The custom of Purdah system among Muslim ladies is more prone to respiratory diseases. The habit of alcohol, smoking, drug dependence may influence the health of a person. Exercise, regular pattern of eating may have positive effect on health. Then lifestyle is an important factor in health and illness.

Education

Studies have shown direct relationship of education and health. Illiterate people have lack of knowledge about maintenance and promotion of health, whereas educated people are more exposed to the varieties of information about health and illness, resulting various diseases are common among poor and illiterate people.

Disease Agent

The disease agent may be defined as "a substance, organism, living or non-living or a force or the presence or lack of which may cause a disease". The agent may be single or multiple to cause the disease. Disease agents have been classified as follows :

Biological Agents

Many viruses, bacteria, fungi, protozoa, metazoas, spirochetes and helminthes are agents in causation of disease.

Physical Agents

Health, cold, humidity, sunlight, have exposure susceptibility to disease.

Chemical Agents

The chemical agents which affect the body may be inside the body (endogenous), i.e., urea, ketones, uric acid, calcium carbonate and outside the body (exogenous), i.e., allergens, metals, fumes, dust, gas, insecticides, toxins, etc. These chemicals may be inhaled, ingested or inoculated inside the body.

Nutrient Agent

All the nutrients, i.e., protein, fat, carbohydrate, minerals and vitamins may be agents to disease.

Environmental Factor

The environment refers to the man's external environment in which he lives. The environment is defined as the aggregate of all external conditions and influences affecting the life of an organism. According to ecological approach, disease is defined as maladjustment between man and environment. The balanced scale with pair of pans represents disease agent and human host and a fulcrum, the environment, health as a state of equilibrium between disease agent and human host (Fig. 12.3a). When this balance is disturbed, the disease occurs (Fig. 12.3b).

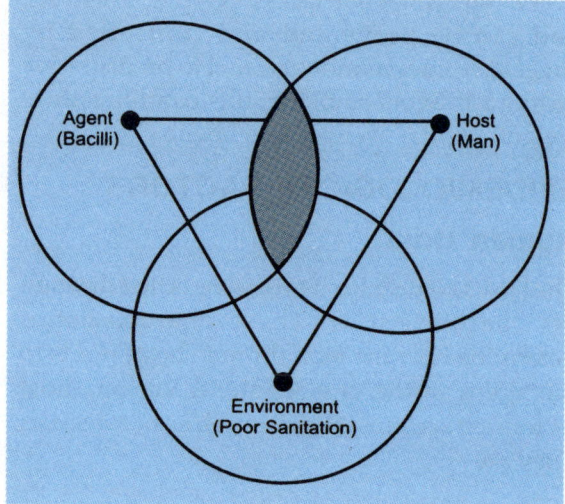

Fig. 12.3(a) : Disease agents and human host

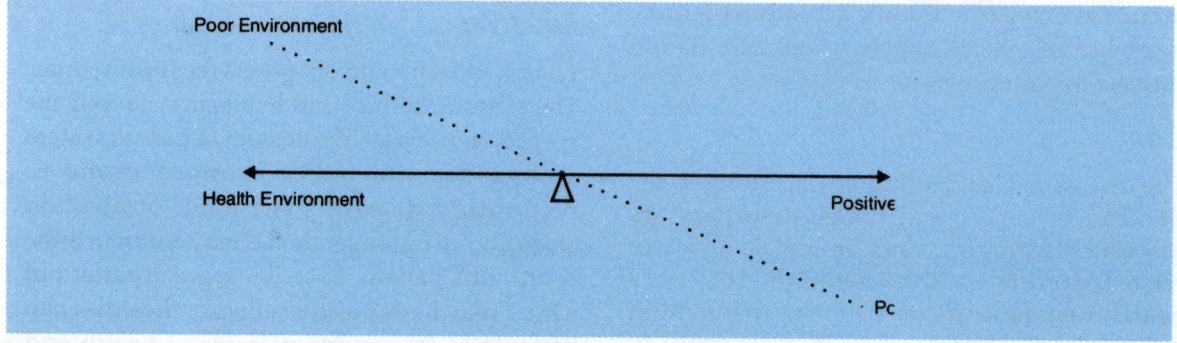

Fig. 12.3(b) : Environment factors of diseases

Man is living in a constantly changing environment due to industrialisation, urbanization and deforestation, which leads to various health problems. Therefore, healthy environment is essential for prevention of numerous diseases. Environment has been divided into three categories :

Physical Environment

This includes : the nonliving things and physical factors like heat, cold, light, radiation, noise, climate, water, air, housing, soil, etc. in which man is continuously interacting. The poor physical environment may affect the health of an individual, excessive heat leads to sunstroke; poor sanitary conditions; and unsafe water supply lead to many infectious diseases. Thus, if the environment is safe, many of the diseases can be prevented.

Biological Environment

Biological environment includes all living things including man himself. These living things are viruses, insects, rodents, animals and plants. There may be agents for causation of disease, carriers of disease, vectors or reservoirs of infections, intermediate hosts. The biological environment plays an important role in prevention and control of various diseases, by maintaining harmonious relationship between man and biological environment.

Psychosocial Environment

Psychosocial environment is another important determinant of diseases. This includes customs, cultural values, habits, attitudes, beliefs, religions, education, occupation, socioeconomic status, etc. Man is a member of social family, where he needs to adjust. There may be conflicts, behavioural differences, which lead to tensions and distress, predisposing mental illness.

ENVIRONMENT		
Physical	**Biological**	**Psychosocial**
Heat	Viruses	Customs
Cold	Bacteria	Culture
Light	Insects	Beliefs
Radiation	Rodents	Attitudes
Noise	Animals	Habits
Climate	Plants	Religion
Air, water		Education

Poverty is closely related to social status, is also closely related to disease. It is very true that poverty leads to sickness and sickness leads to poverty. Man is unable to fulfil the basic needs due to poverty and makes the person unwell and the unhealthy person is unable to earn his living and becomes poorer. Many infectious and nutritional deficiency diseases are prevalent among low socioeconomic group. Poverty predisposes high IMR, MMR, crimes, violence, drug abuse, alcoholism.

The political system also influences the health system while planning the health services and allocation of resources.

Spectrum of Health and Disease
(Fig. 12.4)

The diseases in the community which occur is identical to the spectrum of light, where the colours vary from one end to the other, but difficult to determine where one colour ends and the other begins. In diseases, one ends and the other begins. In diseases, one end of spectrum is subclinical or unapparent infections which are not ordinarily identified and the other end is serious illnesses.

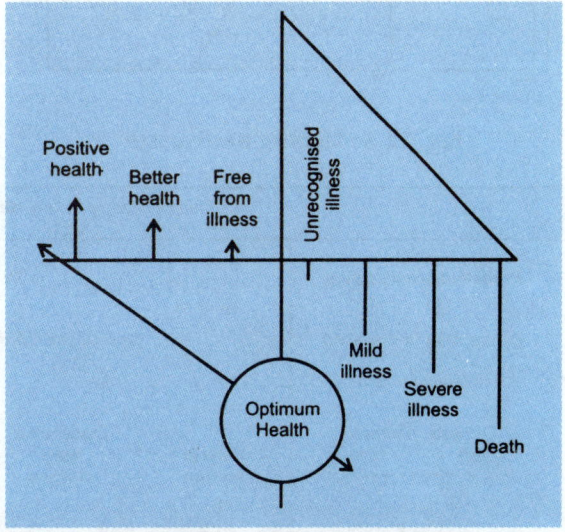

Fig. 12.4 : Spectrum of Disease

The diseases may be found at different levels depending on the occurrence of severity of diseases in the community. When the diseases occur in the community, all the people are not affected with diseases. Some people get the disease and some may be very sick. These variations are due to susceptibility of the host, agent activity and various environmental factors which influence the agent, host and environment. Many people get the infection and remain healthy, but they can transmit the infection, they are carriers of disease and are risk to others which creates major public health problems.

Iceberg of Disease (Fig. 12.5)

The disease in the community may be compared with an iceberg. The diseased people who show the clinical symptoms and can be identified, are apparent in the community, whereas submerged portions of the ice remain inapparent.

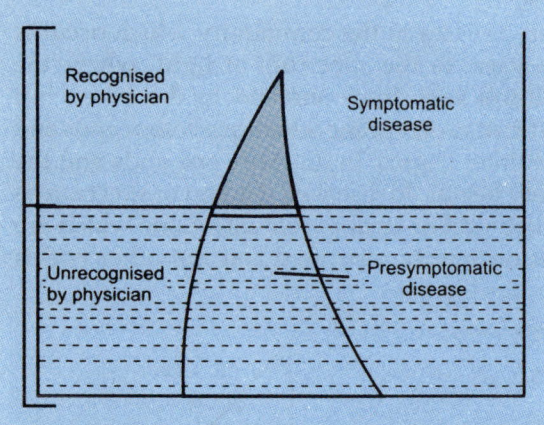

Fig. 12.5 : Iceberg of disease

The inapparent cases are hidden mass of diseases like subclinical carriers and undiagnosed cases are the submerged portions of the iceberg which form the major part of diseases and they may spread the disease in community. These hidden cases constitute an important undiagnosed reservoir of infection and control of such cases is very essential for the prevention of spread of diseases.

NATURAL HISTORY OF DISEASE
(Fig. 12.6, Table 12.1)

The natural history of disease describes the conditions before the onset of disease at the occurrence of disease and the convalescent of the disease.

In order to study the natural history of disease, we have to study the community and epidemiological methods.

The natural history of disease have two phases : Prepathogenesis and pathogenesis.

Prepathogenesis Phase

This phase is before the onset of disease in man, the disease agent is existing in the environment and not yet entered the human host. The factors favourable to interact exist in the environment like poor physical environment, climatic changes, presence of insects, rodents and pests, etc., unhygienic habits, health behaviours, traditional practices, the human host factors like age, sex, marital status, genetic conditions, psychosocial

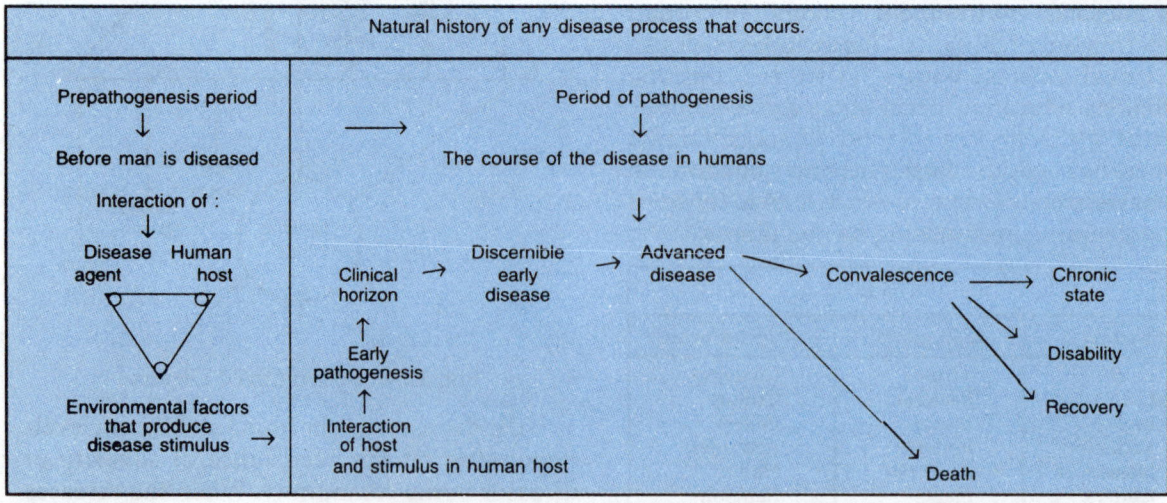

Fig. 12.6 : Prepathogenesis and pathogenesis periods of natural history (Leavell, Clark : 1953, 1979)

status. People living in an environment are always exposed to risk of disease, but the disease starts only when the agent enters the host (susceptible) and there is interaction of agent, host and environment. Therefore, before the interaction the phase is prepathogenesis.

Pathogenesis Phase (Disease Prevalence)

When agent, host and environmental factors interact, the pathogenesis phase starts. This phase begins with the entry of disease agent with human host. The disease agents may be virus, bacteria, parasites, worms, etc. The agent grows and multiplies in the host and brings the pathophysiological changes in the body. These changes are subclinical, that means the patient does not show signs and symptoms, but agent is present in the human host. The host remains healthy and ambulant. After specific period of time for specific illness, the health equilibrium of the body is disturbed, the signs and symptoms of the disease appear. This period is called **incubation period.** The early signs and symptoms, which are difficult to diagnose, is the early pathogenesis phase. Later

when clinical signs become more apparent and clear it is called a stage of **pathogenesis** (disease process) or **fastegium.** The duration of fastegium varies from disease to disease. The end result of the disease may be completely recovered, which refers to as **defervescence or convalescence,** it may even lead to some disability, defect, chronic state or even death.

Example : Tubercle bacilli are existing in the poor environmental conditions and people, susceptible (not vaccinated and in poor health) living in those areas may get the agent. After agent enters into man, he may not show the signs and symptoms immediately after the entry, but it takes around two days for clinical signs to appear, the patient gets cough, fever, sputum and loss of weight, etc. Later, these symptoms are more prominent but with proper treatment and care the patient can be in convalescence stage and if he does not get treatment, he may get complications and die (Fig. 12.6).

LEVELS OF DISEASE PREVENTION
(Table 12.2, Fig. 12.7)

The natural history of a disease provided the basis for community health intervention. The

Table 12.1 : The Natural History of any Disease of Humans

Interrelations of Agent, Host, and Environmental Factor
Factors → Production of **stimulus**
Prepathogenesis period
    Reaction of the host to the stimulus

Early	Discernible	Advanced	Convalescence
Pathogenesis	Early lesions	Disease	

Period of pathogenesis
Health Promotion
Health education, good standard of nutrition adjusted to developmental phases of life. Attention to personality development, provision of adequate housing, recreation, and agreeable working condition. Marriage counselling and sex education
Genetics: Periodical selective examination; healthy lifestyle
Specific Protection
Use of specific immunization *e.g.,* TT. against tetanus, personal hygiene. Use of environment sanitation protection against occupational hazards; protection from accidents; use of specific nutrients; protection from carcinogens; avoidance of allergens
Early Diagnosis and Prompt Treatment
Case finding measures, individual and mass
Screening surveys; selective examinations; objectives: to cure and prevent disease processes; to prevent the spread of communicable diseases; to prevent complications and sequelae; to shorten period of disability
Disability Limitation
Adequate treatment to arrest the disease process and to prevent further complications and sequelae provision of facilities to limit disability and to prevent death
Rehabilitation
Provision of hospital and community facilities for retraining and education for maximum use of remaining capacities; education of public and industry to utilize the rehabilitated; as full employment possible; selective placement; work therapy in hospitals; use of sheltered colony

Levels of Application of Preventive Measures

Primary prevention	Secondary prevention	Tertiary prevention

ultimate aim of intervention programme is to reverse the process of pathological changes as early as possible, so as to prevent complications.

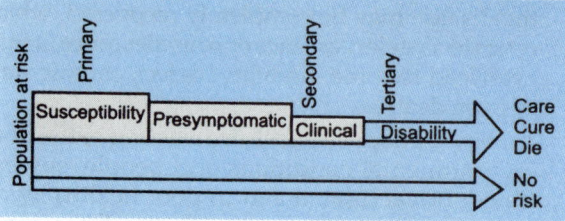

Fig. 12.7 : Levels of prevention

The main objective of preventive medicine is to prevent and control various diseases by different measures which may be done at various levels. These levels may be before the disease starts or after the disease progresses.

Leavell and **Clark** proposed a model of levels of prevention activity that can be superimposed for disease pattern and classified as main disease prevention at mainly three levels. The goals of intervention at each of the three levels are to prevent the pathogenic process from evolving further. These three levels of prevention are called (Fig 12.7) :

- Primary level of prevention
- Secondary level of prevention
- Tertiary level of prevention.

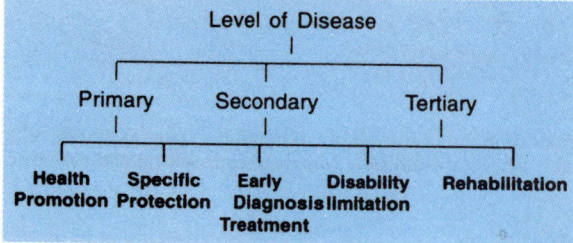

Primary Level Prevention

Primary level refers to the action taken before the onset of the disease to reduce the possibility of occurrence of disease. Primary prevention seeks to keep the agent away from contact with the host or to eliminate the host susceptibility under favourable environmental conditions. Various preventive measures are taken to prevent the occurrence of disease. Primary preventive efforts are of two types :

- General health promotion, and
- Specific protection against diseases.

General Health Promotion

The efforts taken to improve the quality of life and maintain the physical and mental health of a person. It includes all activities that optimize the environment and favour healthy living. Thus, efforts to improve the physical environment, whether at home, outside home, school or workplace, would be included.

Health education aimed at educating the people on various aspects to enable people to live healthier and change their attitudes towards healthy lifestyle. This may include hygiene, good nutrition, sex education, basic education, need for rest and relaxation, harmful effect of smoking, drinking, or drugs, family planning and improving overall standard of living. All these activities can be adopted for health promotion of an individual, with less probability of getting diseases.

Specific Protection

Refers to specific procedures of diseases prevention. Commonly, we say, *"Prevention is better than cure"*. Preventing the diseases are cheaper and easier. Therefore, if more emphasis is laid on primary prevention, major diseases can be prevented. Hence, in specific protection, the measures are taken to protect individual against specific agents such as :

1. Immunization against polio, T.B., diphtheria and tetanus, etc.
2. Attempt to remove the agent from the environment such as sewage treatment, pasteurization of the milk or chlorination of water.
3. Chemoprophylaxis towards various community diseases to prevent their spread, *e.g.*, chloroquine against malaria, D.D.S. against filaria, etc.
4. Protection against accidents and occupational hazards by use of glasses, gloves and helmets, etc.
5. Nutritional supplementation to prevent the deficiency diseases, *e.g.*, vitamin A solution, or iron supplementation to antenatal cases.

Example : To prevent the occurrence of tuberculosis among people at primary level of prevention, the person must have good resistance against disease by balanced diet, hygienic needs, rest and sleep. The BCG immunization against the disease at an early age of life is essential to protect a child or individual against tuberculosis.

The efforts of primary prevention can be seen leading to dramatic reduction in mortality from infectious diseases resulting largely from environmental manipulation and immunization programmes. The reduction in infectious diseases mortality especially infant and child mortality, young women and elderly has led to an increase in population. If the primary prevention is ineffective certain people in community may get illness. These individuals undergo subclinical changes that may lead to acute or chronic disease. Hence, the purpose of secondary prevention is to identify those individuals at earliest immunization programmes.

Secondary Level Prevention

At this level, the disease agent has already entered the host, hence the efforts seek to detect disease at early stage and treat promptly to cure the disease at the earliest, to slow its progression, prevent complication and limit disability when cure is not possible. The secondary level is focused primarily on the stage of presymptomatic disease or very early in the stage of clinical diseases.

Early Diagnosis and Treatment

Screening is the most common form of secondary prevention for early diagnosis and treatment. Many screening tests can detect early physiological indicators of disease before people are aware that they are ill, *e.g.*, VDRL tests for STD, Pap smear for CA cervix or Mantaux test for tuberculosis.

The health care provider's goal is to minimize the number of days of illness and the need for acute or inpatient care.

Secondary prevention is an imperfect tool in control of transmission of diseases. It is often more expensive and less effective than primary prevention. Certain criteria should be met before a screening test is administered.

1. An effective treatment must be available that will change the course of disease.

2. Ensure that test done, will detect the disease before the onset of disease appears.
3. Must be able to detect the positive care.
4. Follow-up services must be available and accompanied by an adequate notification and referral services for those positive on the screening.

It is useful to teach the people regarding early symptoms of disease so that they are alert to the significance to the symptoms that might appear. The early diagnosis of T.B. will help for appropriate treatment with antitubercle drugs, INH thiacetazone, rifampicin, etc. which help in early recovery and less complications.

Tertiary Level Prevention

This level refers not to prevent the disease, but to prevent the disability when the disease has already occurred. It includes limitation of disability at an early stage of illness and rehabilitation in those persons for whom residual damage already exists. Tertiary level activities are focused on the middle to later phase of the stage of clinical disease when irreversible pathological damage produces disability. The goal of tertiary level is :

1. To minimize loss of function and to return to recovered individual to society at an optimum level of health in all aspects like physical, mental, social and spiritual.

2. To limit the disability and help the individual to adjust in case of permanent impairment and disability so as to lead a productive life.

Disability Limitation

Disability may occur when patient reports late. Objective is to reduce the disease progress, by providing timely appropriate treatment and prevent further complications with minimal harm to patient and limited disability, to prevent or postpone death. In case of T.B. patients, if pulmonary complications arise, then surgical intervention may be done, so that patient can recover with minimum disability and helping him to get suitable job for economical support to him.

Disability can be prevented at different levels :

(a) *Primary Level :* By immunizing the child to prevent disability from communicable disease, *e.g.,* polio vaccine.

(b) *Secondary Level :* By specific treatment for a disease for early recovery and prevent damage and complication and reduce disability.

(c) *Tertiary Level :* When complication has already occurred, to handle the physical, mental, social and economical disability by appropriate measures.

WHO defines impairment, disability and handicapped as :

- **Impairment** is any loss or abnormality of psychological, physiological or anatomical structure or function.
- **Disability** is any restriction or lack of ability to perform activity in a manner or within the range considered normal for human being.
- **Handicapped** is a disadvantage for a given individual, resulting from an impairment or a disability, that limits or prevents the

fulfillment of a role that is normal (depending on age, sex, social, cultural factors) for that individual.

The disease, if neglected, may lead to impairment, which may lead to disability and finally a person becomes handicapped (physical, mental, economical or social, etc.).

Various measures are taken to control the communicable diseases and for prevention and spread of infectious agents from neighbouring environment to individuals who are susceptible and who may be exposed. This can be achieved by modifying or eliminating the environment in which the infectious agent lives, by interfering with the means of transmission to the human host, or by increasing the host immunity—all measures aimed at primary prevention. Control is facilitated by maintaining surveillance programmes that quickly identify new cases for follow-up with isolation methods to prevent exposure of those susceptible or by instituting specific treatments to limit the period of communicability and progression

Table 12.2 : Prevention of diseases

Preclinical Period	Subclinical Period		Clinical Period	Resolution Period
Health Promotion	*Specific Protection*	*Early Diagnosis and Prompt Treatment*	*Disability Limitation*	*Rehabilitation*
• Health education • Nutrition • Psychosocial development and support • Adequate housing, recreation, work • Interpersonal relationships • Counselling • Sex education • Genetics • Periodic, selective examinations	• Immunization • Personal health habits • Environmental sanitation • protection against work hazards • Seat-belts • Avoidance of allergens	• Case finding • Screening • Examinations • Intervention at earliest possible at the time of illness	• Adequate treatment to arrest illness and • Prevent further sequela and complications	• Retraining • Assistive devices • Vocational rehabilitation • Occupational therapy
Primary Prevention	Secondary Prevention		Tertiary Prevention	

Table 12.3 : *Example I* : Levels of Disease Prevention of Acute Infectious Hepatitis (Communicable Disease)

Primary Prevention	Secondary Prevention	Tertiary Prevention
For case : Environmental sanitation, especially of water, sewage, etc.	Provision of adequate early treatment.	Patient teaching on levels of damage; avoidance of stressors, toxins, re-exposure; carrier state.
Toilet cleanliness; handwashing facilities available and used.	Encourage development of early differential diagnostic tests for infectious hepatitis.	Adequate convalescent care as long as indicated.
Health education to those who do not use adequate measures for prevention.	Treatment to relieve symptoms, minimizing damage.	Vocational retraining for those whose occupational conditions were causal or would be detrimental to themselves or others.
Isolation from known cases, especially by high-risk persons.	Careful observation of general health of close contacts through duration of incubation period.	
Hygienic measures during food preparation and handling.	Health education on care of sick and indications for professional care when symptoms persist, worsen and danger signs etc.	
Screen all blood donors for virus; test all blood, for virus; tranfusions.	During high-risk times (outbreak) or for high-risk groups, education for signs, symptoms, managements, communication, etc.	
Teach proper sterilization technique for injections.	Professional education to update knowledge of conditions, transmission, prevention and treatment.	
Safe handling of blood-contaminated instruments and equipment.	Adequate acute care to manage symptoms, prevent worsening, secondary infections.	
Regular check-up of health workers involved with patient interiors (surgery, anaesthesia staff); exclusion of carriers.		
For Contacts : Hyperimmune gammaglobulin as passive immunization.		

of pathological changes. Tertiary prevention plays a smaller role in infectious diseases programme than in non infectious programme since infectious diseases less often result in permanent disability.

Rehabilitation

It is defined by WHO as "The combined and co-ordinated use of medical, social, educational and vocational measures for training or retraining the individual to the highest possible level of functional ability".

Rehabilitation has become an essential component of health care system. It involves various disciplines like physiotherapy, occupational therapy, speech therapy, vocational guidance and counselling and placement services. The medical care is not limited to treat

Example II : Levels of Disease Prevention of Hypertensions (Non communicable)

Primary Prevention	Secondary Prevention	Tertiary Prevention
Lower sodium intake for all : infants, children, adults, high-risk groups, etc.	Health education about need for at least regular B.P. check-up and insist on adequate treatment for control of high B.P.	Organise programmes for comprehensive treatment of hypertension through multiple approaches, especially incorporating lifestyle changes for permanent control of high BP.
Improve regular involvement of all age groups in participatory sports, excercise or other strenuous activities.	Screening services at convenient locations at minimal cost to test all populations for BP elevations with reliable interpretation, medical advice and follow-up.	Health education on need to control BP as a primary preventive for stroke, heart attack and congestive heart disease, known hypertensive persons to ensure their continuance with adequate treatment to control their hypertension. This is necessitated by patients tendency to stop taking their medications because they "feel fine" and/or because their blood pressure has been controlled as a result of the medication although this control may not continue without the medication.
Teach pro-heart nutrition at all age levels: eliminate from all schools foods that are high salt, high fat, high starch, at the basic junk foods; consumer education at markets for balanced nutrition.	Education on need to detect and control BP in excess of 140/90; all health workers should be able to screen in their work sites: pharmacists and dentists as well as nurses and physicians.	
Reduce (eliminate?) tobacco smoking; prevent it in children and youth; stop smoking programmes; support groups against back-sliding; assertive behaviour by nonsmokers; push for laws restricting smoking in public.	Physician's education on diagnosis of hypertension, nondrug and drug therapies, contraindications, and adverse effects of drugs used to treat hypertension, on need to teach clients to manage their own treatment and on community resources, especially the community health nurse to work with clients who have hypertension.	
Obesity : Management at all ages		
Stress control programmes: relaxation in work settings; hotlines for harried housewives; T.V. tips on ways to relax.		
Screening programmes to identify risk factors, ego, high blood cholesterol and triglycerides; diabetes; pregnancy, birth control pills; excess salt intake; genetic history; obesity; lack of exercise; high stress levels.		

the patient, but his activity must be restored and retained which will permit them to lead a socially and economically productive life, so that he works within the limits of his disability. The rehabilitation must start as soon as the patient comes in the contact of health personnels.

●●●

13

Concept and Methods of Epidemiology of Diseases

INTRODUCTION

Epidemiology is the scientific and systematic study of occurrence of disease and disease related conditions in population. The most important application of the field is prevention and control of the infectious diseases, but scope also encompasses to non-infectious diseases and disabled conditions, such as accidents, chronic diseases, cancer and malnutrition, etc.

DEFINITION

Epidemiology has been defined in the dictionary as medical science treating epidemics (Webster). The science of epidemiology deals with the study of health-related states and events occurring in a population. As a science, epidemiology not only helps understanding the health concepts, natural history of disease and disease causation, but also helps in planning, implementing and evaluating effective and efficient health care services.

The term **"Epidemiology"** is derived from the term "Epidemic". The meaning of the term is "study among people" (*Epi*-among, *demo* people, *logos*-study). The foundation of the epidemiology was laid in the nineteenth century, when infectious and communicable diseases, *e.g.*, cholera, typhoid and plague were prevalent in the world in the form of epidemic and pandemic. During the nineteenth century and the early twentieth century, the study of frequency, distribution and determinants of infectious and communicable diseases and their prevention and control were primary foci of epidemiologists. There has been considerable reduction in morbidity and mortality from these diseases as a result of epidemiological studies and improved methods of diagnosis, prevention and control. However, the threat of communicable diseases is still present, specially in developing countries, because of poor environmental conditions, poor socioeconomic factors and inadequate health and health-related resources.

Besides, the communicable diseases continue to be serious health problems. Many noncommunicable diseases like cancer, diabetes, cardiovascular diseases, accidents etc. have come up. The focus of epidemiologists have been now towards the prevention and control of non-communicable diseases as well.

As the scope of epidemiology has been expanded, the definitions have also been changed from time to time. Different definitions have been given by various epidemiologists based on facts and changing concepts.

It is defined as *"The study of distribution and determinants of disease prevalence in man"*. The epidemiology is that branch of medical science which deals with epidemics. —*Parkin, 1873*

Epidemiology is the science of mass phenomena of infectious diseases. —*Frost, 1927*

"Epidemiology is the study of disease, any disease, as a mass phenomenon". —*Greenwood, 1934*

Epidemiology is the study of the distribution and determinants of disease frequency in man. —*MacMohan, 1960*

Epidemiology is the study of frequency, distribution and determinants of health-related states, events and morbidity, pattern in population and the application of the study to control health problems.—*Last, 1983*

The principal aim of epidemiology is to understand or discover the cause for risk factors of diseases or controlling its spread, and to provide guidance in planning and implementing the health services.

SCOPE OF EPIDEMIOLOGY

The scope of epidemiology has been broadened during the last few years. The epidemiological methods of studying a disease by its occurrence and distribution, aetiology, prevention and control, are extended to various communicable diseases. The epidemiological approach is now being used in the study of many non-communicable diseases also, such as diabetes, coronary heart diseases, cancer, accidents, alcoholism and congenital defects, etc.

Epidemiology does not only deal with distribution and determinants of diseases studied, but also factors that contribute to the maintenance of health. People, who are high-risk for chronic noncommunicable diseases like cancer and stroke, can also be identified. The behavioural problems like alcoholism, drug abuse, child abuse and suicide can also be studied by epidemiological methodology and evaluation of health services has also been accepted.

This change of epidemiological concept has been due to changing pattern of diseases and methods of control and prevention of health problems.

In order to meet the present and future health care needs of society, problems and needs must be identified—collection and analysis of data to identify the factors, planning, implementation and evaluation for preventing and controlling the diseases. Such processes can be done by epidemiological investigations.

AIMS OF EPIDEMIOLOGY

The main aim of epidemiology is to find the best means of preventing disease or controlling its spread. The ultimate aim of epidemiology is the complete elimination of diseases among people. Formerly, epidemiology was considered to be a science of epidemics and its application was confined to the study of a few communicable diseases such as cholera, smallpox, plague and typhoid fever.

Based on the modern concept of epidemiology, **three main aims** have been identified by International Epidemiological Association :

- To describe the occurrence and distribution of disease problems in human population. That means how disease has occurred and where it is spread and who all are affected.
- To identify aetiological factors in the pathogenesis of diseases which helps to find cause and effect of disease. This describes causative effect of disease.
- To provide information on health-related states and events for planning, implementation and evaluation of comprehensive health care services to deal with health problems and promote health and well-being of the society as a whole. Epidemiology will help to plan preventive measure before the outbreak of a disease.

EPIDEMIOLOGICAL APPROACH

The science of epidemiology deals with the study of health-related events occurring in a population. But, with advancement of science and medicine, epidemiology not only helps in understanding the health concepts, natural history of diseases and disease causation, it also helps in planning, implementing and evaluating effective and efficient health care services.

Epidemiology has its own approach in dealing with the health problems. The unit of study is not an individual, or a patient, but community is studied as a whole or a sample of people is investigated to find out the cause of disease and its modes of transmission, with a view to effective planning for prevention and control. The distribution of disease pattern includes mainly **five questions to find the answer.**

- **When** does the disease occur ? (Time distribution).
- **Where** does the disease occur ? (Place distribution).
- **Who** are the people affected ? (Person distribution).
- **Why** has it appeared ? (Aetiological factors).

- **What** should be done to prevent or control the disease ? (Prevention/control/eradication).

Epidemiologists examine whether there is rise or fall of disease occurrence over a time period, whether significant relationship with sex or age distribution, or lifestyle, etc., that help to find the cause and effect relationship among population. For example, smoking is associated with lung cancer. The cause is smoking habits; the lifestyle of person; will affect the health of a person by causing lung cancer which has been proved scientifically by epidemiologists that "people who smoke have more of lung cancer".

EPIDEMIOLOGICAL METHODS

The epidemiological methods are concerned with the study of the health status of the population at large, identify the mortality (deaths) and morbidity (illness) pattern, determine the factors affecting health and disease, which help in planning, implementing and evaluating the health services which can be done by collecting and analysing the health needs. There are three epidemiological methods. These are : descriptive, analytic, experimental.

DESCRIPTIVE EPIDEMIOLOGY

The first step is to describe the problem in terms of person, place and time. The descriptive epidemiology is related to the study, frequency and distribution of diseases and health-related events in human population in terms of person, place and time. The purpose of this method is to know the extent of health problems and possible aetiological factors (causes) involved. It helps to know who (persons) are affected, what is the source of infection, where it had occurred (place) and when it occurred (time).

Uses of Descriptive Epidemiology

1. It helps in making community diagnosis by describing the extent of disease or health status of a community in terms of incidences and prevalence rates in different subgroups of the population *i.e.*, age, sex, occupation and social class, etc.

2. Provides information on aetiological factors of disease and helps to find further steps to control the diseases.

3. Provides data to plan and implement the health services in an effective and efficient way, within the resources available.

Person Distribution

In this, the epidemiologists collect the information regarding host factors like age, disease, sex, marital status, ethnic group, occupation, educational status, income, dietary pattern, social class, habits.

Age is the most important factor in human host. Certain diseases are more prevalent in certain age groups—measles, chickenpox, polio are more common in young childrens. The disease like cardiovascular, diabetes and cancer in middle age and athrosclerosis in old age.

Some occupations have specific disease prevalence in man and may give rise to different exposures to infections and suspected cause. People working in factories are exposed to the risk of mechanical and physical hazards. Habits like smoking have been related to lung cancer and dietary pattern to athrosclerosis (thickening of arteries), coronary heart disease and obesity. The distribution of diseases in personal factors will help to formulate the aetiological statements.

Place Distribution

This method refers to the areas of high and low incidences related to geographical distribution of cases. Some of the major communicable diseases, *e.g.*, elephantiasis, leprosy, yellow fever and sleeping sickness are endemic in some areas and are not prevalent in other areas. The same phenomenon is applied to various non-communicable diseases also.

This knowledge of place distribution helps to study the disease frequency in various states, *e.g.*, kala-azar in Bihar. It also provides information regarding urban, rural and local distribution of diseases. Accidents more common in urban and worm-infection in rural population.

The study of geographical distribution enables us to know the disease aetiology and helps to find the variations in terms of agent, host and environment. When people migrate from one place to another, preventive measures can be taken to prevent infection to unaffected place.

International Variation

This shows variation in the morbidity and mortality among different countries. The distribution of diseases varies from one country to another country, like yellow fever is more prevalent in South Africa.

National Variations

These are variations in one country but different states are endemic in certain diseases like leprosy, filaria and nutritional deficiency which are more commonly found in south India than in north India. Eye problems are more in north than south India.

The knowledge that a patient comes from a certain geographical area helps in probable diagnosis of the case, in turn it helps for early diagnosis and treatment and to prevent the spread of infection.

Rural-Urban Distribution

Many diseases like worm infestation, malnutrition are more prevalent in rural than urban areas. Some diseases like coronary heart disease, hypertension, diabetes are more common in urban areas due to urbanisation and industrialisation. The death rates, infant mortality and maternal mortality rate are higher in rural than in urban areas.

Local Differences

Particular communities are endemic of diseases within the same community. Therefore, even if the geographical area is the same, but the disease may differ in the same area according to the health hazards. Spread of cholera, measles may be prevalent in a defined community, e.g., slum area of city.

Time Distribution

It is the study of occurrence of diseases by seasonal changes and shows the time distribution by daily, monthly, yearly occurrence, etc.

Seasonal Changes

Some diseases are more common in certain specific season, e.g., spring, summer, winter and rainy season. Upper respiratory infection is common in winter; cholera, malaria and typhoid in summer and rainy season. Measles in spring season, etc. These diseases may show high incidence in these months. Therefore, precautions must be taken before hand so as to reduce the incidences of illness.

Cyclic Changes

The duration of occurrence of disease is in the particular period of time as per cyclic movement. Like measles, shows that every three year cyclic occurrences of disease.

Secular Changes

Some diseases may show upward trend after many years like appearance of plague in Surat in India show a secular trend of illness.

Analytic Epidemiology

Descriptive method describes the aetiological factors of illness and helps in making further investigations in the study. These investigations are further studied and tested to analytic study to determine the association between cause and effect. Analytic study goes beyond the descriptive study by two observational methods.

- Case control study,
- Cohert study.

Case Control Study

These studies are used to test the aetiological factors of disease. These are basically comparison studies. A group of people with the disease is compared with a group of people without the disease. Here the approach used is retrospective, i.e. the disease has already occurred and epidemiologists go back to review the previous records, interviewing the cases and their families to collect the data. This approach has helped in identifying the causative factors of many diseases like association of smoking with lung cancer, rubella in mothers during pregnancy, with congenital anomaly among children, iodine deficiency with hyperthyroidism.

Case control studies are quite commonly done because, they are easy to conduct, less expensive. These studies are usually undertaken as first step to explore aetiological factors.

Cohert Study

This study is done on a group of people having similar characteristics like age, sex, occupation, smoking, pregnancy at the same time and having equal susceptibility of the disease. This is prospective in nature because group under study is free from illness but exposed to risk factors. In this method, epidemiologists select a cohort, *i.e.*, a group of people of the same age group and exposed to similar type of health risk like cigarette smoking, and a group of people of the same age group but not exposed to health risk of cigarette smoking. These two groups are followed up for several years to find that how many people were getting cancer. The first group who are cigarette smoking may show high incidence than the other group which finally concludes that cigarette smoking people are at higher risk than noncigarette smoking people.

These data are statistically analysed and comparisons are done between the incidence among smokers and nonsmokers to determine the association of risk factors to the diseases.

This prospective study is expensive and time consuming, but it has its advantage to study the natural history of diseases estimating risk of getting disease, the groups of people who are exposed to risk factors. It also helps to determine the association between risk factors and diseases by two measures.

Relative Risk

It is stated as the ratio between the incidence among exposed and the incidence among nonexposed. Thus, this measurement helps to identify those people who are exposed will have higher incidence than those who are not exposed.

$$\text{Risk factor} = \frac{\text{Incidence of risk factor}}{\text{Incidence of non risk factor}}$$

For example, the incidence rate of lung cancer among smokers is 3/1000 and incidence among nonsmokers is 0.5/1000.

Relative Risk = 6.

This shows the smokers have six times greater risk of having lung cancer than nonsmokers.

Attribute Risk

Defined as the rate of disease in exposed individuals that can be attributed to suspected cause. It can be determined by finding the difference between incidence rate among exposed and incidence rate among nonexposed *e.g.,*

The incidence rate of smokers = 5/1000
The incidence rate of nonsmoker = 0.5/1000
Difference in incidence of disease = 4.5/1000
Attributed Risk =

$$\frac{\begin{array}{c}\text{Incidence of disease rate among}\\ \text{exposed} - \text{incidence of disease}\\ \text{rate among nonexposed}\end{array}}{\text{Incidence rate among exposed}} \times 100$$

$$= \frac{5-0.5}{5} \times 100 = \frac{4.5}{5} \times 100$$
$$= 4.5 \times 20 = 90\%$$

Attribute risk of disease is 90 per cent.

EXPERIMENTAL EPIDEMIOLOGY

This study is similar to the cohert study except the conditions are under the careful control of investigators.

Experimental study is done to find the cause and effect association for preventive and therapeutic measures. In this study, the preventive and therapeutic measures are given to one group (experimental group) and not to the other group, to find the effectiveness of these treatments. These experiments are done in laboratories usually on animals. Community or clinical trials are done on animals. These experiments involve medical, ethical and moral issues.

Measurements

Rates

Primary measurement used in descriptive epidemiology is the rate, a measure of the frequency of a disease, condition or event in relation to the population in which it occurs, within a specific time period.

Rates are the tools in health care calculations. By using rates it is possible to compare events that occur at different times and places and the different people.

The rate of a disease will help us determine the extent of disease in particular place or specific age group and definite time period of the year, *e.g.*, annual rate of malaria may be high during summer period, among all ages and in slum areas, etc.

The rate consists of two parts, a numerator and a denominator. Numerator is composed of the number of conditions or events of interest that occurred within a specific period of time.

Denominator is the total population at risk during the same period of time. If the time period is long, often the population of risk is estimated at mid-period such as mid-year.

General Principles in Rate Calculation

- Numerator must include all of the events that are being measured, such as deaths of cases and each of these must be in the denominator.
- Everyone in the denominator must be at risk for the event in the numerator. Because a rate is a fraction or a proportion.
- It is necessary to multiply by a base, which is usually a multiple of ten. The procedure removes the decimal points and makes comparison of the rates easier.
- Any base multiple of ten may be chosen that results in the rate above the volume of one. The rate should be a reasonable size, not a fraction.

$$\text{Rate} = \frac{\text{No. of conditions or events occurring in a period of time}}{\text{Population at risk during the same period of time}} \times 1000$$

Using the above formula, the rates can be compared with different countries, states or places, etc.

Example :

Country A

Population at risk of country A	=	2 lakh
Number of pneumonia's cases	=	4800

$$\text{Rate (per thousand)} = \frac{4800}{200000} \times 1000 = 24$$

Country B

Population at risk of country B	=	2 lakh
Number of pneumonia's cases	=	3400

$$\text{Rate (per thousand)} = \frac{3400 \times 1000}{200000} = 17$$

Hence the pneumonia rate of country A is higher than the pneumonia rate of country B.

Incidence Rate

The number of new cases of any disease that occurred in a country in relation to their respective population is called the incidence rate. Incidence rate provides a measure of the rate that people without a certain condition develop during a specific time period. It measures the race at which new illness occurs and reflects factors that affect the development of illness.

For example total number of new malaria cases are 20/1000. The incidence rate is 2 per cent every year.

Incidence rate is defined as the number of new cases occurring in a defined population during a specific period of time. Special incidence rates are :

Attack Rate

It is an incidence rate, used only when the population is exposed to risk to a limited period of time. Such as during an epidemic. It indicates the number of cases in the population at risk and reflects the extent of the epidemic calculated as:

$$\frac{\text{Number of new cases of specific disease}}{\text{Total number of population at risk during a specific period of time}} \times 100$$

Secondary Attack

It is defined as the number of exposed persons developing the disease within the range of the incubation period following exposure to a primary case.

$$\text{Incidence rate} = \frac{\text{Number of new cases or events occurring in a period of time}}{\text{Population at risk during the same period of time}} \times \text{base } 100$$

Prevalence Rate

Refers specifically to all current cases old and new existing at a given time period. The prevalence rate measures total number of people in a given population who have a specific condition at a given point of time. It measures the amount of illness or morbidity that exists in a community.

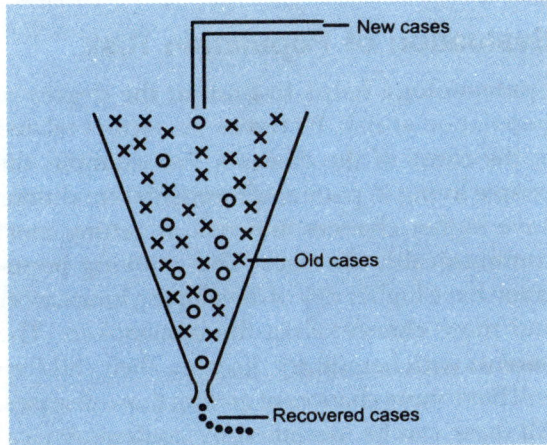

Fig. 13.1 : Prevalence Rate

Prevalence rate is defined as the total number of all individuals who have an attribute or disease at a particular time (or during a particular period) divided by population at risk of having the attribute or disease at this point of time or midway through the period.

$$\text{Prevalence rate} = \frac{\begin{array}{c}\text{Number of existing conditions}\\\text{or events occurring in a period}\\\text{of time (old + new)}\end{array}}{\begin{array}{c}\text{Population at risk during}\\\text{the same period of time}\end{array}} \times \text{base}$$

Prevalence Rate is Influenced by Two Factors

The number of people who have developed the condition in the past (old cases) and the duration of their illness and new people getting diseases.

$$P = I \times D$$

Prevalence = Incidence × Time duration.

The prolonged duration of illness of a condition, the higher prevalence rate will be there in the community. This is best illustrated with the chronic illnesses. Even if the incidence rate is low (new cases) the prevalence rate will be high in the community. For example, there are many more existing cases of cancer in a community.

RATE MEASUREMENTS

A rate measures the occurence of some particular event (of disease or death) in a population during a given period of time. It is a statement of the risk of developing a condition. It also indicates the change in some event that takes place in a population over a period of time.

The rates are usually calculated as per 1000 or per lakh according to the convenience of numbers. Various rates have been described as :

Crude Rates

The actual observed rates, *e.g.*, birth rate and death rate. These are also called as unstandardised rates.

Specific Rates

These are actual observed rates due to specific causes of conditions, *e.g.*, disease specific, age specific and sex specific rates. These can be time specific, *e.g.*, annual, monthly or weekly, etc.

Standardised Rates

These rates are obtained by direct or indirect methods of standardisation, *e.g.*, age and sex.

Ratio

Ratio is described as the relationship in size between two random quantities. In ratio numerator is not a component of denominator. Ratio is the result of dividing one quantity by another. It is expressed in the form of :

$$A : B \text{ or } \frac{A}{B}$$

Examples are sex ratio, doctor patient ratio, doctor nurse ratio, bed patient ratio, etc.

$$\text{Sex ratio} = \frac{1000 \quad \text{(Numerator)}}{927 \quad \text{(Denominator)}}$$

(Denominator is not the part of numerator like rate).

Sex ratio = 1000 : 729.

Proportion

It is defined as a ratio which indicates the relationship in magnitude (intensity) of a part to the whole. Numerator is always included in denominator. A proportion is usually calculated in percentage.

$$\text{Proportion} = \frac{\text{Number of children with ARI}}{\text{Total number of children in the community in defined time period}} \times 100$$

USES OF EPIDEMIOLOGY

These are as follows :

Community Diagnosis

Community diagnosis refers to community identification, which includes health problems and health needs of the community, morbidity and mortality indicators, which determine the health and various factors affecting health. The control of disease is done by priortising the list of health problems, which need immediate attention and those which can be delayed. It also helps to find the disease distribution, causation and measures to prevent the disease. It is also useful tool to identify the community's socio-cultural and environmental characteristics, which help epidemiologist to select the appropriate line of action for prevention and control of disease. Hence epidemiology is one of the diagnostic tool for community health.

Planning and Evaluation

Planning is an essential for equitable distribution of resources and for most effective utilization of health services. For example, the hospitals which are being opened in cities are not according to the health needs of the people. Epidemiological investigation will help to determine the health problems of a particular community and gives further information on the need and type of health services required in the community according to the health needs. This planning will help in maximum utilization of health services, of manpower availability, other resources and facilities, etc.

Evaluation is an important tool to find the effectiveness and efficiency of health services. Evaluation also helps to improve the future health care programme. Any strategy undertaken to prevent and control must be based on evaluation to find out whether the measures taken are effective in lowering the incidence of disease and its cost effectiveness (that means effectiveness in relation to its expenditure).

Evaluation of Population Risk

Epidemiology helps to findout the degree of population at risk. It studies the factors related to the cause of the diseases. For example, the people living in poor environmental conditions have higher chances and risk of getting most communicable diseases. The smoking population have higher risk of developing lung cancer and more chances than the nonsmokers. The parents with hereditary diseases, their children will have more chances of getting those diseases. All these can be identified by epidemiological studies.

To Study the Natural History of Disease

Epidemiology is concerned about studying the disease pattern in the community in relation to agent, host and environment factors and can determine the natural history of diseases, whereas hospital data may not be able to do so, *e.g.*, most of the heart deaths occur due to sudden heart failure of the patient, which may help to develop prompt network for emergency care and availability of CCU in the community. It also helps epidemiology to take precautionary measures before the occurence of disease.

Identification of Syndrome

Some diseases can not be identified and differentiated from one another, study of disease in depth will help to identify the specific disease syndrome. For example, the types of ulcers, duodenal ulcer like gastric and peptic, it was difficult to identify unless depth study were done. Hence epidemiological investigation can be used to define and refine syndromes. By observations of groups these studies have been able to remove misconceptions regarding many disease syndromes.

To Study the Rise and Fall of Disease in the Community

The health of a community is never static, it keeps on changing. Epidemiological study helps to study the decrease or increase of incidence of the diseases during a specific time period Epidemiology provides means to study th disease profile and time trends in human population. By study of these trends, we can make useful projections for future and identify the emerging health problems and their correlations. The study of prevalence of existing health problems will help us to identify the new emerging problems and what steps should be taken to control such diseases and also the effect of control measures.

Identifying the Cause and Effect Relationship

Epidemiology is used to find the cause of a disease and its relationship to effect. Epidemiological studies have proved that rubella infection of an antenatal mother causes congenital anomalies in newborn. Cigarette smoking has correlation with lung cancer. The people who smoke were found to be at higher risk of getting lung cancer than nonsmokers. Premature babies exposed to oxygen cause retrolental fibroplasia. Hence identification of such risk factors will help to remove the causes and risk factors, so as to prevent and control related diseases.

ROLE OF NURSE IN THE EPIDEMIOLOGY OF DISEASES

Using this information, community health nurse can set the priorities for health programmes according to the immediate health needs.

- Establish the health resources more effectively, by giving more emphasis to the urgent health problems needing attention.
- Plan the strategies (steps of action) to meet the new health needs. According to the health problem, she can decide appropriate line of actions or measures to be taken so as to prevent and control the disease ahead of time.
- Evaluate the effectiveness of measures used to control the specific diseases or disorders, community health nurse must evaluate the actions taken to control the diseases, so as to find its usefulness, relevance and appropriateness. It also helps to improve the standards of care and achievements. In case of failures, it gives the scope to improve in providing health care.

Descriptive measurement can tell us what kind of people are at risk of developing certain diseases and disabilities, etc., in the community like leprosy which is more common in which region of India, thus people coming from that place may be the carriers of agent and spread the infection in other areas *e.g.*, filaria is more common in southern part of India. Kala-azar is more among Biharis. The diseases common in age and sex have to be taken specific measures to spread the infections in those people. When we collect data on distribution of diseases, the data must tell that certain diseases are more prevalent in different seasons like measles which commonly spreads from January to March, the diarrhoeal diseases are commonly found in rainy season from June to August, so that precautionary measures can be taken before the incidences occur.

Epidemiology seeks to explain the aetiolgy of specific injuries and diseases, identify and describe factors that contribute to health or illness and provide the basis for developing and evaluating community health programmes to promote wellness and prevent diseases.

Basically, its purpose is to learn why some people get sick and others do not and apply this knowledge to prevent other people from getting sick. Another description is that epidemiology tries to identify the risk factor or variables in an individual's life or environment which give greater risk than average of developing a particular disease thus developing the measures.

●●●

General Measures of Disease Control

14

INTRODUCTION

An outbreak of communicable diseases may be controlled by the following :

1. Eliminating or reducing the source of infection
2. Interrupting the transmission
3. Protecting the person at risk.

It may take sometime before the exact nature of causative agent is known and this will delay the application of specific control measures, such as immunization of person at risk or the treatment of carriers. In an emergency, the first step must be to try to interrupt transmission, since the epidemiological investigations will quickly provide some indications of the possible mode of transmission involved. This may be :

- Person-to-person transmission : Direct or indirect
- Common source of infections
- Combination of both.

TRANSMISSION OF COMMUNICABLE DISEASES (Fig. 14.1)

Person-to-Person Transmission

Communicable diseases are spread by chains of infections through various sources of infection to the host. Mainly, there are three modes of transmission of diseases to the susceptible host, *e.g.*, Direct, indirect and transplacental.

Source of Infection

It is the channel through which the infectious agent passes from reservoir to the susceptible host. These may be a person, animal, object or any substance.

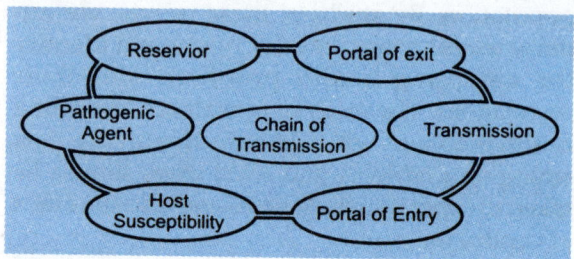

Fig. 14.1 : Transmission of communicable diseases

Reservior of Infection

It is the natural habitat in which agents live and multiply and are ready to enter the host to spread the infection. These can be a person, animal, plant, soil, arthropod and substance.

For example, in case of typhoid, the reservoir is a case or a carrier, but the source of infection is stool, urine, vomitus or contaminated food, milk or water. Source refers to the immediate mode of transmission which may or may not be a part of a reservoir.

Types of Reservior

1. Human,
2. Animal, and
3. Nonliving things.

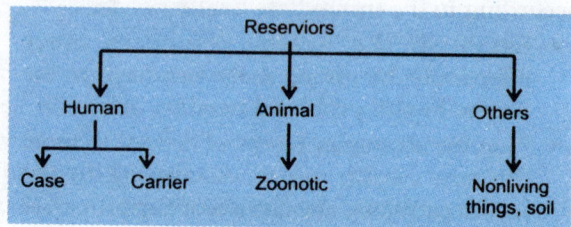

Fig. 14.2: Types of Reservior

Human Reservior

Man is the most important source of infection, in the form of case or carrier. Man is often described as his own enemy, because man is responsible for most of the causation of diseases.

Man as a Case

A case is a person identified as having a particular disease, carries the infection and may spread to other hosts. Presence of infection may be clinical, subclinical or latent.

Clinical case : These cases are identified by their visible signs and symptoms and are diagnosed clinically. The clinical cases may be mild, moderate, typical, atypical, severe or fatal depending upon the degree of illness. Epidemiologically, mild cases are more important sources of infection, because they are ambulant and spread the infection quickly wherever they go.

Subclinical cases : These are inapparent and hidden cases. The patient usually does not show signs and symptoms at this stage. These cases spread the infection either before the occurrence of disease or after the recovery of the disease. The disease agent may multiply in the host but does not manifest itself by signs and symptoms. The disease agent is excreted and contaminates the environment in the same way like clinical case. Subclinical cases play a dominant role in maintaining the chain of infection in the community. Subclinical cases can only be recognised by laboratory tests, *e.g.,* HIV positive patients spread the infection and can be detected by blood examination (ELISA Test).

Latent infection : The case does not spread the infectious agent, but lies dormant within the host without showing signs and symptoms. The clinical symptoms become prominent when the host becomes susceptible and environment conducive to agent, after a long incubation period, *e.g.,* herpes zoster, AIDS and ancylostomiasis.

Carrier

A carrier is defined as an infected person or animal that harbours a specific infectious agent in the absence of clinical manifestations and serves as an important source of infection.

Carriers are usually less infectious than cases, but they are more dangerous than cases because they have hidden infection and escape recognition and continue to live a normal life among people. They readily spread the infection to susceptible host under favourable conditions.

Types of Carriers

These are of three types :
1. Incubatory carriers,
2. Convalescent carriers, and
3. Healthy carriers.

Incubatory carriers : These carriers shed the infectious agent during the incubation period of disease. They spread the disease (infection) before the appearance of clinical manifestation. The duration of communicability depends upon the days of incubation period. Usually the last days of incubation period are highly infectious, *e.g.,* measles, mumps, whooping cough, (pertussis), polio, influenza diphtheria and hepatitis B.

Convalescent carriers : These carriers may spread the infection during convalescent period, that is, after recovery of the disease that is, in case of typhoid fever and cholera who may spread the disease for as long as 6 to 8 weeks. These carriers may cause serious threat to the spread of infection to family members and contaminate the environment. Hence, such infectious diseases should be identified and protected from spread of infection *e.g.,* typhoid.

Healthy carriers : These are carriers of infectious agent, but are clinically healthy. They are the victims of subclinical infection, who have developed infection without suffering from overt disease, but are shedding the infectious agent to other susceptible hosts, and these hosts may get the disease. These diseases may be poliomyelitis, cholera, typhoid, meningococcal meningitis, salmonellosis and diphtheria.

Classification of Carriers by Duration of Time

1. Temporary Carriers : These types of carriers spread the infection for short periods of time. These carriers may be incubatory, convalescent and healthy carriers.

2. Chronic Carriers : They excrete the infectious agent for indefinite time, and may even be for life-long. Chronic carriers occur in many diseases, *e.g.,* typhoid, hepatitis B, dysentery, cerebrospinal meningitis, malaria, gonorrhoea, etc. They are important source of infection in the community. Therefore, their early detection and treatment is essential to prevent the spread of infections.

Classification of Carriers as per Portal of Exit

These carriers are determined by their route of exit to spread the infection.

1. **Intestinal :** Cholera, typhoid, dysentary.
2. **Urinary :** Typhoid.
3. **Respiratory :** Tuberculosis, diphtheria.
4. **Others,** *e.g.,* open wound : Tetanus, etc.

Animal Reservior

Animals are also one of the sources of infections like human sources. The diseases spread through animals are called as **Zoonosis.** There are more than 100 zoonotic infections which may be spread to man, *e.g.,* influenza, yellow fever, rabies, etc.

Birds are also reserviors of infection. When they migrate from one place to another they may carry serious epizootiological and epidemiological risks and spread the infection from one place to another at far distance.

Reservior of Nonliving Things

Soil and other nonliving things also act as reservior of infection and spread the infections, *e.g.,* soil carries the agents of tetanus, and anthrax, etc.

MODES OF TRANSMISSION

Communicable diseases are spread through various modes to the susceptible hosts, depending upon the causative agent. Some of the infectious diseases are spread by single mode, *e.g.,* typhoid fever by vehicle transmission and common cold by droplet nuclei or direct transmission only, whereas some of the diseases are caused by more than one modes, *e.g.,*

measles, mumps and chickenpox are spread by direct as well as indirect modes. AIDS and hepatitis B are spread by multiple routes *e.g.,* (I.V. infusion, placental and sexual routes).

1. **Direct transmission**
   - Direct contact
   - Droplet infection
   - Contact with soil
   - Inoculation into skin/mucosa
   - Transplacental (vertical).
2. **Indirect transmission**
   - Vehicle-borne
   - Vector-borne
     - Mechanical
     - Biological.
3. **Airborne**
   - Droplet nuclei
   - Dust.
4. **Contaminated fomites/articles, clothes, etc.**
5. **Contaminated hands and finger.**

Direct Transmission

Direct Contact

Some of the infectious diseases are caused by direct contact from skin of the patient to the skin of another host which leads to immediate transmission of infectious agents from reservior or source to the susceptible host *e.g.,* by touching, kissing or sexual contacts or continuous close contact. The diseases transmitted through these contacts include STDs, AIDS, leprosy, leptospirosis, diseases related to skin (scabies) and eyes (conjunctivitis, trachoma).

Droplet Infection

The transmission of infection is by direct projection of saliva droplets and nasopharyngeal secretions during coughing, sneezing, spitting, speaking, talking, etc. Particles of 10 μmm (micro millimetres) or greater in diameter can filter in the nose and 5 μmm or lesser can penetrate deeply to reach the alveoli. The droplet infection is usually spread within a distance of 30 to 60 cm between host and case (source) when a healthy susceptible person comes in contact with infected individual within the range, is likely to inhale the micro-organisms and acquire infection.

Diseases spread by droplet infections are mainly respiratory tract infection, eruptive fevers (measles, chickenpox), common cold, diphtheria, whooping cough, tuberculosis, meningococcal meningitis, etc. The droplet infections spread faster in overcrowded places, slums and poor housing conditions, poor ventilations, etc.

Contact with Soil

Some of the infections may be transmitted through direct infected soil contact with body tissues, *e.g.*, hookworm infection, tetanus, etc.

Inoculation into Skin or Mucosa

The disease agents are transmitted directly into skin like rabies virus by dog bite and through contaminated needle and syringes, etc. in case of hepatitis B and AIDS (one of the modes of transmission).

Transplacental Transmission (Mother to Foetus)

The diseased agents are transmitted from mother to foetus, *e.g.*, rubella virus, syphilis, hepatitis B and AIDS and affecting the foetal growth. These disease agents produce malformations of the foetus by disturbing the growth and development.

Indirect Transmission

Transmission of infection is through some modes, *e.g.*, the infective agents spread through fomites, fingers, faeces, flies, food and fluid (water, milk or urine, etc.). It is essential that infectious agents must be capable of surviving outside human host in the external environment and is virulent till it gets into new host. Though this depends upon the characteristics of the agents and other environmental factors, *e.g.*, temperature and humidity, etc. Indirect transmission can occur through:

Vehicle-Borne

The transmission of infectious agents through water, food (including raw vegetables, fruits), milk and milk products, ice, blood, serum, plasma, tissues and organs. Among all these, water and food are the most frequent vehicles of transmission because they are used by everyone and everyday. The infectious agents transmitted through food and water are mainly diseases of alimentary tract, *e.g.*, acute diarrhoeal diseases, typhoid fever, cholera, poliomyelitis, hepatitis A, food poisoning, worm infestation and amoebiasis. The infections spread through blood include hepatitis B, syphillis, malaria, etc.

In case of heavy contamination of food and water, the outbreak will lead to epidemic of the disease. It is not always possible to isolate the infectious agents from the contaminated vehicle, *e.g.*, typhoid bacilli from water. Once the vehicle is controlled, the outbreak of disease, subsides. The common source of infection is usually noticeable.

Vector-Borne

Vector is defined as an arthropod or any living carrier (*e.g.*, snail) that transports an infectious agent to the susceptible individual. The transmission of infection by vector may be mechanical or chemical.

Types of Vector Borne Transmission

Mechanical Transmission

The infectious agent is mechanically transported by crawling or flying arthropods through soiling its feet or by passing the organisms through gastrointestinal tract and passively excreted. There is no development or multiplication of infectious agent on or within the vector.

Biological Transmission

The infectious agent undergoing replication or development or both and requires an incubation period before the vector can transfer. It can be of three types :

Propagative : The agent multiplies in vector without any changes in its form, *e.g.*, plague bacilli in rat fleas.

Cyclopropagative : The agent changes in form and number, *e.g.*, malaria parasite in mosquito.

Cyclo-developmental : Infectious agent undergoes only development but no multiplication, *e.g.*, microfilariae in mosquito.

Transmission Chain of Vector-Borne Disease

1. Man—arthropod—man (Man–mosquito) → malaria.
2. Mammal → arthropod–man → (Dog → rat flea) → plague
3. Bird—arthropod—man– (encephalitis)
4. Man–cyclops–fish—man—(fish tapeworm).

Methods of Transmission of Vector-borne Disease

1. Biting
2. Regurgitation
3. Scratching of infective faeces
4. Contamination of host with body fluids of vectors.

Types of Vectors for Disease Transmission

Invertebrate Vectors

Flies, mosquitoes, fleas, cockroaches, sucking lice, bugs, ticks, mites and cyclops.

Vertebrates

Mice, rodents and bats, etc.

Airborne Transmission

The indirect transmission of infection existing in the polluted environment.

Droplet Nuclei

These are the particles responsible for spread of infection from infected case to susceptible host. They are the tiny particles (1-10 microns) that exist as dry residual of droplets. They may be formed by evaporation of the coughed or sneezed droplets into the air. These nuclei may remain airborne for long period of time, and are liable to be easily drawn into the alveoli of the lungs and will retain there.

The common diseases spread by droplet nuclei are : tuberculosis, chickenpox, measles, and many respiratory diseases.

Dust

The larger droplets are expelled during talking, sneezing and coughing and settle down on floor, carpet, clothes, furniture, beddings, linen and any other objects and become a part of dust. These infectious agents may be bacteria, virus, fungal spores, etc. These bacteria are usually found near the hospital ward and living rooms. Some of them, *e.g.*, tubercle bacilli can survive in dust for considerable time under favourable conditions of temperature and moisture. During sweeping, dusting, bed making, the dust is released into the air and inhaled by the host. Usually, this infection is common for hospital acquired infection.

Fomite-borne Transmission

Contaminated articles or substances other than water and food are capable of harbouring and transmitting the infections to healthy person. These fomites may be clothes, linen, utensils, toys, handkerchief, door handles, taps, books, pencils, lavatory chains, syringes, instruments and surgical dressings. They are important sources of the indirect transmission of various diseases, *e.g.*, cholera, typhoid, dysentery, hepatitis A, intestinal parasites, dyphtheria, measles, eye and skin infections.

Unclean Hands and Fingers (Fig. 14.3)

Hands are considered as most contaminated and most common media to spread the infection. Transmission of infection may be direct (hand to mouth) or indirect. Most common diseases spread through unclean hands are gastroenteritis, typhoid, hepatitis A and intestinal parasites, etc. Unclean hands and fingers and lack of personal hygiene is responsible for these infections.

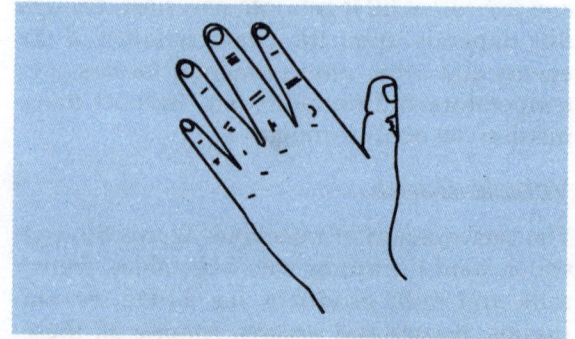

Fig. 14.3 : Uncleaned hand and fingers

PREVENTION OF SPREAD OF INFECTIOUS DISEASES

Special precautions must be taken as soon as an infectious disease is diagnosed. These include :

1. Notification   4. Quarantine
2. Isolation   5. Treatment
3. Disinfection   6. Immunization.

Notification

Certain infectious diseases are notifiable to the medical officer of Primary Health Centres. Not all diseases are notifiable, but certain serious diseases, *e.g.*, smallpox, (eradicated), diphtheria, cholera, typhoid, measles, and poliomyelitis are included in the list. The importance of notification is to allow the health officer to adopt various control measures to prevent the spread of infection. The diseases to be notifiable vary from country to country, and even within same country.

Notification enables early detection of the disease's outbreak, which permits immediate action to be taken by the health authorities to control its spread. Notification is usually done by family members, community leaders, community people, religious, administrative people and teachers. Even on suspicion it can be notified for health authority to verify and diagnose the cases.

Medical officer of health takes steps to trace the source of infection and prevent the spread. He has the power to close schools when necessary, and can issue advice regarding boiling of all water supplies, avoidance of crowd and special arrangement for immunization.

Isolation

This includes isolation of the patient until at risk of infection is passed, as well as isolation of those who have been in contact with the patient until it is certain that they will not develop the disease. Isolation is the oldest communicable disease measure. It is defined as *"Separation, for the period of communicability of infected conditions, as to prevent or limit the direct or indirect transmission of infectious agent from those infected to those who are susceptible, or who may spread the agent to others".*

Infection can be controlled by physical isolation of the case or carrier and treatment (if necessary) until free from infections, provided cases and carriers can be easily identified.

The supervision of contacts varies. Children are usually kept away from school, but adults are not usually excluded from work except in certain serious cases, when the spread of infection is so rapid and widespread that very strict precautions must be taken.

The purpose of isolation is to protect the community by preventing transfer of infection from the reservoir to the possible susceptible hosts. The type of isolation varies with the mode of spread and severity of disease.

Types of Isolation

This is of four types :

1. *Strict isolation*
   • Strict prohibition of visitors and following barrier nursing.
2. *Protective isolation*
   • Preventive measures of items which spread infection.
3. *High security isolation*
   • Complete isolation.
4. *Standard isolation*
   • Required limitations as per diseases.

The patient may either be nursed at home or in hospital. Hospital isolation wherever possible is better than home isolation. Isolation is particularly difficult in rural areas. In some situations the entire village has to be isolated, *e.g.*, in cases of cholera outbreak. The duration of isolation is determined by the duration of communicability of the disease and the effect of chemotherapy on infectivity.

In the home, the room chosen for isolation should be as far away as possible from the living rooms, yet as convenient as possible for the auxillary nurse. It should be quiet and well-ventilated, with as much sunlight and fresh air as possible to help to destroy the bacteria. Easy access to the lavatory and bathroom are a great advantage. All the utensils must be kept separate. The gown must be used inside the room and removed and kept in the room before leaving the isolation room. The hands must be carefully washed and dried before and after attending the patient and after leaving the sickroom.

Visitors are usually not allowed, if permitted, they should wear a protective gown and wash their hands. In respiratory cases, the masks are worn.

Isolation has distinctive value in control of some infectious diseases, *e.g.*, diphtheria, cholera, respiratory diseases, pneumonia, plague, etc. In cases of subclinical and carrier state, the strict isolation will not be able to prevent the spread of disease. Physical isolation is not helpful in cases of tuberculosis, leprosy and STDs. Hence, these cases can be non-infectious by chemical isolation (chemotherapy).

Disinfection

Everything that becomes infected by the patient must be thoroughly disinfected either immediately after use or when the period of infection is passed. The various disinfectants, antiseptic lotions and other measures are used for disinfection of all materials used by patient. Their use ranges from control of communicable diseases to sterilization of sophisticated instruments and treatment of fungal and bacterial infections of skin and mucous membrane.

Definition of Terms

Disinfection is killing of infectious agent outside the body by direct exposure to chemical or physical agents. It can refer to action of disinfectant or antiseptic lotion.

Disinfectant or germicide is a substance which destroys harmful microbes (not usually spores) to prevent transmission of disease. It is suitable to apply only for inanimate objects.

Antiseptic is a substance which destroys or inhibits the growth of micro-organisms. Antiseptics are suitable for application of living tissues.

Deodorant is a substance which suppresses or neutralizes bad odour, *e.g.*, lime or bleaching powder.

Detergent is a surface cleaning agent which acts by lowering surface tension, *e.g.*, soap which removes bacteria along with dirt.

Sterilization is the process of destroying all micro-organisms including spores. This is widely used in medical practice.

TYPES OF DISINFECTION

Concurrent Disinfection

The concurrent disinfection is carried out during the course of the illness. It is the application of disinfective measures as soon as possible after the discharge of infectious material from the body of an infected person. The disease agent is destroyed as soon as it is released from the body and stops the spread of infection. Concurrent disinfection consists of usually disinfection of urine, stool, vomitus, linen, clothes, hands, dressings, apron and gloves, etc. during the course of an illness.

Linen

All infected linen should be received into covered bucket at the bedside. The bucket should contain a suitable disinfectant and the articles should be left to soak for the required length of time before being rinsed and then rounded. Disinfectants which can be used are :

Dettol : 1 Tablespoonful to 1 pint of water for half an hour.

Lysol : 1 Tablespoonful to 1 pint of water for one hour.

Carbolic : 1 : 20 for one hour.

Do not put your hands into disinfectants, as they are skin irritants, but rinse the articles thoroughly in plain water before using it.

Utensils

All utensils handled by patient should be rinsed in running water and boiled for five minutes. Articles which can not be boiled may be soaked in a disinfectant but they must be carefully washed and rinsed properly to be used for food intake.

Excreta

If excreta is a source of infection, it must be covered with a disinfectants, *e.g.*, carbolic lotion 1:20 for four hours and then thrown away. The lavatory pan should be flushed, cleaned and mopped with disinfectant kept for the purpose.

While soaking, the excreta should be left in the bedpan, which is completely covered with a cloth wrung out in the disinfectant.

Discharge

Nasal and throat discharge should be received either into paper, handkerchief or pieces of old linen and be burnt immediately. Similarly, dressings from infected wound must be burnt at once.

Terminal Disinfection

The disinfection carried out when the patient is declared free from infection. It is the application of disinfective measures after the patient has been removed by death or to a hospital or has ceased to be a source of infection. All valuable articles in the room such as cheap toys, clothes, books should be burnt. Terminal disinfection is now scarcely practiced. Terminal cleaning is considered sufficient along with sunning and airing of room, furniture, and beddings, etc.

Patient

When declared free from infection, the patient and the caretaker should take thorough bath, including hairwash, complete change of clothes and patient can be shifted to another room.

Rooms

In majority of cases through airing of room followed by conscientious washing of the room and its furnishings should be sufficient. In certain cases, the rooms are fumigated.

Faeces and Urine

Should be collected in impervious vessels and disinfected by adding disinfectant of equal volume and kept for 1 to 2 hours. Faeces should be broken with the stick to allow proper disinfection. If no disinfectant is available, a bucket of boiled water may be added and allowed to stand until cool. After disinfection the excreta matter may be emptied into laterine and flushed or burried into ground. Bedpans and urinals should be steam disinfected and mopping with 20 per cent of cresol.

Sputum

Sputum can be received in a paper, cloth or handkerchief and destroyed by burning. It may also be disinfected by boiling. Usually the patient is asked to collect the sputum in disinfected liquid (5% cresol) in the sputum cup and when the cup is full, it is kept for one hour and then emptied into running water, drained or disposed off by burning.

DISINFECTION AGENTS

Natural

Sunlight

Sunlight is the natural, easily available and safest disinfectant to kill the micro-organisms. Direct and continuous exposure to sunlight is destructive to many disease producing organisms. The ultraviolet rays of sunlight kill the bacteria and some viruses. Articles such as linen, bedding, furniture may be disinfected by exposure to sunlight for several hours.

Air

Exposure to open air (airing) acts by drying or evaporation of moisture which kill bacteria.

Both the natural agents are useful disinfectants practiced for the purpose.

Physical Agents

Boiling Methods

Boiling and steaming are effective methods of disinfection. Boiling for 5 to 10 minutes will kill bacteria, but not spores or viruses. Boilers provide temperature of 90ºC in an atmosphere of steam. To ensure destruction of viruses and spores, temperature above 100ºC would be required, which can not be achieved in boilers. Boiling is suitable for disinfecting small instruments, tools (dressing sets) which are not used for subcutaneous insertion (needles). Linen stained with faeces, pus or blood should be first washed in cold water (preferably disinfectant, e.g., cresol of 2.5 per cent concentration) and then boil it. Adding soap and 3 per cent of washing soda will be more effective in boiling. Boiling linen, utensils and bedpans require 30 minutes for effective disinfection.

Burning

Burning or incineration is an excellent method of disinfection. Inexpensive articles such as dressings, rags, swabs can be disposed off by burning. Faeces can be disposed of by burning. Burning should not be done in open air, it is best done in an incinerator.

Hot Air

It is one of the effective methods of sterilizing articles, *e.g.*, glass articles, syringes, swabs, dressings, oil, vaseline and sharp instruments. Hot air has no penetrating power and is, therefore, not suitable for disinfecting the bulky articles, *e.g.*, mattresses. Hot air sterilization is done in hot air oven. The temperature of the oven is maintained at 160 to 180ºC for at least one hour to kill spores. Such high temperature can even destroy plastic, rubber and other delicate articles.

Autoclaving

Sterilization at high temperature in excess of 100ºC and 70 pounds pressure is called auto-claving. They generate steam under pressure which is most effective disinfecting agent. Autoclaving is widely used in hospital and laboratory practices. It destroys all forms of lives, *e.g.*, spores, eggs, and viruses, etc. It acts by giving off its latent heat. Autoclaving is the most effective method of sterilization of dressing articles, linen, gloves, syringes, instruments and culture medias. It is not suitable to sterilize the plastic and sharp instruments.

Radiation

Radiation is used to sterilize dressings, bandages, catguts and surgical instruments. The objects are packed in plastic or cloth sheets before radiation and will remain closed until used. The radiations have penetrating power with little or no heating effect. It is one of the most viable, safe and economic methods of disinfection and is commonly used.

Chemical Agents like Physical Agents

Objects which can not be sterilized by physical or natural agents can be disinfected by immersing in chemical disinfectants. Chemical agents are also used to disinfect faeces, urine and other contaminated materials. Various chemical agents can be used for the purpose.

Phenol or Carbolic Acid

Germicidal effects.

Crude Phenol

Mixture of phenol and cresol. It is effective against Gram-positive and Gram-negative bacilli and certain viruses, less effective for spores, used for mopping of floors and cleaning drains.

Cresol

Powerful disinfectant and not more toxic. It is best used for disinfection of faeces and urine.

Dettol (Chloroxylenol)

It is non-toxic antiseptic and can be used safely in high concentrations. It is more easily inactivated by organic matters. It is active against streptococcus, but ineffective against Gram-negative bacteria. Dettol 5 per cent is suitable for disinfection of instruments and plastic equipment, by keeping them for fifteen minutes.

Cetavlon (Cetrimide)

It is an active bactericidal against Gram-positive organisms, but less effective in case of Gram-negative. Cetavlon is soluble in water and has soapy property. The concentration of 1 to 2 per cent of cetavlon is usually effective.

Savlon (Cetavlon and Hibitares)

Commonly used disinfectant for clinical thermo-meters and plastic articles in normal strength for 20 minutes.

Bleaching Powder

Also called as chlorinated lime, is white amorphous powder with a pungent smell of chlorine. It kills most of organisms when used in strength of 1 to 3 per cent. Bleaching powder is widely used in public health practices for disinfection of water, faeces and urine and used as a deodrant. A 5 per cent solution is suitable for disinfection of faeces and urine kept for one hour.

Iodine

Iodine, an alcoholic solution of 1 to 2 per cent, is still one of the most effective skin antiseptics available, but it stains the skin and may produce sensitivity reaction in some people.

Alcohols

Ethyl alcohol is commonly used as antiseptic and disinfectant. Ethyl alcohol (Methylated spirit) is used for skin disinfection and handwashing. Pure alcohol is not effective disinfectant, but when diluted to 70 per cent strength is a good antiseptic.

Quarantine

This is used to restrict the contacts of a well person who has been exposed to a patient with an infectious disease during the communicability period. Quarantine must be adapted to the risk to which the person concerned was exposed and the risk that he represents to the community. The restrictions imposed should not be excessive from either humanitarian or economic point of view.

The Community

The protection of patients and the isolation of the contacts in quarantine will considerably decrease the risk for the community. However, as it may not be possible to identify all patients and contacts, other methods also have to be considered :

Mass immunization: Emergency mass immunization is possible for a limited number of diseases. In case of delay in population protection by the vaccine, other methods may, therefore, be necessary.

Restriction of mass gathering : Such restrictions may be indicated, including closure of schools and even of public places, though the effectiveness is generally limited.

Restriction on travel : This involve the restriction of the entry of infectious persons in the country. The aim is to make sure that unimmunized persons do not travel and thereby carry the disease to other countries.

Epidemiological surveillenc : Case finding, contact tracing and prevention of transmission should all be strengthened in any group in which suspected cases have appeared.

Community participation : Keeping the community informed will reduce the risk of panic. If the community can be induced to participate in the control measures, this will contribute considerably to their effectiveness.

CONTROL OF OUTBREAKS CAUSED BY COMMON SOURCE OF INFECTION

When an outbreak is caused by a common source of infections—whether by arthropod, rodent, direct contact with vertebra animals, food, water, air and soil or a combination of any of these—control method should be based on source reduction and interruption of transmission. The assistance of a specialist entomologist, mammalogist, veterinarian, or sanitary engineer may be required.

Mosquito Borne Diseases

Mosquitoes capable of transmitting diseases to man belong to several species and their control raises technical problem that require the assistance of a specialised team. They constitute the most important group of insect vectors transmitting malaria, filaria, and a number of arboviruses, including those causing yellow fever, dengue and dengue haemorrhagic fever, Japanese encephalitis, etc. They lay their eggs in impounded water, selected according to the preference of species. The time necessary for eggs to hatch and for the larvae they produce to become pupae and adults is reduced at higher temperature. If it is to be cost-effective, mosquito control requires methodical planning of strategy, logistics and field operation. It should be noted that a patient with a mosquito-borne diseases, *e.g.,* dengue or yellow fever in *Aedes acgypti*-infested areas, malaria in *Anopheles* infested areas, should not be moved into an area where such mosquitoes are present. Such movement may be subject to local health regulation.

The method used for mosquito control will vary according to mosquito species concerned. They include insecticide spraying personnel, protection, source reduction and environmental sanitation.

Spraying of insecticides to which the vectors are susceptible is used in emergency measures, mainly to control the mosquito vectors of malaria and epidemic arboviral diseases and can rapidly reduce the density of man biting segment of vector population and thus quickly stops or reduces transmission to man.

Well maintained bed nets and mesh screens fitted to door and windows can give good personal protection against mosquito. Long sleeves and trousers are recommended. Repellents have only a temporary effects.

Environmental sanitation constitutes an important means of controlling mosquito vectors, both in an emergency and long-term. Open drains and ditches frequently provide breeding sites for large number of certain mosquito species. Drains and ditches should be kept in good order so as to ensure gravitational flow and the disposal of unwanted water and effluents. Soakpits require sealed covers and laterines should have well-fitted lids flooding.

Rodent-Borne Disease

Rodents may be the reservoirs of a number of epidermic diseases, including plague, yersiniosis, lymphocytosis, lassae fever, leptospirosis and haemorrhagic fever. Certain rodent-borne diseases may be passed from rodents to man by direct transmission, others through arthropod vectors. Direct transmission occurs as a result of contamination of food and water by rodent urine and can thus also be regarded as indirect.

Epidemiological investigations will determine which procedures, *e.g.*, environmental improvement, rodent proofing and domestic rodent examination by rodenticides, are to be used and in which order.

In an outbreak of plague, the first step in control operations is to use insecticides to kill rat fleas before using rodenticides to kill the rats.

Zoonoses

Different routes of transmission to man are possible :

- Direct
- Through arthropods and rodents
- Through food and the environments.

Direct transmission is mainly an occupational risk of veternary personnel, farmers and hunters and may be more frequent in areas of poor hygiene. Control measures for outbreak resulting from direct contact with animal vary, depending on the diseases and circumstances.

Food-Borne Diseases

Food-borne diseases may be divided into intoxications (food poisoning) and infections. Outbreaks are most frequently caused by *Salmonella, Clostridium perfringens, Staphylococcus, botulism, Bacillus cereus, Camphylobacter, Escherichia coli, Yessinia enterocolitica*. In many cases, the origin of food-borne desease remains unknown and viral agents, including hepatitis A virus, may be more frequently involved than indicated by present data. Food may be contaminated by a large number of toxic chemicals (including pesticides) and their identification and the treatment of those affected require the services of toxicologists.

Outbreak of food-borne diseases usually constitutes an emergency because of the threat that they pose to the life of the individual or to be taken when an outbreak occurs are either general, if the agent is unknown or specific, if it has been identified. The occurrence of an outbreak should serve to stimulate improvements in food sanitation so as to ensure that a repetition is avoided.

Treatment

Many communicable diseases can be controlled by effective chemotherapy, by killing the causative organisms, when they are still in the reservoirs, *e.g.*, before entering the host. Treatment reduces the communicability of disease, cuts short the duration of illness and prevents the development of secondary cases. In some diseases, *e.g.*, syphilis, tuberculosis and leprosy, early diagnosis and treatment is of primary importance in interrupting transmission. Treatment can also be given to confirmed carriers.

Treatment can be applied to the individual, family and community at large, depending upon the type of infections and availability of the medicines. In certain cases, *e.g.*, trachoma, all community people are given prophylaxis, administration of drug, whether they have disease or not.

Interruption of Transmission

Many communicable diseases can be controlled by breaking the chain of transmission or interruption of transmission (Fig. 14.4). For example, water can be a medium for the transmission of many diseases, *e.g.*, typhoid, dysentery, hepatitis A, cholera, poliomyelitis and gastroenteritis. Water treatment will help in preventing all these diseases. Depending upon the level of pollution this may vary from simple chlorination to complex treatment.

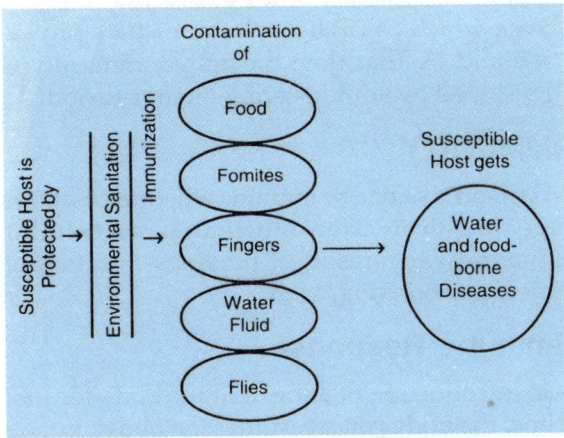

Fig. 14.4 : Interruption of Transmission

Control of Source of Contamination

It is an important long-term measure. Food borne disease is particularly prevalent in areas with low standards of hygiene. Clean practices, *e.g.*, handwashing, adequate cooking, prompt refrigeration of prepared food and withdrawal of contaminated food will prevent most of the food-borne diseases. In case of vector-borne diseases, the control of vectors and their breeding places are of primary importance. In case of droplet and droplet nuclei, it is necessary to control the cases. Environmental sanitation, adequate sunlight will kill the micro-organisms. The cases can be controlled by early diagnosis and prompt treatment of the patient. Personal hygiene and proper disposal of secretions and excretions will help in controlling the spread of infections.

Protection of Susceptible Host

The prevention and control of communicable diseases can be done by protecting the susceptible host (man) by immunization.

Immunization

Immunization is the most effective means of protecting the greatest number of people, by reducing the number of susceptibles in the community. There are some infectious diseases, whose control is solely based on active immunization, *e.g.*, tuberculosis, poliomyelitis, diphtheria, measles, whooping cough and pertussis, etc. Immunization against these diseases is given as a routine programme during infancy and early childhood to maintain adequate level of immunity.

Types of Immunity

Innate or Natural

Immunity developed by child by virtue of his genetic constitutions. This immunity lasts for a short-time, but it protects the baby during the first few months of life, when child is most susceptible, and infectious diseases are most dangerous, if they should occur. Some people appear to be naturally immune to certain diseases, throughout their lives, due to some constitutional factors in themselves. Immunity developed is usually specific in certain species and races, *e.g.*, *S. typhi* produces serious illness in man but non-pathogenic in mice. This is called species immunity.

Acquired Immunity

This is the immunity when a person develops during the lifetime, which may be active or passive.

Active Acquired Immunity

Active acquired immunity may be developed by introduction of natural antigens or artificially administration of antigens to produce anti-bodies. The body is stimulated to produce its own antibodies. Immunity produced is specific for a particular disease.

Natural active immunity is developed by :

• Attack of the disease,
• Subclinical infection.

Artificial active immunity : When antigens of specific diseases are introduced into the body and antibodies are produced by the retinoendo-thelial cells to produce immunity which lasts for long time, *e.g.,* administration of vaccines—toxoids, killed or live.

The active immunity takes time to develop antibodies within the body, but once it is developed will provide immunity for longer period or even lifelong.

Passive Natural Acquired Immunity

When antibodies are prepared in one body (human body or animal) are transferred to another to induce protection against disease is known as "Passive Immunity". Passive immunity of the antibodies are transmitted from mother to the foetus via placenta and mother to newborn via breast milk to protect against various diseases. These antibodies protect the infant during the first few months of life against communicable diseases, *e.g.,* tetanus, chicken-pox, measles and poliomyelitis. The antibodies transmitted to the newborn depends upon the immunity status of the mother. Human milk carries antibodies to protect the child. Thus, it is important to emphasis on breast milk to child and adequate immune system of the mother.

(i) Artificial passive acquired immunity : When readymade antibodies are introduced into the human body, it is called artificial passive immunity, *e.g.,*

(a) *Antiserum :* Passive immunity may be introduced by administering antiserum against specific disease, *e.g.,* tetanus, diphtheria and rabies.

(b) *Human gamaglobulin :* Administration of human gamaglobulin produces passive immunity.

Passive immunity is usually given against certain diseases after exposure to infection, and immediate immunity is required.

Immunity is developed rapidly and is of shorter duration. Thus, in some diseases, *e.g.,* tetanus both active and passive immunity is given which (ATS) helps in immediate protec-tion and by that time the active immunity is developed by administering tetanus toxoid.

IMMUNITY

A person is said to be immune when he possesses specific protection antibodies or cellular immunity as a result of previous infection or immunization (Fig. 14.5).

Immune Response

On introduction of antigen in the body for first time, the body cells react into the body.

Primary Response (Fig. 14.6)

The first time exposure to the antigen introduced in the body, the latent period is 3 to 10 days for

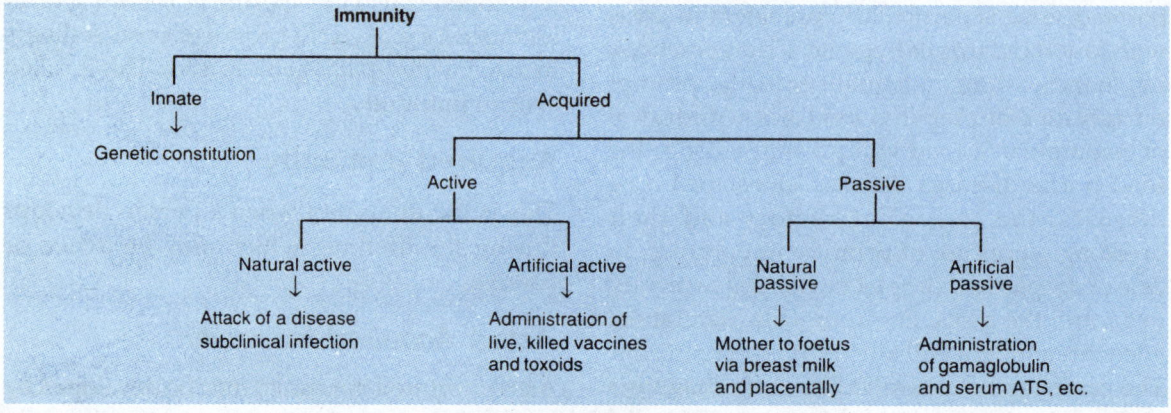

Fig. 14.5 : Immunity

antibodies to appear in the blood. These antibodies rise at the peak in 2 to 3 days and reaches at peak level and then decline fast.

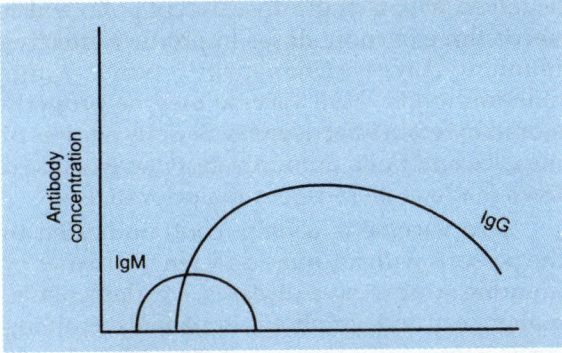

Fig. 14.6 : Primary Response

The first IgM type antibodies appear in the body. If the antigenic stimulus was sufficient, IgG antibodies appear in few days which reaches a peak within 7 to 10 days and gradually falls within weeks or months. The extent of primary response depends upon dose of antigen, nature of antigen (killed or live), route of administration, nutritional and health status of the host. In case of small dose of antigen only IgM type of response may be developed, small doses of antigen at suitable interval may also develop IgM antibodies. To develop IgG antibodies, the dose is required 50 times more than for IgG antibodies, with the primary antigen there is production of 'memory cells' and 'primed cells' by β (Beta) and T (Thymus) lymphocytes. These cells are responsible for immunological memory which becomes established after immunization. The purpose of immunization is to develop immunological memory.

Secondary Response (Booster)

The secondary response has a shorter latent period, production of antibodies is faster and abundant. Antibody response maintained at higher level and for longer period of time.

Secondary response produces IgG and IgM types of antibodies. There is a brief production of IgM and larger and prolonged production of IgG antibody. These responses stimulate the memory cells, thus primary and secondary responses are the basis for immunization by vaccination and booster doses.

Humoral Immunity

It is developed from β-cells (bone marrow) and they produce specific antibodies after antigen enters the body. The antibodies produced are of five types immunoglobulins *e.g.*,

1. IgG   2. IgM   3. IgA
4. IgD and   5. IgE.

They circulate in the blood and neutralize the microbe, or its toxins. These immunoglobulins have the different functions to meet the different types of antigenic challenges. All antibodies are immunoglobulins.

IgG : It is the major immunoglobulin consisting 75 per cent of total serum immunoglobulin. Due to its smaller molecular weight, it can diffuse into interstitial fluid and can also pass through placenta. Antibodies found in IgG are against most of Gram-positive bacteria, virus and toxins of bacilli.

IgM : It forms 10 per cent of serum immunoglobulin. Antibodies of IgM are formed with exposure to antigens. Its production usually appears in recent infections. It has high agglutinating and fixing ability.

IgA : Constitutes about 15 per cent of total serum Ig. Antibody activities are against wide range of bacterial and viral antigens. IgA is found in large quantity in body secretion, *e.g.*, saliva, milk, colostrum, tears, bronchial secretion, nasal secretion, vaginal secretion and intestinal secretion. It provides protection mainly against local infection of the above organs.

IgD : It is estimated as limited quantity in serum and the function is not yet determined.

IgE : It is concentrated in submucous tissues and major antibody response is for immediate anaphylactic reactions.

Cellular Immunity

Cellular immunity is mediated from 'T' cells. They do not produce antibodies, but can recognise antigens and initiate the responses, *e.g.*, activating macrophages, release of cytotoxins. Cellular immunity is responsible for immunity against many diseases, *e.g.*, tuberculosis, brucellosis and for body's rejection to foreign material, *e.g.*, skin grafting. A child born with severe defect in cellular immunity will result in death within 6 months of life.

Herd Immunity

The protection of the whole population against the infectious diseases prevalent in the areas is called herd immunity. It is the level of resistance of a community to a particular disease. Herd immunity can be maintained by:

1. Occurrence of clinical and subclinical infection in community.
2. Mass immunization.
3. Community structure—health status, births, deaths and mobility. Regular immunization programme in the community will keep up the herd immunity at very high level. In community, with sufficient immunity level will reduce the incidence of epidemics and prevent morbidity and mortality due to infectious disease.

Herd structure is not only the population but also animal host and possible insect vector, environmental and social factors that favours or inhibits the spread of infection from host to host. The herd structure also play important role in immunity status of community.

Immunizing Agents

These are active or passive antigens or antibodies prepared and introduced into the body for specific protection against specific diseases. These agents may be classified as vaccines, toxoids and immunoglobulins :

Vaccines : Vaccine is an immunobiological substance designed to produce specific protection against a specific disease. It stimulates the production of protective antibody and other immune mechanisms. Vaccines are prepared either by line attenuated organisms or inactivated by killing organisms and extracting toxins to produce toxoids.

Live vaccine : These are prepared from live attenuated organisms. These organisms have been prepared on tissue culture or chick embryo and become inactive to cause the full blown disease, but are capable of causing immunity in the body. These vaccine are more potent immunizing agents than killed vaccines. In the case of live vaccines, immunization is generally achieved with a single dose except polio which needs three or more doses to produce effective immunity. Live vaccine usually produces a durable immunity. Live vaccine may be properly stored to retain effectiveness. Serious failures of measles and polio immunization have resulted from inadequate refrigeration prior to use.

Live vaccine is usually contraindicated to the persons with immune deficiency diseases or immune suppressive diseases, *e.g.*, leukaemia, malignancy and lymphoma or patients receiving corticosteroids and pregnant women.

The examples of live vaccine are :

Bacterial : B.C.G., typhoid oral and plague.
Viral   : Oral polio, yellow fever, measles, mumps, rubella, influenza.

Killed vaccine : The organisms are killed by heat or chemicals, and introduced into the body to cause immunity. They are usually safe though less effective than live vaccine. Killed vaccine usually requires booster doses at least 2 to 3 times, for its longer effects by producing sufficient antibodies response. Cholera vaccine offers only 50 per cent protection. The 3 doses of pertussis vaccine gives 80 per cent protection for first three years and nil by 12 years. Killed vaccines are usually administered by subcutaneous or intramuscular route. The only absolute contraindication to the administration of killed vaccine is severe local or general reaction to a previous dose.

Examples :

Killed vaccine

Bacterial : Typhoid, cholera, pertussis, plague, meningitis.
Viral   : Polio (salk), influenza, rabies, hepatitis B, Japanese encephalitis, KFD.

Toxoids : Some organisms produce exotoxins, *e.g.*, tetanus, diphtheria bacilli. The toxins produced by these organisms are detoxicated and used in the preparation of vaccines. The introduction of prepared toxoids help in production of antibodies, which help in neutralizing the toxins of specific infectious agents. These toxoids are highly effective and safe immunizing agents.

Example :

Bacterial ———< Diphtheria toxoids / Tetanus toxoids

Cellular agents : Some vaccines are prepared from cellular extracts. These vaccines are usually prepared from polysaccharide antigens of cell wall of organisms or polypeptides, etc. The examples of allulen vaccines are meningococcal, pneumococcal vaccines and hepatitis B vaccine.

Combined vaccine : When more than two or three vaccines are combined to introduce in the body to protect against infection is called combined vaccine. The purpose of combined vaccine is for simple administration, cost-effective and less visits paid by patient.

The examples of combined vaccines are :

Diphtheria Pertussis Tetanus (DDT), Diphtheria (DT), Diphtheria Pertussis (DP), Diphtheria Polio Tetanus (D.P.T.) and typhoid, MMR + DPTP

Adjuvants for vaccines : Some vaccines are prepared as plain vaccines, whereas some as adjuvant vaccines. Adjuvants are the substances that are added to the vaccines to increase the potentiality for immune system, so as to produce greater amount of antibodies with lesser quantity of antigens introduced with less doses of vaccines. The commonly used adjuvants are aluminium hydroxide, aluminium phosphate, water in oil. These vaccines are more effective than plain vaccine.

Freeze dried vaccines : These vaccines are more stable than liquid vaccines. For example, B.C.G., yellow fever, and measles.

Immunoglobulin : There are mainly five classes of immunoglobulins—IgG, IgM, IgA, IgD and IgE performing different functions to produce antigenic effect.

IMMUNIZING AGENTS

Immunizing agents are the readymade preparation of antigens and antibodies. The immunizing may be classified as vaccines, toxoids, immunoglobulins and antisera.

Two types of Ig preparations are available for passive immunity.

1. Human Ig.
2. That is normal human Ig and specific human Ig.

These are used as prophylaxis against viral and bacterial infections.

Normal Human Ig

It is used to prevent measles in highly susceptible persons and provide temporary protections against hepatitis A. The WHO has recommended that these Ig should have 90 per cent of IgG type and low IgA concentration. Live vaccine should not be given for at least 12 weeks after an infections of normal human Ig and if live vaccine has been given then Ig should be deferred for two weeks.

Specific Human Ig

These preparations are derived from plasma of patients blood, who has recently recovered from disease or from individuals who have been immunized against specific infections, thus they provide immediate protection. These are mainly used in case of chickenpox prophylaxis of highly susceptible individuals and for postexposure prophylaxis of hepatitis B, rabies and tetanus prophylaxis.

Ig are usually given intramuscularly. The adverse reaction can be local or systemic. Local reactions, *e.g.,* pain and abscesses are quite common when large volumes are infected. Intramuscularly systemic reaction can be rapid or slow. Rapid reaction can be anaphylactic shock and late can be utricaria, arthrasia, diarrhoea and fever, etc.

Antisera or Antitoxins

The antisera are prepared from non human source, *e.g.,* horses. These are prepared for few diseases, *e.g.,* diphtheria, tetanus, botulism, gas gangrene and snakebite. These are passive immunization. Administration of antisera may cause serum sickness and anaphylactic shock due to sensitivity reaction.

NATIONAL IMMUNIZATION PROGRAMMES

Expanded Programme on Immunization

In 1974, WHO launched a global immunization programme known as EPI with the aim to protect all children of the world against six-vaccine-preventable diseases, *e.g.*, diphtheria, tuberculosis, whooping cough (Pertussis), polio, measles and tetanus which has been now declared as seven including hepatitus B. In India EPI was launched in 1978.

National Immunization Schedule

WHO's EPI Programme (Extended Programme for Immunization)

WHO's Global Advisory Committee for EPI Programme in 1978 had recommended an Immunization Schedule for children and pregnant women. The immunization schedule may be altered to suit the local needs of individuals and groups, keeping in mind the EPI concept. Immunization given in appropriate age as scheduled is very effective means of protecting the child from 7 killing diseases. In case immunization is delayed the child can still be given the appropriate doses of immunization. If the second or third dose of immunization, the immunization schedule has to be repeated again. In case of delayed immunization two vaccines DPT or BCG or measles can be given at the same time but different sites.

WHO has highly recommended BCG and polio at birth or first contact in countries where TB and poliomyelitis are highly prevalent. In other countries routine immunization with DPT and oral polio can be safely and effectively given at 6 weeks of age.

Immunization can be delayed in case child is very sick or malnurished. A child with minor ailment is usually not deprived of immunization *e.g.*, low grade fever, cough, cold, diarrhoea and other minor problems, etc. These children are more in need of vaccine to improve health status.

Universal Immunization Programme

The programme is now called universal immunization programme in 1990; this name was given to a declaration sponsored by UNICEF as a part of United Nations 40th anniversary to the global programme of EPI.

The UIP was launched on November 19, 1985 and is being implemented in the entire country in the memory of Smt. Indira Gandhi. The aim of UIP was to achieve the immunization coverage of the eligible population by 1990. This programme has put upon a high responsibility of rendering quality immunization services to all pregnant women, and infants. To prevent various infectious diseases.

Objectives

(a) Under the immunization programme all infants should be protected against tuberculosis, diphtheria, whooping cough, tetanus, poliomyelitis and measles and all pregnant women against tetanus by vaccination.

(b) Pregnant women should be given two doses of TT, one month interval, as early as possible during pregnancy. If she has received TT during previous pregnancy then she should be given one dose of TT during the current pregnancy.

(c) All infants are to be provided with one dose of BCG, three doses of DPT and OPV and one dose of measles vaccine. These are to be completed before the first birthday of the child.

(d) The children between 16 to 24 months, who have received the above doses, should also receive booster of DPT and OPV.

(e) Children at the age of 5 to 6 years should receive the dose of DT.

(f) Children above one year, if not vaccinated earlier, should also be vaccinated and BCG, DPT, OPV and measles can be given on the same day. But it is desirable that vaccination is completed before first year of child.

WHO EPI IMMUNIZATION SCHEDULE

Global Advisory Committee recommended EPI programme for effective immunization against seven killer diseases, which can be prevented among children. WHO has highly recommended

BCG and polio vaccines to be given at birth or at first contact, in the countries where tuberculosis and polio are highly prevalent and have not been controlled. In all countries routine immunization of DPT and polio can be safely and effectively given at six weeks of age.

The immunization schedule recommended by WHO can be altered according to the needs and resources of the community people. Even if child gets one dose, will give desirable amount of immunity. In case, second dose is delayed, immunization should not restart, but give the second dose. Two or more vaccines can be given in one day, if it is on different routes.

National Immunization Schedule

For Pregnant Women

In early preganancy (at 5 months) T.T. first dose

For infants

Immunization can be given to children with mild health problems or sickness, e.g., diarrhoea, fever, respiratory infection. Giving of immunization will help to maintain the resistance, health and protect from many health problems. If vaccination is not given, they are most likely to die with the disease which are vaccine-preventable.

The Cold Chain

Cold chain is a "system of storage and transportation of vaccines at low temperature from the manufacturer to the actual vaccination site". It is important to maintain the cold chain, to keep the temperature of the vaccine, so as to keep its potency and efficacy. Some vaccines must be kept in freezing temperature e.g., polio, measles and BCG. Vaccine like DPT, tetanus and typhoid must be kept in cold part, but is not allowed to freeze. Polio is the most sensitive to heat and must be kept under –20°C. Vaccines must be protected from sunlight and prevent the contact with antiseptic lotions. Most of the vaccines can

Age Infants and Children	Vaccine	Route	Dose
AT '0' –1½ months	BCG (injection) DPT – 1 (injection) OPV – 1 (oral) HBV. – 1	Intradermal Intramuscular oral	0.01 mL 0.5 mL 2 drops 0.5 mL
2½ months	DPT – 2 OPV – 2 HBV – 2	I/M oral I/M	0.5 2 drops 0.5 mL
3½ months	DPT – 3 OPV – 3	I/M oral	0.5 mL 2 drops
9 – 12 months	Measles OR MMR	Subcutaneous	0.5 mL
16 – 24 months	DPT – Booster I OPV – Booster I OPV – Booster II		
5 – 6 years	DT	I/M	0.5 mL
10 – 16 years	T.T.	I/M	0.5 mL
Pregnant Woman			
Early in pregnancy at 5 months	T.T.	I/M	0.5 mL
7 months	T.T.	I/M	0.5 mL

Children born in institution should receive BCG and OPV – 0 dose at birth.

be stored for 5 to 6 weeks in the refrigerator at the 4 to 8°C temperature. Open vials must be used within 1 to 3 hours and rest should be discarded, not to preserve or reuse.

Cold Chain Equipment

The specialised cold chain consists of the following equipment :

Walk in Cold Room

They are located at the regional level for the purpose of storing the vaccine and transporting to adjoining districts and can be stored for at least three months.

Deep Freezer and Icelined Refrigerator

These freezers are supplied to all the districts and regional centres to store the supplied vaccines. Deep freezers are used for making ice packs and to store polio vaccine and measles vaccine.

Small Deep Freezers

These small deep freezers are supplied to all the primary health centres (PHC), health centres, urban municipal corporation health (MCH) centres. These freezers are used to prepare ice packs, and used for cold boxes, vaccine carriers for transportation of vaccines and use during the vaccination.

A dial thermometer should be placed in the freezer and temperature should be recorded at least twice a day. In case of defrosting the vaccine should be shifted to the cold box to keep up the temperature. In case of electrical failure, the vaccine must be transferred to ice box and then to any other alternative vaccine storage.

Instructions : The equipment must be kept in cool room, away from direct sunlight and some distance away from wall.

- The equipment must be labelled, locked and opened only when necessary.
- There must be voltage stabilizer fixed with equipment.

- It should be defrosted regularly.
- Check the temperature and record twice a day.
- Do not keep any other object on the refrigerator and inside the refrigerator.
- Do not keep other drugs, expired vaccines and stock more than one month's use.

The vaccines in the primary health centre, health centres and municipal corporation health centres are stored in these small deep freezers. These contain two ice packs and can be used for few hours.

Ice Packs

These are packs containing water and not salt added to it. The water should be filled up with the level marked on the side. Make sure that there is no leakage.

The cold chain can not be maintained at subcentres due to electrical and other problems. Hence these vaccines should be stored in the primary health centre and transported daily to subcentres. If cold chain is not maintained, the chances of failures of cold chain is greater and ineffectively and hazards are more.

Cold Boxes

The cold boxes are supplied to transport the vaccines at the peripheral level. The ice packs are kept on the bottom and sides of the box and the vaccine. The vaccines are kept in the poly-thene bags and should not be kept directly with the ice packs. The boxes must be closed tightly.

Vaccine carriers : The vaccine carriers are used to carry the vaccines for the immunization sessions. The ice packs are placed at the sides of the vaccine carriers, or vials should be kept in polythene and not directly into the vaccine carriers. These should be closed tightly.

Day carriers : These carriers are used to carry small quantity of vaccines (6-8 vials) to the nearby place of immunization.

HAZARDS OF IMMUNIZATION

Most of the vaccine carry some sort of hazards to the child. These hazards may be local or generalised, as listed below.

Local Reaction to Inoculation

There may be local reaction at the inoculation site, *e.g.*, pain, swelling, redness, tenderness and formation of small nodule or abscess at the site.

General Reaction of Vaccination

May be headache, bodyache, fever and other associated symptoms. Most of killed vaccine, they cause moderate local and general reaction. Diphtheria, tetanus toxoid and polio have the mild reaction.

Reaction Due to Hypersensitivity

Antiserum (ATS) may cause anaphylactic shock and serum sickness. Though it is rare, but severe complication, which causes dyspnoea, tachycardia, hypotension, cold clammy skin, restlessness, bronchospasm and collapse. The symptoms may appears within few minutes to few hours of injection. Serum sickness is characterised by fever, oedeme, rash and joint pain occurs within 7 to 12 days of injection of antiserum.

Neurological Manifestations

The central nervous system (CNS) involvement due to vaccines may be fatal. These symptoms may be postvaccine encephilitis and encephalopathy especially in cases of antirabis and smallpox vaccine.

Reaction Due to Faulty Technique

The faulty vaccines may result from various causes, *e.g.*, faulty production and transportation of vaccines, improper site and route of immunization, wrong amount of medication, dilutant used, improper temperature, vaccine or dilutant contaminated, incomplete storage, contraindications ignored, use of improper sterilised syringes and needles carry the hazards of infection, *e.g.*, hepatitis B, AIDS and bacterial infection.

Provocative Reaction

After administration of vaccine though rarely but may occur a disease totally unconnected with immunizing agents, *e.g.*, provocation of polio after administration of diphtheria vaccine (APT or PTAP). This may happen when person harbours the disease agents in the body and are provocated due to immunization and produces a disease.

General Precautions

1. Sensitivity reaction should be tested, before administration of antisera or antitoxins. The sensitivity test is done by 0.2 mL of antisera in 1 : 10 diluted in saline, given intradermally.

2. Adrenaline (1 : 1000 solution) should be kept ready while administering serum to prevent adverse reaction of anaphylactic shock, 15 mL of adrenaline solution should be injected intramuscularly in adults.

   Antihystamine drugs, *e.g.*, 10 to 20 mg of chlorempheniramine maleate (Phenargan) can be given intramuscularly. The patient should be observed for 30 minutes after serum injects.

3. The syrings and needles should be sterilised properly.

4. Proper training to the health workers regarding giving immunization to prevent the complication.

5. Discard the open vaccine after immunization session, etc.

EXERCISE

1. Define health. Discuss the determinants of health with examples.
2. Explain the concept of health and diseases. Describe the "epidemiological triad" in causation of disease.
3. Discuss the mortality and morbidity indicators to assess the health status of a community.
4. Explain the concept of disease. Describe the natural history of disease
5. Define epidemiology. Describe the methods of epidemiology.
6. State the aims and uses of epidemiology. Discuss the descriptive epidemiology in detail.
7. Explain the types of immunity. Discuss the immunization schedule from 0 to 5 years and role of nurse in giving immunization.
8. Write short notes on:
   (a) Web of causation of disease
   (b) Dimension of health
   (c) Multiple causation of disease
   (d) Immunization
   (e) Modes of disease transmission.

UNIT V

EPIDEMIOLOGY OF NON-COMMUNICABLE DISEASES

- Cancer
- Diabetes
- Hypertension
- Rheumatic Health Diseases
- Cardiovascular Diseases
- Accidents
- Blindness
- Obesity

15

Cancer

INTRODUCTION

Cancer is the most common term used to designate all **malignant tumours** regardless of their origins. The two main classifications are :

1. Tumours arising from epithelial tissues are called as **carcinoma**, and
2. Those arising from connective or supporting tissues are called **sarcoma**.

Cancer may be characterised by a group of diseases with abnormal multiplication of cells in the body and eventual death of the people suffering from cancer. Cancer can occur at any site or tissue of the body and may involve any type of cells.

HISTORY

Cancer was recognised in ancient times by skilled observer who gave the name 'Cancer'. Its physiological and psychological impact on patients and their families results in profound changes in their lifestyle. Cancer diseases often focus on incurability, feeling of hopelessness and dread, though much progress has been made in prevention, early detection and treatment of cancer.

Problem in the World

Cancer is the **second** leading cause of death in the world next to cardiovascular diseases accounting for 21 per cent (2.5 million) of all mortality. It is estimated that about half a million people die every year from cancer in the SEAR. Cancer contributes to 3.4 per cent of all deaths reported from India, 6.6 per cent from Indonesia and from Myanmar 2.9 per cent, Nepal 0.8 per cent, Sri lanka 4.2 per cent etc. (Tables 15.1 and 15.2).

Table 15.1 : Age and sex distribution (%) of incidents of cancer cases in SEAR countries, 1998

Age (year)	Males	Females	Total
< 9	2.7	1.4	2.1
10-19	2.3	2.1	2.2
20-29	3.3	6.1	4.5
30-39	6.0	17.7	11.0
40-49	12.4	23.3	17.1
50-59	26.3	23.4	25.1
60-69	36.6	18.8	29.0
70-79	10.4	7.2	9.0
Total	**100.0**	**100.0**	**100.0**

Notes : *Based on data from India, Indonesia and Sri Lanka. Among all incident cancer cases, 57.3 per cent are in males and 42.7 per cent among females.*

Table 15.2 : Age and sex distribution (%) of cancer deaths in the SEAR countries, 1998

Age (year)	Males	Females	Total
< 9	1.4	0.9	1.1
10-19	1.8	1.6	1.7
20-29	3.8	5.3	4.6
30-39	8.1	16.7	18.8
40-49	26.0	20.7	23.1
50-59	26.0	20.7	23.1
60-69	34.1	28.6	31.1
70-79	8.9	4.6	6.6
80-89	0.3	0.2	0.2
Total	**100.0**	**100.0**	**100.0**

Note : *Based on data from India, Indonesia and Sri Lanka. Among all incident cancer cases, 57.3 per cent are in males and 42.7 per cent among females.*

In India, the National Cancer Registry Programme of Indian Council of Medical

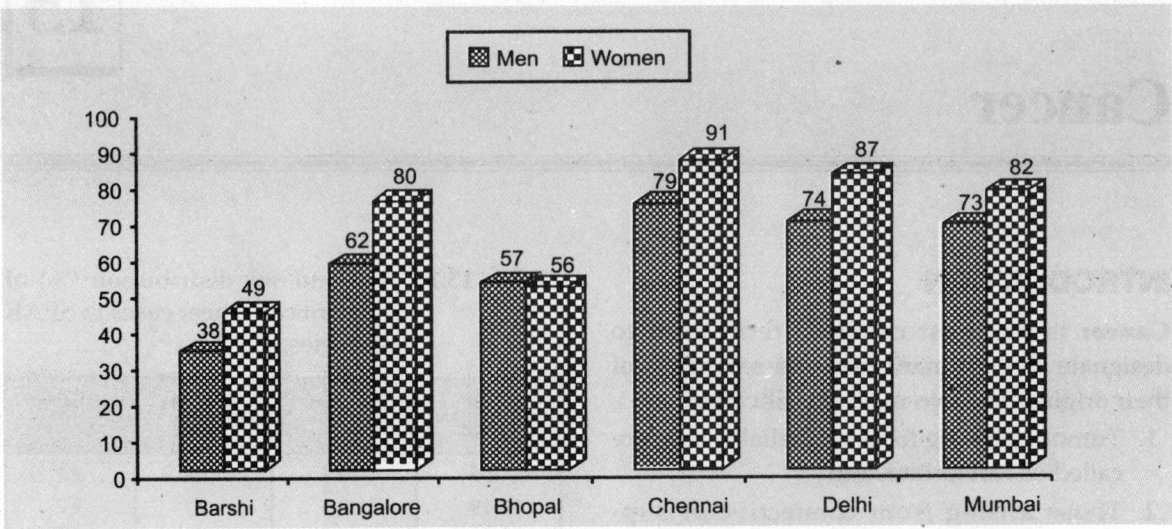

Fig. 15.1 : The chart shows per cent data of Male and Female registry of cancer in India
Source : India, Indian Council of Medical Research, Consolidated Report of the
Population-Based Cancer Registries.

Research provides data on incidence from population based registries and one rural based population registry at Barshi, Maharashtra (Fig. 15.1).

There were 18 million people estimated as suffering from cancer in 1996. Out of these, 10.5 million were women, who had either breast cancer, cervix, colon or rectum cancer. Among men, it was prostate, colorectal or lung cancer. Of the diagnosed cancer cases, 57 per cent occurred in developing countries (Fig. 15.2).

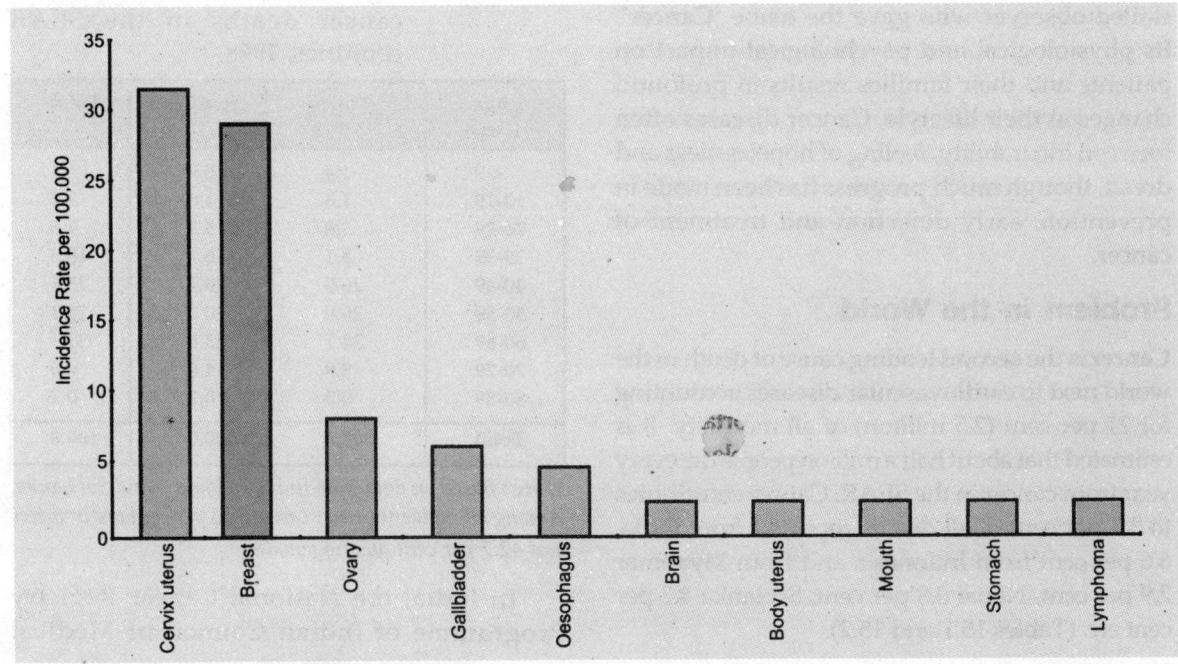

Fig. 15.2 : Bar diagram depicting most common forms of cancer in females (ICMR)

Lung cancer was found to be the most commonly prevalent in both developed and developing countries. Among women, **breast cancer** is the most common.

Problem in India

In India, cancer has become a major public health problem and estimated as one of the ten leading causes of death and the rank is advancing year by year. There are about 20 lakh cases of cancer and 5 lakh new cases of cancer and 3 lakh deaths are estimated in the country.

Epidemiology of Disease

Cancer affects human wherever they live and whatever their race, colour, cultural background or economic status may be.

Cancer ranks second to heart disease as the cause of death, though significant progress has been made in early diagnosis and treatment and

survival rate has been raised to 50 per cent. The success of cancer treatment depends upon :

- **Diagnosis** of more cancers in the early stage.
- **Treatment** of patients within four months of diagnosis.
- **Development** of new diagnostic and treatment facilities especially **chemotherapy**. In spite of these advances, 5 lakh people die of cancer.
- **Sex** : The chances of developing cancer is greater for males than the females. The largest probabilities are **lungs, skin** and **prostate cancers** in **males**. For **women**, the largest probabilities are **breast, colorectal** and **lung cancer**. In both groups (sexes), the largest increases are seen for lung cancer and cancer of colon-rectum (Fig. 15.3).
- **Age** : Fifty-two per cent of all cancers occur in people over 65 years of age. Cancers have been called a **disease** of **ageing**.

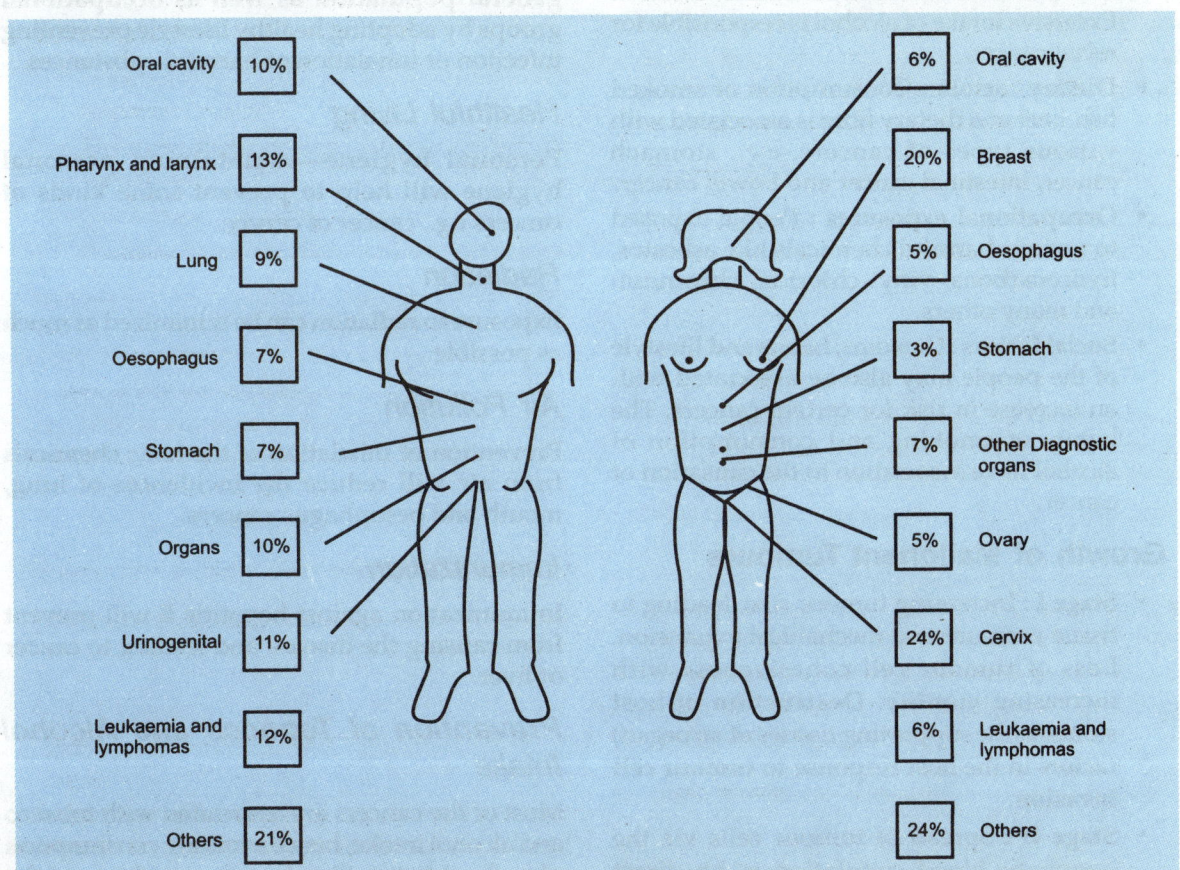

Fig. 15.3 : Cancer incidence by site and sex

Risk Factors

Genetic Factors

In case of cancer, it is difficult to identify the genetic factors but it has been seen that retinoblastoma occurs in children of the same parent. Mongols are more likely to develop cancer (leukaemia) than normal children.

Environmental Factors

The lifestyle is generally held responsible for more than 80 per cent of all cancers. The main causes of cancer are :

- **Tobacco** : Any form of tobacco usage is the major cause of cancer of lung, larynx, mouth, pharynx, esophagus, bladder, pancreas and kidney. It has been estimated as more than one million premature deaths due to cigarette smoking every year.
- **Alcohol** : It has been estimated that a total of 3 per cent deaths are due to alcohol. Excessive intake of alcohol is responsible for rectal cancer.
- **Dietary factors** : Consumption of smoked fish, beef and dietary fibre is associated with various types of cancers, *e.g.*, stomach cancer, intestinal cancer and bowel cancer.
- **Occupational exposures** : People exposed to various harmful chemicals like asbestos, hydrocarbons, vinyl chloride, chromium and many others.
- **Social factors** : Customs, habits and lifestyle of the people may also be associated with an increase in risk for certain cancers. The habits of smoking and consumption of alcohol have association in the causation of cancer.

Growth of Malignant Tumours

- **Stage I** : Increasing tumour size, leading to tissue pressure and mechanical expansion. Loss of tumour cell cohesiveness with increasing motility. **Destruction** of host **stomata** (the supporting tissues of an organ) **factors** in the host response to **tumour cell invasion.**
- **Stage II** : Spread of tumour cells via the lymphatic blood circulation or by direct expansion. Lymphatic system provides the most common pathway for initial spread of cancer cells. The spread may be the lymph nodes draining the region of the primary site.

PREVENTIVE MEASURES OF CANCER

Cancer can be controlled by early detection, and treatment, after care and rehabilitation have reduced the mortality due to cancer.

The basic approach to the control of cancer is through primary and secondary prevention. It is estimated that one-third of all cancers are preventable.

Primary Level of Prevention

Advanced knowledge in the field of cancer has increased the understanding on causation of cancer, hence it has become easier to take preventive measures to prevent the disease in general population as well as occupational groups by adopting healthy lifestyle preventing infection or inhalation of harmful substances.

Healthful Living

Personal hygiene—maintaining personal hygiene will help to prevent some kinds of cancers *e.g.*, cancer of cervix.

Radiation

Exposure to radiation can be minimized as much as possible.

Air Pollution

Prevention of inhalation of the toxic chemicals from air will reduce the incidences of lung, mouth and oesophagus cancers.

Immunization

Immunization against hepatitis B will prevent from causing the disease and leading to cancer of liver.

Prevention of Tobacco and Alcohol Intake

Most of the cancers are associated with tobacco and alcohol intake, hence avoiding consumption of such addicts will reduce the incidence of the disease.

Health Education

Educating people about causation, prevention and control of disease may increase awareness of the people. They must be informed about high-risk groups, precautions for prevention of disease, early identification of disease and treatment to reduce the mortality by the following warning signs :

Seven Warning Signs of Cancer

1. Change in bowel and bladder habits.
2. An ulcer that does not heal.
3. Unusual bleeding or discharge.
4. Thickening or a lump in the breast or elsewhere.
5. Indigestion or difficulty in swallowing.
6. Obvious change in a wart or mole.
7. Nagging cough or hoarseness.

Methods and Medias of Health Education

- Information, education and communication to community.
- Reinforcement of legislative and restrictive measures.
- Smoking cessation activities.
- National and international co-ordination.

Information and Education, Communication

There is a need to change the human behaviour by public awareness about health hazards of smoking through mass media. Health education at large plays an important role in changing the lifestyle of the smokers.

Legislative and Restrictive Measures

The measures should be adopted by controlling production and sale of tobacco products, restriction of smoking in public places, transport buses and places of work. The Government of India has reinforced the Cigarettes Act of 1975, mentioning "Cigarette smoking is injurious to health" on all packets of cigarettes that are put on sale. Government has also reinforced laws in cinema halls, educational institutions, public places and hospitals, etc.

Smoking Cessation Activities

WHO expert committee on smoking control provides information on specific smoking cessation methods such as smoking cessation clinics, nicotine substitutes, hypnosis, etc.

National and International Coordination

Since smoking is a global epidemic, it needs co-ordination between national and international levels to control the smoking epidemics.

Secondary Level of Prevention

The secondary prevention includes early detection and treatment of cancer.

Screening

Screening is an important way to identify the cases at an early stage and help in treatment. It is essential, that early detection programmes will require mobilisation of all available resources and development of cancer infrastructure starting at the level of primary health care and ending at the national central level.

Treatment

The facilities for treatment must be made available to all cancer people. The most neglected problem in cancer is the pain due to cancer. Hence, WHO has developed guidelines on relief of cancer pain—"Freedom from Cancer Pain" is the right of a cancer patient.

Women of all ages now show the importance of reporting any abnormal vaginal bleeding or other discharge occurring between menstrual period or after menopause, for early symptoms of cancer of female reproductive system.

Community health nurse plays an important role in prevention and early detection of genetic cancer. They systematically obtained family cancer history, genetic counselling will help to know the cancer prone family and susceptible family members.

Treatment of Cancer

The most common treatment being used is metabolic therapy, combination of special diet, detoxification, internal cleaning, spiritual and emotional healing and dose of vitamins and minerals. The diet therapy may be a variety of therapies from the grape cure to raw foods to wheatgrass extract. The megavitamins approach involves consumption of large quantities of high dose vitamins believed to increase the body's ability to kill cancer cells.

Other treatment modalities are being practised as irritation chemotherapy, immuno-therapy.

Although cancer is the second most common cause of death in our country. Many forms of cancers are identifiable and are preventable. However, some cancers can not be prevented, from occurring for these cancers there is secondary prevention, or early detection. Dietary modifications are among the important ways to reduce the occurrence of cancer in general.

Three Palliative Care for Cancer Patients in India

The concept of Palliative Care (PC) for cancer patient is the "active total care for those with advanced and incurable disease which includes pain relief, symptom control and psychosocial support".

At present, out of one million newly diag-nosed cancer patients every year, more than 50 per cent will die within 12 months of diagnosis and another one million survives (within 5 years) will show progressive disease. Out of these, 1.5 million require palliative care and less than 0.1 million patients can be covered by existing facilities. Since 1980s, the National Cancer Control Programme has identified that cancer patients with advanced stage require good palliative treatment which emphasises the teamwork of oncologist, nurse specialist, anaesthetist, social worker, psychologist, pharmacist and other supportive staff.

TYPES OF CANCER
LUNG CANCER

Lung cancer is a major public health problem known among the industrial workers from the late 19th century and is the most common cancer in the world, with 51 per cent of cases occurring in developed countries, 85 per cent of cases in

men and 46 per cent in women are due to smoking. If the present situation continues, the lung cancer is likely to be the most common fatal cancer in the world.

It is difficult to assess the problem of lung cancer in developing countries due to lack of accurate statistics. Approximately two-thirds of people in India are smoking below the age of 20 years. Lung cancer accounts for 6.8 per cent of all malignancies, and if smoking is not controlled, the figure is going to be increased in many developing countries.

Epidemiology of Disease
Age and Sex

The incidence of lung cancer is increasing more among females than males, may be due to more exposure to smoking.

Risk Factor
Smoking

Studies have shown the correlation between cigarette smoking and lung cancer. Studies indicate that lung cancer risk for cigarette smoking is 8.6 times more than the nonsmoking.

The risk is strongly related to the number of cigarettes smoked, age of starting, years of exposure, smoking habits (inhalation technique), tar and nicotine content and size of cigarettes, etc. Those who are highly exposed to "passive smoking" (somebody else smoking) are at higher risk of developing lung cancer. The strongest evidence that cigarette smoking is responsible for lung cancer is the incidence of reduction after cessation of smoking.

The most harmful components of tobacco smoke are tar, carbon monoxide and nicotine. Tar is responsible for carcinogenic role. Nicotine and carbon monoxide increase the risk of cardio-vascular diseases, interference with myocardial oxygen supply.

Other Factors

Various other factors that contribute to cancer are air pollution, radioactive substances, occupational hazards (exposure to asbestos, arsenic, hydrocarbons and nickel bearing dust).

Screening for Lung Cancer

Mainly there are two techniques for screening lung cancer. They are chest radiograph and sputum cytology. Mass radiography has been suggested for early diagnosis of lung cancer. Like chest radiograph and sputum cytology, mass radiography has been suggested for an early diagnosis every six months interval.

Prevention of Lung Cancer

Primary prevention is of the greatest importance by controlling smoking epidemic. Since 80 to 90 per cent of all cases of lung cancer in developing countries are due to smoking, various methods can be adopted for controlling the smoking and other measures as described earlier.

BREAST CANCER

Most of female disorders are benign in character, breast one of the two female organs that are primary site for cancer. The breast changes normally during menstruation, pregnancy, lactation and menopause. Although breast is easily accessible to examinations, the detection and accurate diagnosis of breast disease can be difficult.

In both female and male benign lesions of the breast occur more frequently, the malignant lesions (70–30%) out of malignant 99 per cent occur in female, 75 per cent of cancer occurs after 40 years of age, less than 20 per cent occurs at less than 30 years.

Incidence

The incidence of breast cancer (Fig. 15.4) has continued to rise over the past 35 to 40 years, whereas mortality rate has changed very little. This appears to be a hopeful sign in the battle against this disease, higher proportion of women are being treated earlier and method of treatment has improved. Highest incidence is found in the unmarried women, lowest among those who have multiple pregnancies and first pregnancy before 27 years of age. Low incidences also among those who had early menopause.

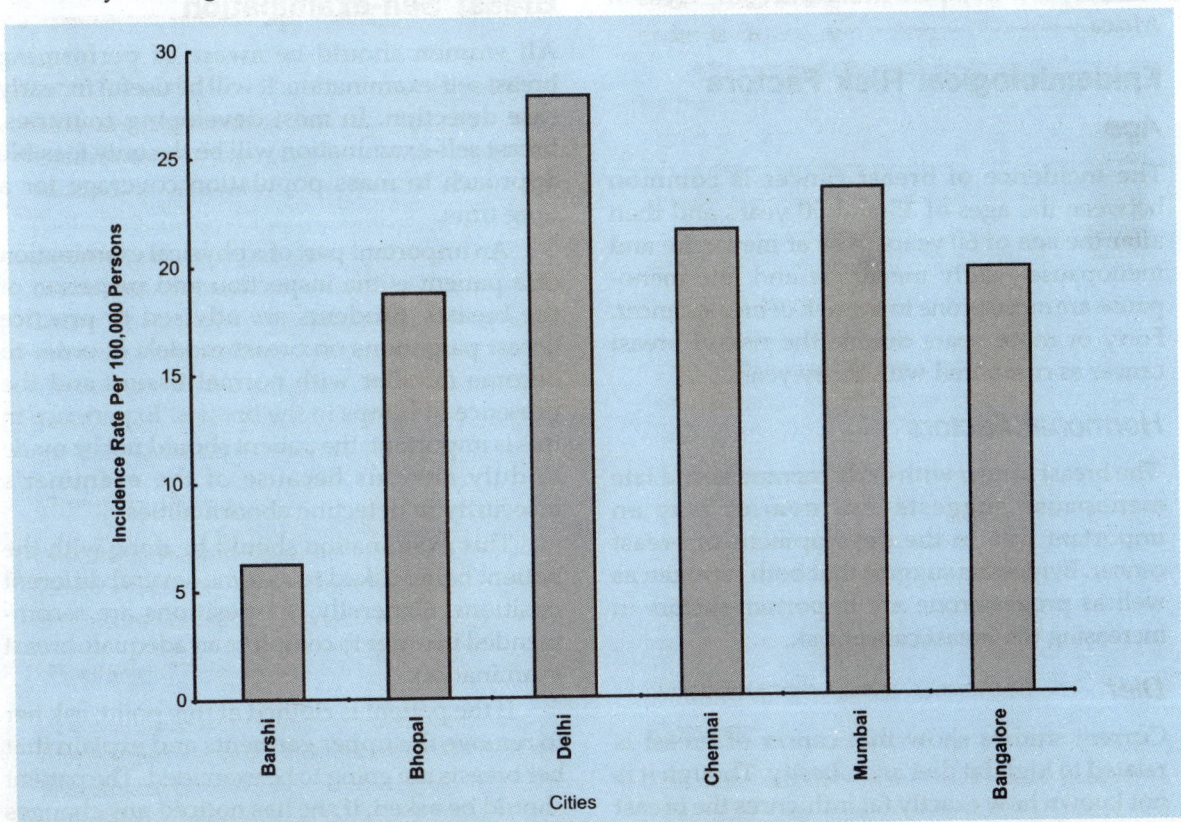

Fig 15.4 : Bar graph showing incidence rate of Breast Cancer per 100,000 persons

Aetiology

Cause is not known. Several factors appear to influence the occurrence.

Genetic

Family history with cancer will predispose more to cancer than the women with no family history. They will develop 10 to 12 years before the cancer than with no family history.

Women who have more menstrual periods are more prone to cancer, while women with children have low incidence of breast cancer.

Cancer of breast is one of the commonest causes of death in most developed countries among middle aged women, and is becoming frequent among women of developing countries as well.

International Variations

The incidence and mortality is high in the USA, Australia, Canada and certain parts of Europe and very low in Japan, India and some areas of Africa.

Epidemiological Risk Factors

Age

The incidence of breast cancer is common between the ages of 35 and 50 years and then after the age of 60 years. Age at menarche and menopause—early menarche and late menopause are more prone to the risk of breast cancer. Forty or more years double the risk of breast cancer as compared with thirty years.

Hormonal Factors

The breast cancer with early menarche and late menopause suggests that ovaries play an important role in the development of breast cancer. Evidences suggest that both estrogen as well as progesterone are important factors in increasing the breast cancer risk.

Diet

Current studies show that cancer of breast is related to high fat diet and obesity. Though it is not known how exactly fat influences the breast cancer risk at cellular level.

Socioeconomic Conditions

Breast cancer is commonly found among high socioeconomic group which may be due to lifestyle.

Others

An increased incidence of breast cancer has been found among women who are exposed to radiation, prolonged use of oral pills, etc.

Screening for Breast Cancer

Early detection for breast cancer has a favourable effect on mortality rate due to breast cancer. It can be detected by the following techniques :

- Breast self-examination (Appendix)
- Breast examination by medical experts (gynaecologists)
- Mammography
- Health education on awareness of lump present in the breast.

Breast Self-examination

All women should be aware of performing breast self-examination. It will be useful for early case detection. In most developing countries, breast self-examination will be the only feasible approach to mass population coverage for a long-time.

An important part of a physical examination of a patient is the inspection and palpation of the breasts. Students are advised to practice breast palpations on breast-models in order to become familiar with normal tissues and the presence of lumps in the breasts. Experience in this is important; the patient should not be made unduly anxious because of the examiner's insecurity in detecting abnormalities.

This examination should be done with the patient being asked to assume several different positions. Generally, six positions are recommended in order to complete an adequate breast examination.

If the patient is clothed at this point, ask her to remove the upper garments and explain that her breasts are going to be examined. The patient should be asked, if she has noticed any changes in her breasts, a patient's awareness of her own body invariably offers valuable information. Elaboration of the procedure, such as stating why there is a need to palpate in each position and the need to express secretion from the nipples helps the patient understand the necessary steps. Giving details of the examination steps and how to recognize signs of abnormalities also teaches her how to examine her own breasts and the value of regular self-examinations (Appendix).

An examination should include systematic inspection and palpation in each of the four quadrants, the tail of the breast and axilla, and beneath the nipple.

In palpation of the breasts, the examiner should use the flats or pads of two or three fingers. Moving the fingers in small circles, pressure should be applied lightly, then firmly and finally with more pressure. Examination of all areas of the breast is achieved by systematically palpating across the breast in "strips" (often described as moving the lawn) or by a "concentric circles" approach.

Position One

Ask the patient to sit on the side of the examination table, preferably the same table which is to be used for the pelvic examination if that is to follow. Her arms should be in a relaxed position at her sides (see Appendix). Observe the breasts for size (one breast is often slightly larger than the other), dimpling, normality of contours, depressions, skin retractions and any deviation of the nipples from their normal position. Always palpate both breasts in each of the four quadrants and tail.

Position Two

Ask the patient to raise her arms high above her head while the same observations, and inspections as above are carried out.

Position Three

Ask the patient to bend her arms and push her elbows behind her back; placing the hands on the hips help to attain this position. The aim is to achieve stretching of the patient's chest muscles. Continue with your inspection. Indicate when this part of the examination is finished, so that the patient can relax for a few minutes.

Position Four

Ask the patient to lean forward from the waist while stretching her arms straight ahead. Continue the inspection with the breasts in the suspended position.

Position Five

This position requires that the patient lies on her back on the examination table. Ensure that she is draped appropriately and feels comfortable. Continue the inspection and palpations. Carefully manipulate the nipples to express secretion and, if secretion is evident, prepare a cytologic smear.

When the breasts have been thoroughly palpated and all areas have systematically been examined, ask her to sit up again.

At this point, palpate the axillae for lymph nodes, including the supraclavicular areas in order to detect any enlarged lymph nodes.

After completion of the breast examination let the patient know that she may cover herself again or get dressed, if there are no more procedures to be carried out. Many patients are anxious for feedback about the findings. If the breasts appear healthy then it is appropriate to share this information immediately. Findings that give cause for concern may be discussed more sensitively in the office when the patient is fully dressed; she can then be told what has been found or noted during the examination and what further tests are needed.

Mammography is the most sensitive and specific in detecting small tumours, which might be missed during palpation, though it requires technical equipments of high standard and radiologists which limit the widespread use of mass screening purposes.

Prevention and Control of Breast Cancer

The aim of prevention of breast cancer is to eliminate the risk factors and promotion of cancer education.

Primary Prevention

The average age at menarche can be increased by reducing childhood obesity by reducing fat intake in diet and increasing physical activity will reduce the incidence of cancer.

Secondary Prevention

Breast screening will help early diagnosis and treatment of cancer and ultimately lowering the mortality due to breast cancer. Self breast examination should be encouraged and taught to mothers for early detection. Early assessment and removal of tumour is more curative than at late stage.

ORAL CANCER

Oral cancer is the most common type of cancer in the world. High incidence is seen in Central and South-East Asian countries, e.g., Bangladesh, India, Indonesia, Thailand and Pakistan. Each year more than 5 lakh new cases and 3 lakh deaths occur throughout the world.

It is a major leading problem in India and accounts for 50 to 70 per cent of all cancers diagnosed.

Epidemiology of Disease

Tobacco Chewing and Smoking

Epidemiological survey shows that 90 per cent of oral cancer is due to tobacco chewing in different parts of country. It was found in Kerala, Andhra Pradesh and Gujarat that oral cancer and precancerous lesions occur almost among those who smoked or chewed tobacco, especially in the part of mouth where tobacco was mostly kept. The other narcotic addictions also have shown the incidences of the oral cancer.

Alcohol

High concentration of alcohol shows the incidence of oral cancer. Alcohol appears to have synergetic effect in tobacco users.

Precancerous Lesions

The presence of precancerous lesions if detected early may prevent the occurrence of oral cancer before they change into cancerous stage. It may result in regression of lesion.

Sociocultural Factors

Prevalence of cancer depends upon the methods of tobacco consumption. It is smoked in the form of manufactured cigarettes or bidi, chutta (cigar), chilum, hukkah or it may be taken by scrubbing tobacco in hands and chewed. Direct chewing has more chances in causing oral cancer.

Prevention

Primary Prevention

The incidences can be reduced by eliminating smoking and chewing tobacco among community people. There is need for mass health education and motivating people to change their behaviours and lifestyles towards healthy living. Legislative measures though can be adopted like banning or restricting the sale of tobacco. But it may not be effective unless people are motivated to change their habits to quit smoking due to its hazards of cancer.

Secondary Prevention

Early detection of precancerous stage especially among the high-risk groups, e.g., tobacco chewers, smokers, alcoholics, etc., may help to treat and cure cancer. In developing countries only 50 per cent of oral cancers are detected at an early stage. Rest of them are detected in advanced stage.

CANCER OF CERVIX

Cancer of cervix is the most common cancer of reproductive system in women. It rarely occurs before 20 years. It is more common between 30 to 50 years, statistics show sexual activity and its relationship to incidence of cancer of cervix, before the age of 25 years. It is more prevalent in those who had many sex partners and several pregnancies.

Cancer of cervix is the second most common cancer after breast cancer among women, estimating more than 5 lakh women in 1995. High mortality and incidence is found among North America, Western Europe, Latin America and South-East Asia, which accounts 80 per cent of the total cases. In most developed countries, the incidence has been declining for last few decades due to availability of latest technology in screening of cancer and treatment, clinically characterised by irregular bleeding and pain on coitus.

Epidemiological Factors

Agent Factor

Human Papilloma Virus (HPV) : Sexually transmitted diseases are possibly causing cancer of cervix. This virus is found in more than 95 per cent of the cancer patients. Though it is said that virus is necessary but not the only cause of a cancer.

Host Factor

Predisposing factors (risk factors) :

- *Age* : Usually young women of 30–40 years, risk increases with increase of age.
- *Genital warts* : Occurrence of genital warts is important predisposing factor in cervix cancer.
- *Marital status* : Incidences have shown that disease is associated with marital status. The prevalence is high among prostitutes and multisex partners, due to its relationship with sexually transmitted infections.
- *Early marriage* : Early marriage, early childbirth are at higher-risk of getting the disease.
- *Use of oral contraceptive* : It has shown a close relationship between use of oral contraceptive and increased risk of cancer.
- *Socioeconomic group* : More common in low socioeconomic group due to poor genital hygiene.

Cancer of cervix is curable in initial stage by complete gynaecological examination and Pap smear will detect premalignant cervical dysplasia, so that women with infections and positive Pap smear are advised regular six months check-up.

Assessment and Clinical Manifestation

Early Stage of Cancer is Usually Asymptomatic

The two chief symptoms of early carcinoma of cervix are leukorrhoea and irregular vaginal bleeding or spotting. Prolonged leukorrhoea may be the only abnormal sign. Discharge increases gradually in amount and becomes watery and finally dark and foul smelling, because of necrosis and infection of tumour mass, bleeding occurs at irregular intervals between periods (metrorrhagia) or after menopause. It may be new site, just enough to spot the undergarments and it is noted usually after some form of trauma (intercourse, douching or defecation). As the disease continues the bleeding may become constant and may increase in amount.

Chronic infections and corrosions of cervix seem to play a significant part in development of cancer of cervix, such pathology becomes evident as a large cauliflower like growths or a deep, ulcerating craters before giving any symptom of its presence.

As cancer advances, the tissues outside the cervix may be invaded, including the lymph glands anterior to sacrum. The nerves in this region get involved producing excruciating pain in the back and legs which is relieved by narcotics. The patient may finally be weak and anaemic, often with irregular fever due to secondary infection and abscesses in ulcerating mass.

Surgical Management

Radiation is the most frequent form of treatment for invasive cervical cancer and surgical intervention for the advanced lesions is usually advised.

Prevention and Control

Primary Prevention

Maintaining personal and genital hygiene may help in reducing the incidence of disease. Safer sex, single partner relationship and sex **education** are important components of primary prevention.

Secondary Prevention

Early detection of cases by diagnosing through clinical manifestation, screening by regular yearly Pap smear will help for early treatment by radical surgery and radiotherapy reduces the incidences of high mortality.

Screening of Cancer of Cervix

- The early detection of cancer of cervix can be done by Pap smear. It has been suggested that all women should have a Pap test every three years.
- The test should be easily available for women with poor socioeconomic status.

CANCER OF STOMACH

It is the world's second most common cancer, with more than 1 million new cases every year and two-thirds occur in developing countries. Symptoms are nonspecific. That is why the disease is diagnosed in the advanced stage. Patient may complain of weight loss, fatigue or gastric discomfort. Diagnosis is confirmed by barium meal, X–ray and tissue biopsy and treatment is done by surgical intervention by the removal of the tumour. The prognosis is very poor even after surgery and chemotherapy.

NATIONAL CANCER CONTROL PROGRAMME

National Cancer Control Programme started in 1975 and was revised in 1984 to strengthen it with the objectives of the following :

Primary Prevention

Health education and prevention of intake of tobacco.

Secondary Prevention

Early detection of common cancers such as cervix, mouth and breast and other tobacco related cancers.

Tertiary Prevention

Strengthening of the existing institutions for comprehensive therapy including pallative care.

STRATEGIES OF NATIONAL CANCER CONTROL PROGRAMME

Regional Cancer Centres

The existing regional cancer centres are being further strengthened to act as referral centres for complicated and difficult cases at tertiary level.

Development of Oncology Wing

A scheme for development of oncology wing in medical colleges has been initiated to fill up geographical gap in early detection and treatment of cancer. It is expected that each of assisted institutions would carry-out outreach programmes for early detection and treatment of cancer.

District Cancer Control Programme

The programme at district level emphasise mainly on health education and pain relief measures.

Cobalt Therapy Installation and Provision for Mammography has been strengthened.

Morphine tablets, Catscan Software and Pap smear kits are supplied to regional cancer centres.

Training of trainees is being held at various states and districts. Twelve training programmes in prevention and early detection of cancer were held for medical officers at PHC/CHC districts in various parts of the country in 1999.

Role of Nurse in Prevention and Control of Cancer

Nurses have major responsibility in the prevention of cancer because of their knowledge about the disease and their opportunity for contact with people in the hospitals and home settings. Nurses have the opportunity to teach about cancer and to motivate patients to seek treatment.

Risk Factors Identification

Risk factors must be identified and moderated. These factors may be :

- **Lifestyle :** e.g., tobacco, diet, alcohol, sunlight exposure and sexual practices.
- **Environmental Factor :** which can not be controlled.

- **Genetic Factor :** Conditions inherited at conception are not usually controllable.

    High-risk families, especially those at risk for breast and lung cancer should be given health education on early detection and treatment.

Activities

- Case finding is the responsibility of community health nurse.
- The nurse must be able to counsel and direct patients to proper sources of help.
- To give information about those conditions that are known to predispose individuals to the development of disease.
- Educate the public about predisposing factors.
- Be sensitive to the needs of patients who may be afraid and embarrassed when confronted with the possibility of cancer.

Early Detection and Treatment

The approach to early detection of cancer is worldwide. General criteria for cancer screening and testing programmes have been taken up by WHO. Multiphasic screening and periodic health examination have been accepted by people. Early detection of cancer can reduce mortality due to cancer. People above the age of 20 years should have a cancer related health check-up every three years and above 40 years every year.

    Women should be taught to examine their breasts each month immediately after the menstrual period or, if postmenopausal, on a designated day each month. Such self-examination is much better method of detecting breast cancer than an annual physical examination.

Research Findings

A virus that has been genetically engineered which destroys cancer cells has shown strong and lasting effects against tumours in patients when combined with standard chemotherapy.

Researchers have found 25 out of 30 patients with head and neck cancer saw their tumours shrink after they were treated with Onyx Pharmaceutical Inc.'s **Onyx-015** along with chemotherapy.

Eight tumours disappeared, Dr. Fadlo Khuri and colleagues at MD Anderson Cancer Centre in Houston, working with teams in Britain, wrote in the journal *Nature Medicine*. "Onyx-015 may be able to sensitize infected and uninfected cells to killing by chemotherapy," they wrote, *"It is very encouraging because this is the first time there has been a phase II trial—a trial with more than just a few patients in it—where the tumours have gone away in a significant number and they haven't come back,"* gene therapy pioneer Dr. William French Anderson of the University of Southern California said.

Every year, 5,00,000 people worldwide are diagnosed with cancer of the head and neck, and about 30 per cent of them die. Such cancers, heavily associated with the use of alcohol and tobacco, are treated at first with surgery, radiation therapy or both. But tumours come back in about one-third of patients. Gene therapy is a possible new approach.

Anywhere between 45 and 70 per cent of head and neck tumour cells have mutations in a gene known as P53, which, when normal, helps repair cancer causing damage. Onyx-015 is an adenovirus, a relative of common cold viruses, that has been genetically engineered to attack cells that lack normal P53. This makes it technically a gene therapy drug.

Khuri's team combined Onyx-015 with two common cancer chemotherapy drugs—5-FU and Cisplatin—to see if it would help them work better. *"Treatment caused tumours to shrink in 25 of the 30 cases evaluated"*, Khuri's team reported. They said only 17 per cent of tumours had progressed 6 months after treatment—which meant the combination of gene therapy and chemotherapy worked better than any treatment alone.

●●●

Diabetes

16

INTRODUCTION

Diabetes mellitus is a long-term complex chronic disorder, characterised by disruption of normal carbohydrates, fat and protein metabolism and the development over time of microvascular and macrovascular complications and neuropathies. It encompasses a heterogeneous group of anatomical and chemical problems predominated by deficiency of insulin or its actions and by glucose intolerance.

World Distribution

Diabetes is one of the leading causes of death in developed countries. The important cause of death is hypoglycaemia and ketoacidosis.

Diabetes is an "Iceberg" disease affecting at least 30 million people throughout the world. In some developing countries, the prevalence has been increasing rapidly due to rapid changes in lifestyle. The chronic diabetes may lead to various complications like, retinopathy, gangrene, coronary heart disease and neuropathy.

Worldwide Problem

Diabetes mellitus is one of the most common noncommunicable disease globally and is one of leading causes of death in developing countries. The important cause of death is hypoglycaemia and ketoacidosis. It was estimated that there were about 135 million adult diabetics worldwide in 1995 and the figure is projected to reach 300 million by 2025 (Fig. 16.1). Nearly two-thirds of world's diabetic population reside in developing countries which are projected to bear 76 per cent of global load by 2025. In some developing countries the prevalence has been increasing due to rapid changes in lifestyle. The chronic diabetes may lead to various complications like retinopathy, gangrene, coronary heart disease and neuropathy.

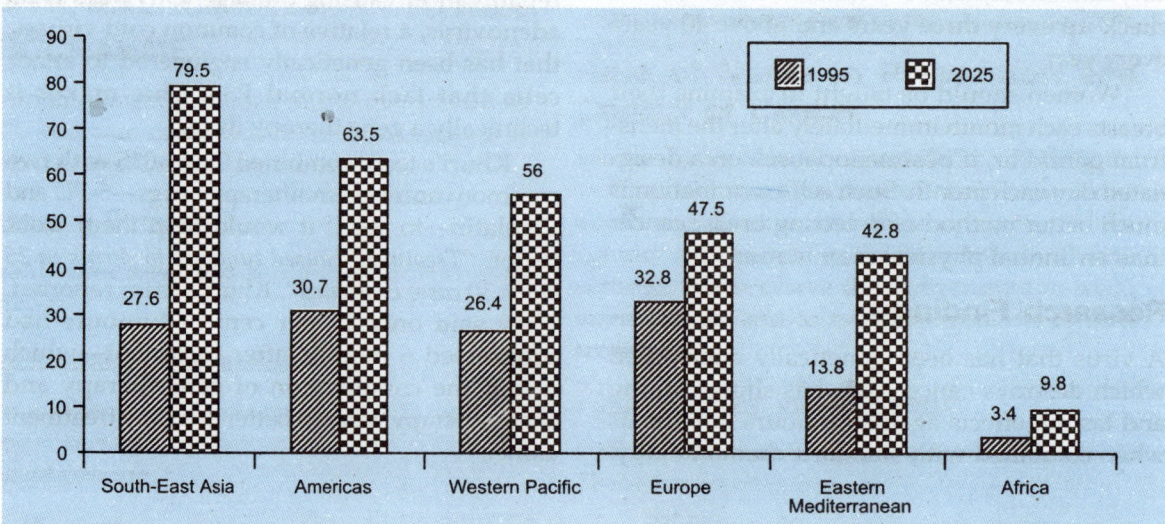

Fig. 16.1 : Estimated prevalence of diabetes mellitus, by WHO Region 1995 and 2025 (expected)

It is estimated that by the year 2025 there will be nearly 80 million diabetics in the region, the highest among all WHO regions. The majority of diabetic patients in South-East Asia region is and will be in the middle age group. This has a substantial impact on the economic and health care system in the countries.

The people are manifesting diabetes in most productive period of their lives and will live upto older age with complications of diabetes with serious demand to health care services.

Problem in India

The population in India has increased suscepti-bility to diabetes mellitus. The prevalence of diabetes in adults was found to be 2.5 per cent in rural and 4 to 11 per cent in urban community. High frequency of impaired glucose tolerance, shown by studies indicate the potential for further rise in prevalence of diabetes mellitus in the coming years. It is estimated that during 1998 about 28,702,100 diabetic cases were found and about 102,000 died of the disease.

The prevalence of diabetes mellitus in India is 1 to 2 per cent.

Epidemiological Factors

It is a major health problem. There are around 6 million known people with diabetes mellitus and every second case is undiagnosed. IDDM accounts for about 10 per cent of all cases, has the peak incidence in the age range of 11 to 14 years of age, affects boys somewhat more frequently than girls. NIDDM accounts for 80 to 90 per cent of all cases, shows a dramatic increase with age, (influences the ageing on the incidence of diabetes mellitus) occurs more frequently in females.

Malnutrition related diabetes mellitus occurs primarily in young adults with histories of nutritional deficiencies, who live in tropical areas. Gestational diabetes mellitus (GDM) occurs in 2 per cent of all pregnant women. Occurrence increases with maternal age but is not affected by race of people with impaired glucose tolerance, 25 per cent will eventually develop diabetes mellitus.

Disease occurs with greater prevalence after 40 years. It is third leading cause of death and increasing at the rate of 6 per cent yearly. Mortality is mainly due to renal and cardiovascular complications. Kidney diseases are 17 times more common among diabetic than nondiabetic. These complications account for 50 per cent mortality among insulin dependant diabetics.

Agent

- Diabetes is caused by deficiency of insulin hormone, which may be due to pancreatic disorders, inflammations, neoplastic and other disorders.
- Defects in the formation of insulin *e.g.*, synthesis of an abnormal and biologically less active insulin molecules.
- Destruction of beta cells may be due to viral infection or chemical agents.

Host Factors

Age

Although diabetes may occur at any age, usually it is common in middle age. Malnutrition relates diabetes in younger group.

Sex

Both male and female are usually affected, though in South-East Asia, it is common among men than women.

Obesity

Obesity predisposes diabetes and risk is related to duration and degree of obesity. Obesity reduces the number of insulin receptors on target cells, but in most cases it produces resistance to the action of insulin. Though all obese people are not diabetic, especially obesity appears to play no role in IDDM pathogenesis.

Sedentary Lifestyle

Sedentary lifestyle appears to be an important risk factor for development of NIDDM. Lack of exercise may alter the interaction between insulin, its receptors and subsequently leads to NIDDM.

Diet

The type of diet does not play important role in causing the disease, but quality food may alter the blood sugar level in the body. Malnutrition among children may result in failure of beta-cell function.

Alcohol

Excessive intake of alcohol can increase the risk of diabetes by damaging pancreas and liver cells. Viral infection like rubella and mumps virus, etc. may destroy the beta-cell of pancreas.

Chemical Agents

Streptozotocin, rodenticide and alloxan. Various chemical agents may also have toxic effect on beta-cells.

Stress Factors

Trauma, surgery and other stress situations may bring out the disease.

Other Factors

Many other factors like occupation, religion, economic status, education, urbanisation and change in lifestyle, have shown variations in incidence of the disease. For example, it is more common in low socioeconomic status, whereas few years back it was among high socioeconomic status, which may be due to change in lifestyle.

Aetiology

The aetiological factors of different types of diabetes mellitus vary. The aetiology of insulin dependant diabetes mellitus supports a genetic or inherited basis that has a permissive role in determining an individual's susceptibility to diabetes mellitus. Environmental factors can trigger onset in susceptible persons. In noninsulin dependant diabetes mellitus, the inherited or genetic factor is dominant, but environmental factors, especially obesity has a major influence on the onset and the clinical course of the disease.

Many factors may disturb the normal insulin formation and cause hyperglycaemia and glycosuria. The instinct enzyme system, pancreatic disease, pituitary disease, adrenal disease, thyroid gland disease, obesity, hereditary, infection, race, nervous system disturbances and others have been postulated as being the causes of diabetes mellitus. The disease shows a marked

tendency to occur in families with a family history of diabetes mellitus, can be obtained in at least 25 per cent of the cases. In identical twins the incidence is 70 per cent, while in non-identical, it is 10 per cent.

Whatever cause, the effect is that there is not enough available insulin to meet the metabolic needs of the individual. There is a failure to store and burn carbohydrate. With the result, glucose is accumulated in blood. When concentration of glucose in blood exceeds the renal threshold glucose is excreted in the urine. When the metabolism of carbohydrate is seriously disturbed, the metabolism of fat and of protein is secondarily affected (weightloss).

Risk Factors

- Obese
- Elderly
- People with family history of diabetes mellitus. Women who have given birth to babies weighing more than 9 pounds.

TYPES OF DIABETES MELLITUS

Insulin Dependant Diabetes Mellitus (IDDM)

Usually begins in childhood, but may occur at any age. In most cases the onset is abrupt weight-loss, weakness, polyuria, polydipsia, polyphasia. Precipitated by environmental factor e.g., viral infections have been associated with suscepti-bility and onset.

Noninsulin Dependant Diabetes Mellitus (NIDDM)

Onset is usually after 40 years without classic symptoms, associated with endogenous insulin level that may be mildly depressed, normal or high and with tissue insensitivity to insulin. Obesity and hereditary have been associated with the onset. Persons do not depend upon insulin, but may be treated with insulin.

Malnutrition Related Diabetes Mellitus (MRDM)

It presents in young adults with histories of nutritional deficiencies. Ketosis is not usually present. Diabetes mellitus is usually found in tropical areas and is treated with insulin.

Gestational Diabetes Mellitus (GDM)

People have the onset of glucose abnormality during pregnancy. Women with known DM who become pregnant are not classified in this group (GDM). After delivery, the woman is reclassified on the basis of blood or plasma glucose testing.

OTHER TYPES OF DIABETES MELLITUS

Diabetes mellitus may be associated with other disorders of pancreatic disease, endocrine, drugs, genetic syndrome.

Improved Glucose Tolerance (IGT)

Persons having glucose level higher than normal, but lower than those who have been diagnosed as diabetes mellitus.

It may be subclassified as obese, nonobese, or include person with other conditions, *e.g.,* injury, infections or drug induction. Persons having past history of glucose intolerance, but now have normal glucose level.

Potential Abnormality of Glucose Tolerance (PAGT)

People having no present history of glucose intolerance, but have a potentially high-risk because of historical factors, *e.g.,* delivering large babies, obesity or family history of diabetes mellitus.

Diagnosis of Diabetes

Urine Testing

It is the simple and convenient method of early detection of diabetes. All those with glucosuria are considered diabetic, though it is not confirmed. High-risk groups can be screened by urine testing. These groups are :

- Above 40 years.
- Family history of diabetes.
- Antenatal women, especially women who show excessive weight gain during pregnancy.
- Patients with premature atherosclerosis.

Blood Sugar Test

Due to inadequacy of urine testing, glucose tolerance test and standard oral glucose test can be done, by taking blood sample on fasting, post meals and random blood sample.

PREVENTION OF DIABETES MELLITUS

It takes place at three levels of prevention.

Primary Prevention

The primary prevention is based on elimination of environmental risk factors as much as possible. These measures may be taken by adopting healthy lifestyle by maintenance of normal body weight, healthy nutritional habits and physical exercises. The intake of balanced diet by taking adequate protein, high intake of dietary fibres and avoiding sweet and fried foods. These measures should be fully integrated into other community based programmes for prevention of noncommunicable diseases and increasing physical activity.

Dietary Changes

The diet must be balanced average calorie, as per individual need. The food with high calorie and less protein must be reduced like simple carbohydrate and fat, whereas fibre content should be increased by consuming *e.g.,* fruits, vegetables, pulses and cereals. The efforts on dietary change remain unsuccessful to reduce the weight. The person needs to have strong motivation to change the behaviour towards reducing weight.

Physical Activity

Regular physical exercise is important in reducing weight. Simple, light and regular exercise, may be simple brisk walking for half an hour daily, will help an individual to maintain the weight and feel physically and mentally relaxed.

Other Methods of Controlling Obesity

Various other methods can be reinforced, though they are not practical and commonly used.

- Appetite suppressing drugs, having been tried to control obesity.
- Surgical intervention like gastric bypass, gastroplasty.

Health Education

Public awareness through health education is important to reduce overweight and obesity. People must be aware of the hazards of obesity and its prevention and control. High-risk people can be identified and given adequate preventive measures to maintain the weight. The health education can be given on diet control, regular check-up, exercises and physical activities.

Hazards of Overweight

Various diseases are associated with obesity and it increases the morbidity and mortality. Obesity is a predisposing factor to diseases like hypertension, diabetes, gallbladder problems, coronary heart diseases. Obesity is also responsible for causing varicose veins, abdominal hernia, osteoarthritis and psychological stresses. Obesity lowers life expectancy and increases the mortality rate among obese people.

Assessment of Obesity

Weight Record : Body weight gives some information about obesity, though it does not exactly measure the excess fat. The weight can be calculated by the following method :

- **Body Mass Index (Ondilitis Index)**

$$= \frac{\text{Weight (kg)}}{\text{Height}^2 \text{(m)}}$$

- **Broca Index**
  Height in cm – 100
  e.g., 175 cm – 100 = 75 kg weight.

Since noninsulin dependant diabetes mellitus (NIDDM) is linked with sedentary lifestyle, overeating and unbalanced diet, obesity, avoid such unhealthy eating, may reduce the risk of diabetes. It is advised to reduce the habit of smoking which may promote atherosclerosis and lead to diabetes.

Secondary Prevention

Screening programme must be carried out in health departments, clinics, hospitals and follow-up of all positive findings is essential, because the number of persons with undiagnosed diabetes and strong association between diabetes mellitus and hypertension, atherosclerotic heart disease and complication is well-known. Hence, once it has been diagnosed, it must be treated appropriately to maintain the blood sugar level and minimize the complications by :

- Diet control
- Diet and antidiabetic medicines
- Diet and insulin.

Proper medical management will help to prevent various complications. Routine blood sugar test, urine for protein and ketones, visual acuity and weight should be recorded regularly. Feet should be examined for defective blood circulation. Protect the feet from injury and observe for any numbness of fingers, etc.

Avoid using tight shoes to avoid injury to feet and foot care.

Self Care

Diabetes is a chronic and lifelong disease. Patient cannot depend upon health care providers forever. Hence self care is an essential component to take care of diabetic patients. The patient must take the major responsibility for his own regimens, examination of own urine, if possible, blood sugar monitoring, self-administration of insulin, controlling intake of alcohol, keeping normal weight, regular exercise, diet control and regular check-up, etc. He must be aware of the early symptoms of glucosuria and hypoglycaemia.

Persons with known diabetes must have access to education, dietary pattern, social support, medical care and nursing care so that prevention and early detection of complications is possible. Services include programmes for hypertension detection and control, smoking cessation, eye care and foot care.

Tertiary Prevention

The neglected diabetes case may get serious complications like retinopathy, nephropathy, neuropathy and cardiovascular complications. It is essential to prevent such complications by providing effective and efficient care through special diabetic clinics, established in towns and cities. The provision must be there to tackle such complications at the early stage to prevent deformities.

Major emphasis will be based on :

- Health education about footcare to prevent ulcer formation, gangrene and amputation.
- Yearly routine ophthalmology examinations to identify eye changes early so that appropriate therapy can be applied to prevent blindness.
- Monitoring the presence of albuminuria to identify the onset of potentially irreversible kidney disease.
- Helping patients control hypertension, improve control of metabolic status and develop low protein diet to preserve kidney functions.
- Educating patients about tests or medications used to control complications.

NATIONAL DIABETIC CONTROL PROGRAMME (NDCP)

The main objectives of National Diabetic Control Programme are :

- To identify high-risk individuals at an early stage and providing appropriate health education.
- Early diagnosis and treatment of diabetic patients.
- Prevention of metabolic and chronic cardio-vascular and renal complications.

A pilot project for strengthening of biochemical laboratories and quality assurance under national diabetes control programme (NDCP) has been initiated in 5 states, namely Maharashtra, U.P., Punjab, Tamil Nadu and West Bengal. The centre will develop manual for technicians, will hold regular workshops for sensitisation and imparting skills to laboratory staffs and will ensure quality control in biochemical laboratories for various investigations required for diabetes. These institutions will provide quality control sera and training to personnel in the laboratories in the state. Automated pipetted devices and quality control

serum will be provided. The computerised record management will be used in these laboratories for the quality assurance.

The focus of the National Diabetic Control Programme (NDCP) would be on a District Diabetic Control Programme (DDCP). The programme will function at three levels : the subcentre, primary health centre and the district hospital level.

ROLE OF NURSE IN PREVENTION AND CONTROL OF DIABETES MELLITUS

Health education is an essential component for prevention, early diagnosis and treatment of diabetes mellitus. Community health nurse must educate the people regarding :

Dietary Control

To emphasise on balanced diet with less calories from carbohydrates (sugar and sugar products) and fats (especially saturated fat). It has been recommended to take all varieties of oil in proportionate amount *e.g.*, groundnut oil, mustard oil, sunflower oil and pure ghee can be consumed in reasonable amount.

Reduce Obesity

By regular exercise and minimise the senile work.

Healthy Lifestyle

By regular eating, sleeping, exercise and avoid smoking, drinking (alcohol), drug abuse, or submeditation, yoga, etc.

Regular Check-up

Especially for the people with family history of diabetes.

Regular Medicines or Insulin Injection

In case of diabetes mellitus, prevent complications like ratinopathy, neuropathy, nephropathy and cardiovascular diseases.

Teach

To take insulin injection at home, at regular intervals and regular doses and prevent hypo or hyperglycaemic shock. Patient should be able to recognise the signs and symptoms of shock, *e.g.*, fainting, giddiness, dryness of the mouth, cold clumsy skin and rapid pulse.

Patients

Is advised to carry identity card and sugar (which can be given immediately to hypoglycaemic patient). In case of hyper-glycaemic patient, refer to hospital for I.V. infusion.

- Patient must take foot care and prevent any shoe bite or injury to prevent diabetic ulcer or involvement of nerves.

- Diabetic patient should not get married to diabetic patient. Chances of getting diabetes mellitus among children is very high if both parents have disease.

●●●

17

Hypertension

INTRODUCTION

Hypertension can be considered as peripheral vascular disorders because they both involve problems of peripheral circulation and are affected by similar risk factors. Hypertension itself is a risk factor in atherosclerosis, the major cause of pheripheral vascular disease.

Hypertension is defined as a consistent systolic blood pressure above 140 mm Hg and or a consistent diastolic BP above 90 mm Hg. Incidence of hypertension increases with age and occurs more in men than in women.

WHO defines hypertension as *"a systolic pressure equal to or greater than 160 mm Hg and or a diastolic pressure equal to or greater than 95 mm Hg"*. Mild hypertension in adults has been defined as a diastolic pressure persistently between 90 to 105 mm Hg.

Worldwide Problem

In developed countries, the prevalence of disease is up to 25 per cent in adults. The prevalence seems to be similar in all developed societies. A few populations either living at high altitudes or belonging to primitive cultures (*e.g.*, a small number of ethnic groups living in the Pacific Islands, Asia, Africa and South America) seem to have exceptionally lower level of blood pressure.

Problem in India

Studies have shown that the prevalence of hypertension was 59.9/1000 in males and 69.9/1000 in females respectively in the urban communities and 35.5/1000 in males and 35.9/1000 in females in rural communities. The incidence is found usually between the age group of 20 to 60 years of age.

Hypertension is the major risk factor for stroke, CHD and renal failure. The higher the pressure, the greater is the risk of complications and the lesser life expectancy. Majority of mortality due to hypertension is due to cardio-vascular illnesses.

Clinical Manifestation

Hypertension is essentially a disease without symptoms. When symptoms do occur, they are usually indicative of advanced hypertension. Signs and symptoms may include early morning headache, unsteadiness, blurred vision, depression and spontaneous epistaxis. The effect of hypertension on cerebral blood vessels and cardiovascular system may include nausea and vomiting, confusion, chest pain and peripheral oedema.

Complications

With prolonged hypertension, the elastic tissues in the arterioles are replaced by fibrous collagen tissues. The thickened arteriole wall becomes less distensible (less elastic) offering greater resistance to blood flow. This leads to decreased tissue perfusion, especially in the target organs of high blood pressure, *e.g.*, heart, kidney, brain. Atherosclerosis is also accelerated in persons with high blood pressure.

In cardiovascular system decrease in coronary perfusion may lead to angina pectoris or myocardial infarction. Congestive heart failure can result from left ventricular hypertrophy, which results as the heart is forced to pump the blood against elevated aortic pressure for long period of time.

When renal vessels thickness and perfusion diminish, the glomerulus is deprived of blood supply. Permanent kidney damage and possible renal failure results.

Cerebral ischaemia and arteriosclerosis can occur as a result of progressive effects of hypertension, strokes can occur as a result of arteriosclerosis or haemorrhage from a leaking cerebral vessel.

CLASSIFICATION

Primary Hypertension

Not associated with any other illness, but occurs due to various predisposing factors, *e.g.*, obesity, old age, lifestyle, food habits etc.

Secondary Hypertension

When hypertension is associated with other disease processes or abnormalities, *e.g.*, kidney, glomerulonephritis, chronic pyelonephritis, tumour of adrenal gland, congenital narrowing of aorta, toxaemia of pregnancy, though 10 per cent of cases are seen as secondary hypertension.

ESSENTIAL HYPERTENSION (IDIOPATHY)

When the cause is not known it is essential hypertension. It constitutes about 75 per cent of cases. The exact cause is unknown.

Malignant

These are severe, rapid progressive elevations of blood pressure that causes damage to small arterioles in major organ systems (heart, kidney, brain and eyes). A primary distinguishing finding is inflammation of the arterioles in the eyes. Retinities and papilloedema occur in later stage. Unless medical treatment is successful, the course is rapidly fatal. The most common causes of deaths are myocardial infarction, congestive heart failure, stroke or renal failure.

EPIDEMIOLOGICAL FACTORS

Age and Sex

The incidence of hypertension increases with age and varies considerably among different groups. Hypertension occurs more often in men than in women, and the rise of blood pressure is greater in those with higher initial blood pressure.

Genetic Factor

It is basically considered as a genetic disease. The evidences of twin studies have confirmed the importance of genetic factors in hypertension. Blood pressure readings of monozygotic twins (single egg) are usually more strongly correlated than those of zygotic (separate eggs) twins. Though no significant correlation has been noted between husband and wife and adopted children and adoptive parents. Hence, hereditary seems to be dominant factor of hypertension.

Predisposing Factors

Dietary Habits

Consumption of high salt intake has shown the high incidence of hypertension and vice versa. Besides sodium, there are other mineral elements such as potassium which also determines blood pressure. Potassium supplements have been found to lower blood pressure of mild and moderate hypertension.

Studies have also found that saturated fat in the food (*ghee*) raises the blood pressure as well as serum cholestrol.

Obesity

Obesity is the major risk factor associated with hypertension. Studies indicate that greater the weight gain, the greater the risk of hypertension. Data has also indicated that when people with hypertension lose weight, the blood pressure generally decreases.

Physical Activity

Hypertension is said to be more among people with sedentary work. Hence, lack of physical activity predisposes hypertension. Lack of physical activity may increase the body weight and then hypertension. Reducing body weight by physical activity may have an indirect effect on blood pressure.

Alcohol

High intake of alcohol is associated with hypertension. Alcohol consumption seems to raise the systolic pressure more than diastolic.

Alcoholic hypertension may or may not be consistent. It may come to normal, when an individual is nonalcoholic.

Stressful Environment

Hypertension has been closely associated with stress and tension in the environmental stimu'. The psychosocial factors affect the ment. I processes by increasing the nonadrenaline level, and supports the overactivity of the sympathetic nervous system, has an important part to play in the pathogenesis of hypertension.

Miscellaneous Factors

Many other factors are also responsible in causation of hypertension. These factors are intake of oral contraceptives, noise vibrations and temperature may also affect blood pressure.

Observer's Error

That can be hearing acuity, interpretation of Korotkoff sounds.

Instrumental Error

Leaking valve, cuffs that do not encircle the arm then too high reading will be observed.

Subject's Error

These include physical environment, position of the subject, external stimuli such as fever, anxiety and so on.

PREVENTION AND CONTROL OF HYPERTENSION

Hypertension is a major risk factor in development of cardiovascular, renal, cerebral diseases. Thus, it is important to control hypertension through primary and secondary prevention strategies, so as to prevent the tertiary strategy by rehabilitation and restoration of patient's general health.

Primary Prevention

Nutrition

Balanced diet with less salt and fat intakes and high fibre diet, restriction of alcohol intake must be emphasized, e.g., fruits, green leafy vegetables, cereals and pulses.

Weight Reduction

The body weight must be controlled to average as much as possible. The prevention and correction of obesity will reduce the risk of hypertension.

Exercise Promotion

Regular physical activity leads to reduction in excessive body weight and reduces the incidence of hypertension.

Health Education

The whole community must be made aware of prevention of hypertension by adopting healthy lifestyle and habits, e.g.:

- Modification of personal lifestyle, yoga and meditation.
- Reduction of mental stress, strain and control of emotions.
- Avoid smoking and consuming alcohol.
- Physical activity in includes regular brisk walk for 20 to 30 minutes which is enough to remain physically fit and sound.

Control of Arterial Hypertension

Arterial hypertension is one of the major causes of CVA; and its early prevention and management is important for the prevention of disease. Control of diabetes, no smoking, prevention and management of other risk factors at community level are approached towards control of the disease. Follow-up of the patients for long-term treatment is essential.

- Balanced diet, rich fibre, low fat and low salt should be advised.
- Regular medical examination and weight checking.
- Prevention and control of other systematic diseases, e.g., kidney, liver and heart, etc.

High-risk Strategy

This is another strategy under primary level of prevention. The main aim is to prevent, the attainment of levels of blood pressure at which the institution of treatment would be considered. Detection of high-risk subjects should be encouraged by the optimum use of diagnostic methods and family history which will help to prevent the disease at an early stage by identifying high-risk individual.

Secondary Prevention

Focussed on identification and control of hypertension in high-risk groups. A major effort should be made for people who have limited access to health care because of economical or geographical constraints.

Objective

The objective of secondary prevention is to identify and control the high blood pressure. Antihypertensive therapy can effectively reduce the hypertension, prevent complications and reduce the mortality due to cardiocerebrovascular and kidney diseases. These measures are :

Early Detection of Cases

The only effective method of diagnosis is to screen the population at large. But it is not possible to take blood pressure of the whole population. However, screening can be done for high-risk cases like obesity, smoking, advancing age, antenatal cases or any other associated problems.

TREATMENT

The aim of treatment is to control the blood pressure till 140/90, though normally blood pressure is 130/80 mm of Hg. Patient with mild hypertension must also be treated. They might benefit in controlling the disease. Control of the hypertension will help in reducing the complication and stroke, etc. Though essential hypertension cannot be treated, we try to maintain the level of blood pressure to normal as much as possible.

TWENTY WAYS TO PREVENT A HEART ATTACK

- Evaluate your family history. Heart attacks, hypertension, atherosclerosis, diabetes and strokes have a strong correlation with family members. If either of your parents suffered with heart attack before the age of 50, you have an especially high degree of risk.

- Stop smoking and avoid passive smoke. The risk of heart attacks as well as stroke is significantly increased with smoking.

- Maintain your ideal weight. Individuals with central or abdominal obesity or those with frequent weight shift have increased risk.

- Diagnose hypertension and treat it appropriately. The risk of heart attack increases as the blood pressure increases.

- Obtain a diabetic evaluation. People with a family history of diabetes and or excessive weight are especially at risk for diabetes. Heart disease is five times more prevalent in diabetics.

- Evaluate your personality and consider a stress reduction programme. People who frequently display aggressive and hostile behaviour, get anger easily and have a low tolerance for frustration have an increased incidence of heart attacks.

- Start a daily exercise programme. Brisk walking has been shown to be adequate. Exercise is one of the few ways to increase HDL or 'good' cholesterol.

- Know your total cholesterol, HDL , LDL, and triglyceride levels. The desirable levels are, for total cholesterol; less than 200 mg/dL, for HDL more than 35 mg/dL, for LDL, less than 130 mg/dL, for triglycerides less than 130 mg/dL. 10 per cent reduction in total cholesterol reduces the risk of heart attacks by 20 per cent.

- Check lipoprotein (*a*) level which is an independent risk factor for heart attack.

- Have your blood antioxidant level checked (vitamin C, vitamin E, beta-carotene and selenium).

- Start supplementation with antioxidant vitamins C, E and beta-carotene. These are important in preventing heart attacks and arteriosclerosis.

- Choose a diet with not more than 20 to 30 per cent of calories coming from fats. Saturated fats must be avoided.

- Have iron and ferritin blood levels checked. There is increased risk for heart attacks with excessive iron intake and elevated ferritin levels.

- Beware of products labelled "low cholesterol" which are high in sugar and other fats.

- Check for a diagonal deep earlobe crease. This is associated with a high incidence of heart attacks.

- Check blood homocysteine levels. It is a amino acid. an independent risk factor for a heart attack.

- Have an "atheriosclerosis profile". It consists of using multisite high resolution blood vessel imaging to assess the status of all peripheral blood vessels.

- Check blood fibrinogen levels. Elevated level has been associated with increased heart attacks and strokes.

- Obtain a glucose tolerance test. Many individuals have subclinical diabetes which is a major risk for heart disease and this cannot be determined with a simple fasting glucose measurement.

- Do you have insulin resistance? Hyper-insulinism is easy to recognise as the basic underlying genetic portion of so called syndrome X. This syndrome or the deadly quartet consists of the following features : Hypertension, central or abdominal obesity, glucose intolerance or type II diabetes, dyslipidaemia, especially elevated triglycerides and hyperuricaemia.

●●●

18

Rheumatic Heart Disease

INTRODUCTION

Rheumatic heart disease (RHD) is an acute inflammatory and crippling disease which leads to continuing damage to heart, increasing disability, repeated hospitalisation and premature death, usually by the age of 35 years or even early. Rheumatic heart disease is one of the most preventable chronic disease, because it is an advanced stage of rheumatic fever (RF). Although rheumatic fever is not a communicable disease, it results from a communicable disease (*Streptococcus pharyngitis*). Rheumatic fever is a febrile condition affecting the connective tissues, particularly heart and joints initiated by throat infection due to *Streptococcus haemolytic*.

Rheumatic heart disease (RHD) is an acute inflammatory reaction. It may involve :

- Lining of heart or endocardium (endo-carditis), including valves resulting in scarring, distortion and stenosis of valves.
- Heart muscles (myocarditis) and
- Outer covering of heart (pericarditis). Usually rheumatic fever and rheumatic heart disease with mild symptoms go undiagnosed or disease may be subclinical with no noticeable symptoms. Careful recall of illness in childhood may include a recollection of "growing pain" confirming the likelihood that patient had rheumatic fever during childhood.

Worldwide Problem

Rheumatic heart disease is a global problem, though the incidence of mortality and morbidity is declining in many of the countries, but it is still a public health problem in developing countries. The prevalence rate in school age children in various parts of the world range from very low to as high as 33/1000. It has been estimated that RF is the most common cause of heart disease in 5 to 30 years of age group.

Problem in India

Rheumatic heart disease is a common form of heart disease among children and young adults in India. It is estimated that over 6 million children are affected by this disease. It accounts for 33 to 50 per cent of all cardiac cases. The regional variations show the highest prevalence of 11/1000 in Delhi and the lowest of 1.8/1000 in Mumbai. Streptococcal infections are very common, especially in children living in underprivileged conditions and rheumatic fever is reported to occur in 1 to 3 per cent of these infections.

Epidemiological Factors of Rheumatic Heart Disease

Agent Factor

The onset of the disease starts from throat infection caused by streptococci. Hence, cases and carriers of the infections may spread the disease.

Host Factor

Age and sex : Rheumatic heart disease affects mainly children and adolescents (5-15 years) and both sexes are equally affected.

Socio-economic status : The disease is more common among low socioeconomic group due to various factors, *e.g.*, poverty, overcrowding, poor housing conditions and inadequate health facilities.

High-risk group : The school children, slum dwellers and people living in closed community are more liable to get the disease.

Environment

Environment : High incidence is among people living in poor sanitary conditions, slum dwellers and crowded places.

Clinical Features

Fever

The onset of illness starts with fever during acute stage followed by profuse sweating. Fever may last for 12 weeks or longer and has tendency of recurrence.

Carditis

Cardiac involvement occurs in 60 to 70 per cent of cases. It starts early in stage of rheumatic fever. All layers of heart—pericardium, myocardium, endocardium and heart—valves are affected. These involvements lead to tachycardia, cardiac murmur, cardiac enlargement, pericarditis and heart failure.

Polyarthritis

Occurs in 90 per cent of patients. Large joints like ankle, knees, elbows and wrists are involved. Smaller joints of hands and feet may also be involved. There is an acute onset of pain and swelling of joints which may subside within 5 to 7 days. There is no residual damage to the joints.

Nodules

Nodules under the skin tend to appear within 4 weeks after the onset of rheumatic fever. They are small in size, painless and non-tender. They last for sometime and disappear, leaving no significant damage to the body.

Brain Involvement

The brain involvement leads to abnormal, jerky, purposeless movement of arms, legs and the body. It gradually disappears, leaving no residual damage.

Skin

Various types of skin rashes appear but have no permanent damage.

Except heart involvement, all other systems come to their normal size.

Diagnosis

WHO recommends throat culture for group 'A' streptococci test to reduce the effect of rheumatic fever.

- Throat culture for group 'A' streptococci.

PREVENTION OF RHEUMATIC HEART DISEASE

Primary Prevention

The aim is to prevent the attack of rheumatic fever by preventing sore throat infection, identification of streptococcal throat infection and treating with penicillin. Many infections are hidden, whereas apparent cases need quick and reliable laboratory services to confirm the diagnosis.

Approach to identify high-risk group, *e.g.,* school age children by taking sore throat swab for culture. The child should be treated with penicillin. Since the facilities are not easily available for culture, it has been justified to treat the children of sore throat with penicillin, which is a less expensive method to eradicate streptococci from the throat.

Secondary Prevention

Identify the cases with rheumatic fever and give them injection of benzathine benzyl penicillin (1.2 million units in adults and 600,000 units in children) at 3 weeks intervals for 5 years. This prevents streptococcal sore throat and the recurrence of rheumatic fever and rheumatic heart disease. The penicillin prophylaxis is a long-term affair, but is feasible, inexpensive and cost-effective, when implemented through primary health care system.

Other Measures

Penicillin alone will not be able to prevent the rheumatic heart disease effectively. Other measures like improving living conditions and socioéconomic conditions will also contribute towards control of the disease.

Prophylactic penicillin is prescribed during acute episodes of rheumatic fever and for several years thereafter. Continuous antibiotics prophylaxis for life may be necessary for those with significant rheumatic heart disease. Patients with carditis during acute rheumatic fever, corticosteroids may be prescribed to decrease cardiac inflammation. If congestive heart failure occur during this period, bedrest, sodium restriction, fluid restriction, diuretics and digoxin are usually prescribed.

Cardiovascular Diseases

19

INTRODUCTION

Heart disease is a major cause of death all over the world. Due to nonavailability of mass diagnostic tests, many people remain undiagnosed under the "iceberg of diseases". Many people are not even aware that they have the disease, until severe symptoms develop. Various cardiovascular disorders, *e.g.*, congenital heart diseases are responsible for newborn deaths. Other cardiovascular disorders with substantial morbidity and mortality include, hypertensive heart disease, rheumatic heart disease, cardiovascular diseases.

Cardiovascular diseases are defined as *"impairment of heart function due to inadequate supply of blood to the heart as compared to its needs due to obstructive changes in the coronary circulation of the heart"*. It constitutes one of the major causes of the death among developed and now in developing countries; reducing the years of the expected life. The people suffering from fatal coronary heart disease are having less years to survive in comparison with the people with mild heart problem or no heart problem. coronary heart disease is held responsible for about 30 per cent deaths among men and 25 per cent among women in most developed countries.

CLASSIFICATION OF CARDIOVASCULAR DISEASE

Cardiovascular diseases may be classified as :
- Angina pectoris
- Myocardial infarction
- Cardiac failure
- Rheumatic heart disease
- Coronary heart disease.

Coronary Artery Disease

Coronary heart disease is a genetic designated, involve obstructed blood flow through the coronary arteries. Coronary atherosclerosis heart disease (CAHD) is the most common type of coronary artery disease.

Epidemiological Distribution of Coronary Heart Disease (CHD)

Many countries pose largest Public Health problem due to coronary heart disease. The incidence of coronary heart disease was very high in Western countries in 1920. And now the incidence rate is catching up in the developing countries like Malaysia, Singapore, Mauritius, Sri Lanka, whereas the countries of higher incidence are declining now, and there is a decline of mortality rate due to coronary heart disease in Australia, Canada and New Zealand. The decline is probably due to change in lifestyle and related risk factor, *e.g.*, diet control, nonsmoking and exercises. It was a disease of higher classes but now all classes.

Worldwide Problem

Coronary heart disease is a worldwide problem, though the mortality rate varies from place to place. The highest mortality due to coronary heart disease is in North Europe, and the lowest mortality is in South Europe.

Problem in India

The incidence of disease in India is higher in the age group between 51 to 60 years, more among males than females. Studies have shown that the prevalence rate is 65.4/1000 among males and 47.8/1000 among females.

International Variation

Highest mortality is seen in North Europe and English speaking countries, *e.g.*, Scotland, Ireland and Finland, Japan has the lowest incidence of coronary heart disease.

Epidemiological Factors

Incidence of coronary artery disease is found much higher in males than females of child-bearing age and older individuals.

Risk Factors

Various risk factors are associated with coronary heart disease. The aetiology of disease is multifactorial. The more rise factor, the more chances. These factors are modifiable.

The exact cause remains unknown. Risk factors help to screen individuals who are at high-risk of developing coronary atherosclerosis heart disease (CAHD). The presence of risk factor does not definitely indicate the occurrence of disease and the absence of risk factor for coronary atherosclerosis heart disease does not mean that an individual will necessarily be free from coronary atherosclerosis. It is felt that three major risk factors are : high blood pressure, hyper-cholestrolaemia and cigarette smoking. Cessation of smoking, lowering of blood lipids by diet and reduction in blood pressure can reduce the risk of coronary artery disease.

Age and Sex

Disease is a major cause of death in man at age of 35 to 45 years. Women seem to be immune until after menopause. The mortality is rapidly increasing with age. Forty per cent of all deaths among men are caused by this single disease at age of 55 to 64 years. The prevalence rate among men is 65.4 and in female is 48/1000. Males have more due to heavy smoking.

Family History

The family history of coronary atherosclerosis heart disease predisposes the risk of disease to offsprings. The family disposition is thought to be due to genetic and environmental factors. The genetic elements are not very clear, but environmental factors, *e.g.*, nutrition, socio-economic status and other risk factors.

Dietary Pattern

The diet with saturated fats, cholestrols, refined sugar and salt is a significant coronary risk factor. The role of fibre in diet reduces the risk of coronary heart disease.

Hypertension

Elevated blood pressure either systolic or diastolic is a significant factor associated with coronary heart disease. They cause atherosclerotic process.

Smoking

Some commit suicide by drowning and some by smoking. The relationship between cigarette smoking and coronary atherosclerosis heart disease is not totally clear, but it has been suggested that the adverse effect of cigarette smoking on the heart and blood vessels involve the effects of nicotine and carbon monoxide. Specific changes include increased myocardial oxygen demand induced by nicotine, interference with oxygen supply by carboxyhaemo-globin and adhesion of platelets. Carbon monoxide causes atherosclerosis and nicotine causes adrenergic *e.g.*, high blood pressure and myocardial infarction. The countries where smoking has been a widespread habit, coronary heart disease is responsible for 25 per cent of deaths under 65 years of age in men. Cigarette smoking appears to be more important in causing sudden death from coronary heart disease especially in men below 50 years. The risk factor of coronary heart disease is directly related to the number of cigarettes smoked per day and method of smoking. The risk of death from coronary heart disease decreases on cessation of smoking. The risk declines quite substantially within a year at stopping smoking and more gradually within 10 to 20 years, it is the same as nonsmokers.

Psychosocial Factors

There is significant evidence of behavioural and other psychosocial influences on coronary artery disease. Smoking behaviour and diet patterns notably change depending on the degree of stress on individual.

Minimum social resources as well as occupation with low autonomy and high demand, are associated with increased risk of coronary artery disease. The stress response plays a focal role between physical and behavioural components.

Serum Cholestrol

The elevation of serum cholestrol greater than 200 mg indicates the increased risk of coronary heart disease. Though increase in serum cholestrol is related to dietary pattern of an individual, but it is not very significant. There are evidences that people with low serum cholestrol also develop coronary heart disease. Hence, it is the level of lipoprotein cholestrol which contributes to the diseases. Low density of lipoprotein cholestrol is directly related to coronary heart disease. Very low density lipoprotein (LDL) has shown association with premature atherosclerosis, which is more strongly associated with peripheral vascular disease. High level of lipoprotein cholestrol is protective against the development of coronary heart disease. Hence, coronary heart disease risk is based on serum lipid level a total cholestrol/high density lipoprotein (HDL) ratio required to be not less than 3.5 for prevention of coronary heart disease.

Physical Activity

Sedentary lifestyle is associated with greater risk of development of early congenital heart disease. Regular exercise increases the concentration of high density lipoprotein and decreases both body weight and blood pressure, which is beneficial to cardiovascular health.

A person has higher chances of developing coronary heart disease with high-risk factors.

Obesity

Obesity is usually caused by a caloric intake that exceeds the energy expenditure. A number of metabolic abnormalities are present in obese persons, but are probably the result of obesity rather than the cause.

When food intake equals metabolic needs, weight remains fairly constant throughout life. A weight gain sometimes accompanies aging because the individual does not adjust food intake to lowered metabolism and diminished activity.

Diet

Obesity is basically controlled with dietary changes. A weight loss diet must provide fewer calories than the person's energy expenditure, while consistently supplying the nutrients necessary for health. Extreme obesity is sometimes treated with fasting or complete abstinence from food. Fasting can be tolerated by repeated periods of 10 to 15 days. If a person is under medical supervision, and fluids and vitamins are provided. An average weight loss of 1 pound/day results from fasting. Complications include postural hypertension, anaemia, cardiac irregularities, decreased uric acid excretion and hyperuricaemia that is reversed when the fast ends, but may result in uric acid neuropathy and fluid retention.

Other Risk Factors

Diabetes mellitus has shown 2 to 3 times higher risk of coronary heart disease than nondiabetic mellitus. coronary heart disease is more found in type 'A' personality.

Angina Pectoris

It occurs when myocardial oxygen demand exceeds myocardial oxygen supply. It is usually caused by atherosclerosis of coronary vessel, but incidence is high in people with hypertension, diabetes mellitus, polycythemia and rheumatic heart disease. Angina is precipitated by exercise, cold or anything that increases the workload of heart and myocardial consumption.

It is characterised by paroxysmal retrosternal or substernal pain, often radiating down the inner aspect of left arm. Tightness of the chest, diffused pain can rarely be pinpointed at the specific sight. Pain is often associated with exertion and is relieved by rest or vasodilation by medications. There may be complications of acute M.I., cardiac arrhythmia, death.

Health Teaching

- Avoid excessive activity in winter
- Avoid overeating
- Sleep in warm room
- Minimum exposure to stressful situation
- Medication if needed
- Regular activity and exercise
- Balanced diet
- Healthy lifestyle : No smoking or alcoholism.

MYOCARDIAL INFARCTION

Acute myocardial infarction is caused by sudden blockage of one of the branches of coronary artery. It may be extensive to interfere with cardiac function and cause immediate death or may cause necrosis of a portion of the myocardium with subsequent healing by scar formation or fibrosis. Coronary occlusion is a term used for blockage of coronary artery. Blockage may be caused by formation of a thrombus in the coronary artery (coronary thrombosis), sudden progression of atherosclerotic changes and prolonged constriction of the arteries.

Clinical manifestations of myocardial infarction are complain of sudden severe, crushing, pain at substernal region. Patient is restless, difficulty in breathing, excessive sweating, nausea and vomiting. 15 to 25 per cent of myocardial infarction may be without pain. The incidence of pain increases with the increase of age. Other less common symptoms may be confusion, arrhythmia, drop in blood pressure sudden loss of consciousness.

Nurse's Responsibilities

- Bed rest
- Provide comfort

- Nutritional rehabilitation
- Relief of anxiety and stress
- Progressive activity
- Home exercise programme
- Counselling.

Health Teachings

- Avoid smoking and drinking
- Eat diet less in calories, saturated fat, cholestrol, *e.g.,* vegetables and fruits
- Weight reduction programme
- Passive exercises
- Avoid stress, anxiety and encourage relaxation and meditation
- Return to work on doctors's advise
- Regular follow-up.

NATIONAL CARDIOVASCULAR DISEASE CONTROL PROGRAMME

The complete statistics about cardiovascular disease and stroke are incomplete. It is estimated that about 8 lakh people die from coronary heart disease and more than 6 lakh from stroke. An increasing trend in cardiovascular disease has been noticed. Survey in India reveals that 10 to 15 adults suffer from hypertension. Estimated deaths due to rheumatic heart disease are 1,41,000 annually.

Since the diagnostic and therapeutic technology required for the management of established coronary and other vascular diseases are highly expensive, preventive action becomes essential. At the same time, cost-effective technology required for the diagnostic and therapeutic interventions needs to be developed and made appropriate use at all levels of health care.

•••

20

Accidents

INTRODUCTION

Accidents represent a major public health problem among noncommunicable diseases. The prevalence of accidents is on the rise due to advancing technologies.

Definitions

Accidents are defined as, *"an unexpected or unplanned occurrence which may involve mild or major injury".*

WHO defines accidents as, *"unpredicted event resulting in recognizable damage".*

Accidents are also defined as, *"occurrence in a sequence of events which usually produces unintentional injury, death or property damage".*

Accidents can be also defined as *"an unexpected and undesirable event, a mishap, anything that occurs unexpectedly or unintentionally".*

THE GLOBAL PROBLEM OF ACCIDENTS

World

Accident is the fourth main cause of death and 8 per cent of deaths are due to accidents. Most of these deaths are among 10 to 24 years of age group. It has been estimated that 4 million people die annually due to injury. Globally one million people die of intentional injury or violence (homicide and suicide) and three million die of unintentional injuries like road accidents, domestic accidents, industrial accidents, fire, drowning, poisons, falls and natural disasters (Fig. 20.1).

More than 8 lac people die of road accidents and two-thirds of them are from developing countries. Twenty-two per cent of mortality among males and females is due to vehicles.

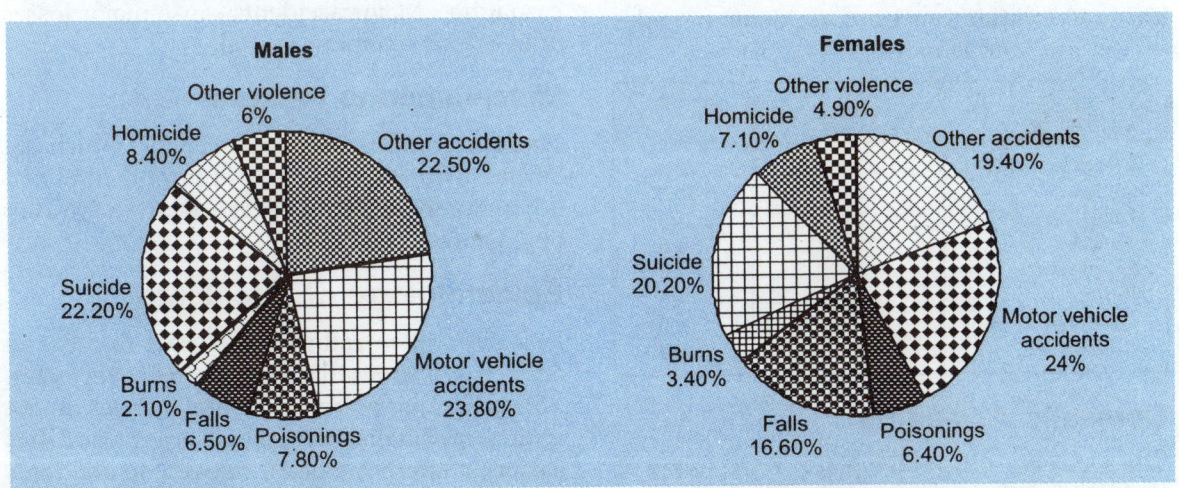

Fig. 20.1 : Global deaths from subgroups of injuries, poisonings and violence

India

Accidents are on the increase in India. Fatality rate due to accident in India is one of the highest rates in the world. It is 20 times more than the developed countries.

India has one of the highest road traffic accident rates in the world. The number of people injured in road accidents has doubled in the past six years. The peak mortality and morbidity from RTA is seen between 15 to 24 years of males. Large proportion of vehicles involved in accidents were mainly two-wheelers, since they provide little protection to their riders in accidents. In some countries more than one-third of all traffic death occur among users of two-wheeler vehicles.

Accidents injury kill thousands of people of all ages every year. Accidents ranked as the third cause of death after cardiovascular diseases and malignancies. Accidents can occur at anytime and in any situation or place, *e.g.*, home, school, workplace, highway and recreation area. Most accidents are the result of carelessness or ignorance and many could be preventable. Therefore, safety education and enforcement are essential to reduce the frequency and seriousness of accidents.

Table 20.1 shows the main causes of accidents in males and females.

Table 20.1 : Main causes of accidents in males and females

Causes of accidents	Male	Female
Vehicular	23.8	23.2
Suicide	22.2	20.0
Falls	8.5	16.6
Violence	5.7	4.9
Homicide	8.4	7.1
Burns	2.1	3.4
Poisoning	7.8	6.4
Others	22.5	19.4

Domestic Accidents

The accidents which take place in the home or in its immediate surroundings, and more generally, all the accidents are not connected with traffic, vehicle or sports. The most frequent cause of accidents are:

- Burns—by electrical, chemical, fire, liquid
- Poisons—drug, insecticide, rat poison, kerosin
- Drowning
- Injury from sharp instrument
- Bites and other injuries from animals
- Others

Domestic accidents are a frequent cause of death or disability at the expense of life.

Industrial Accidents

Every year thousand of workers die and more than 2.5 lac are injured in industries and thousands are crippled in accidents. Due to prolonged working days and no payment for compensation, industrial accidents are a heavy burden on national economy.

Burns

More than one lac people get burnt and scratched in India every year, and 20,000 die due to burns. Ten per cent of all accident deaths are a heavy burden on national economy.

Railway Accidents

More than 11,000 trains carry over one crore passengers everyday in the country. Due to increase in number of passengers and trains, there is increased number of train accidents and casualities. Major accidents cause major losses of lives and economy as well.

Miscellaneous Factors

There are various aetiological factors which can be classified as human and environmental and 90 per cent of causes are due to human negligence.

Epidemiology of Accidents

It is difficult to estimate the exact number of accidental injuries that are sustained every year. This is because many accidental injuries do not require hospitalisation and are unreported. It is easier to determine death rate due to accidents because the cause of death is reported on certificates.

Injuries occur most frequently in males in the age groups 6 to 16 and 17 to 44. In the age group of 65 and above, female have higher risk of accidents (due to osteoporosis).

Most injuries result from motor vehicle accidents involving both cars and motorcycles. Falls and fires are major causes of deaths at home. More deaths occur from accidents in rural areas, due to lack of properly trained emergency personnel and emergency care facilities to transport the victims.

Accidents result in temporary or permanent restriction of activities, hospitalisation and death. The financial impact is experienced through hospital cost, prolonged and expensive care. The impact of accidental injury and death is felt by all groups of society in direct or indirect financial, rehabilitation and social terms.

The epidemiology of accident will be based on gathering precise information about the extent, type and other characteristics of accidents, correlation and environmental factors involved in accidents. It helps in investigating new and better methods of reducing the incidences of accidents.

Planning and Organising Emergency Care

Planning and organising emergency care services should begin at accident site, continue during transportation and conclude in the hospital emergency room. At this point of care, the life may be saved or lost, depending upon the skill of the health care workers and availability of needed emergency equipment. There must be a special trauma care facilities in all major hospitals.

Prevention

Most of the accidents can be prevented by various safety measures. These measures comprise the following :

Data Collection

All accidents must have accurate reporting system. The national data should be supplemented by special surveys and depth studies. These studies will help to identify the risk factors, circumstances and chain of events leading to accidents. Detailed environment data relating to the road, vehicle, weather, etc. must be collected. Adequate data are essential to analyse and interpret the data to rule out the aetiological factors, which help the strategies for prevention.

Safety Education

Safety is defined as freedom from danger, risk or injury, any of various devices designed to prevent accidents. As community health nursing our focus need to be directed towards the reinforcement of safety enhancing activities and extinguishing the accident promoting activities for the individual, family and community. This requires active assessment of environmental conditions in the home, farm, school, occupational setting, health care setting, recreational area and community sites and resources of all kinds. Accidents can be prevented or reduced in frequency through educational activities, safety inspection visits and enforcement of safety laws and regulations. People must be given education about road safety. The road safety and domestic safety must begin with school children. The drivers must be well trained in safe driving. People must be educated regarding risk factors, traffic rules and safety precautions. They should be trained about emergency care and First Aid. It has been truly said that "if accident is a disease, education is its vaccine".

Promotion of Safety Measures

People must use the protective devices to prevent accidents, e.g., seat belts, safety helmets, fire safety, etc. Some countries have introduced laws to use some safety measures on road but more important is people's awareness for using safety devices.

Alcohol and Other Drugs

There should be prohibition of driving after consuming alcohol. Alcohol impairs driving ability and increases the risk of an accident as well as severity of accident. Surveys have shown that 30 to 50 per cent of road accidents are due to alcohol.

Elimination of Causative Factors

The factors which are responsible to cause accidents should be eliminated, *e.g.*, road repairs, speed limit, signal functioning, fire guards, electrical poles and wire management/safe equipments in industries, safe storage of drugs, poisons and weapons, etc.

Legislative Measures

Set of rules must be reinforced in the country to prevent accidents. These laws include driving test, medical fitness to drive, enforcement of speed limit, compulsory wearing of seat belts, use of helmets, checking blood alcohol concentration, regular inspection of vehicles, periodic examination of drivers, factory and industries to ensure safety measures of people at work.

Rehabilitation Services

The rehabilitation services must involve the benefits to injured people so as to make them socially and economically independant. The aim of rehabilitation is to prevent or reduce or compensate the disable and handicapped. There should be social, occupational and medical rehabilitation.

Protective Measure to Control Accidents

Since accident can happen to anyone at any time or place, some attention needs to be given to the kinds and sites of accidents that can occur. At home, injuries result mostly from falls, fires, particularly in the kitchen and bedroom. Poisoning, particularly for children from household cleaning products and various poisonous drugs.

- Various lacerations, abrasions, and fractures from tools, cutting equipments, *e.g.*, knife scissors. Health education to community must focus on improving unsafe conditions in the house and should be according to safety measures.
- Fire hazards such as, combustible materials near heat sources, curtains near cooking stoves, synthetic clothing worn while cooking and electrical inadequacies should be checked, identified and corrected.
- Smoke detectors should be in working order, tested regularly and placed in appropriate places in the house.
- Stairs should be kept clean and have handrails properly fixed. Safety gates should be used in stairs to prevent fall during emergencies, especially for children. Bath tubs or showers should have rubber mats or nonslip floors.
- Drawers of tables, almirahs and cabinets should be kept closed when not in use.
- Sharp instruments, *e.g.*, knives, razor blades, scissors should be kept safely.

All medicines, cleaning products and poisons should be stored safely at higher place so that it is not approached by the children easily.

- Garden equipments require safe storage and should be out of reach of children preventing injuries. To avoid any physical injury and damage caused due to carelessness, one must follow the safety norms and rules. Injury is directly related to our sentiments and emotions and also effects our economic condition. Hence a physical, emotional and economical harm.
- Farm represents another area of safety and concerns. Insecticides, poisons and other harmful materials should be stored safely. Farm equipments must be kept in safe working order to prevent injuries.

The above mentioned hazards to safety can be safeguarded by proper implementaion of safety norms. Precautions can be taken to reduce the potential to injury after proper identification of any expected injury or harm.

Work Place

At workplace the type of accident depends upon the kind of activities carried on. Falls are a source of injury regardless of site, and may be due to water or other liquid on the floor.

Lacerations, abrasions, and various eye injuries occur due to unprotected equipment and machinary, not using safety equipment such as gloves and goggles, improper use of equipment and not following accepted safety protocols.

Additional injuries might result from high noise level, and from various inhalants such as asbestos, coal dust and cotton mill dust. It may be due to long exposure to such area and if delayed the impact will be dangerous and severe. Job stress may cause mental health problem and cardiovascular disease, which can be linked to various accidents and injuries.

Vehicular Accidents

Accounts a large number of injuries and mortalities. Vehicular accidents include, cars, bicycles, motorcycles, trains, buses and aeroplanes, etc. Highway safety is a major source of concern these days. Various safety measures have been investigated and recommended, *e.g.*, speed limit, flight control for aeroplanes, safety regulations for railways to prevent derailments and various train collisions.

It is essential to adopt safety measures for commercial transportation system.

Various safety regulations are recommended on safety belt usage, highway speed limit, signs to alert the drivers to such hazards at hills, corners, and no passing zones.

Motorbikes, scooters and bicycles are involved in many road accidents. Speed limit is applicable to all motorized vehicles.

●●●

Blindness

21

INTRODUCTION

Blindness is one of the major health problem in the world. The number of blind people in India have increased from 9 million in 1971 to 15.69 million in 1980 (ICMR and WHO survey). Thus, the magnitude of the problem has increased despite best efforts, though the pattern of blindness has changed. More than 85 per cent of blind people are curable by modern medical technologies.

Definition

According to WHO definition, blindness is said to be *"visual acquity of less than 3/60 or its equivalent"*. To facilitate screening of visual acquity by nonspecialised personnel, in the absence of appropriate vision chart, WHO has now added *"Inability of a person to count fingers in daylight at a distance of one meter to indicate less than 3/60 or its equivalent"*.

Visual Impairement

A person is considered legally blind when either of the following conditions exist.

- A person's visual field is not greater than 20 degree or,
- Central distance vision in the better eye is 20/200 or worse with use of correct lenses. Loss of visual acquity may range from profound to slight; visual field loss may be peripheral or central; there may be other visual functions affected such as dark adaptation.

Worldwide Problem of Blindness

It has been estimated that more than 180 million people are visually disabled and 45 million are blind. Eighty per cent of total visually impaired are living in developing countries and more than 80 per cent are preventable by prophylactic measures. Majority of them are affected due to inaccessibility of eye care and management of eye problems at an early stage. Blindness leads to economical and social burden on the community.

Magnitude of the Problem in India

The national sample survey conducted by Indian Council for Medical Research (ICMR) (1981) estimated that 1.4 per cent of blinds in total population and 45 millions have been suffering from visual impairement and more than fifteen million are completely blind.

CAUSES OF BLINDNESS

Main causes of the blindness are listed below (Fig. 21.1) :

Cataract 55%
Trachoma 20%
Nutritional deficiencies 2%
Glaucoma 0.5%
Other causes 15.5%
Reflective error 4.0%
Corneal opacity 3%

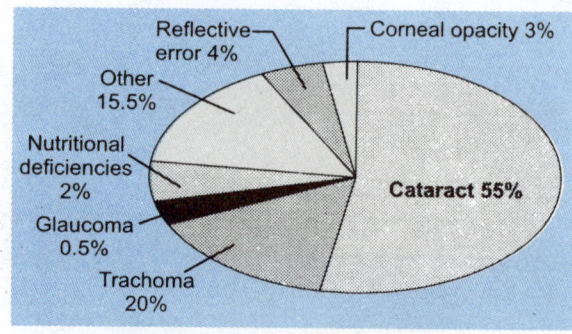

Fig. 21.1 : Causes of Blindness

About 10 million people are blind due to cataract. Considering this, the efforts should be made to reduce the prevalence rate of blindness. This is only possible when serious and systematic efforts are made to tackle cataract problem without further delay.

Prevalence of blindness is high in states like Madhya Pradesh, Rajasthan, Andhra Pradesh, Orissa, Maharashtra, Tamil Nadu, and U.P.

COMMON EYE DISEASES
Cataract

Cataract or opacification of the lense accounts for 55 per cent of total blindness. Most of the cases are senile, and a small number are congenital, developmental or traumatic. Whereas some cases are pathological, associated with systematic diseases, *e.g.*, diabetes, parathyroid, cretinism and other complicated diseases. When cataract is in the immature stage, the changing reflection of the eye needs to be corrected with spectacles. When the decreasing vision starts hampering the daily routine of patients they should be referred for surgery.

Trachoma

Trachoma is a potentially blinding disease caused by *Chlamydia trachomatis* (Fig. 21.2). It usually responds to sulphonamides, acromycin, tetracycline, and erythromycin, etc. Major problem at present is to treat all cases at an early stage not only to prevent loss of vision, but also to eliminate the source of infection. The effective treatment is 1 per cent chlortetracycline or oxytetracycline ointment applied locally twice a day for 5 days in a month at monthly interval for 6 months. Blanket treatment every month for 5 days for six months of oxytetracycline ointment should be applied.

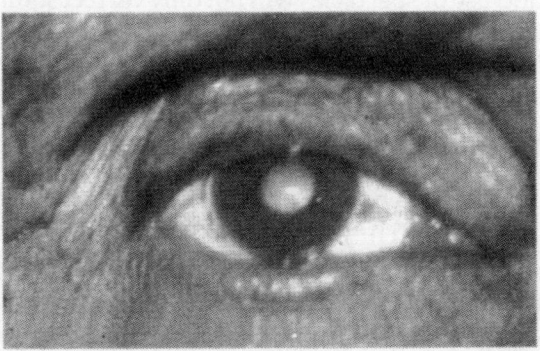

Fig. 21.2 : Trachoma

This should be given as blanket treatment to all children below 10 years. People must be educated regarding cleanliness, face washing, and washing of eyes with tap water will help to decrease the incidence of disease.

Glaucoma

Glaucoma, as a cause of irreversible blindness, has increased in magnitude over the years. It now accounts for 2 per cent blindness in India. Glaucoma is a specific pattern of optic nerve damage and visual field loss (Fig. 21.3). Intraocular pressure (IOP) is the most important risk factor causing glaucoma. The disease is called the *"sneak thief of sight"* because it strikes without obvious symptoms. Person with glaucoma is usually unaware of it until serious loss of vision has occurred. Patients suffering with damage of glaucoma do not even know about it.

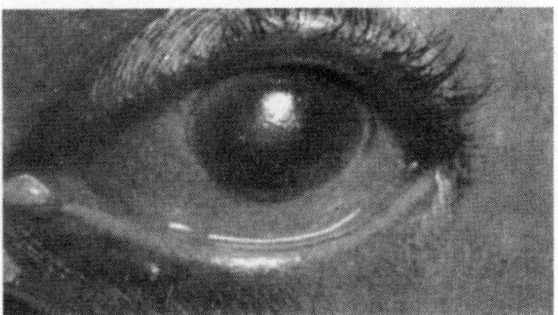

Fig. 21.3 : Glaucoma

Damage caused to the eyesight due to glaucoma cannot be cured till date. People of old age who do not get their eyes tested regularly, those suffering from myopia (near sighted), those with family history of glaucoma, diabetes, migraine, headaches are the one who are at high-risk of having glaucoma. Glaucoma management requires frequent monitoring, so that the doctor can keep check on the effectiveness of the medication taken.

Investigation

Tests which are done to determine if glaucoma is increasing with time, are :

1. Tonometry to measure the IOP,
2. Ophthalmoscopy to evaluate any optic nerve damage, and
3. Perimetry, a test of visual field of each eye.

Early detection and treatment is the only way of combating with this serious disease. This can be achieved by proper survey of population especially in remote areas. All people over the age of 40 years should come for periodical eye check-up.

Nutritional Blindness

Nutritional blindness among young children resulting from vitamin A deficiency is an important public health problem in the developing countries. Xerophthalmia (changes in eyes due to vitamin A deficiency) ranks as one of the important causes of nutritional blindness in children. In India about 40,000 children are permanently blind and 1.2 lac are visually handicapped due to keratomalacia. Multiple factors are responsible for this problem, *e.g.*, poor socioeconomic conditions, poor intake of vegetables, fruits and milk in the diet and recurrent infection like diarrhoea and measles. The affected child is malnurished and may be marasmic and presents bilateral Bitot's spot, corneal and conjunctival xerosis, corneal ulcer and later scaling. Early detection can be done by eye examination of the pre-school and school going children. They should be given a treatment of three injections of aquasol (vitamin A) 1 lac unit intramuscularly, on alternate day, followed by oral aquasol.

Diabetic Eye

20 to 40 per cent of diabetics have affected eyes. At present blindness due to diabetes is not a major health problem due to high prevalence of corneal blindness and cataract. Major cause of blindness in diabetes is due to retinopathy and its associated complications.

Injuries to the Eye

Accident to eyes are seen almost everywhere and happens due to negligence in our daily life. Injuries are damaging the God gifted precious eyes and is considered as perforating injuries caused due to bow and arrow, knife, fall from height, roadside accident, metallic foreign body, etc. In such cases self-medication should be strictly avoided and the patient should be immediately referred to the ophthalmologist. Parents should have strict watch on their children and advise them not to play with sharp objects. They should be extra careful during festivals like Holi, Dusshera and Diwali. Industrial workers are at a greater risk of sustaining injuries. They should be provided with protective goggles, helmets and sheilds as a safeguard against these accidents. In case of chemical injuries, the eyes should be immediately washed thoroughly with tap water and must be referred to the specialist. Workers should also be educated about the advantages of using such protective aids.

Eye Infections

Infections of the eye causes loss of vision and preventive measures are implemented to promptly overcome out of it. A very common problem is conjuctivities which presents *"red eye with excessive secretion"*. Patient is usually advised to use broad spectrum antibiotic drops, wash the eye frequently and wear dark glasses. Some of the infections are highly contagious and their spread can be prevented by avoiding crowds and gatherings. Special precautions should be taken during epidemic of disease such as cleanliness, washing hands time to time and specially before eating anything, separate cloth and towel for infected patient.

Squint

Squint is often considered as a cosmatic problem. It may be the cause of irreversible blindness if not checked at an early stage. Early detection and use of spectacles will not only correct squint but will also prevent the loss of vision. Often it is wrongly believed that squint will get corrected spontaneously with growth of child.

Corneal Ulcer

These ulcers may be of bacterial, viral or fungal aetiology. They cause great inconvenience during active stage and diminished vision after healing. The patient complains of red eye with decreased vision and mucopurulent discharges, pain and photophobia. Many times there may be history of foreign body in the eye, *e.g.*, vegetable peels, coloured powder, metallic powder. Patient must be referred to specialist for treatment.

EPIDEMIOLOGICAL FACTORS FOR BLINDNESS

Host

Age

Thirty per cent of the blind lose their eyesight before the age of 20 and many under 5 years of age, mainly due to trachoma, conjunctivitis and malnutrition. In middle age the causes of blindness are due to cataract, glaucoma and diabetes, etc. Accidents and injury can occur in any age but higher incidence is during 20 to 40 years.

Sex

Higher prevalence rate of blindness is reported in females due to trachoma, conjunctivitis and cataract. This may be due to exposure to smoke, negligence, poor family support, etc.

Occupation

The people working in factories, workshops and cottage industries are more prone to eye injuries due to exposure to smoke, gases, dust, fumes, radiations, electrical flash, airborne fumes etc. Many workers including doctors are known to have cataract due to exposure to X-rays, radiations or heat waves, etc.

Malnutrition

Malnutrition is closely related to blindness, especially among children. Not only vitamin A deficiency causes xerophthalmia but Protein Energy Malnutrition (PEM) causes blindness. Severe blindness, corneal destruction due to vitamin A deficiency (keratomalacia) is common among children from 6 months to 3 years. Malnutrition causes infections diseases, *e.g.*, measles which may lead to complications of blindness.

Socioeconomic Factors

Studies have shown that low socioeconomic people have higher incidence of blindness than among higher socio-economic group. Hence there is close association between social, cultural status and blindness, which can be due to ignorance, illiteracy, poor facilities, cultural practices, low standard of living, poverty and inadequate health care services, etc.

Agent

The different causative agents can be identified among different diseases.

> Trachoma – *Clamydia trachomatis* (Bacterial)
> Cataract – Opacity of lense (Pathology)
> Glaucoma – Increases intraoccular pressure
> Corneal ulcer – Bacterial, viral or fungal
> Xerophthalmia – Vitamin A deficiency
>   (Nutritional).

Environmental

Depending upon the causes, environment plays an important role in causing eye infection, complication which may lead to blindness if ignored. Poor sanitation, heavy smoke, pollution, low personal and environmental conditions can lead to conjunctivitis, corneal ulcer, trachoma, injuries and then blindness if, not treated in time.

Preventive Measures

Eighty per cent of total blindness are preventable. Therefore, it is essential to prevent blindness at all the three levels.

Primary Level

Most of the eye problems can be prevented or treated at primary level by gross root workers, *e.g.*, community health workers or multipurpose workers; who are the first to make contact with community. They should be able to teach the community regarding eye care and should be able to administer medication for minor eye infections. Health education should be given on:

- Cleaning of the eyes with running water at least 4 to 5 times a day and washing at least 20 times.
- Proper nutrition, *e.g.*, green leafy vegetables rich in carotene or fish, liver and meat for vitamin A supplement.

- Regular eye check-up—at least once a year by ophthalmologist.
- Infected eye should be washed with boric acid solution.
- Protect the eyes from injury or any harmful substance by using goggles and protective devices.
- Avoid eye straining by using proper light, especially for children while studying.
- Promotion of personal hygiene, stimulation and safety.
- Vitamin A supplementation to children 1 to 5 years of age.

Secondary Level

Provision for early diagnosis and treatment of all eye problems, *e.g.*, cataract, trachoma, glaucoma, nutritional deficiencies, injuries or any other through :

Eye Camp

Organisation of eye camp at subcentre and primary health centre level will help people for early treatment of any eye ailment and surgical interventions.

Mobile Eye Clinics

Should emphasise on treatment of all infections, making it accessible to the gross root level people. The treatment should be effective and affordable by the people.

- Provision of drug supply through all health agencies.

Tertiary Level

Specialised Care

The specialised care is provided by the medical colleges and nationalised hospitals. They provide sophisticated eye care treatment, such as retinal detachment surgery, corneal grafting and other complex treatment which is not available at secondary level.

Other Measures

Rehabilitation of blind persons by :
- Special schools for blind.

- Provision of employment for appropriate placement so as to make them economically and physically independent. Central Government has opened a National Institute for the Blind at Dehradun (U.P.) to workout new strategies and approaches to improve the conditions of blind.

SPECIAL EYE HEALTH ACTIVITIES

Trachoma Control Programme

Trachoma and other associated diseases are preventable in most of the developing countries.

- Preventive measures include general personal hygiene, environmental hygiene, prevention of hazards, *e.g.*, smoke and other poor health practices (kajal, surma, etc.), prevention of infection and healthy nutrition.
- Early diagnosis and treatment of eye infection and treatment by application of tetracycline.

Vitamin A Supplementation

This is useful prophylaxis against xerophthalmia due to vitamin A deficiency which leads to night blindness. Under the vitamin A distribution scheme in India, 200,000 I.U. (International Units or 5 mL) of vitamin A is given orally to children from 1 year to 6 years of age at every 6 months interval.

School Eye Health Programme

It is essential to protect the eyes of school children who form the major part of community by screening and treating the defects, *e.g.*, amblyopia, trachoma, injuries, squint and refraction error. Health education is an essential component of school health services. Students should be taught about :

- Healthy reading habits like good posture, proper light from back or right side, avoid too bright or glare light, proper distance and angle between books and eyes (Fig. 21.4).

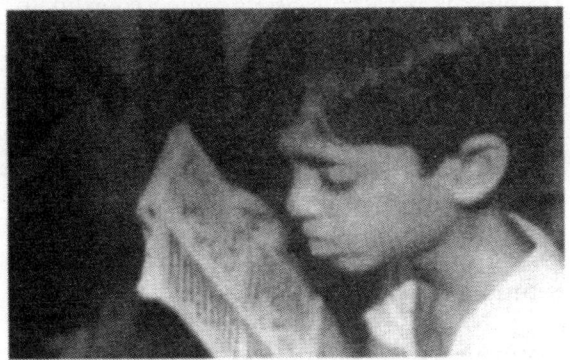

Fig. 21.4 : Unhealthy reading habits

- Protect the eyes from foreign bodies, injury, sharp objects and crackers, etc.
- Good nutrition rich in vitamin A / carotene, *e.g.*, green leafy vegetables, raw vegetables, fish, eggs, etc.
- Regular eye check-up at least every year.

Occupational Eye Health Services

These are special services to prevent the hazards in industries and factories. Special legislative eye health provision has been amended.

HEALTH EDUCATION

- Prevention of occupational eye hazards and use of protective devices in some occupations is essential.
- To improve the safety features of machines, to have proper lighting in working areas, to select people with requisite alertness and good vision and to encourage the use of eye protective devices *e.g.*, goggles.

Eye Health Care for Community

The measures to improve the quality of life and improving the environmental factors are responsible for eye health problems, *e.g.*, proper sanitation, adequate water supply, food rich in vitamin A and personal hygiene, etc. Health education is important component for community awareness of the problems, motivating the people for proper eye care during eye infections and availing the services through eye health camps and mobile vans, etc.

Care of a Blind Person

- Place clothings in specific location in drawer and closets.
- Place food and cooking utensils at specific locations in cupboards and in refrigerator.
- Encourage to be careful when walking.
- Keep furniture and household objects in specific places.
- When assisting a blind person in walking, let the person take help of your arm.
- Provide descriptions of food on the plate using clock placement of food.
- Always persist blind persons to pull out their own chairs and to take their seat themselves.

COMMUNICATING WITH BLIND PERSONS

- Talk in a normal tone of voice.
- Do not try to avoid common phrases in speech such as *"See what I mean"*.
- Introduce yourself with each contact, knock on the door before entering in hospital.
- Explain any activity occurring in the room or what you will do.
- Announce when you are leaving the room, so that person does not keep talking to someone who is no longer there.

NATIONAL PROGRAMME FOR CONTROL OF BLINDNESS AND VISUAL IMPAIRMENT

National Programme for Control of Blindness is centrally sponsored scheme, launched in 1976-77 aiming with the goal of bringing down the prevalence from 1.4 per cent blindness in the population to 0.3 per cent by 2000 A.D. and to provide comprehensive eye care through primary health care.

1956–63 Trachoma Pilot Project in U.P. was started during this period.

1963   National Trachoma Control Programme was initiated by Government for control of blindness.

1977   The name has been changed as National Programme for Prevention of Visual Impairment and Control of Blindness.

Objectives

The main objectives of the programme are :

Immediate

To provide immediate relief by expanding eye care services to the people in far away areas through mobile camp approach.

Ultimate

To establish permanent eye care facilities at community, primary health centre, block level, district and state level through training of manpower of qualified medical and paramedical ophthalmic personnel and equipping institutions at central, regional, state, district and block level.

Mass education on the care of eyes through all available media, *e.g.*, radio, T.V., press, cinema and distribution of health education materials.

Educating groups like teachers, leaders of community and parents under *Community Eye Care Programme.*

Educating individuals specially school children by including chapters in the textbook on formal and nonformal education.

Activities under the National Programme

National Institute of Ophthalmology (Dr. Rajendra Prasad Centre for Ophthalmic Science) has been established for manpower development, research, diagnostic and referral services. To train ophthalmic assistants, 37 training schools have been established in the country. Each primary health centre and district hospital to be provided with at least one ophthalmic assistant.

Since cataract cases constitute more than 50 per cent blindness, therefore, targets have been set for each state for cataract operations.

Voluntary organisations are playing a very significant role in this programme with the success achieved and experience gained through the pilot district project. District blindness control societies have been established throughout the country under the Chairmanship of Deputy Commissioner, District Magistrate.

Training of district blindness control coordinator are being carried out in a phased manner.

Community health education is a built-in component at all levels of implementation. The programme also includes regular check-up and provision of vitamin A prophylaxis and service facilities in rural areas. The Danish International Development Agency (DANIDA) is providing assistance for the mobile units and for equipment of the primary health centres and district hospitals. WHO is assisting in organising workshops and seminars at national and state levels and sponsoring fellowship for regional and extra-regional countries, professional development of man power and supply of sophisticated ophthalmic equipment.

Primary Level

As a part of primary health care services, Primary Eye Care, is being provided at block level primary health centres including community health centre covering a population of 1,00,000. Activities include treatment of simple eye diseases, diagnosis and referral of case needing treatment at intermediate and tertiary level and Eye Care Units. Eye health education survey of local community helps in screening of school children and local industrial workers. Medical Officers working at these centres are being trained in eye care at district hospitals and essential eye care equipment are regularly supplied and checked at these centres.

Secondary Level

Eye care strengthening at all district hospitals have been taken up. Reinforcement of these services have been taken up by attaching a district mobile unit to each district hospital. Minimum of 10 to 15 eye beds are being provided along with essential equipment and instruments, besides curative services at the base hospital. These units also render services in outreach areas, through their auxillary units, which is being attached with them in phased manner.

Tertiary Level

Medical colleges are being strengthened by providing additional influx of modern equipment and faculty strength.

MOBILE SERVICES

Mobile services are intended to provide immediate relief to people in the outreach areas adopting an extended eye camp approach. The services would be comprehensive in nature including outpatient treatment, study of refraction cases using refractometer, surgical cure of cataract, glaucoma, survey of local community, industrial workers and screening of school children. These services also provide diagnosis of cases requiring institutional treatment, and their referral at higher level eye care centres as well as advice on rehabilitation of incurable blinds.

Types of Mobile Services

1. Central mobile units
2. District mobile units
3. Mobile services by voluntary organisations.

Other Associated Activities

Trachoma

National Trachoma Programme was launched in 1963 and later merged with other blindness control activities; measures being carried out as health education, for protection and treatment of disease in 0 to 10 years age group considered as the main reservoir of infection and surgical corrections of trichiasis through mobile services and institutional care.

Nutritional Blindness

Vitamin A prophylaxis programme has been taken up by the maternal and child health (MCH), now RCH department of family welfare. Under this scheme vitamin A prophylaxis solution is distributed through PHC subcentres by Auxillary Nurse Midwife (ANM) and Lady Health Visitor (LHV), during home visiting to cover children from 1 to 5 years with 2,00,000 international units orally every six months. Special preference is given to children living in tribal areas, drought prone areas, other backward areas, integrated child development service (ICDS) blocks and urban slums.

School Eye Health

Some of the states have school health scheme, which includes school eye health services also, the area is being covered mainly through mobile units. These units carryout eye health education and screening of school children for eye diseases and defects.

Control of Corneal Blindness

The Government of India has also taken up strengthening of eye bank infrastructure both in Government and Non-government sectors in a phased manner.

Training Programmes

Thirty-seven training schools, established throughout the country, are conducting two years training course for ophthalmic assistance for posting them at primary-health centres. About 900 ophthalmic assistants are expected to be trained annually. Primary health centre medical officer and ophthalmic surgeon undergo training for continuing education.

Health Education

Some basic concepts on eye care have been included in the school curriculum. Mass education on simple and regular eye care is given through television, radio, newspaper and magazines, etc.

Local health staff and enlightened members of the community (leaders) may play an important role in educating the people. Success in achievement of target of reducing prevalence of blindness to 0.3 per cent by 2000 A.D. (Now 2020) cannot be realised unless health education messages reach every needy person in the country.

CHANGING CONCEPTS OF EYE HEALTH CARE

To provide comprehensive eye health care, the different approach is followed.

Primary Eye Care

Primary health care approach to eye health includes promotion and protection of eye with immediate treatment. For common eye infections and diseases. The prime objective of eye care is to increase the coverage and quality of eye health through primary health care approach and encourage the utilization of health resources and facilities.

Team Approach

The team concept is essential for comprehensive eye health care. The team of eye health care includes ophthalmologist, ophthalmic assistant, health worker (male and female), village health guides and voluntary health agencies.

National Programmes for Blindness

The goal of national programme is to reduce the incidence of blindness and control the preventable blindness. Many of these programmes are concerned with preventable diseases (for blindness), the primary health care approach is to prevent blindness from all causes.

Epidemiological Approach

This focuses on measurement of incidences prevalence of diseases and risk factors among the population at large. The epidemiology of eye diseases will help to find the causes and prevent them from its occurrence of all diseases among all ages.

•••

22

Obesity

INTRODUCTION

Obesity is usually caused by a caloric intake that exceeds the energy expenditure. A number of metabolic abnormalities are present in obese persons, but are probably that result of obesity rather than the cause.

When food, intake equals metabolic needs, weight remains fairly constant throughout life. A weight gain sometimes accompanies aging because the individual does not adjust food intake to lowered metabolism and diminished activity. Obesity is the most common nutritional disorder in the community. It is perhaps the most prevalent form of malnutrition in developed countries both among adults and children. It is associated with increased mortality, predisposes to development of various diseases and decreases the efficiency and happiness of obese people.

Definition

Obesity may be defined as a condition in which there is an excessive amount of body fat.

"It is also defined as an abnormal growth of the adipose tissue due to an enlargement of fat cell size or increase in fat cell number or combination of both".

Excess fat accumulates because there is imbalance between energy intake and expenditure. Obesity is often expressed in terms of Body Mass Index (BMI). BMI more than 30 in males and more than 28.6 in females indicates obesity.

Epidemiological Factors

Host Factors

Age: Obesity is most prevalent in middle age, but can occur at any age and generally increases with age. Infants with excessive weight gain have an increased incidence of obesity in later age. One-third of obese adults have been reported as childhood obesity.

Sex : Studies have shown that men gain in weight between 29 to 35 years, while women gain in weight during 45 to 49 years of age.

Socioeconomic factors : In affluent countries obesity is more common in the lower socioeconomic groups. In developing countries it can occur only in high socioeconomic groups. Some occupations predispose to obesity, *e.g.*, sedentary working conditions.

Genetic factors : A familial tendency exists in many cases, but it is difficult to examine the environmental and genetic component. Patterns of eating and activity are influenced by social, cultural and economic factors, which may be transferred from one generation to another. However, studies involving twins and adopted children indicate the importance of genetic factor in influencing both total body fat and its distribution.

Endocrine factors : An endocrine influence on body fat is seen both in normal physiological situations and in pathological states. Obesity in women commonly begin at puberty, during pregnancy and at the menopause and is frequently associated with hypothyroidism, hypogonadism, hypopituitarism and Cushing's syndrome.

Energy balance : A very small excess of calories, if habitual, can lead to large accumulation of fat. If a person eats a slice of bread that is not needed each day and goes by car instead of walking for 20 minutes, the daily extra 48 kcal will build up over 10 years to 20 kg of fat deposited.

Eating habits : Eating in between the meals, preference of sweets, refined foods and fats, the periodicity of eating and amount of energy derived from it are relevant to aetiology of obesity. A diet containing more energy than needed may deposite in adipose tissue resulting in obesity.

Psychosocial factors : Emotional and stress factors have a close relationship with obesity, overeating may be a symptom of depression, anxiety, frustration and loneliness, excessive obese individuals are usually lonely and secret eaters.

Drugs : The use of steroids, oral contraceptives, antipsychotic drugs and insulin is commonly followed by obesity, mainly due to increase in appetite.

Physical inactivity : It has an important role in causation of obesity. Affluence is commonly associated with reduced energy expenditure. It is well recognised that physical activity is less in obese than in the lean, but this may result from rather than cause, the obesity.

Assessment of obesity : In most cases the diagnosis will be apparent from patient's appearance but the degree of obesity should be assessed, usually by measuring height and weight and reference to a table — obesity must be differentiated from a gain in weight due to fluid retention associated with cardio, renal and hepatic diseases, because oedema can not be clinically diagnosed untill there is increrase of 15 per cent extracellular fluid.

The state of obesity is characterised by an increase in the fatty mass at the expense of the other parts of the body. The water content of the body is never increased in case of obesity.

Methods of Assessment

Body Weights

Body weight, though not accurate measure, but is widely used index for excess fat.

Body Mass Index

It is commonly used for simple measurement.

$$\frac{Weight\ (kg)}{Height^2\ (m)}$$

Broca Index

It is widely used index to measure obesity.

Height (cm) minus 100.

e.g., if height of an individual = 165 cm. his ideal weight is = 165 – 100 = 65 kg.

Ponderal Index

It is given by the following formula :

$$Ponderal\ Index = \frac{Height\ (cm)}{Cube\ root\ of\ body\ weight\ (kg)}.$$

Corpulence Index

It is given by the following formula :

$$Corpulence\ Index = \frac{Actual\ weight}{Desired\ weight}$$

This Corpulence Index should not exceed 7.2.

Skin Fold Thickness Method

Large proportion of total body fat is located under the skin. The skin fold thickness over the triceps muscle can be measured using special spring loaded callipers. Several varieties of callipers are available for the purpose. Measurement may be taken at all four sites, *e.g.*, urid triceps, triceps subscapular and supriliac regions. Obesity is indicated by reading 40 mm in men and 50 mm in women. In extreme obesity, measurement may not be possible.

HEALTH HAZARDS OF OBESITY

Obesity is an important predisposing factor to various noncommunicable diseases, responsible for increased mortality and morbidity.

Increased Morbidity

Obesity is predisposing factor in causation of diabetes, cardiovascular diseases, hypertension, gallbladder problems, etc. Obesity is also responsible for other nonfatal diseases, *e.g.*, varicose veins, osteoarthritis, psychosocial stress and abdominal hernia.

Increased Mortality

The chronic diseases due to obesity increases mortality among people, which is mainly due to increased incidence of hypertension, coronary heart disease and renal diseases, obesity lowers the life-expectancy. There is also evidence that a substantial reduction of body weight of obese people is alone sufficient to reduce the mortality rate.

PROBLEMS RELATED TO OBESITY

Psychological

Obese people often have psychological problems, but it is difficult to distinguish between cause and effect. Many young obese adults are ashamed of their unattractive appearance and develop psychosocial and sexual problems.

Metabolic Disorder

Noninsulin dependent diabetes mellitus, hyperlipidaemia (cholestrol and triglyceride), gallstones, hyperuricaemia and gout are common among obese.

Cardiovascular Disorder

Obesity increases the workload of the heart, which enlarges with increased body weight. Cardiac output, stroke volume and blood volume are increased, leading to hypertension.

Other Problems

Flat feet and osteoarthritis of knee, lumber spine and hips are more common among obese. Abdominal muscles supporting the viscera and leg muscles are less efficient, predisposing to the development of abdominal and diaphragmatic hernias and varicose veins. Adipose tissues around the trunk interferes with mechanism of respiration resulting in exertional dyspnoea and increased susceptibility of respiratory infection. Obesity leads to higher incidences of accidents.

Treatment

Dietary Control

Ultimate cause of obesity is energy imbalance and weight reduction can be achieved only by reducing energy intake or by increasing output, or by a combination of the two. This involves change in lifestyle. The patient must be educated and informed about the disorder and misconceptions.

There is no "slimming food" or 'slimming tablets' for treatment of obesity.

A target weight to aim for and indication of the rate of weight loss is expected. A weekly weight loss of 0.5 kg should be general aim.

Food must be taken in natural form only. Fresh seasonal fruit, fresh green leafy vegetables and sprouts are excellent healthy foods. These diets are classified as juices, fruit raw diet, boiled vegetables rough diets, etc. Being alkaline these diets help in improving health, purifying the body and rendering it immune to diseases.

Theraputic

Fasting

Fasting is a process of giving rest to the digestive system. During this process, the vital energy, which digests the food, is engaged in elimination of diseases. It also helps in treatment of indigestion, constipation, gas, digestive disorder, gouts, along with obesity fasting once a week has good therapeutic effect, long fast should be undertaken under supervision of competent physician. Short fast on fruit or liquid diet may be kept whenever required. Precaution should be observed that total amount of fruit intake a day should not exceed one kg.

Fasting with only water and noncaloric drinks with vitamin and mineral supplements have been recommended in the hospitals for very obese patients who fail to respond to other remedies.

Exercise

Most obese people lead sedentary life, hence regular daily exercise is necessary and beneficial for weight reduction. An hour's walk at due speed of 3 miles/hr will expend about 240 kcal above basal (or more for heavy person). Consult the physician to workout the programme according to physical capacity and other associated problems.

Preventive Measures

The prevention and control of obesity should start in early childhood, because it is difficult to control in adulthood. The children should be taught about healthy lifestyle to maintain normal weight gain, which can be achieved by healthy dietary habits and regular physical activity.

Dietary Changes

Balanced diet with optimum requirements of protein, carbohydrates, minerals, fats and vitamins should be encouraged. Avoid fast foods and habits of eating during meals. Avoid stress among children or adults which predispose the increased appetite. Teach the people to eat less than the required food and consume the quality and not quantity.

Regular Physical Activity

Regular physical activity is the key to an increased energy expenditure. Avoid meals during watching television or reading books, etc. Encourage outdoor games and long walks for children and adults who are prone to be obese.

EXERCISE

1. (a) Discuss the predisposing factors in causation of cancer.
   (b) Describe the role of nurse in prevention and control of cancer.
2. Explain the levels of prevention of cancer. Describe the National Cancer Control Programme in India.
3. Discuss the risk factors for causation of diabetes mellitus. Describe the measures for prevention of diabetes mellitus.
4. Enumerate the role of nurse in prevention of cardiovascular diseases. Discuss the National cardiovascular disease control programme.
5. Write the causes for blindness. Discuss the National Programme for Control of blindness.
6. What do you understand by rheumatic heart disease (RHD)? Explain the epidemiological factors in causation of rheumatic heart disease. Describe its prevention and control.
7. Describe the risk factors in causation of rheumatic heart disease. Discuss the levels of prevention of rheumatic heart disease.
8. A child has come with complaint of fever and joint pain. The throat culture confirms rheumatic heart disease. Describe the role of nurse in providing health education on control of rheumatic heart disease.
9. What are cardiovascular diseases? Discuss the risk factors in causation of cardiovascular diseases. Describe the preventive measures for cardiovascular diseases.
10. Discuss National Cardiovascular Diseases Control Programme. Describe the role of nurse in prevention of cardiovascular diseases.
11. Discuss the worldwide problem of accidents. Describe the predisposing factors in causing accidents. State the role of nurse in prevention of accidents.
12. Plan health education to a group on prevention of accidents and home hazards.
13. Write short notes on:
    (a) Prevention of breast cancer
    (b) Role of nurse in prevention of cervix cancer
    (c) Control of lung cancer
    (d) Risk factors for cancer
    (e) Types of cancers and preventive measures
    (f) Predisposing factors for causing cardiovascular diseases
    (g) Role of nurse in prevention of heart disease.

●●●

UNIT VI

EPIDEMIOLOGY OF COMMUNICABLE DISEASES

- Gastrointestinal Diseases
- Respiratory Diseases
- Vector-borne Diseases
- Zoonotic Diseases
- Surface Diseases
- Emerging and Re-emerging Infectious Diseases

23

Gastrointestinal Diseases

ACUTE DIARRHOEAL DISEASES

INTRODUCTION

Diarrhoeal diseases are associated with unsafe water and poor sanitation coupled with poor food handling practices and bottle-feeding of infant during the first 4 to 6 months of life. The main cause of death from acute diarrhoea is dehydration resulting from loss of fluids and electrolytes. Other causes of deaths are dysentery and malnutrition resulting from incorrect management of diarrhoea along with inappropriate food practices.

Diarrhoea is the passage of loose, watery and frequent stools (Fig. 23.1). The patient passes usually more than 4 to 5 stools per day and acute diarrhoea is the sudden onset of disease, which usually lasts for 3 to 7 days. It is also called as gastroentritis, which is due to infection in the intestine. Though, recent studies indicate the consistency and character of stool rather than the number of stools that are more important.

Worldwide Problem

Diarrhoea is a major public health problem in developing countries. Globally there are an estimated 1.8 billion episodes of childhood diarrhoea each year, including dysentery, claim the lives of 3 million children annually. Household survey carried out during 1994-95, showed that diarrhoea episodes ranged from 0.7 to 3.9 per child less than 5 years of age in South-East Asian Region (SEAR). According to

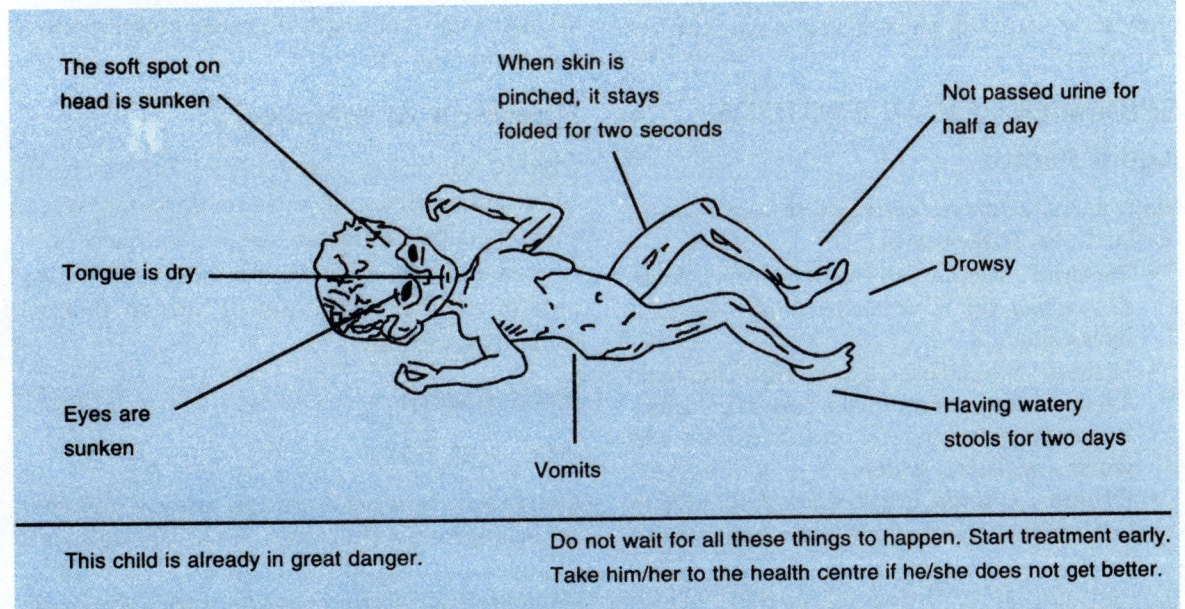

The soft spot on head is sunken

When skin is pinched, it stays folded for two seconds

Not passed urine for half a day

Tongue is dry

Drowsy

Eyes are sunken

Vomits

Having watery stools for two days

This child is already in great danger.

Do not wait for all these things to happen. Start treatment early. Take him/her to the health centre if he/she does not get better.

Fig. 23.1 : A child suffering from diarrhoea

recent reports, oral rehydration therapy may now be preventing about one million dehydration deaths a year, 15 to 40 per cent of all deaths among children under 5 years are due to diarrhoea.

Problem in India

Diarrhoea is a major public health problem among children below five years. One-third of total hospital admission are due to diarrhoea and 17 per cent deaths among children are due to dehydration.

Diarrhoeal diseases cause heavy economic burden on health services as 15 per cent of diarrhoeal cases occupy the beds in hospitals. Though much attention has been paid on prevention and management of acute diarrhoea for last few years and ORS packets have been made easily and freely available.

National Diarrhoeal Disease Control Programme (NDDCP) has made significant achievement in reducing the death rate due to diarrhoea below 5 years of age. SRS report in 1992, estimated 26.5/1000 deaths below five years, out of which 20 per cent were only from diarrhoea which are preventable. Hence, more emphasis since then has been laid to prevent mortality due to diarrhoea with simple procedures.

EPIDEMIOLOGICAL FACTORS

Agent Factor

Many agent factors are responsible for causation of diarrhoea. These can be :

- **Bacterial :** *Shigella, Salmonella, Vibrio cholerae, Escherichia coli, V. parahaemolyticus, Bacillus cereus*, etc.
- **Viruses :** Rotaviruses, astrovirus, calcivirus adenoviruses, enterovirus, coronaviruses.
- **Worm infestation,** *e.g.,* roundworm, pin worm and *Taenia solium.*
- **Others :** *Giardia intestinalis, E.histolitica* (amoebiasis), Trichuriosis and a patient with AIDS.

Bacterial Infection

Among bacterial infections, *Vibrio cholerae* is most common infection causing cholera, other bacilli *salmonella, shigella* and *E. Coli* are most frequent causes of diarrhoea. *Shigella* is a major cause of diarrhoea in India.

Viruses

Many diarrhoeal diseases are caused by a variety of viruses. The rotavirus is considered as singlemost important cause of diarrhoea. It is probably spread from person to person and responsible for about one-half of all diarrhoeal cases in children aged up to two years.

Others

Amoebiasis, giardiasis and worm infestations are also associated in causing diarrhoea. Persistant diarrhoea is one of the major clinical signs of AIDS. According to WHO a child having continuous diarrhoea for 30 days should be investigated for AIDS. Children with measles have tendency of severe diarrhoea episode.

Mode of Transmission

The important mode of transmission of diarrhoea is by faecal-oral route. Faecal-oral route may be water-borne, food-borne or direct transmission via finger, fomites, contaminated food and flies, etc.

Reservoir of Infection

Man is the main reservoir of infection. In bacterial diarrhoea, animals are important reservoirs and transmission originates from both human and animal faeces. For viral infection the role of animal reservoirs in human disease remains uncertain.

Host Factor

Age and Sex

Diarrhoea is most common among children especially below five years of age. Though high incidence is also found from 6 to 11 months, because child starts crawling and unhygienic eating, when child starts picking up and chewing anything from floor. Even the antibodies effect in children received from mother, starts disappearing. It is also common in children under six months of age fed on cow's milk or infant feeding formula due to unhygienic conditions.

Malnutrition also, lowers the resistance and child is susceptible to infection, which causes diarrhoea.

Environmental Factor

Diarrhoea shows seasonal variation. Bacterial infection occurs more frequently during summer and rainy season. Viral diarrhoea is found more in winter. There is relationship between weather and bacterial diarrhoea because flies being the main mode of transmission and flies grow more in summer and rainy season.

Clinical Manifestation

The clinical picture varies from mild, moderate and severe cases.

Mild

Onset is usually insidious with 2 to 5 stools which may be loose, green, offensive and contain mucus and milky curd. Volume may be large or small. The attack may subside in a day or two without any remarkable constitutional manifestation or dehydration.

Moderate

The number of motions is 10 or more and constitutional symptoms like fever, irritability, anorexia and vomiting are usually present. Mild dehydration (3–5%) is associated.

Severe Diarrhoea

The child passes "Too many" loose motions and has severe vomiting to the extent that nothing is retained and oral intake becomes virtually impracticable. Such cases are most often characterized by sudden, rather than gradual onset.

Dehydration Onset

They may have marked constitutional symptoms; moderate (5–10%) or severe (above 10%) dehydration (Table 23.1).

Table 23.1 : Clinical picture of different grades of dehydration

Grade	Clinical symptoms
Mild	Irritability, drowsiness, cry without tears, pallor, sunken eyes, dryness of mouth, tongue and excessive thirst.
Moderate	Lethargic, depressed fontennels (infants), dry and poor elastic skin, sunken eyes, oliguria.
Severe	Shock with unconscious limpness, cold and clammy skin, thin rapid pulse, may not be recordable pulse, oliguria or anuria.

Treatment

Treatment of diarrhoea with the exception of *Shigella* and *Vibrio cholerae* infections and chronic diarrhoea case, antimicrobial drugs are not indicated in the treatment of diarrhoea. Symptomatic drugs are not useful and are a waste of family resources and may even be harmful. National Diarrhoeal Disease Control Programme (DDCP) have issued guidelines to curtail the use of antidiarrhoeal drugs and the routine use of antibiotics.

Recommended treatment for acute diarrhoea is consumption of fluids in increased volume to prevent dehydration, use of ORS and / or I.V. fluids to correct dehydration. Continue feeding to prevent malnutrition. The DDCP is emphasizing on giving increased amount of commonly prepared, recommended, home available fluids (HAF) and continued feeding the child as first line of management. The main preventive intervention is the provision of breastfeeding, including exclusive breastfeeding during first 4 to 6 months of life. Other preventive measures, *e.g.*, handwashing and use of safe portable drinking water and sanitary laterines are also stressed.

ORAL REHYDRATION THERAPY (ORT)

ORT is *"administration of water, sugar, salt solution to patient with diarrhoea to replace the water and salt lost from body"*. The studies have shown revolutionary life-saving solution for diarrhoea, which is one of the main cause of death and is major health problem among children.

The aim of ORT is to prevent dehydration and reduce mortality. ORT is ideal for mild dehydration and majority of children with moderate dehydration.

Indications

- Prevent dehydration, if ORT starts at initial stage of diarrhoea.
- Rehydration of dehydrated patient, so that he does not enter the phase of severe dehydration.
- Maintenance of hydration after severely dehydrated and patient has been rehydrated with I.V fluids.

ORT is based on the facts that glucose given orally enhances the intestinal absorption of salt and water and is capable of correcting the electrolyte and water deficit.

Standard Formula for ORT

The WHO has recommended the standard formula to be followed for ORT :

Sodium chloride	3.5 g	
Sodium bicarbonate	2.5 g	in one litre of
Potassium chloride	1.5 g	clean water.
Glucose	20 g	

The packets are manufactured commercially for sale and are distributed to various hospitals and health centres to be provided free of cost to the people.

Home-made Preparation of ORT

The home-made solution is easiest, cheapest and available at home. The ORT can be prepared as :

- Wash hands before preparation
- Mix one-three finger pinch (¼ teaspoon) of common salt
- Two-four finger scoops (5 teaspoonful) of sugar in one litre of tap or boiled cool water. Lemon may be added for taste.

Instructions of ORS Administration

Oral rehydration solution (ORS) is prepared at least for 24 hours and should be given after each stool, as much as child is able to take. Rest of the solution should be thrown after 24 hours and fresh can be prepared. Never force the child to take the solution.

Prevention and Control of Diarrhoeal Diseases

- Improving water supply, sanitation and hygienic conditions.
- Ensure safe drinking water, hand washing while preparing and eating food.
- Protecting food from contamination and flies.
- Proper and hygienic excreta disposal.

Appropriate Feeding

Breastfeeding should be encouraged during diarrhoea in a hygienic manner. Cleanliness of bottle for children who are bottle-fed. Normal food intake should be promoted as soon as the child is able to eat. Those with moderate and severe dehydration, should receive oral rehydration solution alone during the rehydration phase.

Important Points for Prevention of Diarrhoea

- Low roughage food with small and frequent meals can be encouraged.
- Since staple food does not provide optimal calories per unit weight, these are best to be provided rich source of energy like *khichri*, rice, curd, mashed banana, mashed potatoes.
- Artificially fed infants, milk should preferably be given undiluted during all phases of acute diarrhoea.

Other Solutions

Other solutions like dal water solution, carrot juice, tender coconut water, Bengal gram *kanjee*, weak tea, fruit juice and banana, can be given but under strict hygienic conditions.

Rice Water Electrolyte Solution

Consists of cooking rice water. Salt is added as per need. This may be prepared by taking two-finger scoops of rice powder (boiled rice) in water and boiling it for 3 minutes. Add a pinch of salt, one-fourth medium size lemon juice.

National Diarrhoeal Disease Control Programme (NDDCP)

Acute diarrhoea ranks among "Top Three" causes of death among children. According to conservative estimate almost 500 million children suffer from acute diarrhoea annually and 5 million die every year. In India 1.5 million children die due to diarrhoea every year. Keeping in view NDDCP was started in the year 1978, during Sixth Five-Year Plan with objectives.

- To reduce morbidity and mortality due to diarrhoea among children by promoting ORT.
- To reduce 50 per cent of death among children with diarrhoea by the year 1990.
- To promote ORT at primary levels, *e.g.*, village, subcentre and PHC for early treatment of diarrhoea and prevent dehydration.
- To educate the mothers to enable them to take care of children with diarrhoea by home-made fluids.
- To train the doctors to gain more skills on diarrhoea management.

Components

ORT

The programme had been intensified during Seventh Five-Year Plan to reduce 50 per cent of deaths due to diarrhoea. This was initiated by distributing 200 packets to each subcentres and 100 packets of oral rehydration solution to village health guides at village level. The oral rehydration solution packets were also supplied in sufficient quantity to primary health centre and district hospitals.

Information Education and Communication (IEC)

Health education is an important component of the programme. The mothers are educated about the child care suffering from diarrhoea, about home-made solution, continue feed during diarrhoea especially breastfeed and diet and early recognition of signs of dehydration. To prevent diarrhoea by encouraging breastfeed as long as she can feed, proper weaning and immunization to all healthy children.

- Washing raw vegetable before cooking.
- Proper handwashing after defecation.

Training Programme for Medical Personnels

The doctors should be trained for special clinical skills in prevention and control of diarrhoea, ARI and newborn care, etc. Establishment of training units for diarrhoea control and treatment in medical colleges and district hospitals. At present there are diarrhoea training units in 100 district hospitals and 85 medical colleges (1992).

In 1992, the programme had been integrated with CSSM. ORS packets were supplied along with child survival and safe motherhood kit (CSSM kit). Each kit carried around 150 packets in each subcentre with population 3000 to 5000.

CHOLERA

INTRODUCTION

Cholera is a water-borne acute diarrhoeal disease caused by bacilli *V. cholerae*. The severity of the disease vary from symptom less to severe infections, majority of the cases are mild or asymptomatic.

History

Cholera is an ancient disease in Ayurveda times, it was called as *Vishuchika* and is clearly defined in 'Susruta Samihita' of the 7th century B.C. The history of cholera has been described in four stages :

- **Before 1817 :** It was seen in East and mainly in India.
- **1817-1923 :** Six epidemics were described which originated from India.
- **1923-1960 :** European countries and also a disease of East Asiatic countries.
- **1961 :** In Indonesia suddenly spread off as seventh epidemic.

After spreading in Hongkong and Phillipines, it moved steadily north and westward and reached India in 1964. Then spread to Middle-East, North-East and West

Africa, cases were also seen in Australia, New Zealand, USA and other developed countries.

Worldwide Problem

Cholera is endemic in all the countries except Korea, where cholera has not been officially reported since 1968. 7th endemic is still continuing to spread involving 92 countries in Asia, Africa and Europe. In 1993, it was reported as an endemic in around 80 countries.

In most of the cases food has been found to be the vehicle of transmission. Since there is a large proportion of unapparent clinical cases among El Tor vibrio infected persons, it is not possible to prevent the spread of cholera between countries. However, in most of the cases, outbreaks of cholera can be contained within individual countries.

In October 1992, a new strain of *V. cholerae* serotype 0139 (Bengal) was discovered in India and Bangladesh. It raised fear that this might be the start of a new endemic. However, the 0139 strain has not spread beyond Asia and now seems unlikely to become a global threat. Since the first report in India, *V. cholerae* 0139 has been isolated in China, Hongkong, India, Malaysia, Myanmar, Nepal, Pakistan, Singapore, Sri Lanka and Thailand. In 1994, only sporadic cases of cholera due to *V. cholerae* 0139 were reported from Malaysia, Myanmar, Nepal, Singapore and Thailand.

Although there is no report of a major outbreak of cholera in any country of the region during past few years, new epidemic may occur if the disease is not closely monitored through an appropriate surveillance mechanism. Reporting of cholera cases and deaths in the countries showed a wide variation. In most countries of region reporting is incomplete, irregular or not at all.

Based on the number of cases and deaths reported to WHO from several countries of the region, there had been continued decline in cholera case fatality rate (CFR) from 2.51 per cent in 1991 to 0.8 per cent in 1997. The global and All Asia Case Fatality Rate in 1997 were 4.26 per cent and 1.74 per cent respectively. The low CFR in the region and in Asia may be attributed to the increased access to proper diarrhoea case management.

South-East Asia was traditionally the home for cholera by classical and El Tor strain, the agent responsible for the seventh pandemic in 1961. Many countries, being reluctant to notify cholera for fear of imposition of travel and trade restrictions, tend to report cholera as acute diarrhoeal disease. Cholera remains a global threat and one of the key indicator of social development. Almost every country is facing either a cholera outbreak or a threat of an epidemic. The role of oral cholera vaccine is public health tool to improve cholera control acitivity needs to be further assessed through intervention studies. Efficient cholera surveillance system needs to be stressed with regard to improve risk assessment for potential cholera outbreak.

Problem in India

The geographical distribution of cholera in India has considerably changed since 1964. West Bengal is no more a home of cholera. Many of states which never had cholera or were for from infection for a long-time, got infection and became endemic to El Tor infection. Andaman and Nicobar Islands were infected for the first time in 1966 and Rajasthan in 1969. Recently a large endemic was found in Maharashtra, Tamil Nadu, Karnataka, Delhi and Kerala. These states account for about 80 per cent of reported incidence in the country.

Epidemiological Factors

Cholera is both endemic and epidemic. Global experience shows that cholera cannot be prevented in any country and it creates the problem only in areas with poor sanitary conditions. Epidemic of disease is abrupt and creates acute public health problem. They have a high potential to spread fast and cause deaths. Cholera occurs at intervals even in endemic areas.

Agents/Factors

Cholera is usually caused by *Vibrio cholerae* O group I or *Vibrio cholerae* OI. It is now recognised as new species that are pathogenic for humans *e.g., Vibrio parahaemolyticus,* which has caused outbreak of cholera hydiarrhoea. It is, therefore, necessary to identify *V. cholerae* for specific diagnosis of cholera.

V. cholerae are killed by heating within 30 minutes at 56°C or few seconds by boiling. Sunlight and drying will kill them in few hours. They are easily killed by disinfectants like cresol and bleeching powder. The bacilli multiply in the small intestine and produce exotoxin which causes diarrhoea.

Host Factors

Age and sex : Cholera affects all the ages and both sexes equally. Though children are most affected during 5 to 15 years of age, due to exposure to unhygienic eating from hawkers.

Population mobility : The people moving from place to place may spread infection, *e.g.,* pilgrimage, marriages, fairs and festivals, which increases the risk of exposure to infection. Cases and carriers can easily spread infection to non-infected countries.

Socioeconomic condition : The high incidence of cholera has been found in low socioeconomic group, mainly due to poor hygiene.

Immunity : Once infection gives immunity to the person, though second attacks are found but rare.

Environmental Factors

The poor sanitary conditions are the main cause of spread of disease. Flies may carry *V. cholerae* and spread infection. Human habits, soil pollution, low standard of hygienic, lack of education and poor quality of life are main causes in India.

MODE OF TRANSMISSION

Contaminated Water and Food

Intake of unhygienic food, water or milk are associated with outbreak of cholera. Bottle-feeding could be a significant risk factor for infants and children, fruits and vegetables washed with contaminated water before eating, cooked food may be contaminated by contaminated hands and flies.

Reservoir of Infection

Human being is the only reservoir of infection it may be case or carrier.

Cases

These may vary from inapparent to severe ones. In cholera El Tor most infections are mild and asymptomatic, which play important role in outbreak of the disease. The stool and vomit of the case are the infective materials for spread of infection. The case of cholera is usually infective from 7 to 10 days.

Carriers

They are usually temporary and rarely chronic. The carrier may be apparently healthy person who is excreting *V. cholerae* in stool.

Types of Carriers

These may be as follows :

Incubatory or preclinical carriers : They spread the disease before the appearance of clinical manifestations, which lasts for 1 to 5 days. These carriers are the potential patients.

Convalescent carrier : The patient who has recovered from an attack of cholera may continue to spread the disease for at least 2 to 3 weeks of recovery.

The carriers can often become chronic or long-term carriers.

Contact or healthy carriers : These are healthy individuals who are carrier of *V. cholerae* due to exposure to subclinical infection. The duration is usually 10 days. They also play an important role to spread disease because of their hidden infections.

Chronic carriers : Rarely, but can spread the disease. The gallbladder is infected in chronic carrier and cholecystectomy is the only solution to prevent the spread of infection.

Incubation Period

It varies from 1 day to 5 days, but commonly 1 to 2 days.

Clinical Manifestation of Cholera

The cholera cases are characterized by sudden onset of perfuse, effortless and watery diarrhoea followed by vomiting, rapid dehydration, muscular cramps and suppression of urine.

The severity of disease depends upon the amount of fluid loss. The patient may die due to severe dehydration. The clinical manifestation can be seen in three stages:

Evacuation Stage

Watery diarrhoea and vomiting. The patient may pass 30 to 40 rice watery stools per day.

Collapse Stage

Due to fluid loss, the patient gets dehydrated and may collapse. The patient will have sunken eyes, subnormal temperature, feeble pulse, cold and clammy skin, loss of skin elasticity, shallow and fast respiration. The patient may be restless and become unconscious.

Recovery Stage

The replacement of fluids and electrolyte may help the patient's recovery, otherwise it may be fatal. The patient dies due to renal failure, if aneuria. On fluid replacement the patient shows the signs of recovery. The blood pressure starts rising, temperature returns to normal, urine is re-established.

Prevention and Control of Cholera

Early Case Detection

The cases must be detected in the community for early treatment and prevent the spread of infection. Early detection also helps to identify the household contacts of the patients.

Notification

Cholera is a notifiable disease locally, nationally and internationally. Hence an aggressive search for cases should be made in the community and notify to the nearest health agency. Health workers in the community, *e.g.*, health volunteers, multipurpose workers must be trained to identify the cases of cholera (mild, moderate or severe) and notify to the nearest community health centre. Under National Health Regulation, cholera is notifiable to the WHO within 24 hours of its occurrence, by the National Government, the number of cases and deaths are also to be reported daily and weekly, till the area is declared free of cholera. An area is declared free of cholera when twice the incubation period (10 days) has elapsed since the death, recovery or isolation of the last case.

Identification of the Cases

During outbreak of disease, it is important to diagnose and confirm the cholera cases. For specific treatment of cholera, it is essential to verify *V. cholerae* OI, in the stool of patient, once it has been diagnosed, other cases are considered as cases and carriers of diseases. Hence, precautionary measure can be taken to prevent further spread of cholera.

Treatment

The treatment should be started at the earliest possible time. The treatment must be easily accessible, available to the community people. The immediate treatment can be started at home, by supplementing ORS (oral rehydration solution) to prevent complications and save the life of severely dehydrated patients, requiring intravenous fluids, should be referred to the nearest health centre or hospital. If no health centre is available during epidemic, temporary arrangement of treating the cholera patient should be made. The mobile team at district level should be organised to provide services at remote areas, where endemic is common.

Rehydration Therapy

Lifesaving therapy as rehydration is the most effective treatment of cholera and any diarrhoeal disease. Mortality rate has been brought down to less than 1 per cent by ORS, which can be started immediately at home.

Oral Rehydration Solution

The introduction of oral rehydration solution (ORS) by WHO in 1971, has simplified the treatment of cholera and other acute diarrhoeal diseases. The aim of ORS is to prevent complications (dehydration) and reduce mortality. It has been experienced by workers at Kolkata that 90 to 95 per cent cases of cholera can be treated by oral rehydration solution (Table 23.2).

Table 23.2 : Composition of ORS bicarbonate

Ingredients/items	Amount
Clean water	1 litre
Sodium chloride	3.5 gm
Sodium bicarbonate	2.5 gm
Potassium chloride	1.5 gm
Glucose	20 gm

ORS citrate (Table 23.3) is more effective and stable than ORS bicarbonate. ORS packets are easily and freely available at primary health centres, subcentres, hospitals and other health agencies.

Table 23.3 : ORS citrates composition

Ingredients/items	Amount
Sodium chloride (common salt)	3.5 gm
Trisodium citrate dehydrate	2.9 gm
Potassium chloride	1.5 gm
Glucose	20 gm

Note: 1 packet to be mixed in 1 litre of clean water.

Preparation of Solution

- Wash the hands before preparing the solution.
- Mix the packet in 1 litre of clean water (preferably boiled clean water).
- Keep the solution covered at safe place.
- Administer to the patient as much as possible, after every loose motion.
- The solution can be kept for 24 hours.
- Fresh solution should be prepared after every 24 hours.
- It should not be boiled or sterilized.
- The solution is given immediately when patient starts loose motions and till patient is in mild diarrhoeal condition.
- In case of moderate to severe condition of diarrhoea, the patient is unable to take fluid and must be referred to hospital.
- If child vomits, wait for 10 minutes, then try again, giving the solution slowly.
- The child must be breastfed along with ORS.

The ingredients in the ORS packets are inexpensive, easily available, easy to prepare at home and easy to administer to the patient. The introduction of ORS is a major achievement to fight against cholera and other diarrhoeal diseases.

Intravenous Therapy

In moderate and severe cases, intravenous fluids are administered to the patient who are unable to drink orally, due to excessive vomiting, are transferred to nearest hospital. Timely, intravenous rehydration will prevent the patient from shock. The solutions recommended by WHO are :

- Ringer's lactate, normal saline, etc.
- Diarrhoeal treatment solution is multi-electrolyte solution for I.V. infusion which contain one litre of solution with sodium chloride 4 gm, sodium acetate 6.5 gm, potassium chloride 1 gm, glucose 10 gm.

The initial hours are given more amount of solution, *e.g.,* half of the requirement in first 6 hours and assess the condition of rehydration and adjust the solution accordingly. After 4 to 6 hours all the signs of dehydration should disappear except the urine flow, which may take some time. Too much fluid may also cause pulmonary oedema and puffiness of eyes, hence the fluid intake must be observed carefully. Rehydration must be continued untill all signs of dehydration have disappeared.

Maintenance of Fluid Therapy

After I.V. therapy, the oral fluid should be encouraged to maintain the fluid balance in the body. The patient is encouraged to drink as much as possible to replace the fluid loss.

Sanitary Measures

Provision of safe drinking water : All steps must be taken to provide safe drinking water to the people, to prevent the spread of infection. Chlorination of water and supply of water through intact pipes should be ensured, especially in epidemic areas. The people must be made aware to purify water at household level (small scale) by boiling, chlorination of water.

Disposal of excreta : Community should be encouraged for safe, clean, cheap and effective disposal of excreta, especially the use of sanitary laterines. In the endemic areas this become very essential to prevent the dangers in disposing faeces on the ground and contaminate water, vegetables and hands. It is important to teach about proper hand washing with soap and water instead soil or mud.

Food hygiene : Food is an important source of spread of infection. Community must be educated to maintain food hygiene, while cooking, eating and serving the food. Hygienic measures must be taken for proper food handling techniques. Cooking utensils must be cleaned and dried after use. The food must be covered and kept away from contamination of flies.

Disinfection : The patients stool, urine and all fomites used by patients are contaminated and can spread the disease very fast. Hence concurrent and terminal disinfections must be done. The most effective disinfectant is cresol and bleaching powder. The linen and clothes should be kept in sunlight to kill bacilli.

Chemoprophylaxis : Tetracycline is the effective drug given prophylactically to all the household contacts and nearby community people. Though the effect of the medicine is for shorter period, but still it can prevent the fast spread of disease. Tetracycline is continued for three days (125-250 mg in children) 500 mg twice a day.

Immunization : Cholera vaccine is the specific preventive measure against disease. These are killed vaccines, the organisms are killed and preserved by the addition of 0.5 per cent phenol.

Dose : Cholera vaccine is given in 2 doses subcutaneously, at an interval of 4 to 6 weeks. The dose is given in (Table 23.4).

Table 23.4 : Cholera vaccine doses

Age	I and IInd dose
Adult	0.5 mL
Children 2-10 years	0.3 mL
1-2 years	0.2 mL

If two doses are not possible then one dose, containing vaccine of two doses should be given. The vaccine is usually not given to children below one year. Booster dose is recommended after every 6 months.

Side Effect : The cholera vaccination may have tenderness, mild swelling, redness, mild or moderate temperature elevation. These symptoms may last for 2 to 3 days and disappear. Mild analgesics can be given to the individual. Usually there are no severe reactions.

The vaccine gives 50 per cent protection for 2 to 3 months, hence booster dose is recommended.

Contraindication : The vaccine given during pregnancy has not shown any adverse effect, it is contraindicated among the people with history of sensitivity reaction.

Health Education

Most effective prophylaxis is by giving health education.

Community health nurse must educate the people on prevention and control of diarrhoea and cholera by :

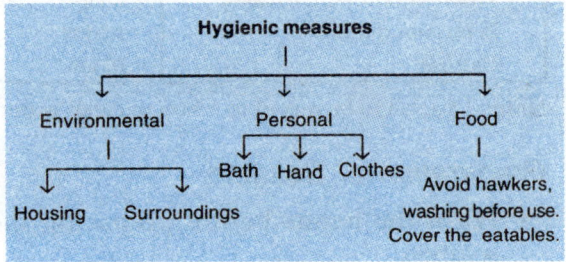

- *Handwashing :* After defecation and before eating.
- *Proper excreta disposal :* Avoid open field defecation and encourage sanitary laterine.
- Safe drinking water by boiling, chlorination especially during summer and rainy seasons.
- Consuming fresh, hot, clean food.
- Effectiveness of ORS during diarrhoea.
- Prevention of dehydration.

TYPHOID FEVER (ENTERIC FEVER)

The typhoid fever is also known as enteric fever, which includes both typhoid and paratyphoid types of fever is a systemic infection due to *Salmonella typhi*, which enters through the mouth to the gastrointestinal tract. It is one of the frequently prevalent infection. The disease may show the endemic, epidemic or sporadic occurrence.

Worldwide Problem

The disease is most commonly found in the places with poor sanitation, unsafe drinking water and substandard ways of living. Typhoid has been controlled in most of the developed countries — UK shows the lowest prevalence in the world, where the disease is almost on eradication. Though it is still common in Africa, Asia and Latin America.

Typhoid fever affects more than 6 million people every year and about 6,00,000 deaths annually. Eighty per cent of these cases and deaths are in Asia and others in Africa and Latin America.

Problem in India

High incidence of typhoid is found in India, with morbidity rate varying from 102 to 2219 per 1,00,000 population in different parts of the country and 1 per cent children below 17 years are infected every year. Average 3,00,000 cases of enteric fever were seen annually in the year till 1986. In 1992 there were 3,52,980 cases and 735 deaths. Typhoid fever is endemic in India.

Epidemiological Factors

Agent

Typhoid fever is water-borne bacterial disease caused by *S.typhi*. The bacilli survive intracellularly in the tissues of various organs. They can be readily killed by drying, pasteurization, heating and common disinfectants.

Host

Typhoid fever affects all ages though, highest incidence is found in the age group of 5 to 20 years. After the age of 20 years the incidence falls, may be due to acquiring immunity by clinical or subclinical exposure to infection. The disease is most severe among young and adult group. It spreads very fast unless isolation techniques are followed.

Sex

More incidences are found among males than females, probably due to exposure to infection. But carrier rate is more in females.

Immunity

All ages are susceptible to typhoid infection. One attack may not give lifelong immunity hence patient can have the second and consequent attacks after exposure to infection. There is no source of natural immunity in man against typhoid infection.

Environmental Factors

The disease is seen throughout the year, but higher incidence is reported during rainy season and increased fly breeding in June–September, because the disease is spread mainly due to flies.

Social Factors

S. typhi are found in water, food, ice, milk and soil for varying period of time, they do not multiply in water, but they survive in ice cream and ice (in freezing). They can survive for 70 days in soil in winter and 35 to 40 days in summer. They also survive and multiply rapidly in milk without spoiling the taste. Eating unwashed and uncooked vegetables are good source of infection. Especially vegetables grown in sewage farms or washed with contaminated water are a positive health hazards.

Drinking unsafe water, open air defecation, poor standard of living, poor hygienic conditions, poor personal cleanliness, housing and food hygiene and poor health knowledge lead to spread typhoid infection.

Reservoir of Infection

The cases and the carriers of typhoid are the only reservoirs of infection.

- Case may be mild, or severe but spreads due to infection till the urine and stool is negative for bacilli.
- Carriers may be temporary which spread the infection during incubation period and those who are in convalescent period (after recovery spread the infection) and convalescence may become chronic and can spread the infection for at least three months or even more.

Source of Infection

The main source of infection is the faeces and urine of the case and the carrier and indirect cause may be food, fly, finger, fomite, faeces, fluid (6F).

Mode of Transmission

The typhoid is spread through faeco-oral or urine oral route. The disease spreads through contaminated hands, by urine or stool of case or carrier or indirectly by ingestion of contaminated food, water, milk, through flies or any other means (Fig. 23.2).

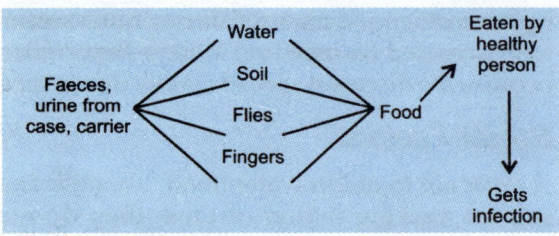

Fig. 23.2 : Mode of transmission of typhoid fever

Clinical Manifestation of Typhoid Fever (Fig. 23.3)

The patient complains of typical continuous fever for 3 to 4 weeks and fever does not touch the normal, relative bradycardia (the pulse does not rise with high temperature in typhoid), lymph node enlargement and the patient feels very sick with headache, diarrhoea and pain in abdomen. The symptoms may worsen in second week and complications like haemorrhage, delirium, epistaxis, intestinal haemorrhage and pneumonia may develop in third or fourth week and if neglected, patient may die. If appropriate treatment is taken, patient may recover. The fever starts coming to normal and other symptoms subside and patient feels better.

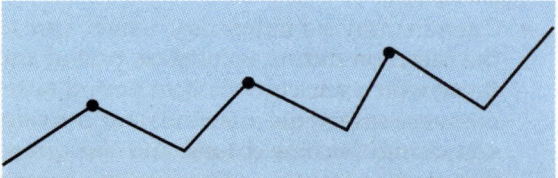

Fig. 23.3 : Pattern of rise in temperature in typhoid patient

The lesions in typhoid are specifically in small intestine, where lymph nodes and lymph tissues become swollen and covered with slough and forms ulceration. These ulcerations may be complicated as haemorrhage through erosion of a vessel or perforation into peritoneal cavity, which may be fatal.

Complications of Typhoid Fever

Haemorrhage

Sudden fall in temperature and pulse, cold and clammy skin, presence of blood in stool may indicate internal haemorrhage. Due to infection, whole blood transfusion is required and nil orally.

Abdominal Distension

Occurs due to paralysis of ulcerated bowel, which is treated by low bowel enema. Nil orally till distension subsides.

Perforation

Caused by ulceration which results in penetration of the intestinal wall. The symptoms are sudden, severe abdominal pain, rapid pulse and collapse. Prognosis depends upon early detection and treatment.

Treatment

Chloramphenicol is the drug of choice in acute typhoid fever and by third day of therapy, patient shows improvement, if incomplete, treatment may lead to relapse of fever and complications. Treatment must be continued for at least 2 to 3 weeks to prevent complications, *e.g.,* relapse and hasten recovery.

Nursing Management of Typhoid Case

- Strict isolation of the case and barrier nursing should be kept to prevent the spread; by putting gown, gloves.
- Complete bed rest and comfort to the patient, because patient may be restless due to illness.
- *Nutrition :* Soft, bland, liquid or semisolid and smoothening, frequent meals are usually advised to the patient.
- Prevent over exertion and mental excitement and restrict visitors as much as possible.

- The patient's activities should be increased gradually after recovery and needs extra care to overcome the weakness in patient.
- *Hygiene :* To maintain personal, environmental and food hygiene. Cleaning the hands before and after feeding the patient, handling of excreta, etc. The clothes must be washed in antiseptic lotion (*e.g.,* dettol, phenol) and dried in sunlight.
- Proper disposal of patient's excreta, flushing the faeces and hand washing after handling excreta. Since it is highly infectious, all things touched by patient should be considered infectious. Faeces and urine of the patient should be preferably disinfected.
- All dishes, bedpans and urinal must be disinfected after each use.

Prevention and Control

Typhoid—A Preventable Disease

Every effort must be taken to kill the bacteria, as they leave the patient and thus prevent the spread of infection.

Immunization

Vaccination is the only specific preventive measure against typhoid. Though it does not give 100 per cent protection, but it definitely lowers both the incidence and seriousness of the disease. It can be given at any age after one year of age. The vaccine is most recommended in endemic areas, household contact of case and school children and health personnel, travellers entering the endemic areas and during fairs and festivals.

Antityphoid Vaccine

It was introduced by Wright in 1896, but its effectiveness was established in 1960. There are mainly three types of vaccines monovalent, bivalent and TAB vaccine.

Monovalent : These are killed vaccines prepared in an **agargrown** heat killed and phenol preserved vaccine. It is prepared by inactivating organisms by acetone and is called as acetone killed and dried vaccine.

Bivalent vaccine : These are prepared by two bacilli *S. typhi* and *S. paratyphi* organisms, killed and preserved by heating at 54°C for one hour and preserving in 0.5 per cent phenol or acetone in dried form.

TAB vaccine : It contains *S. typhi, S. typhi A* and *S. paratyphi B.* Due to its ineffectivity and side effects, it is not recommended as a vaccine for prevention of the disease.

Environmental Sanitation

Purification of water and supply of safe drinking water, improvement of environmental sanitation, to interrupt the transmission of infection, sewage disposal and proper use of sanitary laterine, may be helpful in prevention of spread of infection.

Health Education

People must be educated to change their behaviours to adopt healthy practices by keeping good sanitary conditions at home and environment, washing hands before cooking and eating, washing of raw vegetable properly before eating. Educate children to avoid eating from hawkers, uncovered items. Keep the food covered and prevent contamination from flies.

Control of reservoirs of infection can be done by identification of case, isolation, treatment and disinfection.

Isolation

The cases are usually isolated in the hospital unit to prevent the spread of disease and proper treatment. The isolation is continued till patient shows three bacteriologically negative stools and urine reports.

Treatment

Chloramphenicol remains the drug of choice. Dose is 500 mg/kg body wt/day, 4 to 6 hourly cotrimoxazole, amoxycillin and trimethoprim are equally effective. Seriously ill patients are given injection thydrocortisone 100 mg daily for 3 to 4 days.

Disinfection

Urine and stool of the patient is highly infectious and should be disinfected in 5 per cent cresol for at least 2 hours, linen and patient's clothes, etc., should be soaked in 2 per cent chlorine and steam sterilized or dried under sunlight, if at home. All handlers of patient should wash the hands properly.

Follow-up

The urine and stool examination is done in the follow-up till the patient gets negative reports.

Carriers

Carriers are the important source to spread the infection. They can be identified by blood examination, because they will not show any signs and symptoms of disease. Proper treatment, follow-up is essential to control the infection and treat the patient.

FOOD POISONING

Food poisoning is mainly caused by ingestion of contaminated food or drink. It is an acute infection of gastrointestinal tract caused by living bacteria, their toxins or inorganic chemical substances and the poisons derived from plants and animals. The patient usually gives the history of ingestion of common food and many people affected at the same time showing similar signs and symptoms in majority of cases.

Types of Food Poisoning

Food poisoning is categorised as follows :
- **Bacterial :** Bacteria and their toxins.
- **Chemical :** Fertilizers, pesticides and other chemical agents.

Bacterial Food Poisoning

Most common type of food poisoning is bacterial food poisoning. There are many bacteria involved in causing infection.

Salmonella bacilli : *Salmonella* is primarily a disease of animals. Man gets infection from farm animals and poultry through contaminated milk, food, eggs and their products. Rats and mice are another source, they are highly infected with *salmonella* and contaminate the food by their urine and faeces.

The bacilli enters the intestine and multiply to cause enteritis and colitis. The onset is generally sudden with fever, nausea, vomiting,

watery stool, chills and rigors usually lasts for 2 to 3 days. Mortality is 1 per cent. Prognosis is good if treated at an early stage.

Staphylococci infection : These bacilli are found on the skin, in the nose and throat of the man and animals. Cows suffering from mastitis are responsible to spread the infection through milk and milk products. The spread of infection is usually by eating unwashed raw vegetables and milk. Food poisoning occurs due to toxins produced in the food in which bacteria grow. Since the toxins are heat resistant, it can remain in food after organisms have died. The toxins act directly in the intestine and central nervous system. The patient complains of nausea, vomiting, abdominal cramps and diarrhoea. In severe cases, blood and mucus may appear. The fever usually does not appear in staphylococci infection. The patient recovers in 2 to 3 days with treatment, death is very rare.

Botulism : The causative organism is *Clostridium botulinum* of A, B and E type. They are widely found in soil, dust, intestine of animals and enter into the food as spores. The infection is spread through preserved home food *e.g.*, home-made food, vegetables, smoked or pickled fish, home-made cheese and low foods (pickles). The toxin of bacilli is produced in food under suitable conditions. It acts on parasympathetic nervous system. The clinical features are weakness, dysphasia, diplopia, ptosis, dysarthia and blurring vision. The condition is fatal and death may occur in 4 to 8 days due to respiratory or cardiac failure. In case of botulism, the antitoxin 50,000, 100,000 units I.V. should be given to the patient, as soon as possible. The antitoxin will not be effective, if toxins have already affected the nervous system. Guanidine hydrochloride 15 to 40 mg/kg wt/orally may reverse the neuromuscular block of botulism. Immunization toxins to prevent botulism is also available.

Chemical Food Poisoning

These are non-bacterial food poisoning, in which the food gets contaminated due to various poisonous chemical and cause serious illness. Commonly used pesticides for food production has caused serious public health problem. The fertilizers are used and water gets contaminated with these chemicals and causes hazards to people. The patient usually complains of severe pain in abdomen, nausea, vomiting and feels very sick. Depending upon the type of chemical, the patient may show the signs and symptoms of poisoning.

Prevention and Control

Community health nurse may educate the people regarding :

Food Hygiene

All the food items must be washed thoroughly before consumption.

Especially raw food must be dipped in water for 1 to 2 hours before eating to remove the pesticides or other chemicals.

Food handling must be done hygienically. The food handlers must be free from any type of wound, boils, diarrhoea, dysentery, throat infection, etc.

Preparation and Consumption of Food

The freshly cooked food should be preferably consumed. The food kept for long-time will encourage the growth of bacteria and cause infection. The importance of rapid cooling and storage must be stressed. Milk and milk products, natural or pasteurised, must be safe for consumption. Food must be thoroughly cooked.

Hygienic conditions : The food must be prepared, eaten and preserved under hygienic conditions. Utensils and other equipments must be kept clean and free from flies, rats and dust.

Personal hygiene : People must be taught about clean habits of hand washing after defecation and before and after eating and taking bath daily.

Preservation of food : The food must be preserved under suitable temperature. Food after used must be kept immediately in the refrigerator or in cold storage to prevent the multiplication of bacteria and toxin.

Production : Cook and eat the same day, will help in preventing various GIT infections. The bacteria do not multiply and die below 4°C and refrigeration level should not exceed this level.

Surveillance : Whenever and wherever necessary food sample must be taken from commercial food handlers and laboratory analysis must be done to prevent these infections.

HELMINTHS INFESTATION ASCARIASIS (ROUNDWORM INFESTATION)

Ascariasis is a common helminic infection of intestinal tract caused by *Ascaris lumbricoides*. Clinically manifested is pain in abdomen, nausea, vomiting, loss of appetite or excessive hunger. Roundworms are seen in the stool of the cases. In chronic cases, the worms get accumulated in the intestine and cause intestinal obstruction. The worms if untreated may also affect other parts of the body, *e.g.*, like brain and eye in very late stage.

Worldwide Problem

The helminthic infections are prevalent in all parts of the world. It is estimated that about 25 per cent of world's population is infected with roundworms. The prevalence rate of 50 to 75 per cent has been registered in Asia and Latin American countries; even small parts of America are also affected with infection.

Epidemiological Factors

Agent

Ascaris lumbricoides lives and moves freely in small intestine and brain. The sexes are separate, male and females *Ascaris*. Eggs are excreted through faeces and become embryonated in the external environment and become infective in 2 to 3 weeks. On ingestion by man they develop in the intestine as adults. The larvae penetrate the intestinal wall and enter the liver and lungs through the bloodstream and attack the alveoli of lungs causing cough and respiratory problems.

Host Factor

Children below 5 to 15 years are most affected by ascariasis. Roundworm contribute to malnutrition in children and may lead to growth retardation. Adults seem to acquire some resistance.

Environmental Factors

The eggs remain viable in favourable environmental conditions of soil, *e.g.*, temperature, moisture, oxygen and sunlight radiations. Clay soils are most favourable for development of ascariasis eggs. Open field defecation is the most important factor for widespread of ascariasis in the world. Children play with soil and contaminate houses with soil, may spread infection in houses and surrounding areas. Eggs can easily reach other children, playing in the ground and contaminate hands and food.

Mode of Infection

The faeces of cases are the main source of spread of infection.

Ascariasis spreads by ingestion of infective eggs with food and drink. Food eaten raw as salad without washing and use of contaminated water.

The other means of spread may be contaminated fingers with soil, usually among children playing with mud.

Prevention and Control

Health education may be given on :
- Sanitary disposal of human excreta.
- To prevent or reduce the contamination of soil.
- Avoid open field defecation and use of sanitary latrines.
- Provision of safe drinking water.
- Food hygiene, healthy eating habits.
- Personal hygiene, hand washing habits.

Treatment

The drugs of choice are piperazine, mebandazole, levamisol and pyrantel. The single dose is also available for effective treatment. The drugs paralyse the worms and can be expelled by faeces. Mebandazole is prescribed 100 mg twice a day for three days. A single dose of 100 to 150 mg has been recommended for the treatment and mass treatment.

HOOKWORM INFESTATION (ANCYLOSTOMIASIS)

The hookworm infection is a chronic helminthic disease caused by *Necator americanus* and *Ancylostoma duodenale*. Clinically the disease leads to anaemia, oedema and other complications.

Worldwide Problem

Hookworm infection is more prevalent in hot, moist climate in tropical and subtropical regions, *e.g.*, Asia, Africa, Central and South America. It has been widely distributed throughout the world, it is estimated that in 1996, the prevalence of hookworm was about 151 million cases and approximately 65,000 deaths annually, due to hookworm anaemia.

Problem in India

It is widely prevalent in India and *Necator americanus* are more prominent in South India and *A. duodenale* in North India; another species Aceylanicun has been identified in some villages of India.

The most affected areas of India are Assam, West Bengal, Tamil Nadu, Andhra Pradesh, Kerala, Orissa, Bihar and Maharashtra. More than 200 million people are estimated to be infected in India and 60 to 80 per cent cases from U.P., West Bengal, Bihar, Orissa, Punjab, Tamil Nadu and Andhra Pradesh.

Epidemiological Factors

Agent

The worms appear like hooks, dorsally curved anterior end, measuring 5 to 10 mm (male) and 9 to 12 mm (female). Adult worms lie in intestine of the cases. A female North *Necator americanus* produces 10,000 eggs and *A. duodenale* lay 30,000 eggs per day. The excessive production of eggs indicates continuous exposure to infection. Larvae rapidly develop in the eggs in warm, moist soil in 1 to 2 days. The newly hatched larvae lie in waiting in the soil to penetrate the skin of human host. They can survive in shades, moist soil for up to one month. Infection occurs after entering the body through skin and through the feet. Larvae of *A. duodenale* can also enter through the mouth. They enter the lungs through the bloodstream, enter the alveoli bronchi and trachea, coughed out or enter the intestine through respiratory tract. In the intestine they become sexually mature. They can survive for 1 to 4 years on an average (Fig. 23.4).

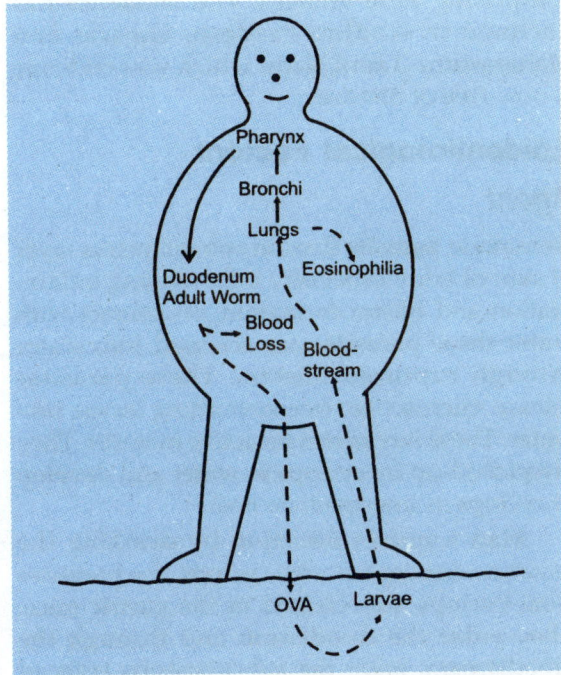

Fig. 23.4 : Ancylostomiosis

Source of Infection

Faeces containing ova and larvae of hookworm are the immediate source of infection, they contaminate the soil and enter the human host by contact with soil. Man is the important reservoir of infection. Since the worm matures in the intestine and passes bundles of eggs through faeces.

Host Factors

Age and Sex

All ages of both sexes are equally affected by infection, though high incidence is found among children below 15 years due to unhygienic eating and playing habits.

Nutritional Status

It indicates that malnutrition is a predisposing factor, hence malnourished children are easily

affected by infestation and vice versa. The worm infestation leads the patient to malnutrition. The chronic disabled disease does not occur in healthy and well nourished individuals.

Occupation

Occupation plays an important role in causation of disease. High prevalence is found among farmers due to agriculture and farming.

Environmental Factors

The favourable environmental conditions for hookworm are damp and sandy soil, under 24 to 32°C of temperature, sufficient oxygen, moisture and average rainfall.

Health Habits

The lack of healthy habits, *e.g.*, open field defecation, barefeet walking, farming practices, with untreated sewage, children playing in the mud with barefeet and hands are responsible in causation of infection. These factors are associated with low socioeconomic, illiteracy and ignorance among people.

Mode of Transmission

Hookworm enters the body by penetrating the skin. *A. duodenal* may also enter through oral route by eating unwashed raw vegetables.

Incubation Period

It is 7 weeks in case of *N. americanus* and 5 weeks to 9 months in *A. duodenale*.

Prevention and Control

Hookworm infection can be prevented by early detection and treatment of the infected people. Stool test and clinical manifestation will help in diagnosing the cases and effective drugs available for the treatment of hookworm infection. The most effective drugs are Albendazole (400 mg/day), mebandazole (500 mg), levanizole, which can be given as single dose or divided doses.

Environmental Sanitation

Hygienic way of disposal of excreta and use of sanitary latrines will prevent the soil pollution.

The farming technique should be modified to avoid handling the soil and protection of feet and hands from spoiling with soil. Children should avoid barefoot walking.

Prevention and Treatment of Malnutrition

The children must be treated for malnutrition and anaemia, because worms affect the healthy children and if child gets anaemia or malnutrition, they must be treated properly with ferrous sulphate and high protein diet.

Health Education

The community health nurse plays important role in educating the public on prevention and control of worm infestation.

- Promotion of use of sanitary latrines and avoid open field defecation to prevent soil pollution.
- Regular use of footwears especially for children playing in grounds and mud, should not walk barefooted.
- Maintaining normal health and prevention of malnutrition and anaemia by taking balanced diet.
- Early diagnosis and proper treatment.
- Consumption of clean and washed food, especially raw vegetables and fruits.

Prevent the spread of infection by orofaecal route by proper hand washing after defecation, before and after eating food and nails should be cut short.

GUINEAWORM DISEASE (DRACUNCULIASIS)

Guineaworm is a vector-borne infection of subcutaneous tissues usually affecting the feet and legs, mainly caused by nematode parasite.

Worldwide Problem

The disease is prevalent in many of the countries. In certain countries, e.g., Brazil and West Indies, it has been eradicated. The incidence has declined by 21 per cent in 1995. Worldwide about 20 million people are affected due to guineaworm infection. Sudan reports around 50 per cent of the total cases, whereas the incidence has declined in many other endemic countries.

Problem in India

It is endemic in India affecting 6 to 8 states comprising 1250 villages. The incidence has declined in Andhra Pradesh, Gujarat and Maharashtra. Tamil Nadu which was endemic is now free of diseases.

Epidemiological Factors

Agent

Nematode parasite lives in subcutaneous layer of skin of body especially legs, causing inflammation and blister formation, on contact with water these parasites are released into water through ruptured blisters. These parasites release microscopic free swimming larvae into water. These larvae remain active in water. They are picked-up by cyclops in water and develop in cyclops as intermediate host.

Man acquires infection by drinking the water contaminated with cyclops, the parasites from cyclops are released in the gastric juice. They enter the duodenum and through the bloodstream, enter the subcutaneous layer of skin and other parts of the body and grow as adults in 9 to 10 months.

Host Factor

Man is susceptible to infection. The habit of washing and bathing near the wells, ponds and surface water contaminated with infection. Hence use of step-well is most desirable to prevent infection.

Environmental Factors

The disease is spread through contaminated water with cyclops. The larvae develop best between 25 to 30°C and will not develop below 19°C, hence disease is more common among tropical and subtropical areas.

Source of Infection

Infected person harbouring the infected cyclops is the main source of infection. The disease is transmitted by drinking contaminated water.

Guineaworm is totally water-borne disease and have no other mode of transmission.

Prevention and Control of Disease

The disease can be prevented by proper education to the people about :

- Use of safe drinking water, boiling of water in the endemic areas.
- Provision of step-wells for use of well-water and chlorination of well-water.
- Educate people to avoid washing clothes, taking bath, putting feet in contaminated water and animal bathing should be restricted.
- Identification of new cases and treatment of the cases with mebandazole, metranidazole and niridazole.

NATIONAL GUINEAWORM ERADICATION PROGRAMME (GWEP)

Government of India launched GWEP in 1983-84, during Sixth Five-Year Plan. It is 50 per cent centrally sponsored programme.

GWEP envisages the efficient implementation of well defined strategies.

- Guineaworm case detection and continuous surveillance through active case funding and regular monthly reporting.
- Guineaworm case management.
- Vector control (cyclop) by application of Temephos in unsafe water source eight times a year and use of fine nylon double layered cloth strainers by the community to filter cyclops in all the affected villages.
- Health education.
- Trained manpower development.
- Provision and maintenance of safe drinking water supply on priority in guineaworm endemic villages.
- Concurrent evaluation and operational research.

NICD with the financial support from WHO has deployed epidemiological surveillance teams in endemic states, which closely monitor the programme and help district/primary health centre authorities in effective implementation of GWEP. Operational component specially surveillance and guineaworm case containment

measures with the goal to eradicate the disease from endemic areas.

Achievements and Current Situation

In 1984 there were around 40,000 GW cases in 89 districts of seven endemic states. During 1996, only 9 guineaworm cases have been recorded in three villages from Jodhpur, (Rajasthan), and rest of the country continue to remain free from guineaworm disease. The states of Tamil Nadu, Gujarat, Maharashtra and Andhra Pradesh were deleted from the list of guineaworm endemic states on being free from guineaworm disease for more than three years. During 1998 till October 1999, no guineaworm case has been reported from any part of the country. Last case was reported in 1996.

Eradication of guineaworm will be another major national achievement of recent times. The country has completed three years of guineaworm disease free in July 1999 and will be eligible for Certificate by the International Commission of Certificate of Dracunculiasis Eradication (CCDE).

National Commission for Certificate of Guineaworm eradication was set-up by Ministry of Health and Family Welfare, comprising eight highly experienced independent experts in the field of public health. The seventh evaluation was carried out in April 1999.

International Certificate Team WHO Guineaworm Eradication Programme visited the country from November 10 to 24, 1999, to assess the status for Certificate of guineaworm Eradication in India.

AMOEBIASIS

Amoebiasis is the condition of harbouring the *Entamoeba histolytica*, the protozoan parasite through contaminated food and water may or may not manifest the signs and symptoms. The severity of the disease vary from symptom less to mild abdominal pain and diarrhoea or acute severe dysentery. Amoebiasis may also cause liver abscess, involve the lungs, skin, brain and spleen, etc.

Worldwide Problem

It is a worldwide parasitic disease infecting the human gastrointestinal tract. It is most common endemic infection in most of the regions of the world, though it is major health problem in China, South-East, West Asia and Latin America. It has been estimated that 500 million people carried infection (*E.histolytica*) in their gastrointestinal tract and one-tenths were infected showing manifestations (40-50 million). In the areas of high prevalence amoebiasis occurs in endemic form as a result of high levels of transmission modes and reinfections. Waterborne infection occurs as an endemic, if there is heavily contaminated drinking water. Prevalence rate vary from 2 per cent to 60 per cent depending upon the favourable environmental conditions.

Problem in India

The prevalence rate is around 15 per cent in India, though the figure is not accurate due to unavailability of reliable source of information and lack of laboratory facilities to diagnose the cases.

Epidemiological Factors

Agent

E. histolytica : These are protozoal group of parasites occurring in two forms—the trophozoites and cystic form. The trophozoites enter the colon and get encysted and cysts are excreted in stool. Some trophozoites cause ulceration in the caecum and colons, rectum and sigmoid. Some may enter the blood and travel in various organs of the body, especially liver.

The trophozoite can not survive for longer period outside the body, hence are not important in transmission of disease. The cysts are infective to man and remain viable and infective for several days in water, soil, faeces and other excretes in the presence of moisture and low temperature. Cysts are not affected by chlorine in normal amount of water chlorination, but they can be killed at 55°C heating, drying or frozen.

Host Factor

Amoebias can affect any age and sex. It is considered to be a family health problem. If one individual gets infection, other members are also infected.

Environmental Factors

The disease is related to poor sanitary conditions and poor socioeconomic status. The incidence of the disease is high during rainy season and wet-dry season. The spread of disease is more common on the use of night soil (faeces as fertilizer) for agricultural purposes. Epidemic outbreaks are often associated with improper sewage system, and poor water supply conditions.

Sources of Infection

Faeces of man harbouring cysts are the main source of infection. Most of the healthy carrier harbouring infection, showing no clinical manifestation spread the disease. The major sources are the food handlers as healthy carriers of amoebiasis.

Mode of Transmission

The Faeco-oral Route

This route is the mode of transmission of disease, unwashed raw vegetables eaten, heavy contaminated water, sewage pollution may spread the infection. This may lead to hand to mouth infection.

Sexual Route

By oral-rectal sexual contact has also been seen as the transmission among male homosexuals.

Vectors

Flies, cockroaches and rodents are capable of carrying cysts and contaminating food and water.

Incubation Period

Lasts for 2 to 3 weeks or as long as 6 weeks.

Prevention and Control

Environmental Sanitation

- Safe disposal of human and animal wastes.
- Proper hand washing after defecation and before cooking and eating food.

Safe Drinking Water

Free from any contaminations should be consumed by people. The cysts are not killed by chlorine, though sandfilters are quite effective in removing amoebic cysts. Water filteration and boiling are more effective than chemical treatment of water for amoebiasis.

Food Hygiene

Protection of food from contamination. Uncooked vegetable can be eaten after washing and disinfecting with $KMnO_4$. Periodical examination of food handlers and education regarding hygienic practices while cooking.

Role of Primary Health Nurse in Health Education

- Hand washing before cooking, eating and after defecation.
- Washing vegetables before cooking and cooking under normal heat.
- Eating raw vegetables after washing properly with $KMnO_4$.
- Use of sanitary latrines.
- Clean and safe drinking water.
- Eating freshly cooked food and avoid contaminated food.
- Early detection and treatment of cases and carriers especially food handlers.

VIRAL HEPATITIS

Viral hepatitis is the infection of liver caused by varieties of viruses, *e.g.*, A, B , C, D and E characterized by mild fever, nausea, vomiting and jaundice in a patient. Hepatitis A virus causes relatively benign disease and is not considered a major public health problem. Hepatitis B is parenterally transmitted and is responsible for severe liver damage and is associated with chronic liver disease and hepatic carcinoma, whereas hepatitis A, C and E are transmitted through the faeco-oral route.

Prevalence of Disease

The increasing incidence of viral hepatitis is a growing public health concern. Although the mortality rate is low, the disease is important because of its easy transmission, morbidity and prolonged loss of time from school or workplace due to prolonged illness.

In India more than four million people suffer every year in some or other form of hepatitis.

Viral hepatitis may be classified into following types :

Hepatitis A

Hepatitis A, commonly known as infectious hepatitis or jaundice, is probably an RNA virus of enterovirus family. It is an acute infection of liver caused by hepatitis A, characterized by headache, mild fever, weakness, malaise and aches followed by anorexia, nausea, vomiting, dark urine and jaundice.

The patient usually recovers in seven weeks with very rare complications of acute liver failure (0.1%) mainly among the adults. The mortality due to this hepatitis is vary rare, may be less than 0.1 per cent.

Prevalence of Disease

The exact incidence is not known due to large number of asymptomatic cases. WHO estimates 10 to 50 persons per lakh are affected annually. The evidences show decline in incidence rate in developed countries, due to good sanitary conditions.

In India the exact incidence is not known, but records show the epidemic of disease in various places of the country. The common source of epidemic, *i.e.*, faecal contamination and drinking water is usually involved.

History

Hepatitis A was described clearly in the late eighteenth century, earlier attributions may be correct, but one poorly substantiated by presumably relevant text "Benign epidemic jaundice" was distinguished by a low fertility rate, in contrast to epidemic disease caused by yellow fever and leptospirosis.

Epidemiological Factors

Agent

The causative organism of the hepatitis A is enterovirus, which only multiplies hepatocytes.

The virus is resistant to heat and chemicals. It can survive for more than ten weeks in water and is not affected by chlorine as per recommendation dose for chlorination. Formalin is an effective disinfectant. The virus can be destroyed by autoclaving or boiling for five minutes.

Reservoir of Infection

Human cases and carriers of the virus are the only source of spread of infection and they are the reservoirs of infection. The case may be mild, or severe one. These cases may play an important role in maintaining the chain of transmission in the community.

Infective Material

The infection is mainly through faeces, blood, serum and other body fluids. Blood serum and other fluids are infective during the brief stage of viraemia and virus is excreted in the faeces for about two weeks before the onset of jaundice and virus may also be excreted through urine.

Mode of Transmission

Faecal-oral route is the major route of transmission, may be direct or indirect, through contaminated water, milk, food, unhygienic ways of living, eating raw vegetables. The virus has been found in the stool of infected patient prior to the onset of symptoms and during the first few days of illness. A young adult acquires the infection at school and brings home, with haphazard sanitary habits, spread it through the family. It is more prevalent in underdeveloped countries, overcrowded areas and poor sanitation. An infected food handler can spread the disease and people can contract it by consuming water from sewage contaminated water; animal handlers can contract hepatitis A from infected primates.

Contaminated drinking water can serve as mechanism of spread of hepatitis. Largest water-borne epidemics have occurred in India, where a high level of the agent may still be formed in general population.

Transmission of Disease

Faecal-oral route : The most common mode of transmission of the disease is due to faecal-oral route, whether direct, person to person or indirect route through food and water contamination. Direct spread of infection is due to poor environment, hygiene and overcrowding.

Parenteral route : Though, spread of infection through parenteral route is very rare, but still infection may spread through contaminated needles, blood and blood products.

Sexual transmission : Infection may occur among homosexual men due to oral and anal contacts.

Host Factor

Age and Sex

People from all ages and both sexes are susceptible to get the infection, though it is more frequent among children.

Incubation period is 1 to 7 weeks, with an average of 80 days, the course of illness is 4 to 8 weeks, generally lasts long and is more severe in the age group above 40 years.

Immunity

Infection with hepatitis A virus provides long-term immunity, which is probably lifelong in majority of instances.

Environmental Factors

The disease may occur any time during the year, but the incidence is higher during the rainy season due to environmental conditions, *e.g.,* water pollution and fly breeding leads to water-borne and food-borne diseases.

Poor environment conditions and overcrowding favour the spread of infection giving rise to hepatitis.

Clinical Manifestation

Mostly patients are symptomless, when symptoms appear, they are mild like upper respiratory infection with low grade fever. The signs and symptoms appear over 24 to 48 hours period. The initial symptoms are loss of appetite, malaise, often generalised muscular aching, nausea, vomiting occur in majority of cases.

Other symptoms includes headache, fever, temperature range 100 to 101°F, abdominal discomfort or pain, usually in the epigastric region or right upper quadrant, heart burn and flatulance. These symptoms persist for 3 to 10 days.

Later jaundice and dark urine may become apparent. The liver and spleen are often markedly enlarged for few days after onset of disease.

Conjunctival mucous membrane and generalized jaundice occur in a typical certain case. The patient complains of weakness, poor appetite and epigastric distress. These symptoms disappear at the peak of jaundice and patient feels quite alright, in spite of biochemical parameters are high.

Treatment

Traditionally the management of acute V. hepatitis was bed rest, diet and vitamin supplements. The patient is advised bed rest, when moderately ill and be ambulatory during convalscent stage. Hospitalization may be necessary for adults to provide adequate rest, especially the mother of small children or living alone.

Small frequent adequate meals, rich in carbohydrate and low fat is usually recommended for the patients.

Vitamins especially vitamin B complex is given for early recovery.

Vitamin K is given to improve regenerate live cells and liver functioning.

Ambulation seems to hasten recovery, provided patient rests after recovery.

Antibiotics and corticosteroids are of no use, therefore, should not be given.

Prevention and Control of Disease

Control of mode of transmission : The disease is transmitted by oral-faecal route. Hence the best way to reduce the spread of infection is by promoting simple measures of environmental and personal hygiene, e.g., hand washing before eating and after toilet, sanitary disposal of excreta which prevents contamination of water, food and milk.

Immunization

- No active immunization is available for hepatitis A.
- Passive immunization : Normal human gammaglobulin prepared from pooled plasma of healthy donors (gammaglobulin IgG preparation) was said to be an effective measure for prevention. Immune gammaglobulin prophylaxis is given either prior to anticipated exposure or after the exposure, provides 50 to 90 per cent of protection. Recommended dose is 0.5 mL intramuscularly for children and 2 mL for adults. It is usually recommended for :
  1. Susceptible people travelling to highly endemic areas,
  2. Control of outbreak in institutions,
  3. Personal contacts of patients with HAV.

Nursing Management

- Bedrest : The patient needs to be provided complete bed rest.
- Diet should be high protein, high carbohydrate and low fat. Food should be served in small, attractive and frequent feeds.
- Disinfection of bedpans, clothings, utensils and other belongings should be done.
- Observation for indication of increasing severity of disease, mental confusion, extreme anorexia.
- Complication of liver damage, recurrence of symptoms, should be prevented by proper rest and diet.

Hepatitis B

Hepatitis B, was commonly known as serum hepatitis. The disease is usually transmitted by parenteral route, characterized by self-limiting infection causing progressive liver disease including chronic active hepatitis and hepatocellular carcinoma.

Worldwide Problem

Hepatitis B is endemic throughout the world, especially in developing and tropical countries. The prevalence of the disease varies from country to country. It has been estimated that

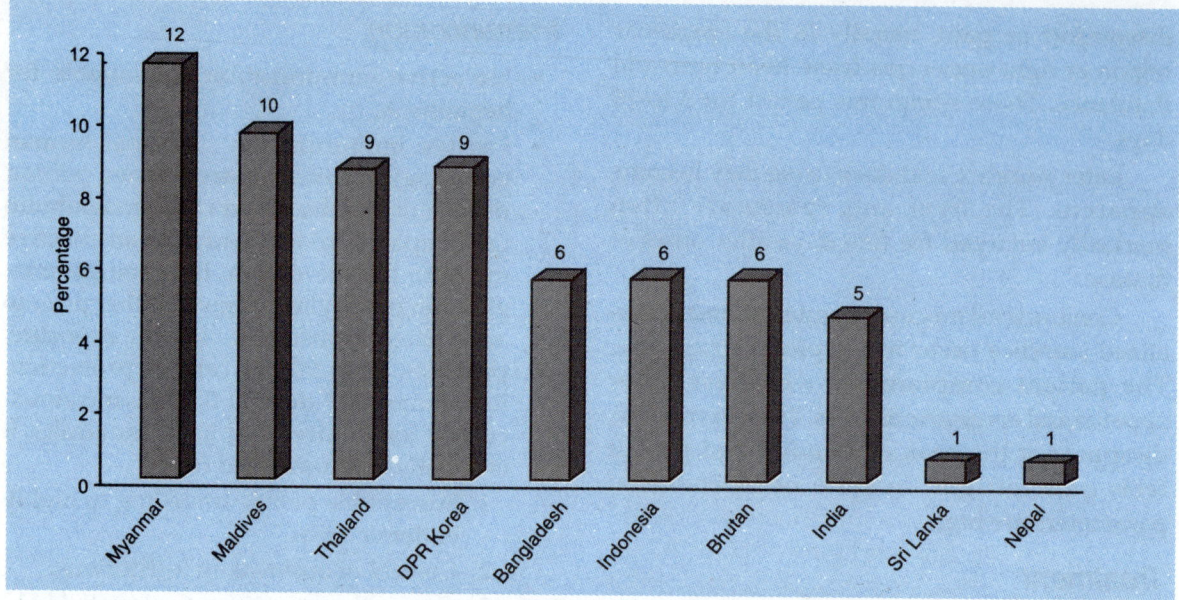

Fig. 23.5 : Hepatitis B prevalence in SEAR by 2000

more than two billion people have been infected with hepatitis B virus and 350 million are chronically infected carriers of the virus, all over the world. HBV infection is directly related to 1 to 2 million deaths per year. Primary liver cancer is a leading cause of death in males.

It is estimated that 400 million people will be carriers of HBV by the year 2000, if HB vaccine is not widely used (Fig. 23.5).

Hepatitis B and Hepatitis C, both are major public health problems of the world. Hepatitis C is not as infectious as hepatitis B. As many as 80 per cent of infected people may suffer serious long-term affects such as liver cancer, which places hepatitis C virus (HCV) among pathogens of primary concern. Based on prevalence rates ranging from 0.1 per cent to 33 per cent in different countries. It is directly related with standard of living and the incidence is the highest in countries where economic level is lower as in South-East Asia particularly India, China and South America.

Problem in India

HBV is a major public health problem in India. Total 98,047 cases and 1,268 deaths due to viral hepatitis were reported in 1992 and 40 per cent of that were due to HBV, though it is not the correct figure due to lack of reporting cases.

There was a major hepatitis B outbreak in Ahmedabad (Gujarat) in 1984 reporting 1783 cases with an incidence of 0.59 per thousand population. Hepatitis A and E are endemic in India and local epidemics keep breaking out now and then. India has largest pool of those hepatitis B causing chronic level diseases. It is the fifth major cause of mortality in the most reproductive years of life (15–45). The spread of hepatitis A and E are linked with personal hygiene and hepatitis B with safety measures during blood and blood product transfusions. There is an apprehension among Delhi Doctors/ Virologists that there is emergence of viral hepatitis B among people, who had received blood and platelet transfusions during the recent epidemic of dengue in Delhi.

History

Hepatitis B virus was the presumptive cause of two epidemic of jaundice in 1883-84. The specific serological technique discovered that hepatitis B is worldwide in distribution with some of the highest prevalence in the medically most underdeveloped population. This fact suggests that it is an old infection rather than recent, mention and detection of hepatitis B was a reaction of serum of a certain aborigine was a source of viral antigen.

Agent

Hepatitis B was first discovered by Blumberg in 1963. HBV is a complex double shelled DNA virus, originally known as "Dane particle". It replicates in the liver cells. HBV has three distinct antigens—a surface antigen or Australia antigen, 'a' antigen and an 'e' antigen. Patients infected with HBV are expected to have one or more HBV markers. HBV would be infected with HIV and global AIDS policy has estimated the figure to be 110 million.

HBV is a DNA virus measuring 42 μm with complex structure consisting of surface antigen (HBgAg).

Reservoir of Infection

Case and the carrier in man is the only reservoir of infection. The spread of infection is mainly due to existence of large number of carriers, estimated as 285 million in the world.

Source of Infection

The infective blood of case or carrier is the main source of infection. Though virus has been found in various other secretions of saliva, vaginal secretions and semen of infected person but there is no spread of infection except blood.

Period of communicability

The period of communicability is several months before the appearance of clinical manifestations.

Host Factor

Age : The countries with higher incidence of HBV is more common among perinatal period and early childhood and the countries with lower incidence have more cases from 20 to 40 years of age.

High-risk group : People who are more prone to get the infection are recipients of blood transfusions, health care and laboratory personnel, homosexuals, prostitutes, percutaneous drug abusers, newborn of HBV carrier mothers and patients who are immunocompromised. Immunization for these high-risk groups and screening has been highly recommended.

Mode of Transmission

- *Sexual transmission :* High incidence of spread of infection has been found through sexual route, particularly among male homosexuals and prostitutes.
- *Parenteral route :* Most common cause of spread of infection is through infected blood and blood products, through contaminated syringes and needles, handling infected blood, dialysis, blood transfusion, skin prick etc.
- *Perinatal transmission :* High prevalence of HBV infection has been found from HBV carrier mothers to their newborn babies. Rarely, the HBV can infect the foetus in the uterus, but most of the infections occur during labour.
- *Incubation period :* The average incubation period is 100 days, though it varies from 45 to 180 days.

Clinical Manifestations

Clinically the patient has similar signs and symptoms like viral hepatitis and chronic liver disease, which may follow infection. Chronic liver disease may be severe and may progress to primary liver cancer.

Prevention and Control of Hepatitis 'B'

Preventive Measure : It is difficult to screen all the patients for HBV, but the high-risk group should get blood test done for positive Australia antigen. Especially, all blood donors should be screened for HBV.

Immunization

Active immunization

Plasma derived vaccine : The antigen is derived and purified from the plasma of human carrier of hepatitis B virus. The vaccine is inactivated with formalin and formulated in an alum adjuvant. The vaccine dose is completed in three doses at 0, 1 and 6 months. An effective antibody response is attained after three doses in 95 per cent of vaccinated people. Immunity continues at protective level for 3 to 5 years. Booster doses are recommended after five years. Both pre-exposed and post-exposed administration of vaccine has been recommended for all health personnel, *e.g.*, doctors, nurses and laboratory workers, protection of newborn infants born of HBV mother and people who are exposed accidently through parenteral route to HBV infection through transfusion, cuts, injuries and needle pricks.

In 1996, the HBV vaccine has been introduced with universal immunization programme. The vaccine will be given to all children of sixth, tenth and thirteenth week of age.

Dose : Three doses with 1 mL each given intramuscularly and 0.5 mL for children below 10 years of age.

RDNA yeast derived vaccine : The vaccine is derived from culture of yeast. The vaccine is safe, effective and is more cost-effective than plasma derived vaccine. The protection of vaccine is at least for nine years and booster dose is usually not recommended.

Dose : Adult—10 to 20 mg and 5 to 10 microgram (μg) for newborn and children.

Passive Immunization

Hepatitis B immunoglobulin is given for immediate protection after exposure, especially health workers, newborn, infants of carrier mothers and sexual contacts with positive cases. The blood test should be done for HBV. If found negative, active immunization should be started immediately in three complete doses, if it is positive nothing should be done.

The dose for immunoglobulin is 0.05 to 0.07 mL/kg body weight, two doses at one month interval. The immunity lasts for three months.

Other Measures

All blood donors should be screened for HBV infection and those positive for Australia antigens should be rejected.

Health personnel should be alerted, the importance of proper sterilization of instruments and practice simple hygienic measures.

Combined Active Passive Immunization

The two immunizations given simultaneously are more effective than the above. The combined vaccine is both for prophylaxis of person's exspoure to HBV and protection against any time exposure.

Hepatitis C

Hepatitis C is an RNA virus, measuring 60 to 70 mm. Hepatitis virus was identified in 1989 and is a single stranded RNA virus. The virus is mainly transmitted through contaminated blood and blood products. More than 50 per cent cases are related to intravenous drug users, who share needles. Less chances of transmission is due to sexual and maternal foetal transmission.

Clinically the disease is characterized with mild illness, later may lead to chronic hepatitis which may lead to cirrhosis of liver or liver cancer, more common in men and alcoholics than in women and alcoholics.

Incubation period 6 to 7 weeks.

Prevention and Control of Infective Hepatitis

- Washing of hands thoroughly after bowel movements.
- Adequate cleaning of toilet.
- Decontamination of food and water before use.

Prevention and Control of Hepatitis C

Health education is essential to inform the general public and health care workers about the risk of transmitting infection with the use of unsterile equipment. Surveillance on a global scale needs to be strengthened in order to improve knowledge of transmission of the virus.

Treatment

Interferon is the only drug that has been found effective in treatment of HCV infection. However, treatment is very expensive and is administered several times a week for several months. It may even cause severe side effects. Due to cost, very few patients can afford to continue the treatment. The treatment with interferon is effective in about 20 per cent of patients. For the remaining 80 per cent international research efforts should focus on combined antiviral therapy. Ninty per cent of people are in need of treatment today can not afford it.

Hepatitis E

The disease is caused by Hepatitis E virus which is a water-borne disease. Water or food supplies contaminated by faeces with virus are responsible for major outbreaks reported all over the countries with hot climate.

POLIOMYELITIS

Poliomyelitis is an acute viral infection caused by polio virus (enterovirus) in human gastrointestinal tract. It affects central nervous system of cases resulting in paralysis and possibly death.

Worldwide Distribution of Poliomyelitis

Polio was highly prevalent in almost all the countries before 1954. With the introduction of polio vaccine, the incidence had declined, very low and almost nil in developed countries like

USA. The last case reported was from Peru in 1991. Though in some countries the decline is spectacular.

The OPV (oral polio vaccine) immunization coverage had gone up in the year 1995 and 83 per cent of children were reported to be immunized by OPV in South-East Asia region (Fig. 23.6).

Problem in India

The annual incidence in India is 2 to 5/1000 in rural and 1 to 3/1000 in urban pre-school children and in south of the country, 3 to 5/1000 is the annual incidence in the whole population.

The first polio epidemic occurred in 1949 in Bombay and many times in Andhra Pradesh, Uttar Pradesh, Gujarat, Maharashtra, Rajasthan, Tamil Nadu and Delhi.

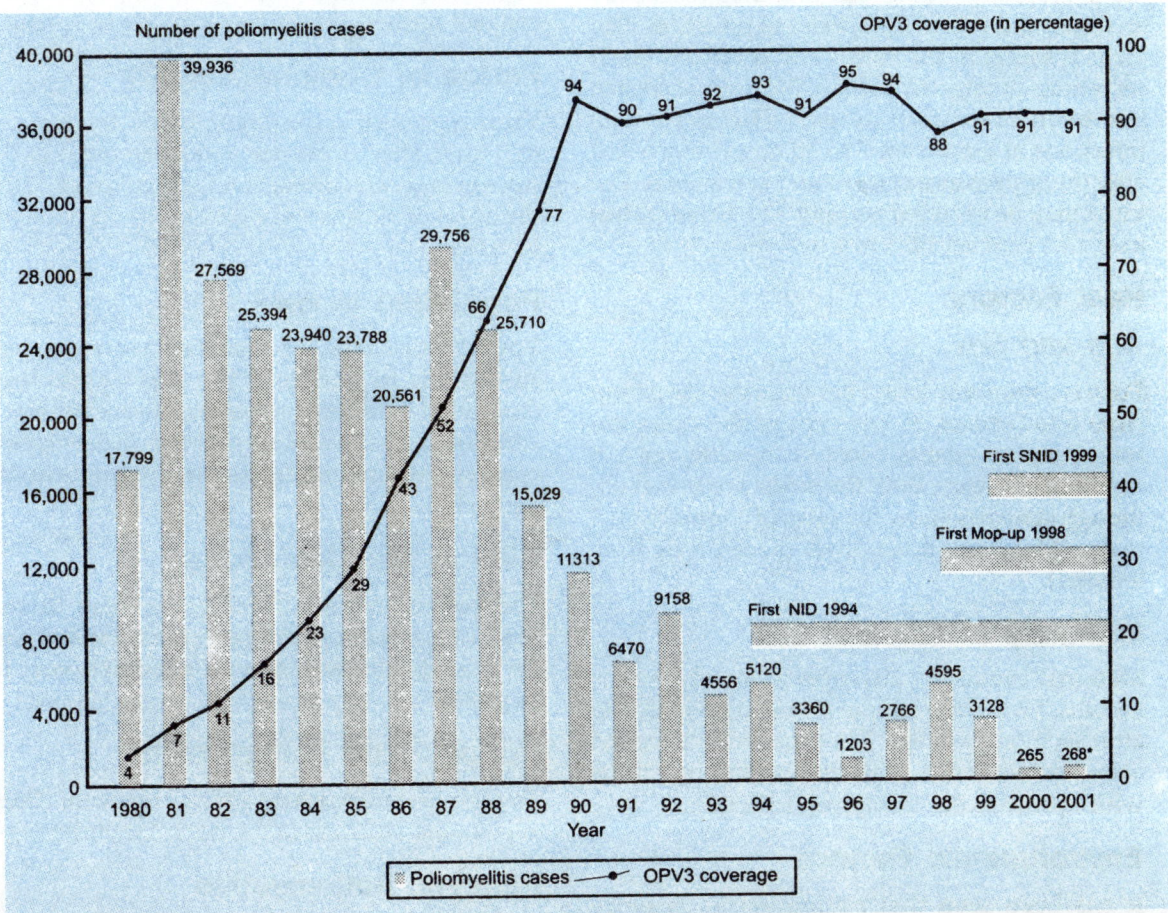

Fig. 23.6 : Trends in reported poliomylitis cases and OPV3 immunization coverage in SEAR in 1980 to 2001

India played an important role in eradication of polio. Since the declining trend is quite satisfactory from 1986 to 1995, the presence of a large number of children under 5 years of age in the country are getting immunized by means of regular immunization and pulse polio.

Epidermiological Factors

Agent

The causative organism for polio is of three types of polio viruses : I, II and III. The most common among these three is polio virus I. It can live for long period in the environment, especially in cold environment, in water and in faeces for 4 to 6 months.

Source of Infection

Man is the only source of infection through faecal-oral route. Subclinical and mild cases play an important role in the spread of infection. The virus is found in the faeces and oropharyngeal secretions of infected person. No animal source has been identified as yet. The person is infectious at least from 7 to 10 days before and after the appearance of signs and symptoms. The virus may be excreted usually 3 to 4 weeks, but may also prolong till 3 to 4 months.

Host Factors

Age and Sex

Polio is commonly found between the age group from 0 to 5 years. 50 per cent of the cases are found among infants. Most vulnerable age is 6 months to 3 years. Both the sexes are involved, though statistics show the ratio of 1 female for 3 males (Males are three times more prone than females).

Immunity

Maternal immunity disappears slowly by six months. Twin child is more prone to get infection after six months of age. The immunity of a child also depends upon maternal immunity status which protects the child from infection.

Environmental Factors

It has been seen that poliomyelitis is more prevalent during rainy season, (May to September) due to environmental factors of polluted water and food. The virus can survive for longer time in a cold environment, overcrowding and poor sanitation provides opportunities for exposure to infection.

Other Factors

Various risk factors have been found to precipitate an attack of paralytic polio like— fatigue, trauma, intramuscular injections, operations like tonsillectomy.

Incubation Period

Usually 3 to 35 days and may even prolong till 30 days.

Mode of Transmission

Polio virus is a wild virus that circulates in the population and multiplies in the human intestinal tract. Direct contact via oropharyngeal route is the principal mode of spread.

Period of Communicability

Virus is present in the throat, blood and faeces 3 to 5 days after exposure and is excreted in the stool in large concentration for 6 to 8 weeks after the onset of abortive nonparalytic and paralytic infection.

Population at Risk

Young unvaccinated children are especially susceptible to infection. The disease has been controlled by effective oral polio vaccine, but is still emerging as a serious problem in developing countries where immunization programmes are ineffective.

Clinical Manifestations

The patient complains of fever, sore throat, headache, nausea, vomiting and abdominal pain for 2 to 3 days, which may be difficult to suspect as polio.

Nonparalytic Poliomyelitis

The above symptoms may be more severe. There is pain and stiffness in the neck, back and legs.

Paralytic Poliomyelitis

The symptoms accompany by weakness and paralysis of one or more muscles, respiratory difficulty may occur in many cases. Site of paralysis depends upon the area of central nervous system (CNS) affected.

Once fever subsides, the spread of weakness and paralysis stops and full improvement on muscle power within two years, the residual defect is usually permanent.

Complications

Management

No specific treatment. The cases may be treated by symptomatic care at home. Enteric precautions are recommended for several weeks.

Prevention and Control of Disease

Immunization

The most effective means of prevention of poliomyelitis is by giving immunization to children, 2 months to 5 years of age (it can start at '0' age in endemic areas).

Types of Vaccination

Mainly two types of vaccines are usually available throughout the world.
- Inactivated (Salk) Polio Vaccine (IPV), and
- Oral (Sabin) Polio Vaccine (OPV).

Inactivated Polio Vaccine (Salk)

In these all the three types of polio viruses are inactivated by formalin. The primary immunization is given in minimum four doses starting after two months of age till five years of age at the interval of 1 to 2 months, as per WHO schedule.

IPV is not commonly recommended for children because the circulatory antibodies protect the person against paralytic polio but does not enhance intestinal or local immunity, because it induces humoral antibodies (IgM, IgG, and IgA Immunogammaglobulins). It cannot be given during epidemic, because immunity is not readily developed due to more than one dose and injections during epidemic attacks are likely to cause paralysis.

Advantages

It can be given to :
- Children with immune deficiency diseases.
- Pregnant women.
- Undergoing corticosteroid and radiation therapy.
- People above the age of 50 and getting the infection first time.

Modified IPV has become available, with 90 per cent effectiveness in first and 100 per cent effectiveness in second dose. It can be stored in refrigeration at 4 to 10°C like diphtheria and tetanus toxoid and can also be mixed with DPT to make it quadraple vaccine for convenience.

Oral Polio Vaccine (Sabin)

It was first discovered by Sabin in 1957. Thus, it is also named as Sabin vaccine for polio. It is a live vaccine, which contains live attenuated, antigenic virus (1, 2 and 3). It should be given to each virus type separately but due to convenience and efficacy, it is given as a combination of these three viruses (Fig. 23.7).

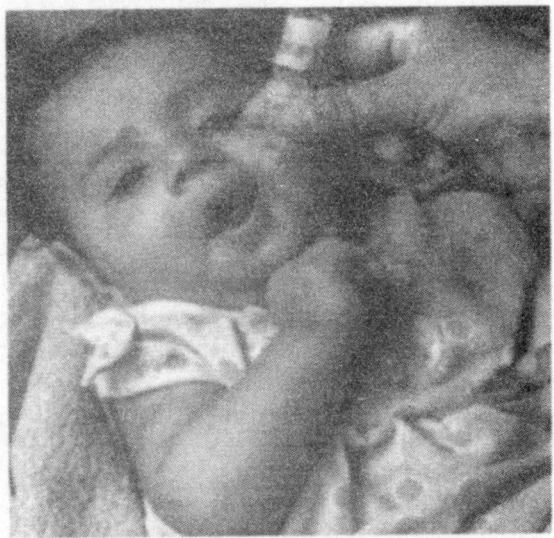

Fig. 23.7: Oral Polio Vaccine Administration

Dose and its Administration

WHO recommended the primary vaccine consists of 3 to 5 doses (depending upon epidemic of disease) at 1 to 2 months interval. Booster dose of OPV is repeated after one year of interval, after the last dose to give adequate immunity. The most effective method of administration of OPV, is by giving three drops by dropper.

The vaccine rapidly multiplies in the intestine and produces humoral and intestinal immunity, thus it produces both local and systemic immunity.

Advantage

The oral polio vaccine is :

- Easy to administer and does not require highly skilled person, since it is given orally.
- Produces local and systemic immunity.
- Relatively inexpensive.
- Can reduce the incidences of occurrence of disease due to effectivity to other people.
- A single dose can protect a large proportion of people.

Contraindication

OPV is not recommended to children with acute infections, gastrointestinal problems, leukaemia, other malignant conditions and children on corticosteroid.

Precautions

The OPV must be given in accurate dose, at appropriate time for its more effective use. The child should not be given breastfeed, hot water, hot feed or hot milk half an hour before and after the vaccination. If child vomites, the dose should be repeated. The mother must be explained about its side effects and management. Though latest study shows that breast milk can be given, but it may cause vomiting and take out the vaccine.

Stabilization

The vaccine can be kept at 4°C for one year and at room temperature for one month.

Nonstabilized Vaccine

The cold chain must be maintained to store, transport and carry the vaccine for non-stabilized vaccine, where it must be kept under –20°C of temperature and while carrying it must be kept either on dry ice or a freezing mixture. During vaccination, the vaccine should not be frozen or too cold to be given. The vaccine bottle must be replaced back in ice after giving vaccine.

The vaccine has to be kept frozen during preservation and cold during transportation.

Epidemiological Survey

A single case seen in a community is considered as an epidemic and preventive measures are expected, within 48 hours of notification of cases. The prompt and immediate epidemiological survey to collect faecal sample of the suspected cases of polio should be done.

The OPV should be provided to all people in epidemic areas, to unimmunized people and whose immunization status is not complete or unknown. For confirmation of diagnosis, serum sample can be collected to identify polio virus and sent to National Enterovirus Units at Mumbai, Coonoor, Chennai, Delhi and Kasauli where sample units have been opened by ICMR.

International Health Regulation Act has declared polio as international notification as soon as possible on occurrence of paralytic polio, number of cases and deaths. WHO has given instructions for Polio Eradication Programme.

Polio Eradication in India

The complete and timely reporting of cases of poliomyelitis is an important element of eradication programme. Even a single case is treated as an outbreak and preventive measures are initiated. All cases of acute flaccid paralysis must be reported immediately to the chief medical officer of the district.

- Obtain highest level of OPV vaccination to all children.
- Active surveillance to detect the new and old cases of polio.
- Pulse polio immunization at least for 3 to 4 years or till eradication of polio.
- Time listing of reported cases to check duplication.
- Reporting of acute paralytic cases to chief medical officer/district immunization officer.

Factors Enabling Eradication of Poliomyelitis

- Polio virus infects only human beings.
- There is no animal reservoir.

- The virus does not survive long in the environment outside the human body.
- There is no long-term carrier state.
- An effective vaccine is available.

Pulse Polio Immunization

Government of India conducted the first round of pulse polio immunization on December 9, 1995, with the objective to eradicate the disease from the country. Immunized children with OPV more than 87 million, and more than 78 million were below the age of 3 and more than 9 million were in the age group of three years and above.

Nearly two million health workers and volunteers conducted immunization, using a network of approximately 0.5 million vaccination posts.

The second phase of Pulse Polio Immunization was conducted on December 7, 1996 and January 18, 1997 immunizing about 120 million children in single day during each round (1998 to 2005).

•••

24

Respiratory Diseases

INTRODUCTION TO ACUTE RESPIRATORY INFECTION

Acute respiratory infection is the infection of respiratory tract which leads to discomfort, disability and increases the morbidity and mortality rate among children, adults and elderly. It causes inflammation of respiratory tract causing variety of diseases *e.g.*, common cold, pharyngitis, bronchitis, bronchiolitis and pneumonia. The disease is clinically characterised as cough, cold, running nose, sore throat, malaise, fever, respiratory difficulties and earache. Usually children start with mild infection *e.g.*, cough and cold, if untreated may develop complications like pneumonia, which is major cause leading to death. In developing countries, the major causes, of severe respiratory tract infections are usually measles and whooping cough. This is more common among urban community than rural, due to exposure to polluted air.

Problem in World

Acute respiratory infection in young children are responsible for an estimated 4.1 million deaths worldwide each year. It is estimated that 40 per cent of global mortality due to acute respiratory infection is only in Bangladesh, India, Indonesia and Nepal (Fig. 24.1). About 90 per cent deaths are due to pneumonia which are usually bacterial in origin. The incidence of acute respiratory infection is similar in developed and developing countries. However, the incidence of pneumonia in developed countries is 3 to 4 per cent, whereas 20 per cent is in developing countries, which may be due to prevalence of malnutrition, low birth weight and indoor air pollution in these countries.

On average children below 5 years of age suffer five episodes of acute respiratory infection per child per year, thus accounting for about 238 million attacks annually. Acute respiratory

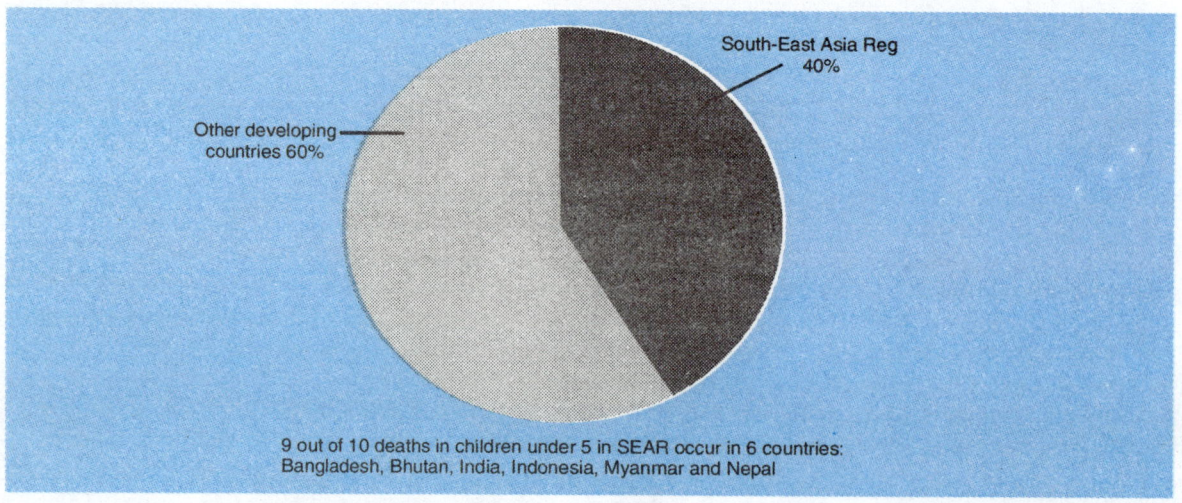

9 out of 10 deaths in children under 5 in SEAR occur in 6 countries: Bangladesh, Bhutan, India, Indonesia, Myanmar and Nepal

Fig. 24.1 : Deaths due to acute respiratory infection in South-East Asia Region countries

infection is responsible for about 30 to 50 per cent of visits to health facilities and 20 to 40 per cent of admissions to hospitals. The incidence can be reduced by proper coverage of DPT and measles vaccines, improved nutritional status, promotion of breastfeeding and control of low birth weight.

Problem in India

Acute respiratory infection is the major cause of high infant and child mortality rate in India. Most of the health facilities are available due to acute respiratory infection among children, 13 per cent of deaths in paediatrics units of hospitals are due to acute respiratory infection.

Epidemiological Factors

Agent Factors

Acute respiratory infection is caused by bacteria and viruses. The severity of the disease vary from type of agent involved and the resistance of the individual. The children who have low resistance due to malnutrition, chronic systemic disease and chronic lower respiratory disease have more severe acute respiratory infection and elderly people are more affected due to this infection. Bacteria usually cause epiglottitis, tonsillitis, bronchiolitis and pneumonia may be severe and cause of death.

The viruses also cause acute respiratory infection. There are also primary causes of great majority of respiratory illness. Rhinoviruses are closely related to cold, parainfluenza virus, bronchiolitis and various virus including pneumonia.

Agents

Bacterial
- *Bordetella pertussis*
- *Corynebacterium diphtheriae*
- *Haemophilus influenza*
- *Staphylococcus pneumoniae*
- *Streptococcus pyogenes*.
  Viruses—
- Adenoviruses
- Enteroviruses
- Influenza A + B + C
- Rhinovirus
- Coronavirus.
- Myxovirus.

Host Factor

Age and sex : The incidence is high in infants and children and elderly of all countries. The rate of acute respiratory infection is higher among children with malnutrition.

Upper respiratory infection *e.g.,* common cold and pharyngitis are higher in children than adults. Adult women experience — more illness than men, due to exposure to polluted air *e.g.,* smoke, cultural purda system, etc.

Environmental Factors

The risk factor for acute respiratory infection are changing climatic conditions, housing conditions, due to increasing industrialisation and socioeconomic development. Overcrowding, poor nutritional status, intense indoor smoke pollution are the poor environmental conditions.

Socioeconomic Factor

Acute respiratory infection is more common among low socioeconomic status children due to living standards. Infection is more common among children attending day care centre due to spread from one-to-other and negligence at day care centre. The infection tends to be more common among urban community than rural due to air pollution, smoking, industrialisation. Maternal cigarette smoking has also been linked to increased occurrence of respiratory tract infection.

Mode of Transmission

The causative organisms are transmitted by airborne route. Most viruses do not survive for long time outside respiratory tract, the disease is mainly spread by direct contact.

Clinical Manifestations

The acute respiratory infection is clinically identified as running nose, cough and cold, fever, unable to take feed, lithargy and excessive crying.

Fast and Irregular Breathing

The respiratory rate may be 40 to 60 breaths/minute. When respiratory rate is :

- 60 and above in child less than 2 months.
- 50 and above in child from 2 to 12 months.
- 40 and above in child 1 to 5 years.

Chest Indrawing

The chest indrawing occurs when child needs more efforts to take breath, the lower part of the chest goes in.

It is definite inward movement of the lower chest wall, while breathing in (inspiration) for observing chest indrawing child should be lying flat on the bed or in mother's lap.

Stridor

Stridor occurs when there is narrowing of larynx, trachea or epiglottis due to congestion and accumulation of secretion, interfering with air entering the lungs.

Wheezing Sound

A wheezing sound is a noise like whistle during breathing out, which is due to narrowing of air passage due to secretions and congestion of the mucous membrane, makes the respiration difficult and noisy.

Drowsy

If the child is not having normal sleep, it shows child is drowsy, whereas he should be alert or awake.

CLASSIFICATION OF ACUTE RESPIRATORY INFECTIONS (ARI)

ARI is often classified by clinical syndromes depending on the site of the infection and is referred to as ARI of the upper (AURI) and lower respiratory infection (ALRI).

AURI cause pharyngitis and otitis media.

Lower respiratory tract infections cause epiglottisis, laryngitis, bronchitis, bronchiolitis, and pneumonia.

Majority of ARI deaths in children are due to pneumonia with the symptoms of cough and difficulty in breathing.

PNEUMONIA

Classification of Pneumonia

No pneumonia — Cough or cold
↓
Pneumonia — Fast breathing
↓
Severe pneumonia — Fast breathing, chest indrawing
↓
Very severe pneumonia. Convulsion, stridor

Table 24.1 : Clinical classification of pneumonia and place of treatment (Age 2 months to 5 years)

Pneumonia	Therapy	Where to treat ?	
Respiratory rate Age (Per minute)		Can be treated at home/ health facility	
50 or more 2–12 months 40 or more 1–5 years	Cotrimoxazole Oral		Advise the mother to give home care — Give antibiotics — Treat wheezing, fever if present follow-up
Severe Pneumonia Chest Indrawing	Antibiotics Intramuscular	Patient should be hospitalised	Refer urgently Give antibiotics Treat fever, wheezing Follow-up
Very Severe Illness Inability to drink Excessive drowsiness Stridor in calm child Respiratory grunting History of apnoea, cyanosis, convulsions Severe malnutrition Hypothermia	Chloramphenicol Intramuscular	Refer immediately and must be admitted and treated at a health facility with provision of oxygen Keep warm Antibiotics	Home care after discharge Keep the child warm Breastfeeding frequently Clear nose if it interferes with feeding Immediately come to hospital if : 1. Breathing becomes faster 2. Feeding becomes a problem 3. Child becomes more sick.

Note : Children less than two months who have fast breathing are always treated as for severe pneumonia and referred to a hospital for treatment.

Table 24.2 : Treatment of Pneumonia (Daily dose schedule of cotrimoxazole for five days)

Age/Weight	Paediatric tablet	Paediatric syrup
	Each tablet : Sulphamethoxazole 100 mg and Trimethoprim 20 mg	Each spoon (5 mL) Sulphamethoxazole 200 mg and Trimethoprim 40 mg
< 2 months (Wt. 3.5 kg)	One tablet twice a day	Half spoon (2.5 mL) twice a day
2–12 months (Wt. 6–9 kg)	Two tablets twice a day	One spoon (5 mL) twice a day
1–5 years (Wt. 10–19 kg)	Three tablets twice a day	One and half spoon (7.5 mL) twice a day.

No Pneumonia

Most children with cough, cold and breathing difficulty do not show any sign of pneumonia *e.g.*, chest indrawing or fast breathing. These children can be treated at home and do not require any antibiotics. Early treatment will help to recover fast and prevent pneumonia. If the cough persists for more than 30 days the child may have tuberculosis, asthma or whooping cough, etc., he needs symptomatic treatment.

Children with fast breathing and no chest indrawing, who comes in early stage which are diagnosed for pneumonia. There are mild cases, which can be treated at home with antibiotics. The mother should be given proper instructions on home care, like how to give medicine and when to come to Health Centre, if the condition of child gets worst.

Severe Pneumonia

The signs of chest indrawing is the only indication of severe pneumonia, and the child is high-risk for death. Some children with chest indrawing also have wheezing (sound in respiration), nasal flaring (widening of nose on breathing) grunting (short sounds when difficulty in breathing).

Cynosis (bluish colouration of the child due to hypoxia).

Very Severe Pneumonia

Very sick child should be referred immediately to the hospital when child shows the signs of :

Convulsions

Abnormal deep sleep and difficult to wake. The child may have severe pneumonia due to hypoxia, sepsis, cerebral malaria or meningitis; meningitis may be developed as complication of pneumonia.

Stridor in Quiet Child

If child has stridor, it is life-threatening obstruction of airway due to swelling of larynx, trachea or epiglottis.

Not Able to Drink

When child is unable to drink could have severe pneumonia, septicemia, throat abscess, meningitis or cerebral malaria, etc.

Severe Malnutrition

When the child is diagnosed for pneumonia, one should always look for signs of malnutrition. If malnutrition is present, the fatality rate increases greatly. In severely malnourished children with pneumonia fast breathing and chest indrawing are widely evident and these children may have an impaired or absent response to hypoxia and a weak or absent cough reflex and they are at high-risk of dying. These children need careful management.

Diagnosis

The diagnosis can be made by physical examination, health assessment and history of illness (onset of illness). Careful assessment and observing the general condition can help in early recognition of pneumonia, which can prevent death. The diagnosis is recognised by increased respiratory rate of child.

History Taking*

Taking history from mother about child's general condition and feeding pattern, fever, drowsy and difficult to wake, convulsions, irregular breathing, short periods of not breathing, child turning blue, any previous history of illness and treatment.

Physical Assessment

Respiratory rate : Count the respiratory rate for one minute. Increased rate according to age is significant sign of pneumonia.

Chest indrawing : Observe the chest indrawing when child breaths in. The child has indrawing if the lower chest wall goes in when child breaths in, it occurs when the efforts required to breath are more than normal.

Observe wheezing : Observe if child makes a soft whistling sound when breathing and shows the sign that breathing out is difficult. This is caused due to narrowing or obstruction of air passage in the lungs. The breathing out takes longer than normal and requires efforts.

Listen for stridor : Child makes harsh noise when breathing in. It occurs due to narrowing of larynx, trachea, epiglottis which interferes with air entering the lungs.

Observe for Drowsiness

If child is sleeping abnormally, and difficult to wake and is drowsy most of the time, when he or she should be alert or awake.

Temperature

Child may have low grade fever.

Severe Malnutrition

Malnourished children are high-risk with pneumonia. These children need careful monitoring and appropriate management.

Cynosis

Difficult breathing may lead to cynosis, which is a sign of hypoxia. It must be observed carefully and utmost care must be taken if child turns blue.

Early recognition of pneumonia will save the life of child.

Treatment of Pneumonia at a Health Centre

Cotrimoxazole is the drug of choice for the treatment of pneumonia. Studies carried out in India have confirmed the efficacy of cotrimoxazole to be similar to ampicillin and procaine penicillin and cure rate of up to 95 per cent have been recorded. Cotrimoxazole is less expensive with few side-effects and can be used safely by health workers at the peripheral health facilities and at home by the mothers.

Children who are less than 2 months old and have fast breathing should be treated as for severe pneumonia and referred immediately to hospital. Similarly, children who show signs of pneumonia and are also malnourished should be immediately referred to hospital.

Children who have pneumonia should be treated with cotrimoxazole in the doses recommended in Tables 24.1 and 24.2.

If at 48 hours or earlier the condition WORSENS, chest indrawing or other signs of severe illness (inability to drink, excessive drowsiness, convulsions or cyanosis) appears, the child should be hospitalised immediately.

Precautions

Children less than two months, cotrimoxazole is not recommended. These children are to be treated as for severe pneumonia. However, in case of delay in referral cotrimoxazole may be initiated.

Contrimoxazole should not be given to premature babies and cases of neonatal jaundice. Such children must be referred to a hospital.

In small children the tablet should be crushed and mixed with milk or other fluids. The mixture should be given to the child with a spoon.

Home Care of Child with Acute Respiraory Infections/Pneumonia

Majority of the cases do not need inpatient care and can be treated at home. Children who are hospitalised have to be taken care by the mother at home after discharge. Mother plays a key role in the treatment of the child with cough and cold. Hence it is very important for mother to understand the basic principles of the treatment.

- How to give antibiotic in proper dose.
- Small frequent feeds, especially breastfeed.
- Recognise the danger signs and bring immediately to health agency.
- Explain danger signs, *e.g.*,
  - ➤ Rapid breathing
  - ➤ Chest indrawing
  - ➤ Refusal to feed
  - ➤ Excessive sleepiness
  - ➤ Convulsions.

Prevention and Control of Acute Respiratory Infection

Many risk factors associated with acute respiratory infection can be controlled to prevent the disease.

- Improve living standard by adopting healthy habits
- Better nutrition
- Reduce air pollution by reducing, smoke in the air
- Maternal child health care
- Immunization to children against seven killer diseases especially measles
- Recognition of early pneumonia referral and treatment.

Role of Nurse in Prevention of Acute Respiratory Infection

Health education to mother about :

- Keep the child in fresh air and free from dust or smoke environment
- Prevent overcrowding
- Avoid spitting and sneezing near the child
- House should be well-ventilated with fresh air
- Keep the infants and young children warm and putting seasonal clothes
- Breastfeed the child as long as possible
- Watch the signs for :

  - ➤ Breathing difficulties
  - ➤ Fast breathing
  - ➤ Unable to feed due to blocked nose
  - ➤ Sickness, fever, lethargy child
- Supplemental feeds rich in vitamin C, *e.g.*, fresh fruit juices.

ACUTE RESPIRATORY INFECTION CONTROL PROGRAMME

The ARI control programme was taken up as pilot project in 14 districts in the country in 1990. In 1992–93 the programme was being implemented as a part of CSSM programme.

The main objective of WHO about acute respiratory infection control programme is the reduction of deaths due to pneumonia using standard case management, which consists of the diagnosis of pneumonia using simple clinical signs like fast breathing and treatment with a safe, effective antibiotic. Education of mother and caretaker, which is mainly achieved through face to face communication, with mass media used only on selective basis. The target of acute respiratory infection control programme was to reduce pneumonia mortality to one-third of the 1990 levels by the year 2000.

Maximum programme impact is seen in countries with high mortality rate (IMR) WHO, recommends priority implementation of programme in countries with IMR 40/1000 and above.

Acute respiratory infection strategy emphasizes inservice training in standard case management for personnel at primary health centre level. Strategy also includes providing adequate supplies of first-line antibiotics to health centres.

Effective reduction in mortality due to pneumonia is possible if children suffering from pneumonia are treated correctly because of difficulty in diagnosing pneumonia in most countries, WHO has given key indication for assessment of correct acute respiratory infection management. A lot has been achieved, the surveys indicate the need for further improvement, especially in the area of training, communicating with caretaker and regular monitoring of national programme.

The treatment of pneumonia by periphery health staff is limited only to CSSM districts. Cotrimoxazole (septran) is included in the kit for health workers, supplied in subcentres and centres.

SMALLPOX

An acute infectious and highly communicable disease caused by variola virus. The clinical manifestations are high grade fever, headache, backache and vomiting. On third day, the rashes appear on the body which is centrifugal. Eruptions are more numerous on exposed area of body and less dense at the hidden areas. It passes through various stages of macule, papule, vesicle, pustule and scab leaving scar.

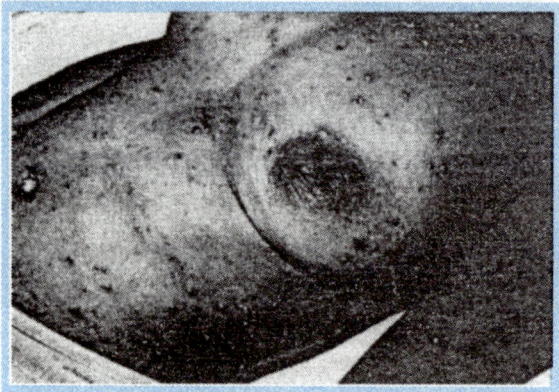

Fig. 24.2 : Smallpox

History

Smallpox was a major communicable disease in early twentieth century affecting all continents of the world. WHO has taken all steps/measures to eradicate the disease. The world's last case of smallpox was seen in 1978 in Somalia (Africa). No further case was seen throughout the world. The WHO declared smallpox free on 8th May 1980. The eradication of smallpox is one of the remarkable achievements in public health and leads to a historical milestone. Eradication has prevented two million deaths, many thousands blindness have been prevented.

Problem in India

India had a long history of smallpox. The main preventive measure was smallpox vaccine. The Government launched National Smallpox Eradication Programme (NSEP) in 1962, but programme failed due to lack of epidemiological basis. The introduction of bifurcated needles in 1969 and potent or stable freeze dried vaccine in 1971 proved eradication very successful. The incidence programme of cases started declining very fast. The Government of India intensified on operation Smallpox—Target Zero. Lastly in April 1977 India was declared smallpox free by international commission.

For assessment smallpox eradication of last case in India was found in May 1975 in Bihar, after that India had no endemic in the country.

Epidemiology of Disease

Agent Factor

The causative organism of smallpox is variola virus, which is one of the most dangerous viruses.

Host Factor

Age and sex : It can occur at any age and to any sex.

Immunity

An attack of smallpox gives life long immunity. Second attack is very rare.

Source of Infection

Smallpox is spread mainly by either direct (droplet infection) face to face contact with infected person or indirectly through contaminated fomites. Fomites include clothes, beddings, etc., of the patient.

Reservoir of Infection

The virus is found in human host and not the animal host which has been eliminated at present. The remaining reservoirs are 4 viruses kept in research laboratories.

Incubation Period

It may vary from 7–17 days, but mostly it is observed to be 12 days.

Clinical Manifestation

Smallpox begins abruptly, with a high temperature, varying between 102° and 105°F and is associated with headache and severe bodyache. The patient complains of severe backache, nausea and vomiting. Abdominal pain may also be present in severe cases. These prodromal symptoms continue for 2 to 4 days.

The typical smallpox eruption appears between 2nd and 4th day of prodromal symptom. The temperature of the patient subsides on appearance of eruptions. The lesions are visible initially on the face, neck and upper chest, hands, forearm and lower limbs. Later on they appear all over the body. The eruptions are more numerous on the exposed area of the body. Distribution of eruptions is away from the centre (Figs. 24.3 and 24.4).

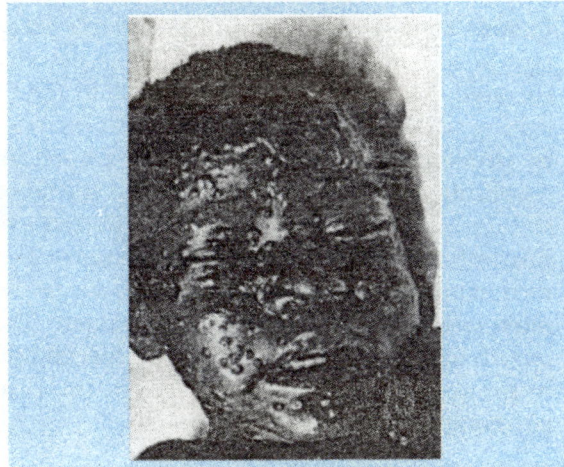

Fig. 24.3 : Numerous eruption on face

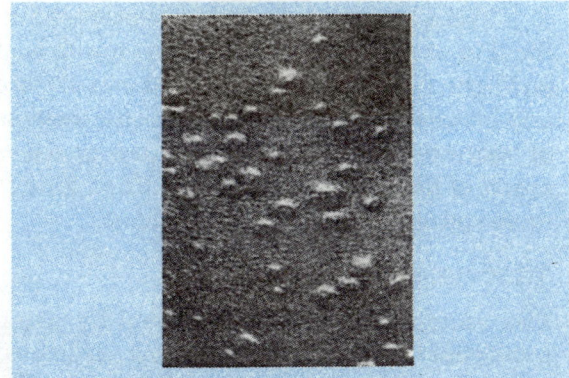

Fig. 24.4 : Less dense eruption on hidden areas

The eruption first appears as red macules, which turn into papules by second day. The papules are filled with a clear fluid called as vesicles. They are firm and deep, within 4 to 5 days lesions appear all over the body, *e.g.*, palm, sole, etc. The lesions increase in size. The hardness of vesicles may persist during pustules stage. The last stage that is crusting stage begins from 8th to 10th day of the rash. The content of the pustules dry, producing a thick crust. The crust remains intact for few days on the skin surface of the body and extremities, they dry and then drop off all over the body except palms and soles, where the skin is quite thick, the rash is present for a longer period of time, unless the hands and feet are soaked to remove the lesions; the rash may persist till 12th to 20th day after it first appeared. The smallpox mark remains as permanent spot on the face. The crust removed from patients eruption is highly infectious.

The temperature might arise again on formation of pustules and temperature may again come down after 10th to 12th day, if no complication. Itching is present which is troublesome symptom, especially during the pustules and crusting stage.

The blood sample shows leucopoiesis with the appearance of the rash and during the pustule stage, leucocytosis is noted. Moderate anaemia may also be seen but not very frequently.

Home to home surveillance was done to identify any case of smallpox and had to be internationally notified, so as to control the disease, and the patient to be treated adequately to prevent him/her from complications, etc.

Complications

The complications occur due to secondary infection of the skin with subsequent septicaemia, furunculosis, abscess formation, cellulitis and gangrene. Pneumonia is one of the common respiratory complications among the groups including laryngitis, pleurisy and empysema. Lesions may occur on the conjunctiva and cornea of the eye with conjunctivitis, keratitis, iritis and sometimes panophthalmia. Visual defects and blindness were the common complications of smallpox in India and Africa. Otitis media may also occur, though central nervous system complications are very rare.

Treatment

Symptomatic treatment can be given to the patient, *e.g.*, analgesics for fever, etc.

Care of Skin

Skin must be kept clean, with application of potassium permanganate ($KMnO_4$) 1:10,000 dilution; a betadine lotion and not to scrub with soap and water. Itching can be reduced by application of magnesium sulphate. Boric acid compresses and glycerine water application will relieve discomfort. Cleaning and washing of eyes with boric acid is done for the patients with conjunctivitis and photophobia.

Nutrition

The patient may be given liquid diet, glucose water, skimmed milk in adequate quantity. If patient is unable to take, then gastric intubation is recommended.

In mild cases there may not be any difficulty in swallowing, semisolids and fluids should be offered.

Antibiotics

The antibiotics are not given to cure the illness, but to prevent the complications or for the treatment of complications like pneumonia, abscess formation and septicaemia. Penicillin is usually given intramuscularly. 600,000 units of procaine penicillin once a day.

Preventive Measures

Strict Isolation

Since smallpox is highly communicable, the patients are to be completely isolated, to prevent the spread of infection. All fomites, and clothes to be disinfected. Avoid face to face interaction with the patients. The door of room should not be left open.

Concurrent Disinfection

All fomites and clothes used by the patient must be kept separate and disinfected in Dettol or Savlon lotion. The beddings must be kept out in sunlight. The smallpox virus is found in upper respiratory tract discharge, urine, tears, skin and mucous membrane lesions, hence must be carefully disinfected. The disease can spread by direct or indirect contact through air-borne transmission. Therefore, the gown, cap, mask should be worn while giving care to the patient.

Though hand washing and use of disposable shoe covering may prevent the spread of infection, use of sterile gloves, clothing and linen should be used for reverse isolation to prevent complication.

The vaccinated personnels should give care to the patient.

The patient must be given physical comfort, therapeutic, nutritional and supportive care. Prevention of complications is an essential role of the nurse. Patients with numerous lesions, use of sterile gloves and frequent change of linen are indicated. Barrier nursing should be followed.

Care of Skin and Mucous Membrane

Pustule stage is the most uncomfortable stage and at that time the temperature is usually elevated, patient looks toxic, severe burning or itching will be there. Scratching of lesions may be prevented to avoid secondary infection. Application of the deodorants like boric acid or sodium bicarbonate are effective and also relieve discomfort due to eruption. Mild sedative and recreational therapy will be helpful to divert the attention and provide comfort to patient. The mouth lesions may be present. The special oral hygiene may be given with potassium permanganate.

Active Immunization

Smallpox vaccine discovered by Edward Jenner in 1798 is a live attenuated vaccine prepared on the skin of sheep. The virus is sensitive to heat and light, therefore, must be stored in cool place and handled with care, since the effectiveness of vaccine depends on an adequate concentration of living virus. The freeze dried form is more stable than glycerinated vaccine.

Vaccination Reaction

The vaccine is given intradermal by using multipuncture technique by using bifurcated needle inserting live virus into the skin. The papule appears in 3 to 5 days, which becomes vesiculated, soon it changes into pustule and surrounded by erythema and induration. The erythema occurs between 8th to 10th day. There may be fever and general malaise associated with vaccine. The erythema and swelling subsides and crust forms, which falls off within 21 days, leaving a peculiar scar.

Contraindications of Vaccination

- The children with immunodeficient problem should not be given vaccine.
- Skin problems like eczema, chronic dermititis.
- Blood disorders like leukaemia, lymphoma and reticuloendothelial malignancy.
- Dysgammaglobulinaemia.
- Patient receiving immunosuppressive drugs such as steroids or antimetabolic or radiations, should not be vaccinated.
- Pregnant woman should not be given primary vaccination, because the virus may pass through the placenta and affect the foetus.

Time of Vaccination

The vaccination can be effectively carried out in first week of life, with revaccination at one year of age. Vaccination is best performed on the upper arm over the insertion of deltoid muscle. No preparation of skin is needed unless it is very dirty. Site should be gently cleaned with water and not spirit, because antiseptic lotion may interfere with live virus and decrease the effectiveness.

Methods of Vaccination

Multiple Pressure : The needle is held to the skin surrounded with up and down movement for 6 to 10 pressure in primary vaccination. The bifurcated needle is dipped into vaccine and then, held on the surface of the skin with 1 to 2 pressures. The appearance of blood spots after 20 to 130 seconds indicates adequate penetration of the needles.

CHICKENPOX (VARICELLA)

Varicella is one of the most prevalent acute highly infectious childhood disease caused by virus varicella-zoster. Most of the children are affected by the disease, adults who have escaped in childhood may develop it in more severe form. The disease is clinically manifested by fever, headache, general malaise and eruptions of rashes on the abdomen may indicate the first sign of disease.

History

Silicon physician Ingrassia differentiated it from smallpox in 1553 and Morton introduced the word chickenpox when he found it in common use. Chickenpox is caused by a virus which attacks a large majority of children.

Varicella is an acute highly infectious disease caused by virus varicella-zoster and characterized by high fever and malaise.

Worldwide Problem

It is a worldwide problem and occurs both as an endemic and epidemic form. In 1553, chickenpox was first time differentiated from smallpox by the Silicon physician, Ingrassia and Morton introduced the word chickenpox when found in an identical form.

Epidemiological Factors

Varicella-zostor is the causative organism of chickenpox. The virus can be grown on the tissue culture. The causative organism of chickenpox is also called Human Herpes Virus.

Host Factors

Age and Sex

Chickenpox usually attacks the children below ten years of age of both sexes. Adults if escaped in childhood, may get infection later.

Immunity

One attack usually gives immunity to prevent further attack, thus second attack is very rare. If mother is protected against chickenpox by getting an attack the newborn gets protection for first few months of life.

If mother gets infection during pregnancy may affect the foetus or newborn. The condition is known as congenital vericella.

Environmental Factors

The disease shows seasonal variation, the disease usually occurs during winter season. The incidence is very high in the months of January–

March. Overcrowding is the predisposing factor in spread of infections.

Source of Infection

Oropharyngeal secretions and skin lesions of the case (patient) are the main sources of spread of infection. Chickenpox is transmitted by :

- Direct contact with the patient and patients infective material.
- The disease is also spread by droplet and droplet nuclei. The portal of entry of the virus is respiratory tract of the host. Indirect spread may be through contaminated fomites, beddings and skin lesions of the patients.

Modes of Transmission

The disease is transmitted mainly by droplet infection and droplet nuclei. Most patients are infected by direct contact with the case.

Period of Communicability

May be 2 to 3 days before the patient develops the signs and symptoms of chickenpox and patient remains infective for 4 to 5 days during manifestation.

Incubation Period

The usual incubation period is 14 to 16 days. It may vary from 4 to 27 days.

Clinical Manifestation

The clinical features in chickenpox may vary from mild illness with few scattered lesions to severe febrile conditions with widespread rashes. In majority of cases, disease tends to be mild.

The chickenpox usually occurs in two stages :

Prodromal stage (Pre-eruptive)

Oneset is sudden and the initial symptoms of chickenpox are fever, headache, maliase, cold, cough and running nose. These symptoms are marked in adults, but may be absent in children. This stage lasts for 24 hours. In adults this stage is more severe and may last for 2 to 3 days.

Eruption Stage

The first sign of chickenpox in children is appearance of eruption. The rashes consist of red maculopapule spots which appear first on the abdomen and soon spread all over the body.

Characteristics of Eruption in Chickenpox

The eruptions are scanty on the exposed area. Axilla may be affected but palms and soles are usually not affected. The rashes undergo the development of :

- Macula
- Papula
- Vesicle
- Scab.

In all four stages, development is so sharp that all stages can be seen together simultaneously, in the same area (pleomorphism). The vesicles filled with clear fluid which contain virus, they form crust after drying and form the scab. The scabbing starts from 5 to 7 days of eruption stage.

Centripetal Distribution

The rashes are more dense and appear first on the abdomen and hidden areas of the body. They are less on the exposed areas, e.g., arms, hands, legs and face, etc. Mucous membrane of the mouth may also be affected. Axilla, palm and soles are usually not involved. The density of the eruption diminishes centrifugally (Periphery first and then centre).

Rapid Evolution of Rashes

The rashes appear rapidly through the stages of macule, papule, vesicle and scab. The evolution of all stages of rashes is so fast, that the first to attract the attention is when vesicles appear. These vesicles are filled with clear fluid and look like "dew drops" on the skin (Figs. 24.5 and 24.6). After 12 hours the fluid becomes turbid and may even become purulent in cases of secondary infection. After 2 to 3 days these vesicles dry up and are covered with scabs that remain on the

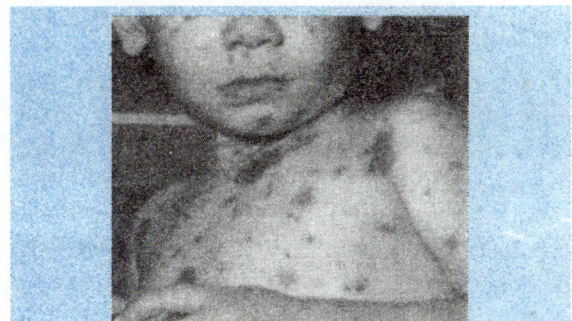

Fig. 24.5 : Chickenpox

skin for several days, when the scab falls off they do not leave scar, unless the vesicles have become infected.

Pleomorphous or Polymorphous

In chickenpox, all stages of rashes appear at the same time due to rapid evolution. Hence when macule, papule, pustule, vesicle are seen at the same time they are called polymorphous or pleomorphous. This is due to skin lesions develop at intervals of few hours.

Complications

There are few complications for chickenpox. The most common and important is skin infection due to scratching. The scratched vesicle may result in extensive lesions resembling impetigo.

Chickenpox is known to be a wild disease with high morbidity, but very low mortality.

Though rarely found but it may have serious complications among patients especially in children with malignancy and immunosuppressive patients. The complications like pneumonia, encephalitis, acute cerebeller ataxia and haemorrhage may occur.

The infection during antenatal period may cause still births and birth defects to children.

Varicella haemorrhage is rare but fatal form of chickenpox.

Prevention and Treatment

Early Detection of Case

To prevent the spread of infection, it must be identified and notified to the nearest health agencies to take preventive measures.

Isolation

The case must be isolated till the eruptions have dried and scab is removed. The school children, if suffering from chickenpox, should not be allowed to attend the class. All the useable items or articles of the patient must be kept separate and handled with precautions.

Disinfection

The soiled articles of the patient, *e.g.,* linen, clothes and discharges should be disinfected in antiseptic lotion, *e.g.,* Dettol. The scab must be disposed off carefully.

Immunization

The chickenpox has been considered as a mild disease, hence active immunization is not given much attention. The live vaccine against chickenpox may postpone the disease in childhood and if developed in adulthood may be serious. It is also objectionable to give vaccine because of its latent infection which may produce virus in later years which may be more severe than the natural occurrence of chickenpox. Therefore, the vaccine is not much useful for prevention of disease.

Passive immunization

Immunoglobulin given within 72 hours of exposure is recommended for prevention of infection. It is recommended to administer a dose of 1.25 to 5 mL intramuscularly, though it is not given to immunosuppressive patients of acute case or newborns.

Nursing Management and Treatment

- Isolation of the patient and complete bed rest are essential.
- The liquid and semisolid soft diet is usually recommended.
- Application of soothening lotions on the skin to prevent itching, *e.g.,* calamine lotion or cold creams are advised.
- Symptomatic treatment helps to reduce the discomfort in patient. The treatment is based on antipyretics and sulphonamides to prevent secondary infections.

- Disinfection of all articles during and after the illness of the patient. All the linen should be kept in the sunlight.

MEASLES (RUBEOLA)

Measles is an acute, infectious and highly communicable disease of childhood, which can cause severe morbidity and serious complications. The disease is caused by a specific group of myxoviruses, and clinically characterised by fever and prodromal symptoms.

History

The Arabian physician Rhazes (865–925 AD) had identified measles. Although it had been observed and described previously by several others, Koplik was first to diagnose the spot appearing in the mucous membrane of the mouth and the spot has been identified on his name. In 1958 measles vaccine was first used in a clinical trial and live measles vaccine was used in 1963.

Worldwide Distribution of Measles

The disease is universal and endemic in urban communities and generally epidemic in rural communities. In developed countries, the disease is relatively mild in large communities, in small communities and rural areas the disease may be moderately severe. In developing countries, case fatality rates range from 2 to 15 per cent as compared to less than 0.2 per 10,000 cases in developed countries. The annual incidence of the disease has declined after the measle vaccine has become available. Before vaccine became available there were 7 to 8 million deaths every year, which has come down to 1 to 2 million deaths all over the world, though still there are 40 to 50 million cases every year worldwide.

Many countries had initiated the Mass Immunization Programme (MIP) to reduce the disease, where case fatality is very high. A fall in incidence of measles is already noticed in several developed countries where overall incidence has declined from 10/1000 to 1/1000 cases, as a result of mass vaccination against measles. Region of America had implemented mass immunization strategy to eradicate the disease.

Problem in India

Measles is the major cause of morbidity and mortality among children. The high incidence of the disease is seen every alternate year during the months of January to March. Though there is reduction of cases with increased immunization coverage levels, still several outbreaks have been reported in rural and slum areas.

Epidemiological Factors

Measles is mainly caused by a group of myxovirus, which can not survive outside the body. The virus is RNA paramyxovirus with one antigenic type. It is stable at room temperature for 1 to 2 days. The measle virus is present in blood, urine, and nasopharyngeal secretions in infected case. The virus can not survive outside the human body.

Modes of Transmission

It is spread by direct transmission in most of the cases by means of droplet infection. Articles freshly contaminated with nasal or throat discharge are highly infectious.

Period of Communicability

A person is noninfectious during the incubation period except for 2 to 4 days before the appearance of symptoms. Measles is highly infectious during prodromal period and at the time of eruptions and declines after 4 to 5 days after appearance of rashes. Hence the patient must be isolated at least for 7 days after eruption stage.

Host Factor

Age and Sex

Disease may attack at any age and sex, though high incidence among children of 3 to 5 years have been seen. In crowded urban areas, infants and pre-school children have high incidence. In less populated areas school age children have the highest incidence. Infants under 4 to 5 months of age whose mothers had measles, rarely get the disease due to passive immunity transmitted via placenta. Infants of mothers who never had measles are susceptible to infection.

Immunity

All unimmunized people are at risk, though one attack of measles infection generally produces permanent immunity. Infants are protected by maternal antibodies up to six months of age. In some instances it may persist more than nine months. Immunity after vaccination is long-lasting.

Nutrition

Malnourished children are more prone to measles and the attack is very severe than healthy children. Mortality due to malnutrition is very high, which may be due to poor cell mediated immune system. Adversely measles lead to malnutrition.

Environmental Factors

Seasonal Pattern

Disease has seasonal variation with cyclic incidence. Peak incidence occurs during winter and spring seasons. In the past, the epidemic appeared at 2 to 3 years interval and this had reduced after introduction of vaccine in 1963.

Socioeconomic Condition

The socioeconomy has no direct relation with occurrence of disease, but malnourished children are more prone to infection which indicate poor socioeconomy.

Incubation Period

Usually 9 to 14 days from time of exposure to appearance of symptoms.

Clinical Manifestation

The manifestation of symptoms show the pre-eruptive and eruptive stages.

Pre-eruptive Stage

The period before the appearance of rashes over the body of the patients. This is characterised by moderate fever, around 102 to 104°F, malaise, running of nose, respiratory infection, redness of eyes. After one or two days purulent bluish white spots appear on the mucous membrane of the buccal cavity called Koplik spots (by the name of scientist who discovered it) during this stage the child may feel extremely uncomfortable and look miserable (Fig. 24.6).

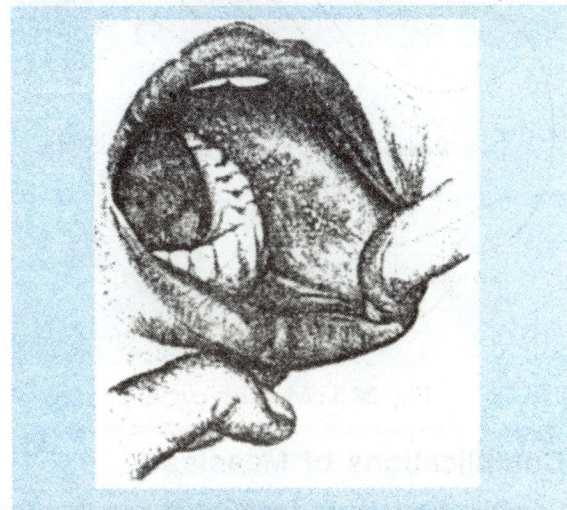

Fig. 24.6 : Koplik's spots in measles

Eruption Stage

Bright pink or red colour rashes appear first on the face and neck (Fig. 24.7), and then on the chest and all over the body including upper and lower limbs. After 5 to 6 days the rashes begin to disappear leaving the brownish discolouration.

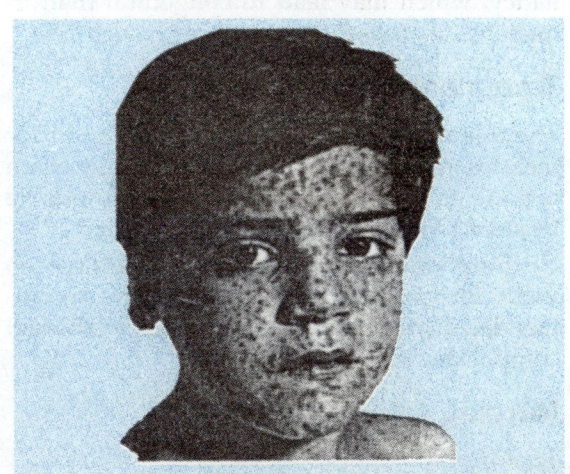

Fig. 24.7 : Early measles eruption

Cervical lymphadenitis, splenomegaly may be noted. Otitis media, pneumonia and gastroentritis symptoms are more common in infants. Liver enlargement may be common in adults.

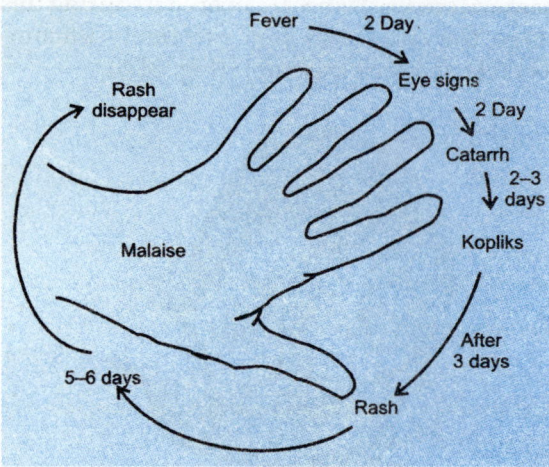

Fig. 24.8 : Measles cycle

Complications of Measles

Complications result from extensive viral or secondary bacterial infection. Otitis media is one of the most common complications, other respiratory complications include mastoiditis, and pneumonia.

When infection becomes more severe heamorrhagic measles is most serious, which is highly fatal form of infection. Measles may complicate pregnancy, at or near full-term pregnancy, which may lead to congenital malformation. Rubella is the main cause for such defect.

Treatment

There is no specific therapeutic treatment for measles, symptomatic treatment is usually given to patients. The patients may have photophobia by strong light, which should be avoided.

Sulphonamides and antibiotics have no value for cure of illness, but they are recommended to prevent the secondary infections and complications.

Nursing Intervention

Isolation

The patients can be kept in isolation, comfortable, good ventilation and darkroom, because they are sensitive to light. Acute stage patient should be on bed rest. The concurrent and terminal disinfection should be done for nasal, throat or skin discharges.

Care must be taken in handling secretion and contaminated articles.

Comfort Needs

Physical, emotional and therapeutic needs of the patient.

Care of Skin

Bathing, oral hygiene, eye care should be given, by avoiding chilling and irritation. Soap should be omitted during eruptive stage. Bicarbonate may be added in water to give bath to patient, to relieve itching, protect the eyes from strong and direct light which is irritating. Eyes should be kept clean.

Preventive Measures of Measles

Measles is highly infectious disease among children. It can be prevented and controlled by :

Isolation

Measles can be prevented by isolating the case *e.g.*, its fomites, toys and utensils. The clothes must be disinfected in disinfectants like Dettol, etc., or kept under sunlight. Visitors must be restricted.

Early Detection and Treatment

The early detection is essential to give appropriate care and treatment to the patient. Preventive measures may be taken, which includes symptomatic treatment, adequate diet and nutrition.

Active Immunization

Measles is one of the seven killer diseases, taken up under expanded programme for immunization and universal programme for immunization, children can be protected by giving measles vaccine. It is live vaccine, which is frozen dried. A single dose of the reconstituted vaccine, *i.e.*, 0.5 mL, should be given intramuscularly. The vaccine must be stored under 2º to 10ºC in the refrigerator. It should be used within one hour of reconstitution. The measle vaccine is safe and very effective, which gives 95 per cent protection for 15 years.

Contraindication of Vaccination

Measle vaccine should not be administered during :

- Pregnancy
- Leukaemia, lymphomas and other generalised malignancies
- Patient on steroids, radiations and anti-metabolic therapies
- Febrile illness
- Tuberculoid patients
- Marked egg sensitivity, etc.

Passive Immunization

With the availability of active immunization all children should be protected by the live measles vaccine. In circumstances where unprotected people exposed to infection can be given immunoglobulin soon after exposure within 4 to 6 days for protection. Measles vaccine can be given after 6 weeks for future safeguard.

RUBELLA (GERMAN MEASLES)

Rubella or German measles is an acute disease of children caused by a virus and is characterized by mild symptoms of respiratory infection, fever, lymphadenopathy and rashes all over the body. Most patients are children from 3 to 12 years of age and one attack gives lifelong immunity. Younger children are immune. Incidence of the disease increases during the first half of the year and epidemics occur every 3 to 4 years. It is a worldwide disease and occurs in epidemics. Infection in early pregnancy may lead to various congenital defects in newborn.

History

Rubella was discovered in 1941 by Norman Gregg an ophthalmologist, as an association of congenital cataract to newborn of rubella infected mothers. In 1962, rubella virus was discovered. In 1967, the vaccine was developed.

Epidemiological Factors

Agent Factor

The causative organism is RNA virus of togavirus family. The virus is found in the nasopharyngeal secretions, blood and cerebrospinal fluid (CSF) and urine of the cases and carriers of rubella. Postnatal mother as a carrier is not definite, but newborn of rubella mother spreads the infection for some months.

Host Factor

Age : Women of childbearing age are susceptible to infection. Children around 15 years of age are accountable for about 70 per cent of cases. One attack gives lifelong immunity.

Environmental Factors

The people living in low socioeconomic conditions with poor housing conditions, overcrowding, poor ventilation and ignorance predisposes the disease.

Incubation Period

Remains for 10 to 15 days.

Spread of Infection

The virus is spread by direct contact with droplet and droplet nuclei through respiratory route especially nose and throat. The virus can also transmit from infected mother to the foetus through placenta, causing neonatal congenital rubella.

Clinical Manifestations

The patient develops the symptoms of respiratory infection and fever but are less severe than in measles. There may be complaint of a stiff neck due to swelling of lymph glands.

On the second day, a popular rash consisting of well defined oval areas usually appear on the face. It may first appear on any part of the body, but later spreads all over the body. Rash is the first indication of the disease in children. It is a minute, discrete pinkish, macular rash and not confluent as in measles. The rash spreads rapidly, remains for two days and then fades faster than the rash of measles. They leave some disquamation but not discoloration of the skin as in measles. The lymph gland swelling also subsides by this time.

Complications

Complications seldom develop and almost all patients show complete recovery without relapse.

In rare cases during nine months to one year arthralgia may occur in adults. There may be encephalitis, thrombocytopenia purpura, and congenital malformation, can occur.

Preventive Measures

Isolation

The patients with rubella must be isolated for a day or two before the appearance of rash, if exposure is known.

Immunization

Live attenuated vaccine developed in 1979 is the effective preventive measure against rubella. The vaccine is administered 0.5 mL subcutaneously as single dose. It is usually combined with measles, mumps and given to children during 9 months to 1 year as measels-mumps-rubella vaccine. Mild reaction, e.g., fever, malaise, headache may be developed but it subsides within 1 to 2 days and there is no serious reaction due to vaccine.

Congenital Rubella

There is much evidence of a relationship between rubella in pregnant mother during first trimester and congenital defects in the newborn.

Rubella infection inhibits cell division and this is probably the reason for congenital malformation and low birth weight babies. The most common congenital defects are deafness, cardiac malformation, mental retardation, congenital cataract. The incidences of these cases is about 50 per cent. Other resulting defects include glaucoma, retardation, hepatosplenomegaly. These are referred as congenital rubella syndrome.

The rubella infection during the gestation period is a major factor for the foetal infection and congenital malformation. The congenital rubella is a chronic infection which continues in the foetus during pregnancy and lasts for months and years after birth, whereas acquired rubella (noncongenital) is an acute infection.

If mother gets infection during first trimester, there may be stillbirth, spontaneous abortion or child may develop multiple defects, e.g., ductus arteriosis, (congenital heart disease), cataract and deafness (congenitally). Since the foetus organs are developing in first three months and virus interferes in normal development. But if mother develops infection after 3 to 4 months, there may not be major defect in child.

MUMPS

Mumps is an acute infectious disease caused by paramyxovirus group, a virus that has affinity for glandular and nervous tissues. It is characterized most commonly by enlargement and tenderness of one or both the parotid glands. Other organs may also develop the infection in 30 to 40 per cent of patients.

Distribution of the Disease

The disease occurs throughout the world. Epidemics are most frequent in late winter and spring. The incidence of natural infection in developed countries has decreased as a result of immunization. The morbidity rate tends to be high, whereas mortality due to the disease is very rare.

Epidemiological Factors

Agent

Paramyxovirus group is the virus, which can be isolated from saliva or swab taken from the surface of Stensen's duct or the mouth. It is also found in urine, blood, human milk and cerebro spinal fluid (CSF) of the case.

Host

Age and Sex

It can occur at any age and sex depending upon previous immunity status. Generally it is more common in the age group of 5 to 15 years. The highest incidence is among nonimmunized children. Transplancental antibody protects infants from infection in the first 6 months of life. One attack usually results in lifelong immunity, rarely second attack may occur.

Environment

Incidence is higher during winter and spring seasons, though it may occur anytime during the year due to overcrowding, because the disease is spread by droplet infection through upper respiratory tract and through fomites.

Mode of Transmission

The infection is spread by direct contact, respiratory secretions and fomites.

Period of Communicability

It is less communicable than measles, pertussis and chickenpox. The period of infection is uncertain but may be from 6 to 9 days after the appearance of parotid swelling. In a person with inapparant infection the virus has been recovered in saliva between the 15th and 24th day after exposure.

Incubation Period

It is usually 16 to 18 days but may extend up to 3 to 4 weeks.

Clinical Manifestation

Usually, the disease starts with prodromal symptoms like fever, headache, malaise, anorexia and pain around the ears and jaws. Mumps mainly affect parotid and salivary glands, followed by swelling which reaches maximum by 1 to 3 days. One or both parotid glands may be affected with severe pain and tenderness (Fig. 24.9). It may also affect testes, pancreas, nervous system, joints, eyes, ears, ovaries, prostate, breast and heart, etc.

Patient usually complains of pain and stiffness on opening the mouth. The swelling and pain may subside within three weeks of infection but weakness and fatigue may persist for longer period.

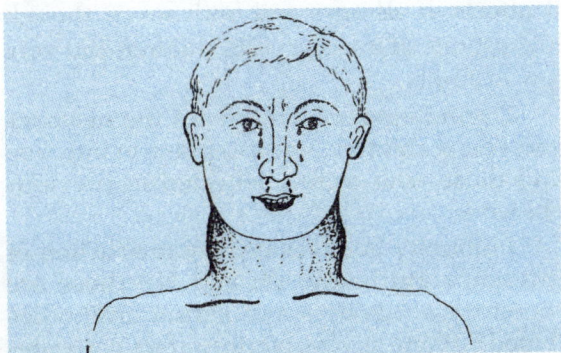

Fig. 24.9 : Patient with mumps affecting both parotid glands

Complications

Severe cases may be associated with severe dysphagia, dyspnoea, myocarditis, hepatitis, meningitis, otitis, orchitis (may lead to sterility.), ovaritis, encephalopathy, etc.

Management

No treatment is available except supportive care.

Prevention and Control

Isolation

Mumps is highly infectious disease with long incubation period, thus it is difficult to control the spread of disease. However, the cases should be isolated till the clinical manifestations subside. And all the articles should be disinfected. Contacts should be kept under observation. Respiratory precautions are recommended until swelling subsides.

Children may return to school after the first week of illness.

Supportive Care

Pain may be relieved by administering analgesics, hot and cold compresses.

The patient must be given bed rest to prevent complications. Adequate comfort, therapeutic, nutritional and emotional needs must be considered.

Diet

No restriction of diet except in acute stage, when patient may find it difficult to swallow and is painful to child; soft and semisolid food is more easily managed. The diet should be increased as the swelling subsides. Acid foods, *e.g.,* fruit juices may increase discomfort, hence should be avoided.

Passive Immunization

Mumps immunoglobulin is available for the patients, and should be given soon after the exposure to infection. There is no evidence that passive immunization will prevent the disease after exposure to infant.

Active Immunization

A live attenuated mumps virus vaccine was licenced in 1967. This vaccine is now available in combination with measles and rubella vaccines. The appropriate recommended age is usually after 6 months of age and before child gets susceptible to infection, it should be best given between 9 to 12 months of age. A single dose of 0.5 mL intramuscular produces 95 per cent mumps antibodies.

Morbidity due to mumps vaccine has not been recorded, no significant systematic and local reactions were observed. Thus, it is one of the most effective and safe vaccines.

Mumps live vaccine must not be given during pregnancy and patients receiving immunosuppressive therapy or severely ill-patients.

INFLUENZA

Influenza is an acute disease of the respiratory tract caused primarily by influenza virus A, B and C. The viruses vary in their antigenic stability and several distinct strains of type A and B exist. The disease is characterized by sudden onset of chills, fever, malaise, muscular pain and cough.

History of the Disease

The name influenza is said to be given by Italians during epidemic of 1358, though association of infectious agents began with pandemic of 1889 in which **Pfeiffer's influenza A-2** antibodies had been found in sera of persons who experienced that pandemic and similar viruses caused the illness during 1889 to 1957.

Influenza began with isolation of influenza 'A' in 1933 by Smith, Andrews and Laidlaw. Another influenza 'B' occurred in 1954 made the problem more complex and influenza 'C' was first described in 1949 by Taylor. Influenza 'C' behaved somewhat different from influenza 'A' virus and its role in respiratory disease is less significant.

Distribution of the Disease

Characteristically influenza occurs in epidemic form and affects millions of people in all the countries.

The first pandemic occurred during 1918–1919, affecting around 500 million people and 20 million were killed. In India, 6 million people died due to influenza pandemic.

Recent outbreak of influenza was in 1957–58 caused by influenza 'A'. Influenza 'B' shows the annual cyclic occurrence and influenza 'C' is seen as sporadic outbreaks. Because the viruses have the ability to change dominant antigenic properties, cyclic epidemic is expected.

Epidemiological Factors

Agent

There are three main viruses namely influenza A, B and C. Influenza A and B are responsible for epidemics throughout the world. Both influenza, A and B viruses have 2 surface antigens, the haemagglutinin (H) and neuraminidase (N) have been associated with influenza in human. Specific antibodies to these antigens are important determinants of immunity.

Modes of Transmission

The virus is spread through airborne droplet infection and direct contact with the case or subclinic transmission from person to person or by articles contaminated by nasopharyngeal secretions.

Period of Communicability

The personal communicability symptoms begins within 24 hours and continues till 5 days infectious period.

Host Factor

Age and Sex

It affects at all ages and both sexes; though highest rate of infection is in children and very low in adults.

During epidemic outbreaks the newborn and young children are susceptible to infection and those who were uneffected in previous epidemic.

Immunity is developed by production of influenza antibodies (H and N), those are secretory antibodies and serum antibodies (blood). Immunity respiratory tract correlates better with secretory antibody than with serum antibody, although the latter is associated with protection. Antibodies appear in seven days after exposure and reaches to peak level in 15 days. The person comes to preinfection state after almost one year.

Environmental Factors

Epidemic of influenza occurs during winter in northern hemisphere and in India epidemic has been found in summer and rainy seasons.

Attack rates are high in overcrowded places.

Mode of Transmission

Influenza is spread mainly from man to man by droplet infection or droplet nuclei created by sneezing, coughing or talking. The virus enters the body through respiratory tract of the host person.

Clinical Features

The influenza virus enters the respiratory tract and causes inflammation and necrosis of the mucosa of respiratory system. The disease is clinically manifested by fever with chills, bodyache and general weakness, fever usually lasts for 1 to 5 days. If neglected, patient may develop pneumonia as complication of influenza.

Prevention and Control of Influenza

Isolation

Influenza can be controlled by isolation of the influenza cases. Avoidance of crowded places especially during epidemics, encouraging cases to cover their mouths with handkerchief while coughing, sneezing and talking. They should be encouraged to stay at home, especially school children. Proper ventilation at public buildings can prevent the spread of disease.

Immunization

Influenza vaccine provides effective means of preventing the disease. WHO recommends vaccination every year and the results are highly effective. To be successful, vaccine must be administered at least two weeks before the onset of epidemic or preferably 2 to 3 months before influenza is expected. Influenza vaccine does not control epidemic, hence it is only recommended in the selected population groups, *e.g.*, industries, police, transport and medical personnel. It is also recommended to specific age groups, *e.g.*, elderly and people with chronic diseases are considered as high-risk groups.

Influenza Vaccines

Killed vaccines: Most of the immunization is based on killed vaccines. The vaccine is prepared in aqueous or saline suspension. The vaccine is administered subcutaneously, a single dose of 0.5 mL is given. After vaccination, the serum antibodies increases within a week and reaches the peak by two weeks. The protective value of the vaccine varies between 70 to 90 per cent and immunity lasts for only 3 to 6 months. Revaccination is also recommended annually.

The killed vaccine may produce fever, local inflammation at the site of injection. There may be allergic reactions due to egg, since the vaccine strains are grown in eggs.

Live attenuated vaccines : These may be administered as "nasal drops" into respiratory tract. They stimulate local as well as systemic immunity.

Split virus vaccine : It contains 'N' antigen, which produces antibodies only to the neuraminase antigen of the prevailing influenza virus. Antibody to neuradiminase reduces the amount of virus replicating in the respiratory tract and the ability to transmit virus to contacts. It also reduces the clinical symptoms in infective people.

Chemoprophylaxis

Antiviral drugs have been tried for the prophylaxis, *e.g.*, amantadine and rimantidine. These drugs block penetration of influenza A virus in the host cell and prevent virus replication. These compounds shorten the duration of fever, headache, cough, sore throat, general malaise and also reduces virus spread to other hosts. Amantadine or rimantidine, a dose of 100 mg, twice daily for 3 to 5 days have been found effective treatment, side effects are lesser with rimantidine. These drugs have not been used for public health measures for widespread control of influenza.

DIPHTHERIA

Diphtheria is an acute communicable disease, spread by toxins of *Corynebacterium diphtheriae*, involving respiratory system characterized by formation of greyish or yellowish membrane (false membrane) commonly found over the tonsils, pharynx or larynx. Congestion, oedema or local tissue destruction, enlargement of regional lymph nodes and patient may show the signs and symptoms of toxaemia.

Distribution of Diphtheria

Worldwide Problem

Geographically diphtheria is prevalent throughout the world, but it occurs in clinical form principally in the temperate zone. The subtropical and tropical areas show a high proportion of immune adults as gauged by **Schick test**, but clinical cases are uncommonly seen. Epidemic of disease is usually local and not widespread in state or country. The incidence of diphtheria (diphtheria is not commonly found in most of the developed countries) has declined to a marked degree in most developed countries due to effective immunization, but in most of the developing countries it still remains the serious problem, with high mortality among children due to unavailability of adequate immunization. The affected children may show serious illness and develop malnutrition—kwashiorkar and marasmus.

In developing countries, the disease still continues to be endemic due to lack of availability of adequate immunization. The exact number of diphtheria cases and deaths are not known due to incomplete information available from most countries where disease occurs.

According to WHO, there are 1,00,000 cases of diphtheria every year and 8000 deaths due to infection and complications. In 2000, 4554 cases of diphtheria were reported in SEA Region and DPT coverage was 90 per cent (Fig. 24.10).

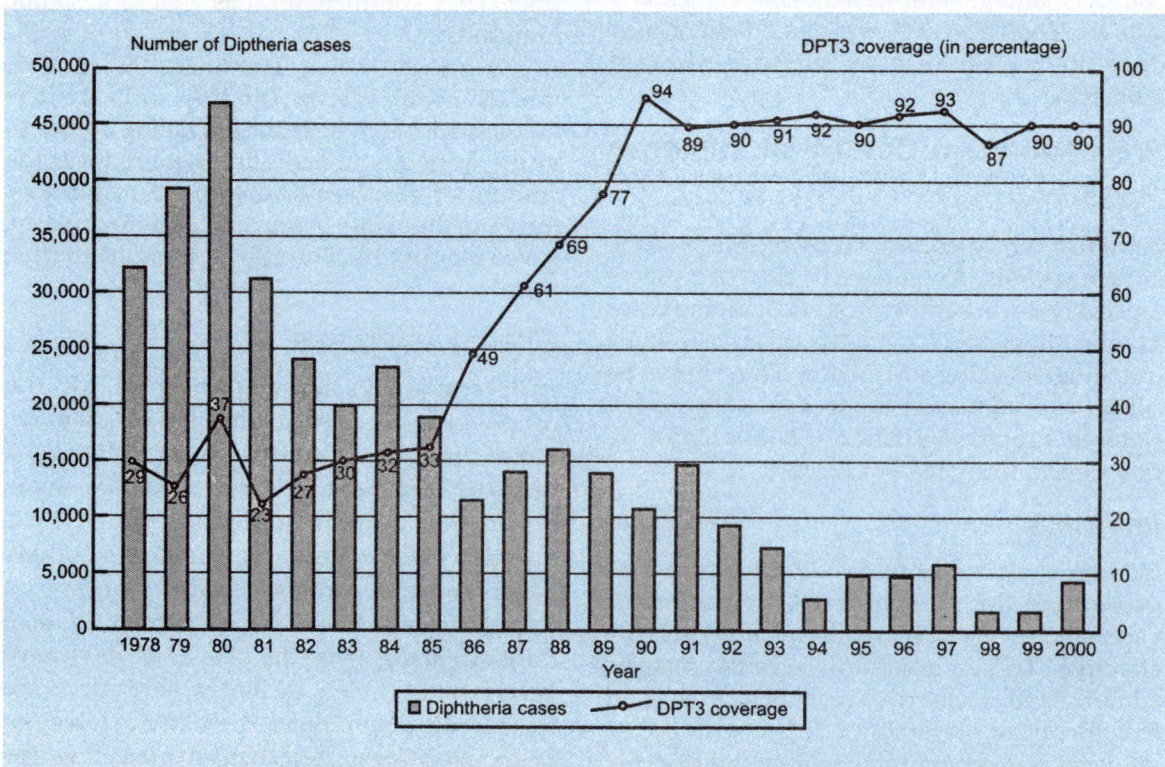

Fig. 24.10 : Number of Diptheria Cases and DPT3 Coverage

Problem In India

Diphtheria is still prevalent in India, though the incidence has declined from 9426 cases in 1986 to 1257 cases in 1995. This may be due to effective immunization coverage among children.

Epidemiological Factors of Disease

Agent

The causative organism of diphtheria is *C. diphtheriae* which is a Gram-positive rod like nonmotile, and of varying shape and size. It produces a powerful exotoxin. Three types of organisms have been identified as **gravis, mitis** and **intermedius**. All of them are pathogenic to human host, these toxins can affect the heart and cause myocarditis or nerves leading to paralysis. These bacilli are sensitive to pentamidine and are readily killed by heat at 60°C and chemical agents but may survive in freezer.

The patient usually complains of sore throat, difficulty in swallowing, low grade fever.

Mode of Transmission

Transmission is by direct contact via coughing, sneezing and talking with a person who has disease or is a healthy carrier.

The infection can be spread mainly by droplet infection through nasopharyngeal secretions, discharge from skin lesions and contaminated fomites.

The patient may spread the infection for 14 to 28 days from the onset of illness.

Communicability and Transmission

Cases and carriers are the sources of infection in diphtheria. Carriers are more numerous and are the cause of most of clinical cases. Period of communicability varies from 2 to 4 weeks in untreated individuals. Few patients remain carriers of virulent bacilli for as long as 6 months.

Population at Risk

This depends upon the immunization status of the population. Infants born of immune mothers are relatively immune for about six months.

Host Factor

Age and Sex

It rarely occurs among children below six months of age and not common above middle age. Diphtheria is most common in the age group from 1 to 5 years. Both the sexes are equally affected. It has been found that maximum incidence takes place among school children.

Immunity

One attack of the disease generally leads to lifelong immunity. Infants get immunity from immune mothers for few months of their life. People also develop active immunity due to inapparent infection. Survey in India has shown that 70 per cent of children above 3 years and 99 per cent above 5 years of age have developed immunity against diphtheria. A high immunity of 70 per cent is necessary to prevent the epidemic of the disease.

Though immunity status of the community is largely determined by the size, incidence of cases and carriers and the proposition of individuals who have been inoculated against the disease.

Environmental Factors

Disease may occur at any time of the year but higher incidence is seen during winter season. Different parts of the country have shown different variations in the incidence of disease like more cases are seen from August to October in Delhi and November to January in Mumbai (Fig. 24.11).

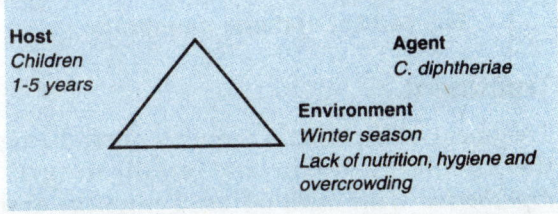

Fig. 24.11: Epidemiological factors of diphtheria

Economic status appears to extend some influence on the incidences of disease, particularly in colder months. Lack of proper nutrition, inadequate facilities and overcrowding appears to favour the transmission of disease.

Incubation Period

Incubation period varies between 1 to 10 days, with average between 2 to 5 days.

Clinical Manifestation

The manifestations of diphtheria depend upon the location of infection, immunization status of the host and whether toxins enter the systemic circulation.

Onset is rarely sudden and symptoms are rarely severe. The patient usually complains of headache, temperature, sore throat and malaise. The membrane begins to form at one side of tonsils and spreads over to the other side. The diphtheria membrane is white greyish or greyish green in colour (Fig. 24.12). Sometimes there is bleeding particularly if an attempt is made to remove the membrane. The patient usually complains of difficulty in swallowing.

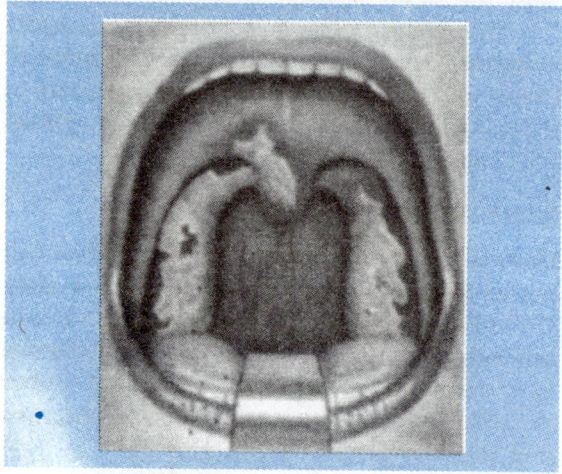

Fig. 24.12 : Diptheria membrane

Treatment

Treatment of diphtheria requires neutralizing the circulating toxin and eradicating *C. diphtheriae* with antibodies. Penicillin and erythromycin are effective against infection. Supportive care is an essential part of treatment.

Bed Rest

The patient must be provided bed rest at least for 4 to 6 weeks. Particularly for patients who have extended tonsillar involvement.

Soft Diet

If the patient is unable to swallow, in severe cases, the patient is provided liquid diet and transfusion may also be recommended. Patient is given soft bland diet for easy swallowing like milk, *dal*, soup or *khichri*, etc.

Antitoxins to all the patients unless they are serum sensitive, in such instances they should be desensitised. In mild case, antitoxin is given intramuscularly, but for severe cases 40,000 units are given I.M. and rest is given intravenously diluted with glucose or saline solution.

Steroid Therapy

Corticosteroids are also prescribed to prevent myocarditis. No local treatment is useful. Membrane should not be peeled off, it may cause bleeding.

Prevention and Control of Diphtheria

Early Detection

Cases and the carriers must be detected at the earliest from within the families and schools. Carriers can be detected by taking nasal and throat cultures for diphtheria bacilli.

Isolation

All cases and carriers should be isolated preferably in the hospital till at least two nasal and throat cultures show negative results. If the patient is at home, contact should be quarantined till the patient is isolated.

If the patient has recovered, still he may harbour infection, therefore, modified isolation may be necessary. The outbreak of the disease might occur due to premature isolation of convulscent carriers. Precautions must be taken for contacts at home to minimize the visits to patient untill he has two negative reports.

The bacilli are sensitive to penicillin, therefore, the cases can be treated by giving 2.5 lakh units of penicillin or 250 mg of erythromycin.

Schick Test

Schick test is used to test susceptibility for diphtheria. Material for the test consists of highly purified diphtheria toxin in buffered human serum albumin. The test dose introduced subcutanously is 0.1 mL because allergic or false positive reaction may occur. Control fluid (Schick toxin heated at 65°C for 15 minutes) may be used particularly if the tests are to be read within 72 hours. Heating destroys toxins but not bacteria protein content.

A positive Schick test results in an area of uniform redness which varies in size and is called positive if it is at least 1 cm in width. The reaction occurs first within 36 to 72 hours, soon after the bright red changes to red-brown, with pigmentation usually occurring later and noticeable for 2 to 6 weeks.

Active Immunization

The disease can be prevented by active immunity by giving diphtheria toxoid along with pertussis and tetanus (combined DPT) for infants and children. The initial dose is 0.5 mL given intramusculary in three doses, at the interval of 4 to 6 weeks within 6 months of child's age. Booster dose is repeated after one year of last dose of DPT (at around 1½ years of age).

Passive Immunization

Antitoxin adds in the prevention of diphtheria. People exposed to disease, should be protected by giving 10,000 units of antitoxins.

All suspected patients should be given diphtheria antitoxin, 10,000 to 80,000 IM immediately.

The carriers can be given erythromycin for 5 to 10 days to control the disease and spread its infection.

Contacts

All contacts must be assumed to be the carriers of infection, hence they must be examined for throat swab and immunity status. They must be placed under medical surveillance and examined daily for the evidence of infection at least once a week against disease.

Mass Immunization

The children can be protected by giving immunization to large population and repeating booster to give lifelong immunity.

Diphtheria Vaccines

Diphtheria vaccines are available in various forms like:
- APT (Alum Precipitated Toxoid).
- PTAP (Purified Toxoid Aluminium Phosphate Precipitated).
- TAF (Toxoid Antitoxin Floccules).
- FT (Formal Toxoid).
  APT and PTAP is given:
  Dose : 0.5 mL at the interval of 4 to 6 weeks in 3 doses, intramuscularly.

TAF is given 1.0 mL after the age of 10 years.

Diphtheria vaccine should be given, preferably PTAP after Schick test. APT is not recommended because it is pure and gives rise to undesirable reaction. Primary vaccine for adults is advised to give TAF and FT.

Combined Vaccine

The most effective method of administering immunization is with combined vaccine. Children can be immunized against diphtheria, pertussis and tetanus. The vaccine has purified diphtheria and tetanus toxoid and killed pertussis bacilli. Absorption is carried out on mineral carrier like aluminium phosphate. The absorption increases the immunological effectiveness of the vaccine and reduces the generalized reaction.

Storage

DPT/DT vaccines should be kept under the temperature of +4 to +8°C and should never be kept under freezing point (0°C in frozen). The vaccine should be used before the date of expiry mentioned on the vial. If the temperature of the vaccine is not maintained, it may loose its potency (effectiveness).

Age of Giving Vaccine

Primary vaccine should be started at the earliest by two months of age, as recommended by WHO schedule in EPI programme of immunization. To complete the primary course, it is recommended to give three doses at 4 to 6 weeks interval before the infant completes one year and booster dose may be given after one year of the last dose, as the child reaches one and a half years of age. If child is unable to complete within this time period, the DPT immunization may be completed within 5 years of age. If in any case child is unable to take second or third dose within two months the whole course may be repeated.

Mode of Administration

DPT is given intramuscularly in the upper and outer quadrants of gluteal region. DPT is not given subcutaneously, because it may cause granuloma.

Side Effects

The child may get slight pain at injection site, malaise, mild fever, sometimes high fever and convulsions which are rare. Slight analgesics may be advised along with the vaccine.

Contraindications

Immunization should be given only, if the child is healthy. It should not be given to sick children, with history of convulsions, infections, urticaria or eczema, any previous history of severe hypersensitive reaction and children who are on steroid therapy. Though immunization can be given to child with mild fever and illness.

WHOOPING COUGH (PERTUSSIS)

Whooping cough is an acute, highly infectious and communicable disease of respiratory tract. It is caused by *Bordetella pertussis*, clinically characterized by severe attack of coughing ending in a whoop. The whoop may be absent in mild cases. In young infants, episodes of cyanosis occur rather than whoop.

Geographical Distribution

Whooping cough occurs in almost all the countries. Though there has been a marked decline in the incidence of the disease, it is still a serious disease with high mortality in many of the developing countries.

It may occur as endemic or epidemic. The affected children may show serious illness and develop malnutrition, kwashiorkor and marasmus. The reported DPT3 coverage in SEAR is high, but survey in several countries indicated that there is over reporting and actual coverage may be lower. In 2000, countries of SEAR reported 39,656 cases of pertussis, which may still be under reported. Difficulty in diagnosis and poor quality of routine reporting may account for under reporting. Estimated incidence in the region to be as high as 8.5 million cases each year causing 90,000 deaths (Fig. 24.13).

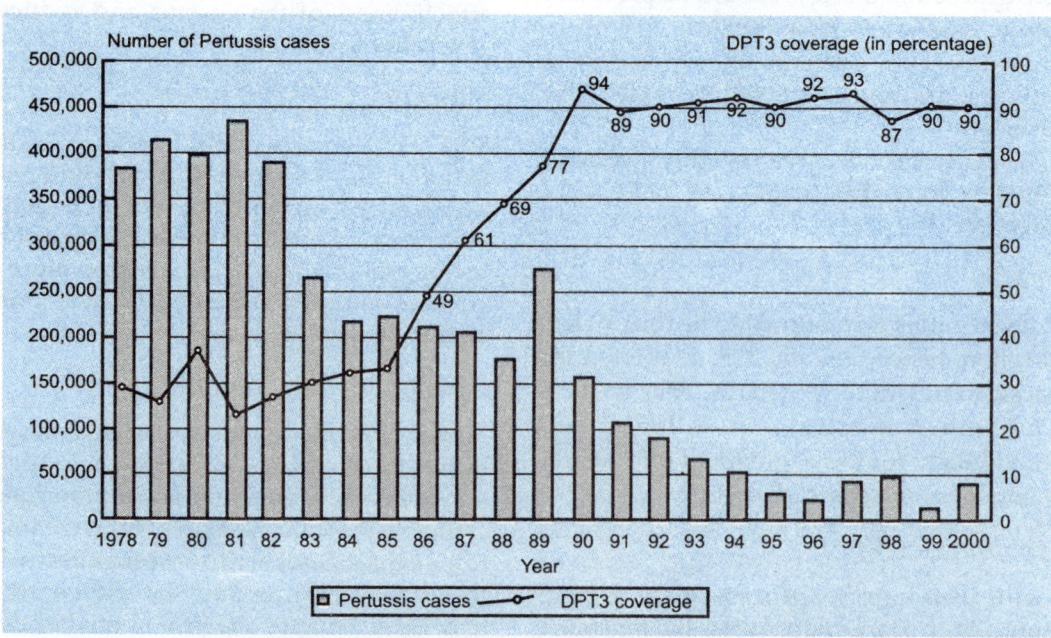

Fig. 24.13 : Number of Pertussis cases and DPT3 coverage

Epidemiological Factors

Whooping cough is caused by *B. pertussis*, one of the smallest bacteria. It occurs in smooth and rough phases, capsuled, noncapsuled forms and elaborates an exotoxin and endotoxin. The disease is mainly spread through an infectious nasopharyngeal or bronchial secretions of case.

Case of Pertussis

The infection is mainly spread through a mild, missed or unrecognised case. The pertussis is highly communicable during later part of incubation period, early clinical symptoms, and period of infectivity may vary from one week to three weeks.

Communicability and Transmission

The spread of infection is primarily by the airborne route, by droplet and droplet nuclei. The *bacilli* can readily be destroyed by drying, exposure to ultraviolet rays and temperature of 50 to 55°C.

The infection is spread mainly by clinical cases, unrecognised carriers and prodromal stages.

The period of infectivity may vary. Usually the infection disappears in five weeks.

Host Factor

Whooping cough is more common among infants and children. Most of the cases are found below five years of age. The mortality is highest during first year of life due to severity of disease. Though in adults it may not be very serious, but it causes unpleasant and prolonged disability.

Sex

Both the sexes are equally affected, though severity is observed more in female than in male children. There is no exact cause known for it.

Immunity

Infants are susceptible to infection from birth. There is no natural maternal immunity for children. Immunity can be developed only by immunization. The person who gets first attack may develop second attack also.

Environmental Factors

The disease occurs in all seasons, though the highest incidence is seen during winter and spring seasons. The incidence is lower in tropical countries as compared to cold countries.

Mode of Transmission

Whooping cough is mainly spread by droplet infection or direct contact, when the patient coughs, sneezes or talks. The children get the infection from playmates mostly during the early stage of illness.

Incubation Period

Usually the incubation period of pertussis is 7 to 14 days.

Clinical Manifestation

The clinical symptoms appear after incubation period of 7 to 10 days. Usually, there are three stages of clinical manifestation.

Preparoxysmal or Prodromal or Catarrhal Stage

Characterized by malaise, anorexia, serous or mucoid rhinorrhea, sneezing, lacrimation and conjunctivitis, mild fever. The symptoms are similar to respiratory infections. During this stage the disease is highly communicable. The early diagnosis is very difficult due to mild symptoms in the initial stage. The cough is initially dry and troublesome, appears late in catarrhal stage and is marked by consistent, severe and more frequent at night.

Paroxysmal Stage

In this stage the characteristics of whoop appear after 7 to 14 days of first stage. Infants may have cyanosis due to inability to provide a forceful inspiratory effort needed to produce a whoop. The paroxysmal symptoms are provoked by external and internal stimuli (temperature, emotional and physical stress, poor ventilation, airborne irritants), characterized by persistent cough. In severe cases, epistaxis is common. There may be scleral haemorrhage. Vomiting at the end of cough may aid in removing of the mucus from the respiratory tract. The patient is a febrile unless some complications occur.

Convalescent Stage

Occurs after the acute onset, usually within four weeks. The convalescent stage usually lasts for 3 to 4 weeks. In partially immunized child, the cough may be mild, paroxysmal symptoms may be shortlived. Whooping, emesis and even loucocytosis may be absent. It is essential to recognise the disease, because such patients might serve as source of spread of infection among children.

Prevention and Control of Pertussis

Cases and Contacts

The disease can be controlled by early detection, isolation and early treatment of cases. Early diagnosis can be done by examination of nasal and throat secretions. Treatment helps in shortening the duration of illness and also reduces the period of infectivity.

Erythromycin 30 to 50 mg/kg body weight in divided doses daily for 14 days is an effective drug against *B. pertussis*. Other drugs are septran, chloramphenicol or tetracycline.

Immunization

Pertussis vaccine is an essential means to protect infants and children against the disease. The vaccine can be given intramuscularly in three doses of 1 mL each during the third, fourth and fifth month of age. The vaccine is prepared from freshly isolated virulent phase I strains of *B. pertussis*.

Side Effects

The children may get prostration, convulsions and screeming, which may disappear in few hours of vaccination.

Combined DPT Vaccine

Combined vaccine of DPT is an effective and the most convenient means of giving immunization. Therefore, combination of DPT is commonly practised in the immunization schedule. Absorbed DPT carries mineral adjuvant which reduces the number of reactions to pertussis.

Three doses of DPT vaccine are given from the age of two month till one year of age.

Passive Immunization

An unimmunized child exposed to whooping cough may be given passive immunization to get temporary protection.

Single attack give lifelong immunity. Second attack is very rare. Natural immunity to pertussis is unknown. Pregnant woman with pertussis does not transmit the infection to foetus. The protective antibodies are IgG (Immunogammaglobulin G).

Treatment of Case

The antibiotics are useful in controlling the secondary infections and complications, though they may not reduce the frequency or severity of spasm nor do they shorten the illness.

Isolation

Patient should be isolated first untill considered to be noninfectious. Infants and children should be kept away from patient.

Health Education

The family or community must be aware about the spread of infection. All contact children must be immunized for DP. The child with whooping cough expels large quantity of organisms from nose and mouth while coughing and sneezing for at least four weeks. All fomites of patient contaminated with sputum or vomitus should be disinfected with dettol, phenol, etc.

Adequate Nutrition

The patient can be encouraged to take high protein liquid/soft and bland diet.

Care of Children

Most of infants need to be hospitalised, to be cared by experienced personnel. An infant, on the onset of severe symptoms should be placed on his/her abdomen, head down on the lap of the attendant. This reduces the risk of vomitus aspiration. Older children are best handled at home, unless complication occurs. Isolation and restriction of contacts should be according to instructions.

Complications

The bacterial infection may cause otitis media or pneumonia. Bronchiectasis is rare, whereas atelectasis is quite common complication of the disease.

Haemorrhage is common, epistaxis, scleral haemorrhage are seen frequently.

Complications involving central nervous system are few and uncommon, but they are usually serious and fatal.

Most frequent complications that occur within two years of age are convulsions. These may be associated with high grade fever.

Other complications resulting from increased intra-abdominal pressure are umbilical or inguinal hernia or rectal prolapse.

MENINGOCOCCAL MENINGITIS (CEREBROSPINAL FEVER)

Meningococcal meningitis is an acute bacterial disease caused by *Neisseria meningitidis*. The disease is clinically characterized by severe headache, fever, nausea, vomiting, pain in the neck, stiffness of the neck and progresses to coma within few hours. If untreated morbidity and mortality is as high as 80 per cent and if treated in time, it comes down to 10 per cent.

Worldwide Distribution of Disease

Meningococcal meningitis is a significant cause of mortality and morbidity in most parts of the world. Frequent epidemics have been recorded in North of the equator in tropical Africa affecting the regions and also temperate zone of other continents, *e.g.*, Europe, America and Asia. During recent years, outbreaks of this disease have been reported in Bhutan, India, Nepal and Myanmar. These outbreaks as well as majority of sporadic cases of meningococcal meningitis have been associated with serotype A and C. Only in a few, sporadic cases have serogroups B and Y been identified.

It has been estimated that about one million cases of meningitis all over the world with 2,00,000 (2 lakhs) deaths. Since 1988, all countries of the region have been immunizing Haj pilgrims with bivalent (serogroup A and C) meningococcal vaccine before their pilgrimage.

This strategy has been effective since a significant reduction in meningococcal meningitis cases have been reported in pilgrims returning from Saudi Arabia. In addition, the timely introduction of chemoprophylaxis (single dose of ciproploxacin) to close contacts of patients has also played an important role in preventing secondary cases among Haj pilgrims during and after their stay in Saudi Arabia.

Meningococcal meningitis has the potential to develop into explosive if not diagnosed and treated early and can cause very high death rates. During an outbreak in Myanmar in 1995, there were 65 cases, with case fatality rate (CFR) of 35.4 per cent. Generally CFR is high during the early stage of an epidemic when cases are often diagnosed late and patients are, therefore, hospitalized in critical condition. A classic example is meningococcal meningitis epidemic in Delhi, India, during 1987, when a total number of 3,061 cases with 677 deaths were reported giving CFR of 22.1 per cent.

Between 1994 to 1997 few cases of *M.meningitis* were reported from Indonesia. A study of aetiology of meningitis cases during 1996 to 1997 in major hospitals in Jakarta, showed that cases of bacterial meningitis were mostly associated with *Haemophilus* influenza (type B) and *Staphylococcus pneumoniae*, but not with *Neisseria meningitis* in children as well as in adults. Low incidences of meningococcal meningitis have also been reported from Sri Lanka (61 cases in 1995 and 68 in 1996) and Thailand (71 cases in 1996 and 60 in 1997).

Epidemiological Factors

Agent Factor

N. Meningitis is Gram-negative diplococci. The organism produces a polysaccharide capsule which is the basis of serogrouping. At least 13 serogroups of the organism (A, B, C, D, X, Y, Z, W135, 29E, H, I, K, and L) have been identified and the risk of epidemic disease differs by serogroups. Serogroups A, B and C have been responsible for epidemic outbreaks. While serogroups A and B are main cause of large epidemics, serogroup B usually causes less intense epidemic. These three groups account for 90 per cent of meningococcal meningitis cases.

Host Factor

Age and sex : The disease occurs in all age groups and both the sexes; but majority of cases have been reported in children under six years of age.

Immunity : All age groups are susceptible to infection. Younger age groups are more susceptible than adults, because adults may acquire the immunity by exposure to subclinical infection.

Environmental Factors

The high incidence of disease is found during dry and cold months of the year (October and February). There is association between poor socioeconomic condition and prevalence of disease, because it predisposes to overcrowding, poor environmental conditions and ignorance.

Source of Infection

Man is the reservoir of infection. The disease is spread mainly by direct contact through droplet from nose and throat of infected persons and the carriers. Clinical cases (diagnosed ones) spread only negligible source of infection. Carriers (unnoticed / undiagnosed) are the most important source of spread of infection.

Incubation Period

2 to 10 days, usually 3 to 5 days.

Clinical Manifestation

The patient complains of headache, pain and stiffness of the neck, backache, nausea and vomiting. Patient may be irritable and develop convulsions and coma. Herpes and petechiae are suggestive of meningitis. Nausea and vomiting, headache and convulsions are due to increased intracranial pressure. Muscle spasm indicates meningeal irritation. There is positive Kernig's sign.

Treatment and Nursing Management

- The specific organism must be identified and diagnosed.
- Streptomycin and pencillin are given intramuscularly. It can be given orally or intravenously.
- Fluid replacement and adequate nutrition with high protein diet.
- Bed rest and keep the patient in quiet darkroom.
- Accurate intake-output to be maintained.
- Observe carefully the signs of increased intracranial pressure or other complications.
- Rehabilitation during convalescent period.
- Prompt care of patient during convulsions and coma to protect from injuries.

Complications

Visual impairment, hearing difficulties, personality changes, headache endocarditis, paralysis, etc.

Prevention and Control

Surveillance

The surveillance must be carried out in community where the cases are seen with clinical manifestation of meningitis and these should be identified for treatment.

Early Diagnosis and Treatment

Early detection can reduce the mortality and spread of infection. All the cases must be treated with antibiotics and can save the life of 90 per cent of cases. Pencillin is the most effective to control the infection and chloremphenicol can be given to pencillin sensitive patients. Isolation is usually not much useful in prevention and control of disease.

Chemoprophylaxis

All the contacts and carriers (if diagnosed) must be given chemoprophylaxis as rifampicin 600 mg twice a day for two days. The mass chemoprophylaxis to all exposed people is recommended to reduce the incidence in the endemic areas. The reduction in cases depends upon the people covered with chemoprophylaxis.

Immunization

Meningococcal meningitis vaccine is very effective, prepared from purified group A, C, Y and W135 meningococcal polysaccharide. The vaccines are monovalent, bivalent and polyvalent. The immunity lasts for three years, hence booster dose of vaccine is recommended every three years. The vaccine is usually not given to children below 2 years and to antenatal mothers. Raising health education on improving the standard of living, avoid overcrowding and clean environment, good nutrition wil prevent the spread of infection.

WHO provides technical guidance for surveillance, laboratory diagnosis, case management and prevention and control of meningococcal meningitis. Technical support has also been provided for intercountry and national training courses, meetings and seminars. Diagnostic reagents have been provided to Bangladesh, Bhutan, India, Myanmar, Maldives and Nepal.

TUBERCULOSIS

Tuberculosis is a major public health problem in most of the countries. It is an infectious disease caused by *Mycobacterium tubercle*. It primarily affects lungs causing pulmonary tuberculosis. It may also affect other systems like bones, intestine, brain, etc. The disease may be acute or chronic, general or localised.

History

Tuberculosis is as old as mankind and has taken heavy toll of human lives from ancient times. Tuberculosis became more prevalent in Europe in eighteenth century.

1882 : **Robert Koch** discovered tuberculosis bacilli, which was one of the most important discovery in bacteriology and in the history of medicine.

1895 : **Rontgen** discovered X-Ray which was helpful for diagnosis of tuberculosis.

1907 : **Van Pirquet** discovered the tuberculin test.

1921 : BCG vaccine was discovered by **Calmette and Guerin.**

1944 : Discovery of Streptomycin.

1946 : PAS and

1949 : BCG vaccine was introduced in India.

1955 : Were successful in controlling the disease.

Geographical Distribution

Worldwide Problem

The disease is found almost everywhere. It is a major public health problem in many parts of the world, inspite of availability of highly effective drugs and vaccines. The statistical figures available show that there are 15 to 20 million infectious tuberculosis cases available all over the world. There are 4 to 5 million new cases and three million deaths due to tuberculosis every year.

In developed countries the death rate has declined from 199/1,00,000 to 0.5/100,000 (1980). The morbidity rate has also declined due to availability of BCG and chemotherapy and improvement in standards of living and quality of life.

The problem is still acute in most of the developing countries. Many of the cases are undiagnosed or diagnosed at later stages; resulting in increase of the cases. Reliable data shows 95 per cent cases are from the developing countries and 80 per cent of the cases are reported in the economically productive age group of 15 to 49 years. Drug resistant tuberculosis is a growing threat worldwide. Cure rate

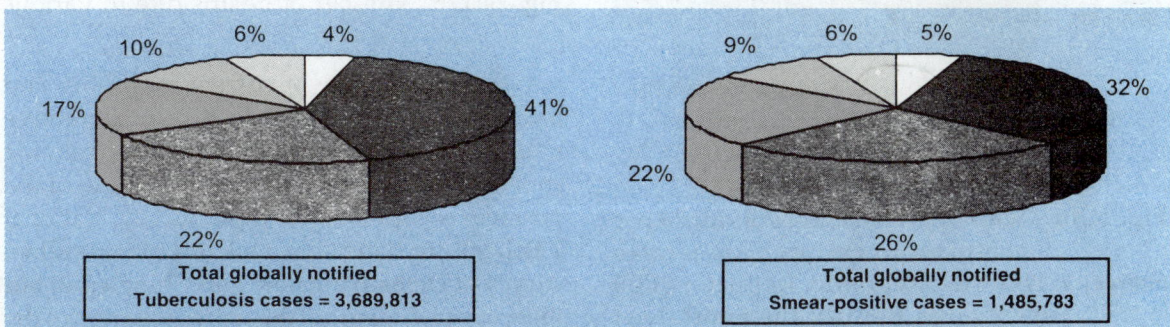

Fig. 24.14 : Tuberculosis cases, by WHO Region, 1999

has fallen from 95 per cent to 56 per cent and among AIDS patients infected with bacilli resistant to both drugs, the death rate is 91 per cent. 3.8 million cases of tuberculosis were reported during 1990 to 93, whereas 2.9 million was in 1984 to 86 (Figs. 24.14 and 24.15).

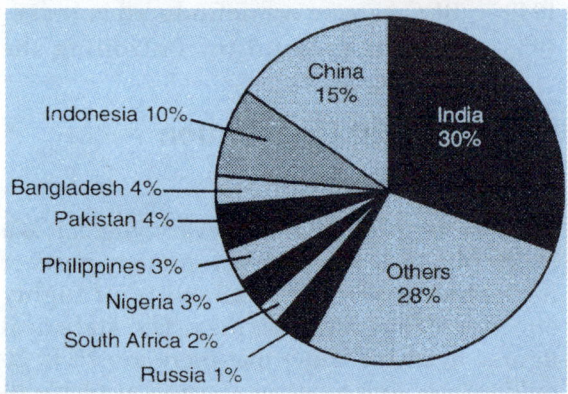

Fig. 24.15 : Burden of Tuberculers—India alone accounts for almost one-third of global burden

South-East Asia : T.B. is the biggest killer among adults in SEAR. Nearly three million cases of T.B. and one million deaths occur yearly. Since nearly 80 per cent of deaths occur among economically productive age group, the disease has a serious impact on economic development of country. Poor socioeconomic conditions and inadequate T.B. control measures are a vicious circle, each one accounting the other. In 1995, 88 per cent cases reported in the region were from India (Fig. 24.16).

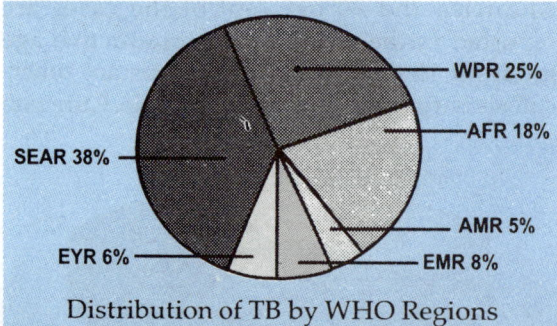

Distribution of TB by WHO Regions

Fig. 24.16 : South-East Asia accounts for 38 per cent of the world tuberculosis cases
Source : WHO The Regional Report : 2003 Tuberculosis Control the South-East Asia Region

Unless effective action is taken, the T.B. situation is expected to worsen with the emergence of multidrug resistant T.B. and HIV / T.B. co-infections. The emergencies of multidrug resistent T.B. is of serious concern to regional countries, due to high mortality.

T.B. is the most important life-threatening opportunistic infection associated with HIV in SEAR. HIV and T.B. each speed-up progression of the other of the 4.5 million people who were HIV positive in 1997 about one-third were also infected with T.B. Between 56 to 80 per cent AIDS cases diagnosed in Thailand, India, Nepal and Myanmar have had T.B. T.B. accounts for at least one-third of AIDS deaths worldwide and 40 per cent in SEAR.

Problem in India

In India 14 million people are estimated to be suffering from active tuberculosis of which 3 to 3.5 millions are highly infectious. About 0.5 million die of the disease every year. An estimated 2 to 2.5 million cases are added every year.

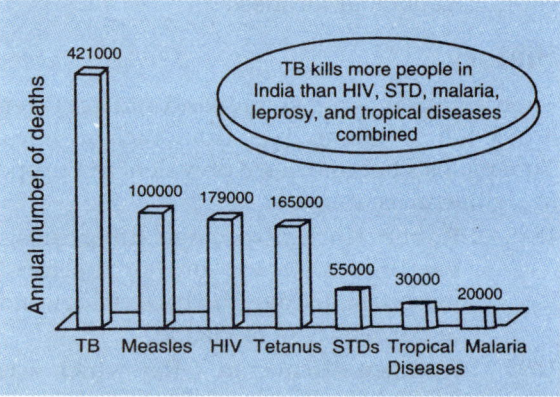

Fig. 24.17 : Number of deaths due to various diseases

The exact figure of current morbidity and mortality is not available due to defective national reporting system, the only reliable source of information on the magnitude of the problem is Population Sample Survey. National T.B. Institute, Bangalore, took three longitudinal survey at Delhi, Bangalore and Chingleput, but these surveys were not the representatives of the entire country (Fig. 24.18).

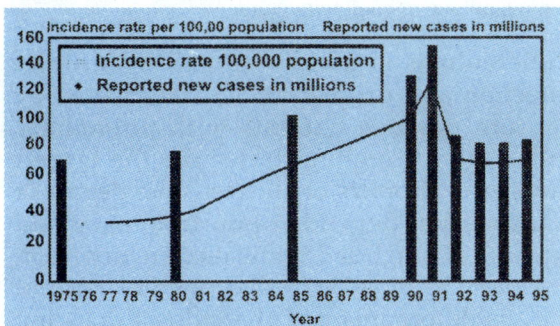

Fig. 24.18 : Regional trends in Tuberculosis incidence

Tuberculosis affects the socioeconomic and emotional security of the entire family, when the father of the family is affected due to disease.

Epidemiology of Disease

Agent Factor

The causative organism for tuberculosis is *Mycobacterium tuberculosis* and *mycobacterium africanum*. It is referred to as human and bovine strains. The human strain is responsible for the vast majority of cases, the bovine strain mainly affects the cattle and other animals.

The tubercle bacilli are nonspore forming rods. They are nonmotile, slender slightly curved acid fast bacilli. They can be readily destroyed by heat, but are resistant to chemical disinfectants and drying. They can be readily destroyed by sunlight and can survive for months in cool dark places.

Source of Infection

There are two sources of spread of disease, that is bovine and human source.

Human source is the most common in man, where the spectrum is positive for tubercle bacilli. These bacilli are carried out to healthy host by direct contact. When a person has positive sputum, and coughs, sneezes and talks, the organisms are discharged in air by droplet and droplet nuclei. These bacilli may enter directly into healthy individual or through the infected air. Bacilli may also be found in pus, pleural and peritoneal fluid, urine, faeces and gastric contents. It does not transmit through fomites, clothes and utensils.

Sputum of the patient is the most common source of organism. Pus from T.B sinuses, urine from T.B. kidneys, milk and other daily products from T.B. cattle are rare sources of infection. The bacilli are sensitive to heat and sunlight but resistant to drying.

Two most frequent ways of entry of bacilli are inhalation and ingestion.

Inhalation

Large number of bacilli are found in sputum. Coughing spreads the infection in the air.

Ingestion

It is another mode of transmission especially among children, because they frequently place contaminated objects in the mouth. The tubercle bacilli may be swallowed and passed through intestinal mucosa and produces early lesion in mesenteric nodes.

Host Factors

Age: Tuberculosis affects all ages. More than 80 per cent of T.B patients are in the age group of (15 to 54 years), which is productive population and causing major burden to socioeconomic development in developed countries, the disease is now more common in the elderly.

Sex: T.B is more prevalent in male than in female.

Hereditary: It is not a hereditary disease. T.B spreads among family members due to high communicability. However, the twin studies indicate that inherited susceptibility is an important risk factors.

Nutrition: Malnutrition is believed to be predisposing factors for tuberculosis but studies have shown the nutrition has no influence on causation of disease.

Immunity: Man has no inherited immunity against T.B. However, the immunity may be developed by virtue of natural exposure to infection or B.C.G immunization. Post-infection with a typical mycobacteria is also credited with certain amount of naturally acquired immunity.

Socioeconomic Factors

Tuberculosis (T.B.) is considered as social problem with health problem. The poor standard of living of people is a major factor that helps in spread of infection. Poor socioeconomic condition, overcrowding, poverty, illiteracy, ignorance about causation of disease, malnutrition, large families, early marriage, habits of spitting anywhere and everywhere, industrialisation and social customs like *Purdah* system in Muslim women, all these factors are predisposing to the presence of tuberculosis. The habits of sharing *hukkah* is a common practice in rural area which contributes to spread of infection.

Social stigma : People consider this disease as a social stigma, thus they do not want to disclose the fact, resulting in late diagnosis and increased risk of spreading of the disease. Disease also leads to poverty due to chronicity of disease.

Environmental Factors

Environment is important in spread of disease, since *mycobacterium* can live for longer period in dark and damp places. The disease is more prevalent in the slum areas, with poor housing condition, lack of environmental sanitation, poor ventilated and congested houses where there is less sunlight, etc.

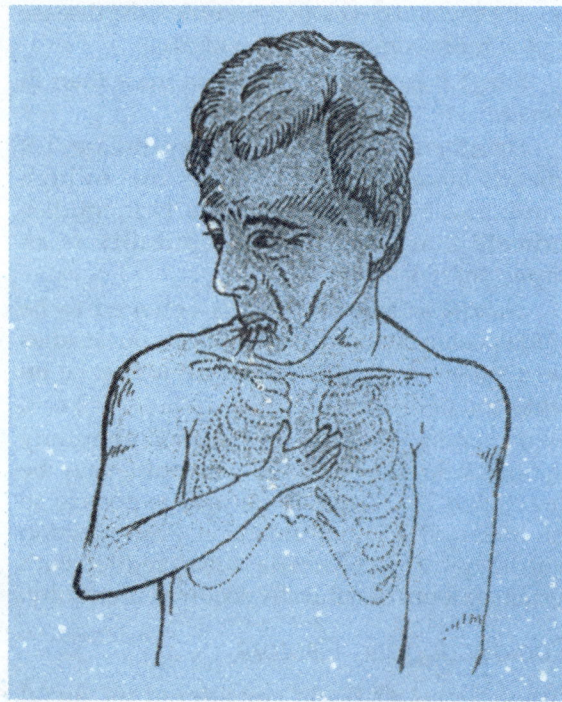

Fig. 24.19 : Patient suffering from Tuberculosis

Modes of Transmission

Tuberculosis is mainly spread by droplet infection and droplet nuclei transmitted by sputum positive patients with pulmonary tubercular. Coughing transmits the largest number of droplets of all sizes. The degree of transmission depends upon frequency and intensity of cough and ventilation environment. The particles must be fresh enough to transmit the viable organism. Tuberculosis does not spread by fomites like dishes and other articles used by patients. Mode of disease transmission is very rare by the extra pulmonary tuberculosis patients or sputum negative patients.

Incubation Period

Incubation period ranges from 3 to 6 weeks, even though it depends upon the closeness of contact, extent of disease and sputum positivity of case.

Pulmonary tuberculosis is mainly an airborne disease, although the infection may also spread by ingestion of contaminated milk. The bovine source of infection is usually infected milk. There is no evidence of bovine tuberculosis because of the boiling of milk before consumption.

The patients remain infective as long as they are untreated and not treated completely. Effective antituberculosis drugs reduce 90 per cent infectivity within 48 hours. Period of infectivity is as long as the bacilli are excreted by the infected host and this period may last from months to years.

Though it was believed that malnutrition predisposes the infection due to susceptibility to diseases, but studies have shown no evidence of such relationship between nutritional status and tuberculosis.

Diagnosis of Tuberculosis
Case History

A systematic case history helps to decide whether or not the patient requires diagnostic tests to confirm T.B. (Fig. 24.20). Patient must be asked whether he or she has been exposed to T.B. or whether they have spent time with someone who T.B. infection has Patients with pulmonary T.B. may complain of one or more of the following symptoms.

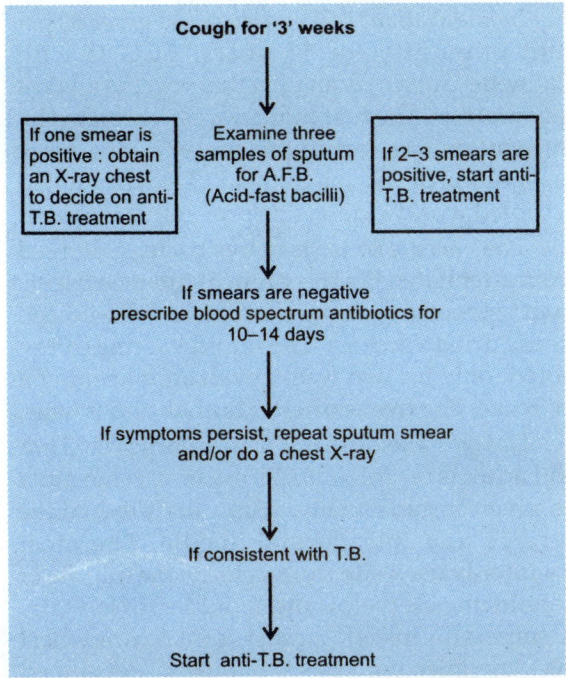

Cough for '3' weeks

If one smear is positive : obtain an X-ray chest to decide on anti-T.B. treatment

Examine three samples of sputum for A.F.B. (Acid-fast bacilli)

If 2–3 smears are positive, start anti-T.B. treatment

If smears are negative prescribe blood spectrum antibiotics for 10–14 days

If symptoms persist, repeat sputum smear and/or do a chest X-ray

If consistent with T.B.

Start anti-T.B. treatment

Fig. 24.20 : Diagnosis of T.B.

- Persistent cough with or without expectoration
- Pain in chest during breathing or coughing.
- Shortness of breadth
- Coughing out sputum or blood.

There may be loss of appetite, weight loss, malaise, fatigue, fever and night sweats, etc.

Physical Examination

Physical examination will provide information about patient's overall condition and other factors that may influence the treatment of T.B., if it is diagnosed.

Sputum Microscopy

Take three specimens of sputum and the most reliable way of making a diagnosis is to find T.B. bacilli in a smear of sputum. The technique is simple and inexpensive, during the course of treatment and it helps to assess the response to determine cure.

Radiology

Chest X-Ray has a limited role in diagnosis of pulmonary T.B. Chest X-ray usually appear abnormal revealing infiltrates, fibrosis or cavities, but could also appear normal. Chest X-ray also help identify other lung abnormalities that may be presents (Fig. 24.21). When the sputum smear reveals acid-fast bacilli, a chest X-ray may be superfluous. However, chest X-ray becomes necessary when there is suspected complication, such as pneumothorax, massive or bilateral pleural effusions or a pericardial effusion.

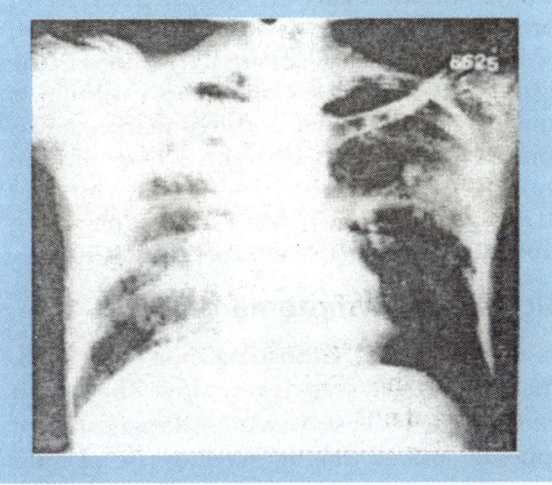

Fig. 24.21 : Typical chest X-ray findings in a patient of tuberculosis

- There is frequent or severe haemoptysis If pulmonary tuberculosis is suspected.

Tuberculin Tests

It is an important diagnostic aid and should always be used whenever the diagnosis is doubtful. It was discovered in 1907 by Van Pirquet, the positive result of which indicates the presence of infection. Mainly three types of tests identify tuberculosis are as follows :

1. Mantoux intradermal test
2. The heaf test
3. Tine multipuncture test.

Heaf Test

It is done for people in large groups, because it is quick, cheap, reliable and easy to perform.

Tine Test

It is not recommended due to its unreliability.

Mantoux Text

It is preferred when more precise measurements are required.

The antigen used for the test is tuberculin which are of two types, old tuberculin and purified protein derivative (PPD). The PPD is commonly recommended due to purer preparation and has less side effects.

Mantoux test is carried out by injecting antigen intradermally on the outer surface of forearm, dose 0.1 mL. The result of the test can be seen after 3 days (72 hours). Reactions in the form of erythema developed above 10 mm is considered as positive, and less than 6 mm is considered negative, between 6 to 9 mm are considered as doubtful. Individual showing 20 mm and more have greater chances of getting tuberculosis than those who are having 10 mm.

Signs and Symptoms of T.B.

Pulmonary T.B is the most common type of T.B. The onset of the disease is very slow. The person complains of malaise, weakness, fatigue, loss of appetite, loss of weight, evening rise of mild temperature, later on producing cough with expectoration. In some cases, haemoptysis can occur, which gives the warning signal about seriousness of the disease. In advanced stage the patient becomes bedridden with high fever, night sweats, dyspnoea, chest pain and hoarseness of voice. Children usually get lymph adenitis.

Complications

- Bronchial or tracheal ulcer
- Laryngitis pleurisy
- Pneumothorax tuberculous emphysema
- Bronchiectasis
- Intestinal tuberculosis by ingesting sputum.

Preventive Measures of T.B.

- Immunization—preventive treatment
- Surveillance
- Early diagnosis and treatment of cases
- Chemotherapy
- Rehabilitation.

Immunization : BCG vaccination gives 80 per cent immunity for 15 years. BCG (Bacilli Calmette Guerin) is an effective vaccine against tuberculosis. The first human was vaccinated by intracutaneous technique in 1927. But more recognition of vaccine came in 1948 when it was accepted worldwide as safe preventive measure.

The vaccine consists of live bacteria derived from attenuated bovine strain of tubercle bacilli. Two types of vaccines are available — liquid and freeze dried vaccines. The liquid vaccine can be potent only for two weeks even after keeping it in freeze. The freeze dried is human and bovine.

Dosage : The dose to the newborn is 0.05 mL and adult is 0.1 mL or 0.075 mg of vaccine must be given intradermally, using the tuberculine syringe and intradermal needle. The most commonly used site for vaccine is the middle of deltoid muscle (below the shoulder) of left arm. A successful injection must form 5 mm wheel over the injection site. A papule is developed after 2 to 3 weeks of administration of vaccine, which increases in size till 8 mm in 5 weeks. It then breaks and subsides in an ulcer form which heals and leaves a scar. The injection may penetrate tissues subcutaneously, it may develop an abscess.

Age for Vaccination

The BCG is advisable to be administered from at birth to 40 days. The early vaccination gives effective protection against meningitis and generalized tuberculosis.

Direct BCG Vaccination

BCG can be given directly without Mantaux test to all people at birth to 20 years of age. Revaccination can also be given to those groups of people who have not been vaccinated adequately, *e.g.*, vaccine with low potency, wrong technique, even new borns who received less dosage may not have significant level of protection against the disease.

Vaccine is more widely used, because it is more stable quality than liquid vaccine. If kept in refrigerator, it can remain potent for one year. If kept in icebox, it can be used within three months. It can also be kept at room temperature for 10 to 30 days with favourable climatic conditions, ten to fourteen days during April to August and 30 days from November to February. The vaccine must be protected from sunlight. Normal saline may be used to dilute the vaccine.

Surveillance

It is an essential component of control programme, to find out whether problem is increasing, decreasing or static. It is also essential for control measures to give BCG vaccination and chemotherapy.

Early Detection and Treatment

Early detection of sputum positive cases, who are spreading the disease in the community. The 'WHO' defines a 'case' of pulmonary tuberculosis as a "person whose sputum is positive for tubercle bacilli". Early detection involves:

(a) Sputum smear examination of all the people who have :
 1. Persistant cough for three to four weeks
 2. Continuous fever with night sweating
 3. Unexplained chest pain
 4. Haemoptysis at later stage.
(b) Screening of the people at risk, by doing mass X-ray photography.
(c) Bacteriological examination of the sputum for confirmation.

Chemotherapy : Case finding must be followed by appropriate treatment by antitubercle drugs, which should be easily available, free of cost, to every detected patient.

Antitubercular drugs : The combination of bacteriostatic and bacteriocidal is very effective treatment (Multi-drug therapy).

Rifampicin : It is a powerful bacteriocidal drug. It has special advantage when the bacilli are resistant to other drugs. In combination with isoniazid (INH), it can cure the extensive tuberculosis within nine months. Drug must be given empty stomach in one daily dose of 450 to 600 mg.

INH (Isoniazid) : A very effective drug used in tuberculosis. It acts rapidly on multiplication of bacilli. It can penetrate the cell membrane and gets widely distributed in the body including cerebro spinal fluid (CSF). The daily dosage is 5 to 10 mg/kg body weight.

Thiacetazone : It has bacteriostatic action and combination with INH makes completely therapeutic. These drugs stop the multiplication of bacilli.

Ethambutol : It is bacteriostatic and is used in combination to prevent the emergence of resistance to other drugs. It is given orally. Ethambutol has replaced para-aminosalicylic acid (PAS) in the treatment of adults.

Streptomycin : It acts entirely on multiplying bacilli and is given intramuscularly. It acts only on extracellular bacilli. The daily dose is 0.75 to 1 gm for 90 days.

Pyrazinamide : It is effective on slow multiplying bacilli. Its daily dose is 20 to 30 mg/kg body weight.

Domicillary Treatment

Domicillary treatment is an effective approach due to prolonged disease. It has been universally accepted that good chemotherapy, and domicillarly treatment has been proved to be more successful than hospital treatment. It is seen that patients treated at home have no hazard of spreading of disease, because those receiving the proper treatment are unlikely to transmit the infection. The patients under treatment are sputum free from bacilli. It is a cheaper method of treatment and can be managed at primary health centre level.

Rehabilitation Treatment Regimen Chart According to Category

The tuberculosis patients need rehabilitation due to their chronic illness. Because of the successful treatment of the patients with domicillary treatment they can lead a normal life and work, except for the group who are seriously ill.

National Tuberculosis Control Programme

This programme was started in 1962 and is integrated with general health services. The programme aims at early detection of cases and treatment in districts, the programme is implemented through District T.B. Centres

(DTC) and number of peripheral Health Institutions. The District T.B. Programme (DTP) is supported by state level organisation for coordination of T.B. activities in states. The programme provides free services to the people.

Activities

The main activities under this programme are case finding, treatment, and B.C.G. vaccination. Immunization has been included in expanded programme of immunization. Multipurpose workers have been trained to give B.C.G. vaccine.

All sputum positive cases are sent to District T.B. Control Centre and records are maintained.

Achievement

National T.B. Programme has been given high priority by the government. At present, out of 460 districts, 390 DTB centres have been established. Medical and paramedical teams duly trained are available at these centres. Besides these centres, 330 T.B. clinics, 17 T.B. training and demonstration centres and about 47,000 T.B. beds are functioning in the country.

Detection of new T.B. cases have been doubled within last few years and more than 18 lakh cases are detected annually. Short course chemotherapy containing more effective drugs is being introduced in the country.

International Assistance

The international agencies like UNICEF, WHO, DANIDA and Swedish International Development Agency (SIDA) have provided necessary support and assistance to the Project in the form of supplying X-ray equipment. X-ray rolls, laboratory equipment, vehicles, short course chemotherapy drugs and operational research.

Revised National T.B. Control Programme (RNTCP)

RNTCP was reviewed in 1992 by an expert panel. Based on the findings and recommendations, revised strategy was evolved with objectives of curing at least 85 per cent of smear positive cases and detection of at least 75 per cent of sputum positive cases should be done.

The strategy was extended to a population of 202 million people in 102 districts and 15 states.

Ever since WHO declared T.B. a global emergency in 1993, the region has made considerable progress towards achieving the targets. All member states have now adopted the DOTS (directly observed treatment short-course) strategy for control of T.B. and are implementing DOTS in parts in most of the country (Fig. 24.22).

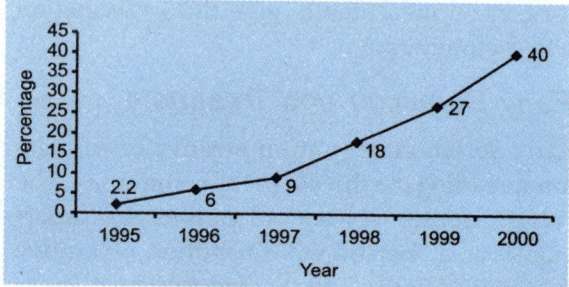

Fig. 24.22 : Trend in population coverage with DOTS in the SEA Region, 1995–2000

Benefits of DOTS (Fig. 24.23)

- DOTS more than doubles the accuracy of TB diagnosis
- DOTS results in success rates of up to 95 per cent
- DOTS prevents the spread of tuberculous bacilli, thus reducing the incidence and prevalence of TB

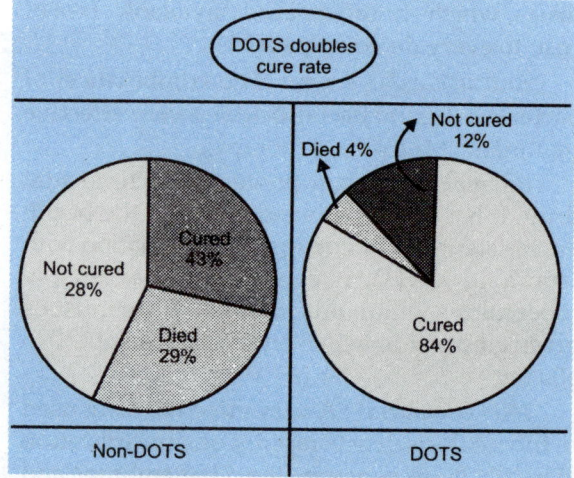

Fig. 24.23 : Benefits of DOTS

- DOTS helps in alleviating poverty by saving lives, reducing the duration of illness and preventing new infectious cases; thus, losing fewer years of employment
- DOTS improves the quality of care and overcomes stigma
- DOTS prevents treatment failure and the emergence of MDR-TB by ensuring patient adherence and an uninterrupted supply of anti-TB drugs
- DOTS lends credence to TB control efforts
- DOTS provides a model for strengthening health services.

DOT Therapy

Direct observed treatment is WHO recommended strategy for global T.B. control. This strategy emphasizes adequate and efficient diagnosis and treatment. It means short course chemotherapy given under direct observation to at least all

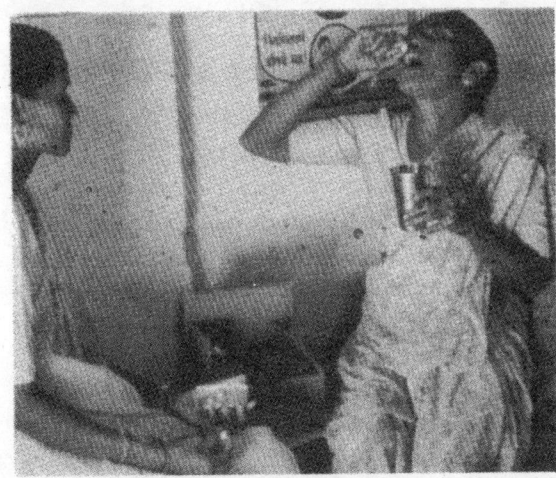

Fig. 24.24 : DOTS therapy

identified smear positive T.B. cases. Globally the DOT strategy has been recognised as the best approach to T.B. control to achieve a decrease in the disease burden and a reduction in the spread of infection.

Treatment Under DOTS

The WHO recommended treatment regimen for DOTS is short course chemotherapy. It is divided into two phases—the Intensive and the continuation phases. In India the treatment regime is as follows :

- In the intensive phase (2–3 months), each dose given thrice a week is administered under direct observation.
- In the continuation phase (4–5 months), at least one of thrice a week doses, is administered under direct observation.

The actual treatment regimen and duration depend on the category of treatment of the patient. The categories of treatment are given in the Table 24.3.

Table 24.3 : Treatment under DOTS

Category of treatment	Type of patient	Regimen
Category I	New sputum smear-positive Seriously ill sputum smear-negative Seriously ill extrapulmónary	2 (HRZE)$_3$ 4 (HR)$_3$
Category II	Previously treated Sputum smear-positive Relapse Sputum smear-positive Failure Sputum smear-positive Treatment After Default	2 (HRZES)$_3$/ 1 (HRZE)$_3$/ 5 (HRE)$_3$
Category III	New sputum smear-negative, not seriously ill Extrapulmonary, not seriously ill	2 (HRZ)$_3$/ 4 (HR)$_3$

In spite of significant achievements DOTS coverage in the region is still very low and has currently reached only about 12 per cent of total population. This limited coverage has been attributed due to lack of priority and difficulties in expanding DOTS coverage. Difficulties are, however, to be overcome to implement the programme successfully by training the staff, establishing diagnostic and treatment centres.

WHO considers T.B. as one of the most important health problems in the region and accords top priority for its control. Support is provided to all countries to assist them in the formulation and strengthening of National T.B. Control Programme. Priority intervention is needed to strengthen national responses have been identified. These include continuous, improved advocacy efforts to increase political committment at all levels, human resource development with special emphasis on strengthening managerial capacity at national and intermediate levels.

Success of DOT depends on five components :

- Political commitment
- Diagnosis by sputum microscopy

- Standardised short-course in chemotherapy taken under observation, for at least all sputum smear-positive cases of T.B.
- Establishment of a system of regular supply of drugs
- Accountability.

Targets and Achievements

RNTCP project is being implemented in a phased manner to ensure that quality of services is maintained. 740 million population have been provided RNTCP services under World Bank assisted Project and rest of the country by DFID, DANIDA, USAID and GFATM assitance.

By March 2004, 851 million of the country's population in 466 districts were covered under the programme. Thirteen States/Union Territories are fully covered under RNTCP. Remaining states/districts are preparing to start RNTCP services and the entire country is expected to be fully covered by 2005.

Major Achievements

- By March 2004 nearly 76 per cent of the population in 26 States and Union Territories were covered under RNTCP.
- India is the second largest country in the world in terms of population coverage under DOTS.
- In 2003 India placed more than 9 lakh cases on DOTS, more than any other country in a single year.
- Since the inception of the programme in 1993, nearly 28,00,000 patients have been placed on treatment thus saving about 5,00,000 additional lives.
- Diagnostic facilites in about 7800 laboratories throughout the country have been established.

Training : RNTCP training programme for medical and paramedical staff working under the programme are regularly held at National T.B. Institution, Bangalore. These institutions are rendering training to district and state level officers in RNTCP.

Tuberculosis and HIV : Involvement of NGO's, private practitioners, Indian Medical Association are being worked out and is proposed to involve them at appropriate level in planning, programming, implementing and IEC and evaluation of RNTCP.

In coordination with WHO, local supervisors have been hired to work under the direction of respective State Governments to ensure effective implementation and monitoring of RNTCP.

Support Department For International Development (DFID) has agreed with Government of India to support RNTCP. Area of support includes strengthening of central T.B. division, training activities, implementation of revised NTCP in Andhra Pradesh. The project was expected to be implemented in 2000 to 2001.

DANIDA : Assistance has been sought to implement the revised strategy or NTCP in state of Orissa. Government of Denmark has agreed to provide grant for implementation of RNTCP in 14 tribal districts of Orissa. The services have already started in some of the districts.

Role of Nurse in Care of TB Patient

Transmission of T.B. is mainly by the airborne spread of infectious droplets. The source of infection is a person with T.B. of the lungs (pulmonary) who is coughing. A single cough can produce thousands of tiny infectious droplets which can stay in the air for several hours particularly in location with poor ventilation and no direct sunlight.

Tuberculosis is a social problem. A T.B. patient and the family are very sensitive and do not wish their neighbours to know about the presence of T.B. in the family. T.B. is a chronic long-lasting disease, hence most of the cases are treated at home. A nurse must keep in mind the principles of home visiting and priortising the case selection and care of the patient at home.

- Motivate the patient to take regular treatment, when the patient defaults in taking drugs, a visit must be paid and repeated till the patient becomes regular and involve the family members.
- In case of newly diagnosed patients, visit the home for initial motivation, instituting procedures designed to care for the patient and to prevent the spread of infection.

- Frequent visit to the patients to ensure the proper disposal of sputum and precautions regarding protection of other members.
- *Contact examination* : All household contact must be advised for screening for the exposure by X-ray chest, sputum test and Mantaux test. If the members do not show any infection, they can be given BCG and those who show early sign of infection, may be treated by small doses of isoniazid (INH) and thiacetazone, etc.

●●●

25

Vector-borne Diseases

INTRODUCTION

Vector-borne diseases are those disease or infections that are transmitted by invertebrate vectors namely, malaria, dengue, filaria, etc. In this chapter we learn about these diseases.

MALARIA

Malaria (*Mala* means bad and *aria* meaning air) is an infectious disease caused by parasite belonging to *plasmodium* (Sporozoan parasite) and transmitted from man to man by bite of species of infected female *anopheles* mosquitoes. The disease is clinically characterized by recurrent fever, splenomegaly and anaemia. It is the most persistent, the most destructive, the most widespread and the most difficult to control among all the tropical ailments.

History

Hippocrates has been called the **"Father of Medicine"**, but he might also have been called as the first malariologist, because no one before and after him described the malaria fever. In 1880, **Laveran** recognised the parasite in blood smear.

In 1897, **Macalliun** discovered the process of fertilization that explained the two types of parasites in circulating blood, the sexual and asexual. After two years, **Ross** in England and **Bastianelli** and **co-workers** in Italy proved that the malaria is carried by mosquitoes. The quinine was a recognised drug for malaria in 1940s.

Worldwide Problem

Malaria is worldwide problem and occur mainly between latitudes 45°N and 45°S. Malaria is one of the most widespread diseases in all countries of the world. These countries include almost whole of USSR and Europe, North-East countries, the USA, most of the Caribbean, large areas of northern and sourthern parts of South America, Australia and China.

300 to 500 million clinical cases of malaria occur every year. It continues to be one of the biggest contribution towards morbidity and mortality of world's population, which in turn contributes to social and economic development of the country.

All the South-East Asia Region countries except Maldives have been reported as malarious areas. There were more than 23 million incidence estimated in the region in 1998. Although significant advances have been made in malaria vaccine development, there is no effective vaccine as yet. Malaria control is based on vector control and case detection and treatment.

Revised malaria control strategy has been implemented to reduce the mortality and morbidity in the malaria endemic regions. **Roll Back Malaria** initiative was launched by WHO, UNICEF, UNDP and World Bank with strategy.

1. Strengthening health system to ensure effective health care services at all levels.
2. Effective use of insecticide treated mosquito nets.
3. Training of health workers.
4. Effective and simpler means of administering medicines with help of grass root level workers of trained births attendents, village health guides.
5. Development of more effective antimalaria drugs.

Problem in India

Malaria was a major public health problem in 1953 in India. Annual incidence of 75 million cases, with 8 lakh deaths directly due to malaria, were reported.

As a result, National Malaria Control Programme (NMCP) was initiated. The annual incidence of malaria came down to two million per year. Looking at the success rate of control programme, the Government of India initiated National Malaria Eradication Programme (NMEP) in 1958. It was thought that disease could be eradicated. But adversely, the incidence of malaria rose to a peak of 6.4 million cases with 59 deaths. Hence eradication programme was again renamed as Modified Plan of Operation to control the disease and was launched in 1977. As a result, the number of cases came down to 2.1 million in 1984. In the year 1995, there were 2.8 million cases reported with 106 deaths due to malaria.

Existing Situations

Malaria is still a public health problem in several parts of the country and the major endemic areas are in north-eastern states and Andhra Pradesh, Chhattisgarh, Gujarat, Jharkhand, Madhya Pradesh, Maharashtra, Rajasthan and Orissa, besides a few focal areas in other parts of the country. About 80 per cent population of India live in low endemic zones with malaria prevalence of less than 2 cases per thousand population per year (Fig. 25.1 and 25.2).

The state health authorities reported 1.65 million cases in 2003. Of these, 0.70 million cases were caused by *Plasmodium falciparum* (*PF*). 943 deaths were reported during the year. The annual malaria incidence in the country has recorded a consistently declining trend since 1997 except a marginal increase in 1999. The yearwise number of reported cases and deaths since 1996 is given in Table 25.1.

During 2003-2004, an increase of 35 per cent in total malaria cases and *Plasmodium falciparum* (*PF*) incidence were recorded.

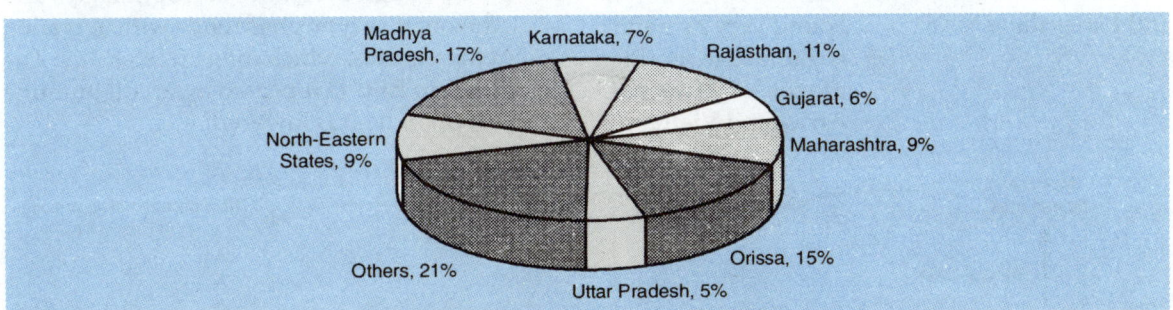

Fig. 25.1 : Per cent distribution of total malaria cases during 1997

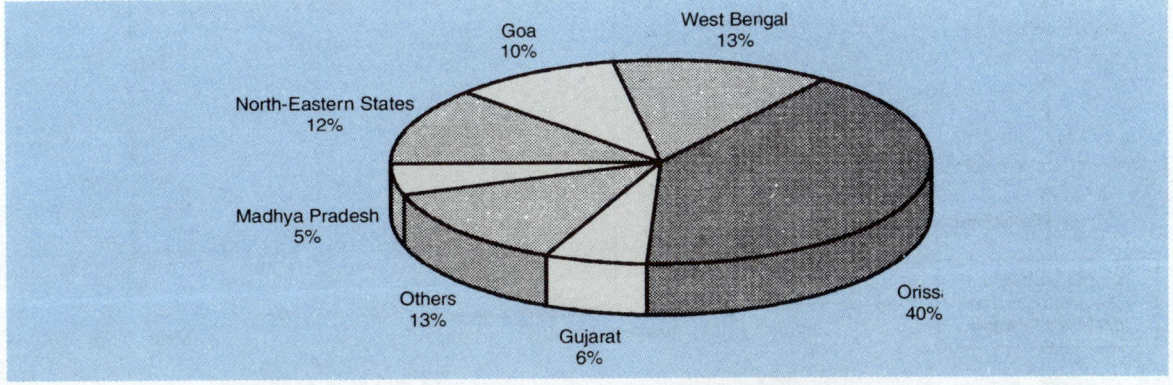

Fig. 25.2 : Per cent distribution of deaths during 1997

Table 25.1 : Deaths and cases of malaria since 1996 to 2003

Year	Cases (in million)		Deaths	API*
	Total	*Pf*		
1996	3.04	1.18	1010	3.48
1997	2.66	1.04	879	2.86
1998	2.22	1.03	664	2.44
1999	2.28	1.14	1048	2.41
2000	2.03	1.05	932	2.09
2001	2.09	1.01	1005	2.06
2002	1.84	0.89	973	1.80
2003	1.65	0.70	943	1.62

*Annual parasite incidence (API) is number of laboratory confirmed cases per 1000 population

Epidemiological Factor

Agent Factors

Four types of agent species of malarial parasites that cause malaria in man are :

(*i*)   *Plasmodium vivax*   70%

(*ii*) *Plasmodium malariae*   1%

(*iii*) *Plasmodium falciparum*   29%

(*iv*) *Plasmodium ovale*   Found very rare and is confined to specific places of tropical Africa and Vietnam.

Life Cycle of Plasmodium

The malarial parasite undergoes two cycles of development, which are : Human cycle (asexual) and mosquito cycle (sexual cycle). Man is the intermediate host and mosquito is the definite host (Fig. 25.3).

Asexual Cycle (Human)

Intermediate host: When an infected mosquito (female *anopheles*) bites a man, it injects the sporozoites of parasite.

• The sporozoites disappear within 60 minutes from peripheral circulation. Some of them are destroyed by WBC (phagocytes) and some reach to liver cells. After 1 to 2 weeks of development, they change into merozoites and are released in blood circulation. Some of merozoites remain dormant in liver cells for years and release in blood, later in life and cause relapse of malaria.

• These merozoites attack the RBC in blood, pass through the stages of trophozoites and schizont. Erycytic phase ends with liberation of merozoites, which infect fresh RBCs. The attack to RBC is repeated again till immune system of host is lowered.

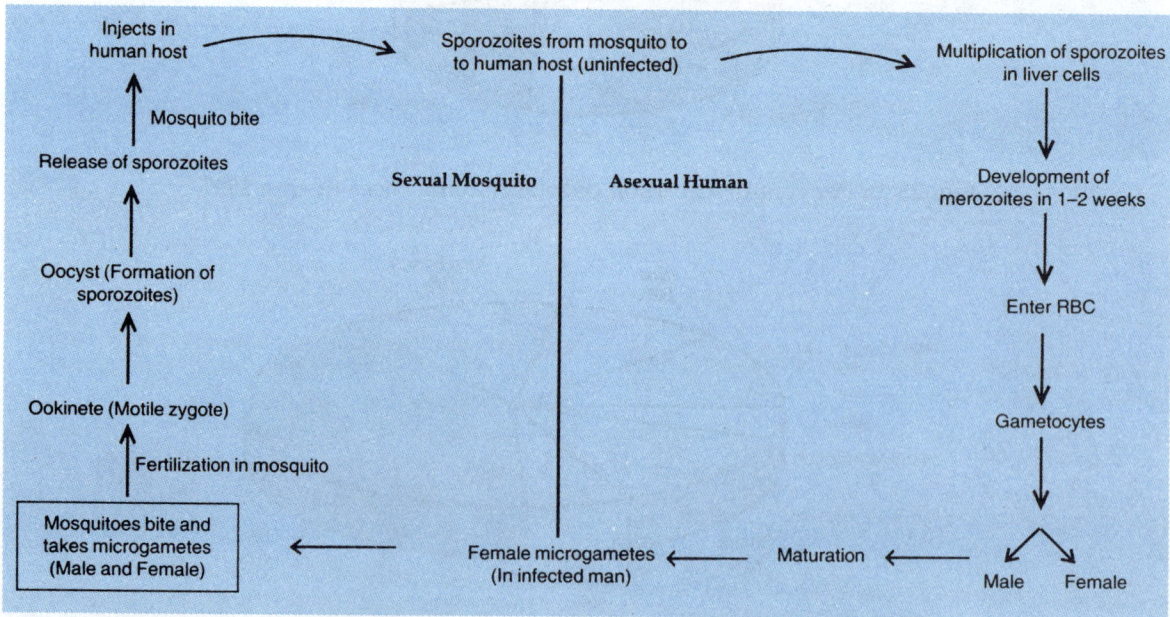

Fig. 25.3 : Life cycle of Plasmodium

- The gametocytes become male and female gametocytes. These are sexual types of parasites which are infectious to mosquito.

Sexual Cycle (Mosquito) — Definitive Host

When a mosquito bites the infected person, gametocytes (male and female) are ingested by the mosquito (vector). Further development of gametocytes takes place in mosquito.

In stomach of mosquito the male gametocytes develop 4 to 8 thread like filaments called microgametes and the process is called "exflagellation". The female gametocytes undergo the process of maturation and change into gametes or microgametes. The male microgametes are attracted towards female microgametes, with the process of chemotaxis and one of which causes fertilization of female gametes resulting into zygote. Zygotes are motionless bodies and become motile within 18 to 24 hours. This is known as ookinete. They penetrate the stomach wall of mosquito (vector) and develop as oocyst on the outer surface of stomach. Oocyst grows rapidly and develops into various sporozoites within oocyst, when it bursts and liberates sporozoites into body cavity of mosquito and migrates to salivary glands and mosquito is ready to transmit sporozoite through the buccal cavity by biting the healthy host (uninfected).

Host Factors

Age

Malaria can affect any age group, though newborns are seen to be resistant to infection with P. falciparum, which may be due to high concentration of haemoglobin during the first few months of life, which suppresses the development of P. falciparum.

Sex

Males are more frequently exposed to the risk of getting disease than females probably due to more outdoor exposure for them, which may not be true in today's world.

Immunity

There is no natural immunity. The infant, if protected, may get immunity for 3 to 5 months. Immunity to malaria in human is acquired only after repeated exposure over several years. Certain people living in malaria infected areas develop the natural immunity though it is not confirmed.

Human Habits

Habits of the people like sleeping outside the houses, thereby giving more chances for mosquito bite.

Population Mobility

Movement of people from one place to another, transmit malaria disease. Tourists also spread the infection.

Occupation

Malaria is associated with the agricultural occupation, hence it is more of a rural disease.

Housing Conditions

The types of houses people live in play an important role in causing the disease. People living in poorly ventilated and dark houses are more exposed to malaria.

Reservoir of Infection

Human reservoir is one who carries sexual form (gametocyte) of Plasmodium. Children are more likely to carry gametocytes, hence children are better reservoirs than adults. A person can serve as reservoir only when :

- Person harbours both sexes of gametocytes in blood for further development.
- Gametocytes must be mature. Immature gametocyte do not undergo further development. They may take 2 to 4 days to mature after entering blood.
- Gametocytes must be viable, if it starts taking antimalarial drug, gametocytes lose their viability.
- Gametocytes must be present in sufficient density to infect mosquitoes. The number of gametocytes necessary to infect mosquitoes is not definitely known.

Period of communicability : Malaria is infectious till gametocytes are mature and viable in the blood in sufficient density.

Gametocytes are the most numerous during early stages of the infection and they also tend to occur in peripheral blood.

Environmental Factors

Malaria is highly associated with the environmental conditions.

Seasonal Variations

Malaria is a seasonal disease, because it is related to rainy season, which causes collection of water which is favourable for mosquito breeding. Rain also increases the atmospheric humidity which is conducive for mosquito to survive. The highest incidence is from July to October.

Temperature and Humidity

The favourable temperature is 20 to 30°C and relative humidity 63 per cent or more which is favourable for malarial parasites to grow, temperature affects the life cycle of malarial parasite. If there is a large variation in temperature and humidity, the mosquitoes do not live long.

Reservoirs of Water

Open drainage, pits, garden pools, coolers, irrigation channels, all man-made reservoirs lead to mosquito breeding and hence high incidence of disease.

Modes of Transmission

Vector Transmission

Malaria is transmitted by the bite of female *Anopheles* mosquitoes. Mosquitoes are only infective and harbour infection when sporozoites are present in their salivary glands. The important vectors which are responsible for causing malaria in India are :

Anopheles culicifacies, Anopheles fluviatilis, Anopheles minimus, Anopheles stephensi, Anopheles maculatus, Anopheles sandaicus, Anopheles phillipinensis. The important vector in rural community is *anopheles culicifacies* and *anopheles stephensi* in urban areas (Fig. 25.4).

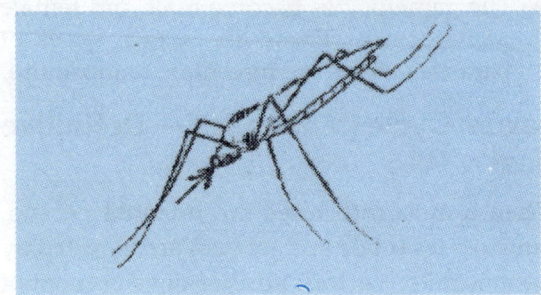

Fig. 25.4 : Anopheles mosquito transmits malaria

Factors Affecting Causation of Malaria

Density

Species must be present in sufficient quantity near human habitat.

Lifespan

The vector mosquito must live for at least 10 to 12 days after an infective blood meal to become infective. To control malaria, the lifespan must be shortened to less than ten days by insecticides.

Breeding Habits

The breeding habits vary in different species. Some mosquitoes breed in moving water and some in the wells, fountains or overhead tanks. Antilarvae measure must be adopted based on their breeding habits.

Time of Biting

Usually mosquitoes bite at night. Except *Aedes* mosquito, *Anopheles* mosquitoes have nocturnal feeding habits.

Vectorial Capacity

It is the effect of various factors, *e.g.*, density of vector population, susceptibility to infection, lifespan of mosquito. Susceptibility of infection is the physiological capacity of transmission of infection.

Resistance to Insecticides

When mosquitoes are resistant to insecticides, it is difficult to control the breeding of mosquitoes and hence to control the disease.

Direct Transmission

Malaria may also be transmitted through hypodermic, intramuscular and intravenous injections to man, especially blood transfusion, because the infective parasites remain at least for 14 days in the bottle of infective blood. People living in endemic areas taking antimalaria prophylactic and those who had an attack should not donate blood at least for three years afterwards.

Congenital Malaria

The infected mother may transmit the infection through placenta, though it is rare.

Incubation Period

The incubation period varies with the species of mosquitoes. Average I.P. :

P. falciparum	9–14 days (12 days average)
P. vivax	18–40 days (28)
P. ovule	16–18 days (17)
P. malariae	8–17 days (14)

Clinical Manifestation

After incubation period patient may complain of anorexia, headache and fever with or without chills. The pyrexial stages are usually characterised by these stages. The malaria is characterised by high grade fever which may or may not be with chills and rigors, nausea and vomiting and loss of appetite. The fever may be irregular or continuous. The typical malarial fever shows high grade irregular fever with hot and cold stages.

Cold Stage

The sudden onset of rise of temperature up to 39°C to 41°C with chills and rigors, patients feel extreme cold accompanied by shivering, severe headache, nausea and vomiting. In the beginning the skin is cold, but becomes hot later. The pulse is rapid, feable and weak. This stage continues till one and half hours.

Hot Stage

The patient feels very hot and wants to remove all clothes, the skin is hot and dry to touch, severe headache continues. Pulse and respiration are rapid. This stage continues for two hours.

Sweating Stage

Fever comes down with profuse sweating. Body temperature comes down rapidly to subnormal and skin is cold and moist. The pulse rate decreases, patient feels relaxed and often falls asleep. This stage lasts for 2 to 4 hours.

There may be rise of temperature every alternate day; there may be enlargement of spleen, secondary anaemia due to RBC destruction.

Clinical features of malaria vary from mild to severe and complicated according to the species of parasites present in the patient's state of immunity, the intensity of infection and malnutrition. Headache, nausea and vomiting are usually severe and patient has the tendency to develop delirium, haemolytic jaundice and anaemia.

Diagnosis

It is essential to exclude malaria in all cases of fever of doubtful origin in the tropics. The differential diagnosis is usually from typhoid fever, tuberculosis, influenza, urinary tract infection, septicaemia, liver abscess and hepatitis.

Suspicion of the diagnosis is aroused by epidemiological and clinical evidences.

Blood smear

Two types of blood slides, thick film for identifying the parasite and thin film for identifying its type of species to be prepared on single microscope glass slide.

Blood smear for malarial parasite has a failure rate as high as 99 per cent, since it is seldom made at the peak of the fever and also it is not properly prepared or carefully examined.

Fluorescent antibody technique may be employed for detecting species specific IgG antibodies which are known to persist for many months after cure of malaria.

Complications

The incidence of complication in *falciparum* infection is fairly high.

The pernicious malaria is particularly seen in the age group of 6 months to 3 years and may cause :

Cerebral Malarias

Characterized by meningeal sign, convulsions and coma. Cerebrospinal fluid is more or less normal in most of cases. Cerebral malaria is believed to be a hypersensitivity reaction to cerebrospinal fluid to antigenic challenge of malarial infection.

Gastrointestinal Malaria

Which is characterised by diarrhoea, dysentry and vomiting.

Hyperpyrexia

(a) Patient may go into convulsion, delirium and unconsciousness
(b) Haemoglobinuria and shock
(c) Severe anaemia
(d) Acute nephritis
(e) Splenomegaly.

Chronic Malaria

In which patient gets repeated attacks of malaria, leading to growth retardation.

Relapse in Malaria

In which patients may get malaria after a gap which is more than normal periodicity of malaria pyrexia.

Treatment

Administration of antimalarial drug is the only specific treatment for malaria, after diagnosis. The regimen recommended by the WHO and adopted by the National Malaria Control Programme (NMCP) is given as below :

Presumptive Treatment of Malaria

Presumptive treatment means all fever cases are assumed as malarial cases and administration of a single dose of chloroquine phosphate in 600 mg (4 tablets) to adults and proportionate dose to children is recommended (Table 25.2). Before administration of chloroquine, blood smear is obtained to confirm the diagnosis and determine the type of malaria.

Table 25.2 : Agewise dosage of chloroquine as recommended by WHO and adopted by NMCP

Age	Dose (mg)	No. of tablets
Below 1	75	1/2
Above 1–4	150	1
Above 5–8	300	2
Above 9–14	450	3
Above 14 and above	600	4

The aim of presumptive treatment is to reduce fever and other symptom which may be due to malaria, before confirmation and to reduce the mortality, morbidity and its complication. In most of the cases, single dose of chloroquine can save lives of all types of malaria.

Presumptive treatment is given to all age groups. Even pregnant women in any month of pregnancy or during postpartum period should receive presumptive treatment. Presumptive treatment should also be given in fever cases, where microscopic blood examination is not possible.

Radical Treatment (for Confirmed Case)

Radical treatment is given when malaria slide is found positive for malarial parasite to ensure complete cure of malaria, prevention of relapse, prevent complications and to make the patient infection free to mosquitoes, which prevents further spread of the disease.

Drug Regimen

(a) Single dose of 600 mg of chloroquine for adult on first day (Not to repeat if presumptive treatment has been given) and 15 mg primaquine (8 aminoquinoline) followed by 15 mg of primaquine for another four days (total primaquine $15 \times 5 = 75$ mg).

1st day   600 mg chloroquine + 15 mg primaquine.
2nd–5th day   15 mg of primaquine daily.

(b) In *P. vivax* 600 mg of chloroquine and 15 mg of primaquine for five days is found quite effective. But administration of dosage of radical treatment according to age, as per NMCP (WHO) is (Table 25.3) :

Table 25.3 : Agewise dosage as recommended by WHO in NMCP

Age	Dose (Primaquine)	Tablets
Below 1 year	—	
Above 1–4 years	2.5 mg	1
Above 4–8 years	5.0 mg	2
Above 8–14 years	10 mg	4
Above 14 years	15 mg	6

The doses can be given in divided doses/ day, *e.g.*, twice a day.

The chloroquine is given as a start dose on the first day only. Primaquine is started on the second day and given for a period of five days.

Primaquine should not be given to infants and pregnant women due to its side effects.

Radical Treatment for P. falciparum : On confirmation of species of *Plasmodium falciparum*, the dosage for chloroquine should be 600 mg and primaquine 45 mg for adults, the doses can be suitably adjusted according to age.

Radical Treatment for P. vivax : WHO recommends a total dose of 1500 mg of chloroquine to adult (first and second day 600 mg and third day 300 mg).

Radical Rx for *P.falciparum* in areas of resistance strain. The revised drug therapy for *P. falciparum* is as follows :

• Sulphalene–1000 mg (single dose) and Pyrimethamine–50 mg then, primaquine 45 mg (single dose).

These drugs should be given under caution and not on the same day, because they precipitate haemolytic crisis in sensitive cases. The dose should be adjusted according to age (Table 25.4).

Table 25.4 : Agewise dosage as recommended by WHO in NMCP

Age	Sulphalene	Pyrimethamine
Below one year	—	—
Above 1–4 years	250 mg	12.5 mg
Above 4–8 years	500 mg	25 mg
Above 8–14 years	750 mg	37.5 mg
15 years and above	1000 mg	50 mg

Toxicity of Chloroquine

Chloroquine has few side effects like nausea, vomiting, blurring of vision, headache, though they are mild and for short duration.

Chloroquine should never be given empty stomach to avoid the toxicity of the drug. It is advised to administer the medicine in between the intake of milk.

In case any toxic effects, *e.g.*, cramps, nausea, vomiting, cyanosis occur, it should be stopped immediately.

Mass Drug Administration

Mass drug administration has been highly recommended under the revised strategies of NMCP or WHO with extensive antimosquito, antilarvae, other protective and preventive measures for interruption of transmission of disease, though mass therapy has not been recommended for children below five years; due to its toxic effect, *e.g.*, retinopathy and less feasibility and accessibility.

Chemoprophylaxis

Chemoprophylaxis should be complemented by personal protection where feasible and by other methods of vector control under National Malaria Eradication Programme (NMEP). No regular chemoprophylaxis is recommended except in the following situations :

Pregnancy and Infants : Chemoprophylaxis is still desirable for pregnant women living in areas where transmission is very intense and leads to parasitaemias, causing low birth weight and anaemia or to high-risk of life-threatening malarial attacks. Chemoprophylaxis should be given at least one week before entering the endemic area and continued at least for 4 to 6 weeks after leaving the area.

New Drugs for Malaria : New drugs for malaria like mefloquine and halogantine have been developed. The injectable traditional Chinese herbal medicine called artemisinin, extracted from artemisium, is also very effective and faster in clearing the blood from malarial parasites.

NATIONAL MALARIA CONTROL PROGRAMME (NMCP)

Due to high incidence of malaria among people, the Government of India started National Malaria Control Programme (NMCP) in 1953.

Objectives

- To reduce the incidence of malaria cases in the country by DDT (Dichlorodiphenyl trichloroethane) spray
- To lower the morbidity and mortality rate due to malaria.

Implementation of the Programme

The programme was very successful, showing declines in malarial cases. In 1958, the incidence of malaria dropped from 75 million cases to 2 million cases.

Looking at the splendid improvement in 1958, Malaria Control Programme has been changed to Malaria Eradication Programme. The main objective of the programme was to completely eradicate (root out) the disease by total ending of the transmission, elimination of reservoir of infection. The results of this programme were satisfactory till 1961, when the incidence of malaria declined to 0.5 million cases. The disease was eradicated in many parts of the country by 1965. But there was a sudden rise of the incidence up to 6.45 million cases with 59 deaths in 1976.

NATIONAL MALARIA ERADICATION PROGRAMME (NMEP)

Due to successful NMCP there was sharp decline of malaria incidence. Hence WHO recommended Malarial Eradication Programme as an International Programme in 1957.

Malaria Eradication

Eradication means pulling out by the root, malaria eradication applies to immediate effects for the elimination of malarial parasites from the human host, so that there is no source of infection.

OBJECTIVES

NMEP is a centrally sponsored national health programme, operating on a 50–50 sharing basis. The centre provides material assistance to states, including antimalarial drugs and insecticides. Hundred per cent cash assistance is provided to the North-Eastern states.

With the implementation of modified plan of operation (MPO), the total malaria cases came down from 6.45 million in 1976 to 2.18 million cases in 1984. The malaria situation since then has been contained around 2 million cases annually.

The main objectives of the programme are as follows :

- Elimination of reservoirs of infection
- Prevention of recurrence of malaria
- Ending the source of transmission of malaria
- Early case detection and prompt treatment
- Selective use of insecticides
- Promotion of personal prophylaxis
- Capacity building and epidemic preparedness.

Epidemiological Situations

In 1998, a total of 9,37,536 malarial cases including 4,05,210 *P. falciparum* cases were reported from various states. Malarial incidence declined by 17.05 per cent. Malarial cases increased in Goa, Madhya Pradesh and Orissa. In the rest of the states, there was a decline in total number of malarial cases.

Malaria in Urban Areas

The Urban Malaria Scheme (UMS) was launched in 1971 with the objective to control malaria by reducing the vector population in the urban areas through recurrent and antilarval measures and detection and treatment of cases through the existing health services.

Passive surveillance and antilarval measures are main components of UMS strategy. In this scheme, all the towns having more than 40,000 population are to be covered and the scheme was implemented in 181 towns distributed in 17 states and two Union territories.

Strategy for Malaria Eradication

Strategy

Spray of insecticides, *e.g.*, DDT, HCH and malathion to kill mosquito (vector) and hence interrupting transmission of malaria in all human habitants where mosquitoes rest.

Surveillance from house to house for search of malaria cases by :

- Finding out all fever cases
- Malarial parasite blood smear for all fever cases
- Presumptive treatment to all fever cases
- Radical treatment to all the cases of malaria.

The National Malaria Eradication Programme, was divided into four phases namely :

- Preparatory phase
- Attack phase
- Consolidation phase
- Maintenance phase.

National Malaria Eradication Programme Strategy

The programme was divided into four phases.

- *Preparatory phase :* This phase was not given much attention, because it was covered during the National Malaria Control Programme. All preparations for control were taken up for eradication programme.
- *Attack phase :* During this phase complete insecticidal coverage was the main objective of the programme. The spray of DDT twice a year during malaria transmission period (rainy season) for 3 to 4 years was taken up to eradicate the mode of transmission. During the later part of attack phase, a programme on case detection and treatment was carried out in which, each fever case was identified, blood smear was taken and presumptive treatment was given. If blood smear was positive radical treatment was continued.
- *Consolidation phase :* During the phase spraying was stopped, but surveillance was continued. The main activities were active and passive surveillance, presumptive and radical treatment of malaria cases

epidemiological investigation of cases and remedial measures to eliminate the causes of malaria.

- *Maintenance phase :* When no more indigenous cases of malaria appeared despite careful search during a period of three years of which two years were in the consolidation phase, the antimalaria units went into maintenance phase and were handed over to the state governments for continuation of malaria vigilance activities.

Achievements

In the initial stage, malaria eradication was highly successful. But soon there was setback and outbreak in a number of states.

Causes of Setback

Various factors have been classified and are given below :

Administration : Due to high cost and shortage of insecticides and antimalarial drugs, inadequate budget provisions for states, inability to manage workers for insecticide spray, diversion of workers and funds towards family planning and neglecting malaria covering contributed towards failure in malaria eradication.

Technical cause : Technical problems like resistance of mosquito vector to insecticides and resistance of malaria parasites to antimalarial drugs, were serious obstacles for malaria eradication.

Operational cause : Inadequate surveillance, inadequate coverage by residual insecticides during the attack phase leaving many houses unsprayed and incomplete consolidation and maintenance phase.

Revised Strategy of Malaria

Due to failure in malaria eradication programme, it was essential to control the rising incidence of malaria, the Government of India, Ministry of Health appointed an expert committee on malaria to review the situation. Based on their recommendations, modified plan of operation (MPO) to control the malaria was initiated and put into operation in April 1977.

Modified Plan of Operation—1977

Modified plan of operation came into force from 1st April 1977, mainly with the objective to prevent deaths due to malaria. The malaria incidence began to decline and in 1987 the incidence came down to 1.7 million cases. There was again a rise of malaria in 1991 and came down by 1992 to 1.4 million.

The report of experts suggested that in order to control the malaria situation in India, the affected areas must be sprayed by DDT, HCH and malathion at least three rounds every year.

Objectives

The main objectives of modified plan of operation were as under :
- To reduce the mortality and morbidity due to malaria
- To undertake the antimalarial measures in the intensive areas
- To measure the extent of achievements of planned programme.

Classifications of Endemic Areas

The areas were classified according to Annual Parasite Incidences (API) :

Area with API More than two

All the areas with API two and more were brought under regular insecticidal spray with two rounds of DDT, HCH or malathion.

Early Diagnosis and Treatment : Active and passive surveillance activities for collection of blood smear are important components of MPO, in the areas with API 2 and above. Presumptive and radical treatment of all fever cases.

Areas with API less than two

Spraying : No regular insecticidal spray, but spray is limited to areas where cases have been identified during surveillance.

Early diagnosis and treatment : Regular follow-up for early detection and treatment in these areas fortnightly.

Strategy

Antimalarial Drugs and Fever Treatment Centres

The antimalarial drugs as well as fever cases will be given by all health centres, malaria clinics and health workers in the rural community. It has been decided to utilize the community health volunteer for distribution of drugs for malaria and to take up blood smear.

Urban Malaria Scheme

The urban malaria scheme was launched in 1971 to reduce the transmission of malaria in the urban areas by vector control by intensive antilarval measures and drug treatment. The urban malaria scheme covers around 181 cities and towns including Delhi, Mumbai, Kolkata and Chennai.

Plasmodium Falciparum Containment

An additional component of *"P. falciparum Containment Programme"* has been initiated in October 1977 with the assistance of Swedish International Development Agency (SIDA). The main purpose of this programme was to prevent or control the spread of *P. falciparum* infection.

Research

Studies had been conducted by Indian Council of Medical Research (ICMR) that revealed chloroquine resistant in many parts of the country, *e.g.,* Orissa, Bihar, North-East region, U.P., Assam, Andhra Pradesh, Delhi, M.P., Andaman and Nicobar Islands.

Surveillance

Surveillance is defined as case detection through laboratory services and providing facilities for proper treatment. The timely collection of blood smear for malaria and examination of blood smear is the key element in the modified plan of operation.

If all the detected cases are given radical treatment, it will certainly lead to depletion of human reservoir. The surveillance is of two types defined as under :

Active Surveillance : The surveillance carried out by basic health workers known as Malaria

Surveillance Workers (MSWs), who are named as Multipurpose Workers (MPWs) to cover a population of 10,000 and supervised by health assistant. The MPWs will visit every house once in fortnight and enquire :

- If any fever case is there in a house, including any guest or visitor.
- Any case during the first and previous visit.
- Collection of blood smear for fever cases and giving presumptive treatment single dose of chloroquine (600 mg for adult and 300 mg for children), collects the slides from subcentres and send them to laboratory at PHC.

Passive surveillance : The malaria cases reported at health agency, *e.g.*, hospital, PHC, SC, dispensaries or private practitioners are known as *"passive surveillance"*. These health agencies take blood smear, give presumptive treatment, but radical treatment for positive case is only done by health worker (Malaria) HW (M) by active surveillance.

Malaria Clinics

Under modified plan of action, malaria clinics were started to identify the fever cases by taking the blood slides, detecting the malaria cases and administration of antimalarial drugs. Priority was given to the areas which were difficult and inaccessible, especially tribal and poor socio-economic areas. The urban malaria control programme comprised intensive antilarvae measures and drug treatment.

Health Education

The emphasis has been given to educate people on causation of disease, treatment and preventive aspects. The people have to be made aware of the programme because without their cooperation the programme cannot be successful; because of their role in spray of insecticide, avoiding stagnant water and avoiding white wash after spray for at least 2 to 3 months.

Treatment

Presumptive Treatment

This is given to all fever cases, assuming them to be malarial cases. After blood smear is taken, a single dose of chloroquine 600 mg for an adult and proportionate doses for children are given.

Radical Treatment

This is given to those patients whose blood smear is positive for malarial parasite. The standard treatment in India is given for five days.

Adult Doses

- 1st day 600 mg of chloroquine 15 mg of primaquine.
- 2nd to 5th day 15 mg of primaquine daily for four days.

Preventive and Control Strategy

Early Case Detection

All fever cases are presumed as malaria cases and given presumptive treatment with chloroquine.

Treatment

Appropriate treatment of all positive cases of malaria with antimalarial drugs to reduce the morbidity and mortality.

Presumptive Treatment

The aim of presumptive treatment is to relieve symptoms possibly due to malaria and to reduce complications due to malaria. Single dose can save the lives of all types of malaria.

Radical Treatment

If the blood smear is positive for malaria parasite, the health worker must administer radical treatment for malaria; so as to completely cure the disease to prevent the recap, to make the patient noneffective and to prevent the spread of disease.

Chemoprophylaxis

Chemoprophylaxis is recommended for travellers from non-endemic areas and as a short-term measure for police, soldiers and labour forces living in high endemic areas. Chemoprophylaxis should be complemented by personal protection where feasible and by other methods of vector control.

Chemoprophylaxis is necessary for pregnant women living in endemic areas, chemoprophylaxis should start a week before the arrival at endemic areas and continue for at least 4 to 6 week after leaving malarial area.

Other Preventive Measures

Health Education on Prevention and Control of Malaria

Malaria is a complex disease and its distribution and intensity vary from place to place. Neither chemotherapy nor chemoprophylaxis will be able to reduce the malaria prevalence or transmission. It can be obtained only with proper antimosquito and antilarval measures.

Vector Control Measures

Vector control is the most effective measure to control malaria in endemic areas. This can be done by :

Anti-adult Measures

By residual spray of dichlorodiphenyl trichloroethane (DDT), malathion, hexachlore hexane (HCH) and fenitrothion are most effective measures to kill adult mosquitoes. The discontinuity of spray in the houses will lead to resistance to these insecticides, hence spray should be continued for an indefinite period. Malathion and fenitrothion are organophosphate insecticides which are being used with increasing frequency for malaria, following the development of vector resistance to DDT.

Space Application

It involves the application of pesticides in the form of fog or dust using special equipment. The ultra-low-volume method of pesticide dispersion by air or by ground equipment has been proved to be an effective and economic means of control.

Personal Protection

Protection against mosquite bite—the individual protection against mosquito bite by use of repellents, protective clothes, bed mosquito nets, mosquito coils, screening of houses, etc. The methods of personal protection are of great value when properly employed. However, they are not much used at large scales due to its cost.

Household methods, e.g., application of mustard oil and fumes of burning Neam leaves also helps in control of mosquitoes.

Antilarval Measures

Destroying the mosquito larvae by using larvicides, both biological and clinical, in stagnant water.

Environmental sanitation by avoiding the water collection, especially during rainy season, to keep the areas clean and dry and to avoid larvae development. The kerosene oil spray on the water collection areas prevents the larvae to grow. The antilarvae measures, e.g., putting kerosene oil on the collection of standing water and use larvicide, e.g., temphos is widely used. However, larvicides must be repeated at frequent intervals and hence it becomes more costly.

Elimination of Source

The mosquito breeding places can be removed by filling the pits and avoid stagnation of water. Measures must be taken to maintain the environment sanitation.

Integrated Control

All the measures must be adopted as much as possible to control the spread of malaria. It is important to assume the prevention of spread of malaria.

Malaria Vaccine

Many vaccines in controlling malaria are currently under development. Any effective malaria vaccine approved by large scale application would be used as part of intepreted National Malaria Control (NMC) measures.

Existing Situation

With the implementation of modified plan of operation (MPO) in 1977 (consequent upon malaria resurgence reaching its peak of annual incidence of 6.47 million cases in 1976), the annual incidence declined to 2.18 million cases in 1984. Since then annual malaria incidence has been contained between 2 to 3 million cases in spite of population growth, rapid and unplanned urbanization, developmental

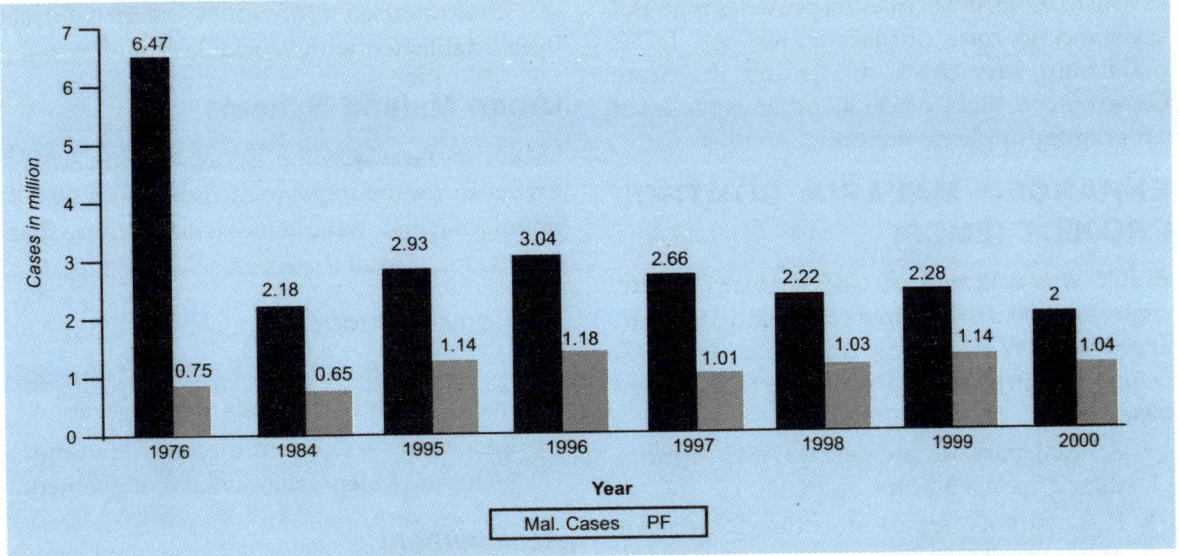

Fig. 25.5 : Malaria trend in India

activities, etc., that led to increased malariogenic potential in country. Coupled with escalation in cost of insecticides, vector resistance to conventional insecticides and drug resistance in parasite in some areas.

During the year 2000 there was decline of annual incidence of malaria by 12.37 per cent and decline in *Plasmodium falciparum* incidence (The malignant variety of malaria) by 9.13 per cent. The malaria specific mortality also declined by 7.25 per cent.

During 2001 a decline of 3.42 per cent of total malaria cases and 11.09 per cent in *P. falciparum* incidence has been reported as compared to the corresponding period of the year 2000.

Malaria has been a serious problem in North-Eastern states mainly due to :

• Topography and climatic conditions being congenial for perennial malaria transmission.
• Prevalence of highly effecient malaria vectors particularly *Anopheles minimus, Anopheles fluviatilis,* and *Anopheles dirus,* predominance of malignant variety of malaria parasite *i.e., P. falciparum,* and
• Drug (chloroquine) resistant *P. falciparum* in some areas.

These states contribute 8.5 to 11 per cent of total malaria cases reported and 13 to 15 per cent

of total malaria mortality cases in the country. Assam reports maximum cases of malaria followed by Arunachal Pradesh, Tripura and Meghalaya.

NATIONAL ANTIMALARIA PROGRAMME (NAMP)

This programme is operative in the country with central assistance with the following :

• Cent per cent central assistance to North-Eastern states that includes material, equipment and monetary assistance towards operational cost since 1994.
• Material assistance, *e.g.,* insecticides (DDT and synthetic pyrethroids), medicine and money assistance through distric malaria control society for malaria control in 1045 hard case tribal primary health centres of 100 districts of eight states, *e.g.,* Andhra Pradesh, Chhattisgarh, Gujarat, Jharkhand, Madhya Pradesh, Maharashtra, Orissa, Rajasthan, covered under Enhanced Malaria Control Project (EMCP) with World Bank assistance since 1997. Nineteen high-risk urban areas are also covered in EMCP for enhanced control support.

Fifty-fifty sharing cost between central and states in other malaria prone areas of the country in which Government of India provides material assistance in form of insecticides, *e.g.*, DDT, malathion, larvicides, drugs and the State Governments have to bear all other expenses of programme implementation.

ENHANCED MALARIA CONTROL PROJECT (EMCP)

EMCP was initiated in 1045 primary health centres of 100 districts in 8 states and 19 urban areas with World Bank assistance in 1997. Selection of primary health centres (PHC) were based on :

- Annual parasite incidence (API) of more than 2 for last 3 years.
- *P. falciparum* cases are more than 30 per cent of total malaria cases.
- 25 per cent or more population of PHC being tribal.
- Reported deaths due to malaria from PHCs.

Components

The main components strengthened under the project include :

- Early case detection and treatment
- Selective vector control and personal protection methods including insecticide treated mosquito nets
- Epidemic planning and rapid response
- Intersectorial co-ordination, institutional and management capabilities strengthening.

The project facilitated strengthening of surveillance including malaria microscopy and introduction of rapid diagnostic kits to ensure early case detection. Newer medicines like artemisinine derivatives have been introduced in the programme for management of severe and complicated malaria besides use of synthetic pyrethroids, biological control agents and insecticide treated mosquito nets. The project also facilitated capacity building for endemic preparedness and response and manpower development at various levels of programme implementation. Progress has been intensified for Information, Education and Communication (IEC) activities.

Computerised Information System (CIS) has been established with World Bank support.

Urban Malaria Scheme

Urban malaria scheme is functioning in 131 towns in the country with more than 40,000 population and malaria incidence of more than 2/1000 for at least three years.

Strategy Includes

- Early diagnosis and treatment through malaria clinics, hospitals, dispensaries
- Recurrent weekly antimalarial operations including bioenvironmental management.

Achievement

There was decline of 17.8 per cent in malaria cases and 52.47 per cent of *P. falciparum* incidence in 2000 as compared to 1999 in towns covered under urban malaria scheme. The declining trends were continuing during 2001.

LYMPHATIC FILARIA (ELEPHANTIASIS)

Lymphatic filaria is a common mosquito-borne disease transmitted by *Haemophagus arthropodes*, characterized by acute and chronic clinical manifestations like lymphadenitis, lymphangitis, filarial fever, elephantiasis of the genitals, legs or arms, hydrocele, etc. Though not fatal, the disease is responsible for considerable suffering and disability. The disease has been specified as lymphatic filariasis due to lymph node's involvement mainly, caused by helminthic worms inhibiting the lymphatics.

History

The word 'Filariasis' is derived from "Filar" which means "Threadlike". The name has been given to a group of diseases caused by specific nematodes belonging to filariadae family and transmitted by mosquito (*Haemophagus arthropodes*). Its existence in India is marked since 6th century.

Table 25.5 : History of Filariasis

1709	Clark in Cochin gave the name Malabar legs to filariasis.
1866	Wucherer in Brazil found microfilariae in chylous urine. Hence the name is given as *W. bancrofti*.
1872	Lewis working in Calcutta found micro-filariae in peripheral blood.
1876	Bancroft in Brisbane discovered adult female.
1878	Manson working in China discovered the development of *W. bancrofti in* 50 per cent mosquitoes. Filariasis was the first disease proved to be transmitted by insects.
1927	Bruge discovered the microfilariae by *B. malayi* in Indonesia.
1940	Rao and Maplestone discovered adult of *B. malayi* in India.
1946	Diethyl Carbamazine was discovered.
1955	National Filaria Control Programme was launched by the Government of India.

Worldwide Distribution of the Disease

Filaria is a worldwide major public health problem. Millions of people are already infected and many are at risk of getting the infection all over the world. Countries like African countries, Caribbeans, Latin Americas, Islands of Southern and Western Pacific Ocean, India, China, Indonesia, Malaysia, Korea, Philippines and Vietnam are affected by filaria.

It has been estimated that around 300 million people throughout the world are infected with *B. malayi* and *W. bancrofti* more than 1,100 million people live in endemic areas. Of these, two-thirds of the world's estimated infected people are found in China, India and Indonesia. Global burden of lymphatic filariasis – 2000 (Fig. 25.6).

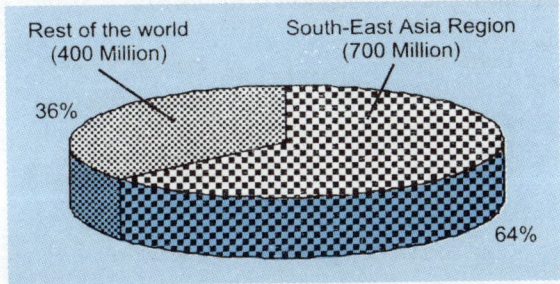

Fig. 25.6 : Total population at risk (1100 Million)

Problem in SEAR

Lymphatic filaria is one of the major public health problems in SEA Region. Except Bhutan and Domincan Public Republic Korea, the other countries are endemic with filaria, National Filaria Control Programmes are in operation in India, Indonesia, Mynmar, Sri Lanka and Thailand (Fig. 25.7).

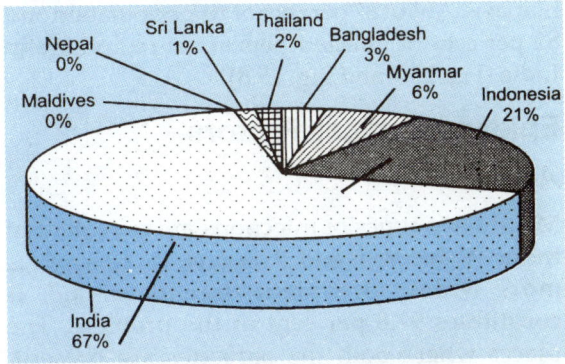

Fig. 25.7 : Filaria situation in SEA Region, 2000

It is estimated that about 700 million people are living in endemic area. Total global population of nearly 1.1 billion. People (64%) are at risk of developing the disease in the countries of SEAR. About 60 million are harbouring microfilariae or suffering from clinical manifestations of the disease, this represents about 50 per cent of global burden. All three lymphatic filaria parasites, *e.g.*, *Wuchereria bancrofti*, *Brugia malayi* and *Brugia timori* are prevalent in the region.

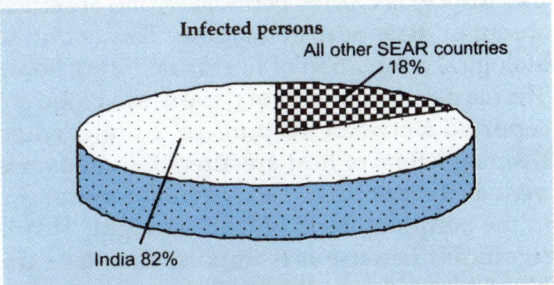

Fig. 25.8 : Filariasis situation in the SEAR and India, 2000

Problem In India

Filaria is a major public health problem in India, next to malaria among mosquito-borne diseases.

The disease is prevalent all over the states except Punjab, Haryana, Himachal Pradesh, Delhi, Meghalaya and Jammu & Kashmir. Severely infected areas are U.P., A.P., Bihar, Kerala, Orissa and Tamil Nadu. It has been estimated that at present 420 million people live in endemic areas, out of which two-third live in rural areas and one-third in urban areas. About 29 millions harbour microfilariae and 20 millions are suffering from filariasis. About 67 per cent of risk population and 82 per cent of infected persons in region are in India (Fig. 25.7 and Fig. 25.8).

Epidemiological Factors

Agent

Mainly two types of infections are prevalent in India. *W. bancrofti* and *B. malayi*. *W. bancrofti* is more widely prevalent than *B. malayi*. It constitutes 97.8 per cent of the problem. The places where both the parasites are present, mixed infection occurs.

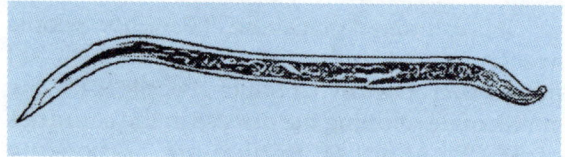

Fig. 25.9 : Microfilariae

Periodicity of the Diseases

The microfilariae (Fig. 25.9) of *W. bancrofti* and *B. malayi* appear in large number at night, hence they display nocturnal periodicity, and are either absent or disappear in daytime. This is due to biological adaptation of nocturnal biting habit. The maximum numbers of parasites in blood are reported between 10 p.m. to 2 a.m., when sleeping habits of host are altered and adverse periodicity is noticed. The microfilarae are seen in the periphary food of host at night. This is significant because it is important to take the blood smear during this period.

Life Cycle

The adult parasites are found in lymphatic system of human host. They give off larvae or microfilariae in the bloodstream of man. The mosquito cycle starts on ingestion of these microfilariae by bite of female mosquito. These microfilariae undergo three stages of development in mosquito alimentary canal. The final stage of larvae is active and may be found in any part of the mosquito. When it reaches the mouth of the mosquito, they are ready to transmit the infection to new host, under favourable climatic conditions. Hence the definite host is man. Intermediate host is mosquito.

Reservoir of Infection

The nematodes are transmitted from man to man through bite of infected mosquito. Infected persons with circulatory microfilariae in periphery blood are the reservoirs of infection. Most of the carriers are usually without any recognisable symptoms of illness. Those people, with advanced stage, may turn out to be negative for microfilariae.

Incubation Period

The incubation period is considered from the time interval from invasion of infective larvae to the development of clinical manifestations. This period is 10 to 12 months but can be as long as 16 months and even longer.

Mode of Transmission

The saliva of mosquito carrying Microfilariae (MF) is the mode of transmission from one person to another.

By bite of infected mosquito, it passes through the punctured skin and penetrates the skin on its own.

Filariasis is transmitted by bite of the infected mosquito (*Culex fatigans*) which carries the microfilariae and inserts into the human host through punctured skin (Fig. 25.10).

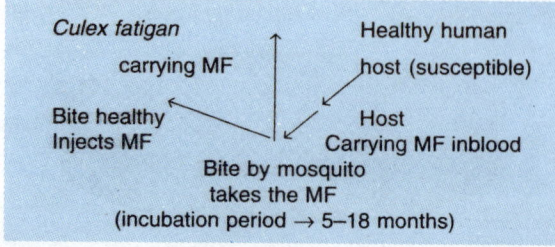

Fig. 25.10 : Mode of transmission of filariasis

Vectors of Filariasis

Mosquitoes are the only vectors of spread of all three types of parasites—*W. bancrofti*, *B. malayi* and *B. timori*.

Culex, Anopheles and Aedes

Vectors are the mosquitoes which serve as vector for *W. bancrofti*.

Mansonia Mosquito

Chief vector for *B. malayi* infection. The breeding for mansonia mosquito is associated with certain aquatic plants like Pistia plant. The mosquito breeding can be controlled by removing such plants.

Host Factors

Age and Sex

All ages and both sexes are susceptible to filariasis. More common among 20 to 30 years of age.

Migration of People

Movement of people has spread the infection from one place to another. Nonepidemic areas also harbour infection due to people who come from endemic areas like Kanpur, Andaman and Nicobar, etc.

Immunity

Person may develop immunity against infection after longer duration of exposure.

Social Factors

Illiteracy, poverty, industrialisation, urbanisation, people movement, etc. influence the causation of disease.

The swelling of the legs and other parts of the body causes suffering, disability and reduction in work capacity leading to social stigma for the patient.

Environmental Factors

Environment plays an important role in spread of infection. The *Culex fatigans* can survive in temperature 70° to 100°F with 70 per cent humidity. Filarial disease is associated with poor drainage system. The vectors breed in polluted water. The common breeding places are pounds, drains, septic tanks, open ditches, burrows, pits and soakage pits.

Climate

The parasites are more prevalent during hot climatic conditions. Rainy season influences the breeding.

Clinical Manifestation

The clinical manifestation can be classified as:

Stage of Invasion (Asymptomatic)

The infective larvae growing excess in the body undergo development. The triad of eosinophilia, lymphadenopathy and positive intradermal test and history of the residence in endemic areas, would probably be the best criteria to diagnose early filaria.

Symptomless or Carrier Phase

The person is harbouring the microfilariae in the blood but does not show any clinical symptoms. Hence, it is difficult to diagnose and they may spread further infection. Usually night blood may help in detecting the cases.

Stage of Acute Manifestation

The stages of acute manifestation are filarial fever, lymphangitis, lymphadenitis, elephantiasis of genitals, legs or arms and hydrocele in man. The lower extremities are affected more than upper extremities (Figs. 25.11 and 25.12).

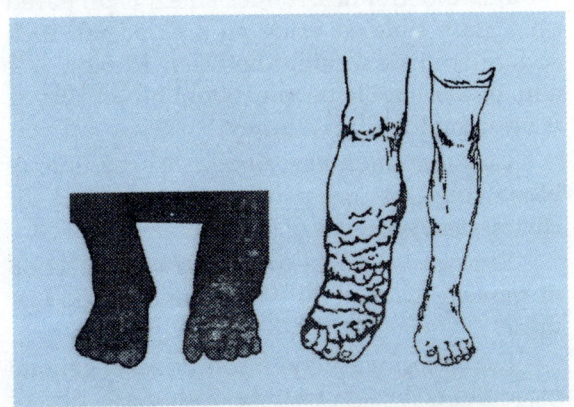

Fig. 25.11 : Elephantiasis of legs

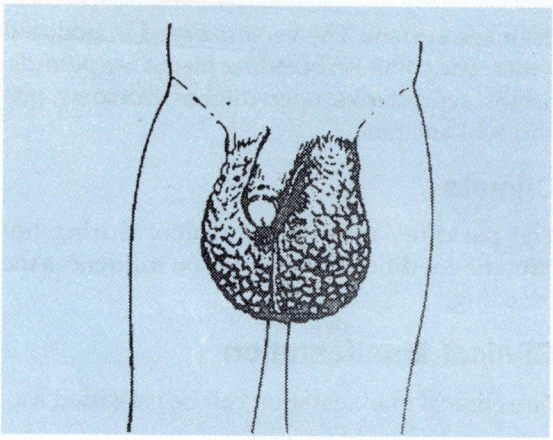

Fig. 25.12 : Elephantiasis of genitalia

Stage of Chronic Manifestation

Clinical features are elephantiasis of legs, arms, genitals, hydrocele which usually occur after 10 to 15 years of acute stage, due to fibrosis and obstruction of lymphated vessels causing permanent disability.

Filarial Survey

Filaria survey is essential to assess the prevalence of disease in a community. The sample for survey must be representative of the whole population covering all ages and both sexes. Sample can be obtained at random and statistical advice should be obtained. WHO Expert Committee Report on filariasis gives the following elements for survey.

Mass blood survey : Once the filaria cases are present in an area, a mass survey should be done for thick blood slides. A thick smear is prepared on a glass slide covering an area of half inch square or circle at night between 10 p.m. to 2 a.m. of susceptible people. Night blood survey is important in filaria survey.

Clinical manifestation survey : At the time of blood collection the people are examined for clinical manifestations of filariasis are recorded.

Serological test : The focus on direct detection of parasite antigens in the patient's blood or urine.

Entomological survey : It comprises of general mosquito collection from houses, dissection of female vector species for detection of develop-

mental stage of parasite, to study the extent and type of breeding places of mosquitoes. The data is compiled to express in certain parameters like clinical parasitological and entomological survey.

ASSESSMENT OF FILARIA CONTROL PROGRAMME

Filaria control is necessary to evaluate for further action. The effects of filaria control can be assessed by using clinical parasitological and entomological methods given below :

Clinical Parameters

These parameters are incidences of acute menifestations, *e.g.*, lymphoedema elephantiasis, hydrocele, chyluria etc.

Parasitological Parameters

Microfilarial Rate

The percentage of persons showing MF in the peripheral blood (20 cu.mm) in the sample population. One slide taken from each person specifies the species of parasite.

Filarial Endemiaty Rate

The percentage of people examined showing MF in their blood, or disease manifestation or both.

Microfilarial Density

The number of MF per unit volume (20 cu.mm) of blood in samples from individual persons. It indicates the intensity of infection.

Average Infestation Rate

The average number of MF per positive slide, each slide being made from 20 cu.mm of blood. It indicates the prevalence of microfilaraemia in the population.

Entomological Parameters

These comprise :

(*a*) vector density per 10 man per hour catch,

(*b*) percentage of mosquitoes positive for all developmental stages,

(*c*) percentage of mosquitoes positive for infective larval (stage III),

(d) annual biting rate,

(e) types of larvae breading places etc.

These parameters help to measure the conditions existing before and after control measures start to assess the progress of control campaign against vector as routine.

Filaria Control Measures

Different strategies need to incorporate to control the spread of filaria, since the mode of transmission is being mosquito and integrated approach is needed to control the diesease. Filaria can be controlled by mosquito control and chemoprophylaxis treatment in the endemic areas. The current strategy of filariasis control is based on :

1. Chemotherapy
2. Vector control measures.

Chemotherapy

Diethyl carbamazine (DEC) is the only effective and safe drug against filarial parasite. It kills microfilariae and reduces the parasite density in the blood of host and prevents further spread of infection.

The total dosage recommended by WHO Expert Committee in 1974 is 72 mg of DEC per kg body weight for *W. Bancrofti* filariasis and 30 to 40 mg per kg body weight for *B. malayi* infection. DEC is most generally accepted as 6 mg/kg body weight daily in divided doses after meals. DEC is rapidly absorbed after oral administration, reading peak blood level in 1 to 2 hours. DEC causes rapid disappearance of MF from the blood and is effective in killing MF. The effect of drug on the adult parasite is uncertain, probably no effect on infective stage larvae.

Toxic Reaction

DEC may produce two kinds of reactions :

(a) Due to drug, *e.g.*, headache, nausea, vomiting dizziness etc. These effects may be seen after few hours of first dose of DEC and usually do not last for more than three days.

(b) Allergic reactions due to destruction of microfilarial and adult worms, *e.g.*, fever, local inflammation around dead worms, orchitis, lymphadenitis, lymphoedema and hydrocele.

These reactions disappear spontaneously and interuption of treatment is not necessary.

Filarial Control in the Community

Filaria does not cause explosive epidemic because:

1. The parasite does not multiply in the insect vector
2. The infective larvae do not multiply in the human host
3. The life cycle of the parasite is relatively longer. These are favourable factors for successful control of filaria.

Chemoprophylaxis

DEC is effective drug used as chemoprophylaxis as well as chemotherapeutic for control of filaria DEC can be administred in various ways :

Mass Drug Therapy

DEC is used in highly endemic areas. DEC is given to almost everyone in the community irrespective of harbouring the MF or not, menifesting the clinical symptoms or no sign of infection. The drug should be taken by 80 per cent of the population in endemic areas to control the further spread of infection. Mass treatment control projects using DEC have markedly reduced the prevalence of *W. bancrofti* in many of the pacific islands, whereas the results of mass chemotherapy in India in 1960 had shown little success, due to floor population compliance. For successful mass chemotherapy community participation is essential requiste; which can be done by intensive health education to public to ensure their co-operation.

Selective Treatment

The treatment (DEC) is given to infective people only, may be more effective in the areas of low endemicity of disease. The strategy is based on detection and treatment of filaria cases and human carriers. The recommended doses is 6 mg DEC per kg. body weight daily for 12 days and to be completed in twelve weeks. Dosing once a week or once a month has also been recommended but it is practically difficult. In endemic areas treatment must be repeated at specific intervals, usually every two years, because MF clearance with DEC is usually incomplete even after adequate treatment and also people living in endemic areas are susceptible to reinfection.

DEC Medicated Salt

The DEC medicated salt is a strategy of mass treatment using very low doses of DEC for a long period of time. The common salt medicated with 1 to 4 gm of diethyl carbamazine (DEC) per kg has been recommended for filaria control in endemic areas of *W. bancrofti* and *B. malayi*, particularly after an initial reduction in prevalence has been achieved by mass or selective treatment of MF. carriers. Treatment should be continued for at least 6 to 9 months.

Ivermectin

Ivermectin is a broad spectrum antibiotic ectoparasites. Studies have shown that ivermectin 20 to 400 μg/kg body weight, single dose were effective in completely destroying MF in blood in all cases within weeks, but within three weeks the infection recurred in most patients.

There is no drug toxicity, but there may be reactions due to inflammatory response triggered by dying of Microfilariae.

Vector Control Measures

Filaria can be controlled by mosquito control particularly in the areas where mass treatment by diethyl carbamazine is not feasible in population to reduce the transmission of MF, which can be done by vector measures involved in the prevention of breeding of mosquitoes by closing the open drainage and providing the underground waste water disposal system. This may not be possible because of financial involvement. But other temporary methods may be adopted for this, which includes.

- Antilarval measures
- Anti-adult measures.

Antilarval Measures

These measures should include the elimination of breeding places by providing adequate sanitations and underground waste water disposal system which may not be feasible in developing countries, hence it must have some temporary or recurrent alternative. The other activities may include the followings :

Chemical control measures

- *Mosquito larvicidal oil :* Mosquito larvicidal oil (MLO) is an effective measure against pre-adult stage. It has been proved to be less effective and more expensive than other chemical preparations, therefore has been replaced by pyrethrum oil, haemephos and fenthion.
- *Pyrosene oil :* This is pyrethrum based emulsifiable larvicide. The emulsion concentrate contains 0.1 to 0.2 per cent pyrethrins by weight and is diluted in water in the ratio of 1 : 4.
- *Organophosphorus larvicides :* Organophosphorus larvicides like haemophos, fenthion have been widely used with successful results. However, mosquitoes have developed resistance to these larvicides. The frequency of application is once a week in all breeding areas.

Removal of pistia plant: Mosquito breeding can also be controlled by removing the pistia plant from the water collection areas.

In case of Mansonia mosquitoes, breeding is best controlled by removing the supporting aquatic vegetation such as pistia plant from water collections and converting the ponds to fish or lotus culture. Certain herbicides, *e.g.*, phenoxylene may be used to destroy aquatic vegetations.

Engineering Measures

These are very effective measures by filling up of ditches, avoid water being stagnant. Proper maintenance of water tanks and soakage pits may help in control of mosquito breed.

Anti-adult Measures

The mosquitoes have become resistant to DDT, HCH and dieldrin, thus it has become difficult to kill the adult mosquito. Application of malathion has been effectively used recently to kill mosquito.

Social Measures

Avoiding the bite of mosquito by protecting with mosquito nets, repellents and adequate clothes, etc.

Periodical night blood examination for people living in endemic areas. If positive for microfilariae, they should take diethyle carbamazine.

Surveillance of endemic areas for follow-up of the known cases and carriers to prevent the spread of infection.

Prevention of mosquito breeding places nearby areas of human dwellings.

Health education to motivate people to participate in all antifilarial activities.

Integrated Approach

No single control measure is likely to control the spread of disease. An integrated approach is needed to control filaria using all possible strategies and measure to bring optimum results.

Primary Health Care Approach

The primary health care at grassroot level in endemic areas to control filaria is essential. Single dose of DEC is very effective even two years after treatment. A combination of DEC and ivermectin have proved to be equally effective by reducing the microfilaraemia more than 95 per cent, two years after treatment. Intensive local hygiene on affected limbs, with or without the use of antiseptic lotions have shown dramatic effect in reducing the disability. Finally there have been development of insecticide sprays and polystyrene beads to seal laterines and storage tanks to reduce the population of culex mosquitoes.

NATIONAL FILARIA CONTROL PROGRAMME

Filaria is a major public health problem. About 420 million people living in the endemic areas are exposed to the risk of infection and 19 million people already carry the infection. 25 million people have microfilarial in the blood.

National Filaria Control Programme started in 1955 to undertake the following measures in the programme :

- Delimitation of the problem in hitherto unsurveyed areas.
- Control measures for urban areas through recurrent antiparasitic measures by control units and clinics giving treatment with diethyle carbamazine (DEC) to clinical cases and microfilariae carriers.

- Number of microfilaria (MF) carriers and disease cases detected during last four years by control units and filaria clinics.

So far, 238 out of 300 districts in endemic areas have been surveyed and 175 have been found to be endemic for filaria.

Filaria Day

During 1997, in view of the recommendation made in support of revised single day DEC mass therapy as a supplement to existing National Filaria Control Programme (NFCP) strategy in highly endemic areas, it was proposed to implement the strategy in 13 districts on pilot basis. However, eight districts were covered in the states of Kerala, Orissa, U.P., West Bengal during November 1997. Approximately 49.7 to 94 per cent coverage (achievement) was observed in these districts by giving eight day DEC therapy. Filaria day observance is a continuing five years project implemented by the states in high endemic districts.

DENGUE FEVER AND DENGUE HAEMORRHAGIC FEVER

Dengue fever is a viral disease which is transmitted through the bite of female *Aedes* mosquito. Dengue viral infection may remain asymptomatic or manifest either as undifferentiated febrile illness (viral syndrome). The primary infection leads to classical dengue fever for that particular serotype. Subsequent fever by any other serotype may sometimes precipitate dengu haemorrhagic fever (DHF) which is usually more prevalent among children and may cause fatality in some cases.

Dengue fever and dengue haemorrhagic fever (DHF) are caused by four antigenitically related but distinct dengue arbovirus serotypes (DEN 1, 2, 3 and 4) types. Dengue viruses are transmitted by *Aedes* mosquitoes of subgenus stegomyia with *Aedes aegypti* is the major vector.

Worldwide Distribution of the Disease

Dengue is a disease of tropics and is one of the most emerging disease affecting nearly half of the world's population. It is estimated that there are between 50 to 100 million cases of dengue fever and about 5 lakh cases of dengue

haemorrhagic fever which require hospitalisation every year. Dengue affects more than
100 countries in the world except Europe and is
rapidly spreading in many areas. In 1995, the
worst dengue epidemic in Latin America and
the Caribbeans for 15 years struck at least
14 countries causing more than 2 lakh cases of
dengue fever and almost 6000 cases of dengue
haemorrhagic fever.

Dengue epidemic is increasing due to
urbanisation, overcrowding, poor housing
conditions, poor environmental sanitation and
increasing slums (Fig. 25.13).

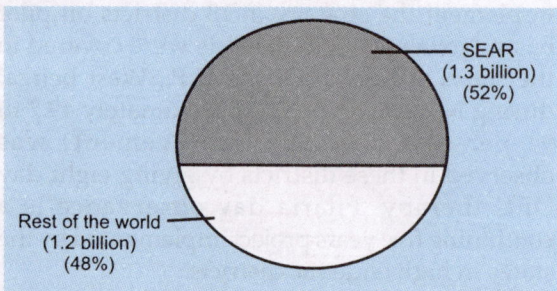

Fig. 25.13 : Population at risk of dengue fever/
dengue haemorrhagic fever, 2000

South-East Asia Region

In 1950, Thailand was the first country in South-
East Asia Region to experience a dengue fever
epidemic.

1997, most countries in the region, especially
India, Indonesia, Myanmar, Sri Lanka and

Thailand had experienced large outbreaks.
Currently dengue fever/dengue haemorrhagic
fever is endemic in seven countries of the region
(Bangladesh, India, Indonesia, Maldives,
Myanmar, Sri Lanka and Thailand) and 1.3
billion people live in endemic area are at risk of
infection. Dengue is a notifiable disease in
Indonesia, Myanmar, Sri Lanka and Thailand.

Causes for Epidemic in SEAR

The causes for epidemic in South-East Asian
Reginos are as follows :

*   Unprecedented human population growth.
*   Unplanned and uncontrolled urbanisation.
*   Inadequate waste management and water
    supply.
*   Lack of effective mosquito control.
*   Increased spread of dengue viruses.

Problem in India

In India first recorded outbreak of dengue fever
was in 1812. Serological survey was first carried
out in 1952, showing DEN_1 and DEN_2 were
widely spread. Further outbreaks occured in
1967, 1970, 1982. An explosive outbreak of
dangue haemorrhagic fever in Delhi in October
1996 with 10,000 cases and 400 deaths reported
isolation of DEN_2 from serum samples, whereas
in other states and UTs only 3,064 dangue
haemorrhagic fever cases and 60 deaths were
reported (Fig. 25.14).

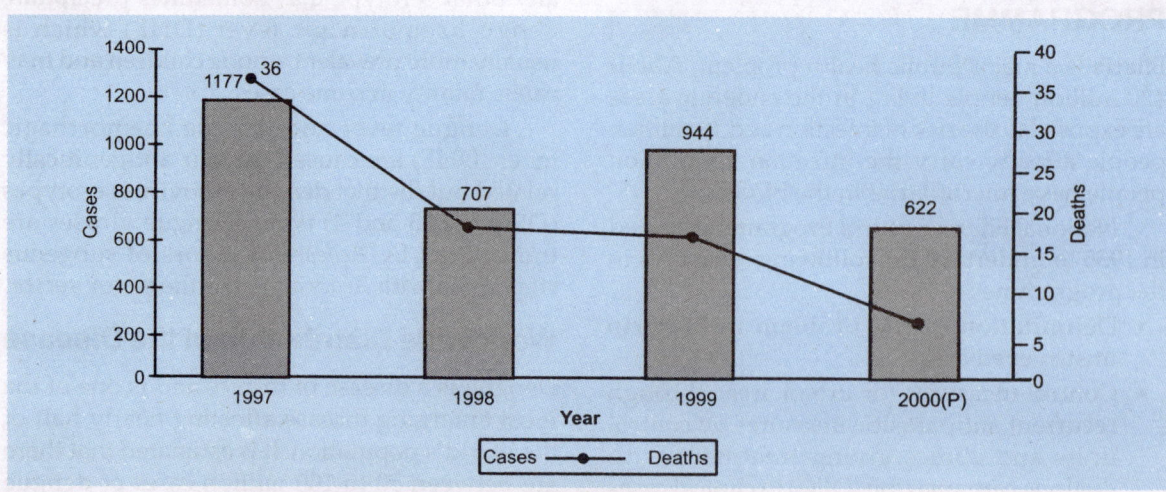

Fig. 25.14 : Dengue/Dengue haemorrhagtic fever in India

Dengue/dangue haemorrhagic fever has been reported from 15 states/Union Territories since 1996. Total numbers of 12,750 cases and 217 deaths were reported in the country during 2003, however, 203 cases and 2 deaths have been reported up to March 2004.

Dengue haemorrhage fever is a severe form of dengue fever, caused by infection with more than one dengue virus. The serious illness is probably due to double infection with dengue viruses.

Clinical Manifestation

The patient will have sudden rise of temperature, haemorrhagic condition, *e.g.*, purpura, ectostosis, epistaxis, gum bleeding, haematemesis and/or melaena, enlarged liver.

Stages of Severity of Illness

- Fever with acute onset, continuous and lasts for 2 to 7 days, unless bleeding indicates dangue haemorrhagic fever.
- Frequent bleeding disorders in the skin and other organs through different parts of the body.
- Cardiac failure menifested by slow, rapid and weak pulse, hypotension with the cold and clammy skin and restlessness.
- Patient undergoes shock with undetectable blood pressure and pulse.

Investigations

The blood examination confirms the clinical diagnosis.

- *Haemoconcentration :* Haematocrit increased by 20 per cent or more of baseline value.
- Thrombocytopenia (100,000 mm^3 or less).

The patient might undergo the stage of shock due to loss of blood.

Treatment

Usually symptomatic and supportive treatment is recommended.

- Antipyretics are perscribed to reduce high fever. Aspirin should be avoided, since it may cause gastric irritability, bleeding and acidosis.

- *Plasma supplementation :* Due to blood loss, the plasma replacement can be given as per requirement.
- Intravenous fluid therapy should be continued for at least 12 to 24 hours. Isotonic type of fluid can be infused.
- Haematocrit should be determined every 6 to 8 hours, vital signs should be recorded frequently to assess the general condition and adjust the fluid replacement. Over-rehydration should be carefully examined because excessive fluid may cause respiratory distress due to pleural effusion ascites, pulmonary congestion and oedema.

The type of fluid used may be five per cent dextrose in Ringer lactate or five per cent dextrose in normal saline.

Management of Shock

The patient may get shock due to loss of blood and hyperpyrexia. Replacement of fluid and plasma is the immediate management of patient with shock. Replacement of plasma loss with isotonic solution of five per cent dextrose in Ringer solution or 5 per cent dextrose in normal saline at the rate of 10 to 20 mL/kg body weight per hour can be given. Blood transfusion is recommended in serious conditions, when condition of the patient improves the I.V. fluid replacement is reduced subsequently. Children should be given 5 per cent dextrose in half strength normal saline (5% dextrose in ½ NSS) when vital signs are stable, I.V. fluid should be discontinued. Urine output improves and the patient feels good appetite, shows the sign of improvement.

Nursing Care of the Dengue Haemorrhagic Fever Patient

- *Complete bed rest :* The patient must be given complete bed rest during acute febrile condition.
- *Cold sponging :* The high temperature can be reduced by cold sponging, along with antipyretics.
- Oral fluids and electrolyte can be given to the patients with excessive sweating, vomiting or diarrhoea.

- Precautions must be taken during I.V. infusion or blood transfusions and while discontinuing the fluids.
- Frequent vital signs recording is essential especially when the patient is in shock.
- Reassurance and psychological support.

Prevention and Control

Dengue fever and dangue haemorrhagic fever, a viral infection, is widely prevalent in India and all the four serotypes are found. Since 1996 NAMP has been monitoring dangue fever/dangue haemorrhagic fever situation in India.

There has been decline in dangue fever/dangue haemorrhagic fever incidence after 1996 outbreak in Delhi. During 2001, outbreaks had been reported from Rajasthan, Tamil Nadu, Karnataka, and Gujarat.

Strategy for prevention and control of dangue fever/dangue haemorrhagic fever includes :

- Surveillance for disease and vectors.
- Early diagnosis and prompt case management.

- Vector control through community participation and social mobilization.
- Capacity building.

There is no separate programme for prevention and control of dangue fever/dangue haemorrhagic fever and states tackle the problem with their own resources. Need based assistance is being provided for outbreak containment within resources available under National anti-malaria Programme (NAMP).

- Dengue fever and DHF can be prevented by :
  ➤ Protection from mosquito bite control.
  ➤ Mosquito breeding places, *e.g.*, stagnant water collection should be avoided and keeping the surroundings clean.
  ➤ Antilarvae and antiadult measures.
- *Vaccine :* No affective vaccine is available to prevent dangue fever or dangue haemorrhagic fever.
- *Isolation :* May be helpful in preventing, the spread of infection. The case of dangue fever can be kept under nets to avoid bite and spread of disease.

●●●

Zoonotic Diseases

6

INTRODUCTION

Zoonotic disease includes the two types of diseases namely rabies by dog, monkey biting and plague by rat killing.

RABIES (HYDROPHOBIA)

Rabies is an acute viral disease that primarily affects animals, but is occasionally transmitted to human beings invariably as a result of a rabid animal (dog, monkey) bite. Clinically the disease is characterised by a variable incubation period, an acute neurological illness, progressing to coma in 4 to 10 days, and complications that interfere with neurological, pulmonary and cardiovascular functions.

History

Rabies was first recognised by Aristotle in 335 B.C. who mentioned that the disease was spread by a rabid dog. Pasteur showed that rabies virus could be modified by passage in animal brains and inactivated by drying. His studies were helpful in development of antirabies vaccine in 1885.

Geographical Distribution

Rabies is an almost invariably fatal viral disease transmitted to human through animal bite, the most common animal being dog.

Dogs cause the majority of human rabies except in the place where effective dog Rabies Control Programme is existing. Rabies is a worldwide zoonotic disease. Some countries are free from rabies and few have eradicated the disease. According to the WHO experts, in many countries, rabies is spreading in spite of various preventive and control measures.

In India, few Union Territories like Lakshadeep and Andaman and Nicobar Islands are free from the disease (no indigenous case of rabies has occurred in man or animal species for the last two years). Three million people in the country receive antirabies prophylaxis every year. The incidence among animals is higher than humans.

India has an estimated dog population of 25 million. Most of these dogs are unprotected against rabies. Studies conducted by National Institute of Communicables Diseases (NICD) Delhi, gave a projection of annual incidence of 2.12 million animal bites and estimated that 30,000 people die of rabies annually. India produces nerve tissue culture vaccine and about 3.25 million doses are consumed, offering protection to 0.65 million people against rabies.

Epidemiology of Disease

Agent

The disease is caused by rabies virus named Lassa virus type I which belongs to a group of Rhabdoviridae and is a neurotrophic virus. Rhabdovirus is called neurotrophic virus because it affects the nerve cells of the brain and spinal cord.

Rabies virus maintains a zoonotic cycle involving wild or domestic carnivores. In the absence of effective control measures, the virus is endemic in dogs, passes from dog to dog by bite. Although most mammals are susceptible to infection, the virus is known to be enzootic in a few wild animal species.

Virus is excreted in the saliva of affected animals. It multiplies in salivary glands, secretory glands, corneal cells, kidney, muscles and lungs. The virus can be inactivated by heat,

337

sunlight, formalin, phenol and other disinfectants.

Mode of Transmission

Man is exposed to rabies by bite from rabid domestic or wild animal. The saliva of the dog must contain virus at the time of bite to cause the disease. Small number of nonbite human rabies cases have been associated with the exposure to environments that contain rabies virus in higher concentration (hot breath of rabid wolf).

Man-to-man transmission, although rare, is possible. The transmission by child bite to breasts, by corneal and organ transplantation has also been reported.

Dogs secrete rabies virus in their saliva up to five days before their death. The risk of developing human clinical rabies depends upon a variety of factors including the site and severity of bite and species of the animal biting. These differences are related to the quality of virus inoculated in the number of nerve fibres in various parts of the body.

Healthy animals may secrete rabies virus in their saliva and such animals are sometimes called as "rabies carriers". These animals will develop clinical rabies in almost all cases within a short period of time, depending upon species like three days for dogs, two days for rats and several months for bats. The short period of secretion found in dog and cat is the basis for quarantine of these animals after a bite. If animal remains normal within ten days of bite and does not die, it is not considered as risk of developing rabies, even if the dog develops rabies.

Immunity

Natural immunity is developed in many species of animals including human beings. Serological immunity develops after natural exposure in both men and animals and may be used to diagnose both clinical disease and animals recovered from rabies. In man, the antibodies are first detected in serum 8 to 10 days after onset of symptoms (unless prior vaccine has been given). Serum antibodies rise rapidly to high levels, remain elevated (if recovery occurs) for months or years.

Host Factors

All warm blooded animals including man are susceptible to rabies. Rabies in man is a fatal disease, though risk of infection and complications depend upon the amount of infection in the body and site and severity of bite.

Incubation period may be as short as ten days or as long as one year or more. It has also been seen as long as 19 years. More than 90 per cent cases develop between 20 to 90 days after exposure.

Clinical Manifestations

The prodromal symptoms consist of fever, malaise, headache, sore throat, sometimes cough and abdominal pain. The prodromal symptoms usually last for 2 to 4 days and are followed by neurological symptoms like aseptic meningitis, encephalitis and cranial or peripheral neuropathies. Cerbrospirnal fluid (CSF), at this stage, does not reveal any abnormality. The acute neurological phase is accompanied by hyperactivity, excitability, and hydrophobia increased salivation. The patient may have pharyngeal spasm followed by generalised hypertonic activity.

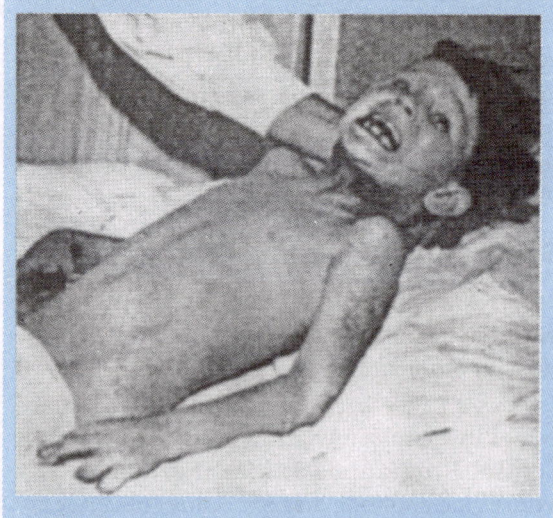

Fig. 26.1 : Rabid child with hydrophobia

Paralytic signs may develop during the acute neurological stage. Paralysis may be maximal in the bitten extremity. The temperature ranges from 100 to 104°F. The acute neurological stages last for 2 to 7 days and ends with the onset of coma. In coma, variety of complications can develop, *e.g.*, irregular respiration, hypoventillation and respiratory arrest, cardiac arrythmia, most commonly atrial premature contractions and sinus bradycardia precipitated by hypoxia or external stimulus. Increased intracranial presence has been reported and hypothermia, hypotension and gastrointestinal bleeding are common during coma.

Management

There is no specific treatment for the patient. The patient should be kept in a quiet room protected from external stimuli such as bright light, noise, or cold draught which may precipitate convulsions. Relieve anxiety and pain by sedatives.

Nursing Care

Careful nursing care is essential because patients are potentially infectious. The patient should be isolated and mask, gown and gloves should be worn by all persons contacting him. Strict concurrent and terminal disinfection of all articles contaminated by the patient is necessary, though there are not much cases found from human to human.

Prevention and Control

It is the most important and significant from public health viewpoint. Prevention of spread is by control of the disease among domestic animals. That is done by active vaccination of animals. Both killed virus and modified live virus are available for animal use, but live vaccine may cause clinical rabies in some animals, and should not be used for approved species.

Rabies can be prevented among high-risk groups, like veterinarians, animal handlers, or laboratory workers; by immunization before exposure.

Rabies may be controlled by interrupting the chain of transmission at any situation of the arrow indicating, *e.g.*, The wild animal bite can be prevented by domestic animals. Man should prevent getting bitten by animals or by infected

host (man). The infection may also spread from dead infected man, etc. The prevention should be as in Fig. 26.2.

```
                    at (1) ↓   Point
Rabid domestic animal⇐Rabid wild animal
  →Exposed host← usually carry the virus
        (2)   (Man)   (3)
              (4) ↓
      Infected case (Rabid patient)
              (5) ↓
           Rabid man
              (6) ↓
           Dead man
```

Fig. 26.2 : Prevention and control of rabies

The important aspect of control is to prevent the spread of rabies in domestic animals by active immunization and elimination of the stray dogs.

High-risk groups like veterinarians, animal handlers or laboratory workers can be given immunization before exposure. The vaccine with fewer side effects such as duck embryo rabies should be used with three doses of one week interval and booster after three months.

Post-exposure prophylaxis :
- Local wound care
- Active vaccination
- Most situation passive immunization.

Wound Care

The wound should receive prompt and thorough cleaning with soap and water. After rinsing, wound should be scrubbed with an antiseptic lotion; either alcohol, tincture or 0.01 per cent aqueous solution of iodine.

Such local care alone has shown significantly reducing the risk of rabies. Leaving the wound unsutured decreases the risk of rabies and is recommended when practical (may be 24–48 hours) and with minimum stitches. Prophylaxis against tetanus should be done by administering Tetanus Toxoid.

Post-exposure Immunization

The first antirabies vaccine was discovered by Pasteur in 1883, though many new vaccines have been developed in recent years.

Antirabies vaccine is the only vaccine given after exposure to infection. The ARV helps to produce the immunity in infected man and antibodies are produced within 5 to 10 days of ARV before incubation period which protects the person from getting rabies.

Indications for Antirabies Vaccine

Antirabies vaccine should be given to the person when :

- Dog or animal cannot be located.
- Animal dies within ten days of bite.
- Laboratory examination shows that the brain cells of biting animals are positive for rabies.
- All bites by any wild animal.

Antirabies Vaccines

Duck embryo vaccine : The vaccine is prepared from duck-embryo. The vaccine helps to eliminate the neurological problems. Though the neurological hazards have been seen to be reduced, but there are chances of allergic reaction to the lesion. Therefore, the vaccine is not recommended for these.

Nervous tissue vaccine : The schedule and doses of vaccine depends upon the degree of rabies risk due to which person is exposed, whether slight, moderate or severly bitten.

Dosage for children is 2 mL and adult 5 mL usually daily for 7 to 14 days.

Site of Administration

The ideal site is anterior abdominal wall, because of enough space for large dosage of vaccine to be injected. It is given deep subcutaneously by folding the skin between two fingers. The area is divided into quadrants and different sites are selected for daily injection. Aseptic techniques should be maintained to avoid other infections and complications.

Human diploid cell : One mL of vaccine is given intramuscularly in six dosages on the day of bite — 0 day, 3, 7, 14 and 30 days — and booster dose is given after 90 days, on the gluteal muscles. These vaccines are more effective, convenient and safe with no serious side effects. Since these vaccines are very costly, each dose costing Rs. 300, these cannot be administered to a large population. Hence nervous tissue vaccines are still practised for the people who cannot afford human diploid cell (HDC) vaccine.

PLAGUE

Plague is an acute infectious disease caused by *Yersinia pestis*, the plague bacillus is essentially a disease of rodents and their fleas. Plague is primarily and basically a zoonotic disease and transmitted by infected flea. People get infection when bitten by an infected flea and handling the infective material as well as by airborne droplets from pneumonic variety of plague. Plague may appear as an epidemic (*e.g.*, Surat) or sporadically in the community.

History

Plague is an ancient disease known as *Mahamari* (the great death). Plague has been described in Christian's Holy Book Bible and Hindu's Holy Book Bhagwat Puran. It has been mentioned that as soon as rats die in homes the cleanliness must be done to prevent plague.

First plague epidemic took place in the year 542 with 100 million deaths. Second, in the year 1346 lasted for three centuries and claimed 25 million lives and third in 1894 continued till 1930. The danger still exists that plague may spread over into human population, as it appeared in India in 1994 after 28 years.

The sudden reappearance of human plague in India in 1994, caused global concern. It created a sense of panic, both within and outside the country and led to the imposition of unwarranted trade and travel restrictions by several countries. There is need to be vigilant since the natural foci of infectious plague exist in India, Indonesia, Myanmar and possibly Nepal.

Worldwide Problem

The plague had been one of the major public health problem in the world, taking heavy toll of human lives. At present the global fatality rate is 9 per cent, ranging from 14 per cent in Africa and 6 per cent in America. The high rate persists instead of availability of effective preventive and control measures and treatment against the disease. Some countries in America, Asia and Africa report the cases every year. Cases also occur in areas which are free from infection for many years. Peru experienced a major epidemic of plague in 1984, 1990 and in 1992.

Natural foci of plague in South-East Asia exist in India, Indonesia, Myanmar and Nepal. Hence, there is need for vigilance about this disease. There are no reports of plague in recent past from Bangladesh, Bhutan, DPR Korea or Maldives. The last case of plague is recorded in Sri Lanka in 1938, Thailand in 1952, Nepal in 1968 and in India and Myanmar in 1994. In Myanmar during 1994, six bubonic plague cases with no deaths were reported. Spread of disease was prevented by the inplementation of early treatment and prompt control measures.

Problem in India

Plague was a serious public health problem in India. The sudden outbreak of human plague in India caused a global concern. Bubonic cases in the Beed district of Maharashtra and pneumonic cases in the city of Surat in Gujarat were seen.

A total of 4780 suspected clinical cases, 167 presumptive (seropositive) cases and 54 deaths due to plague were reported between 19 September and 22 October 1994. Outbreak of Surat created local panic and international concern. Effective measures taken by India brought Surat outbreak rapidly under control and the disease did not spread to other states of the country and other countries. However, the economic loss suffered by India during this outbreak was estimated to be 1.75 billion US dollars.

The first recorded outbreak of plague in India appeared in 1032, 1325 and 1403. In the year 1617, it was reported during Mughal emperor Jahangir's rule from Punjab, Ahmedabad, Surat and Deccan. In 1895, it appeared as pendemic in Calcutta and Bombay and spread all over country. Plague reached its peak in India in 1907 and continued till 1918. It was considered a major health problem till 1950, then it declined due to application of DDT for malaria control. Uttar Pradesh and Madhya Pradesh which were major areas for plague became plague free in 1950s and 1960s. The last reported case was seen in 1966 and there was no laboratory confirmed case of human plague in India, till it appeared in 1994, when four persons tested positive for bubonic plague and pnemonic in Surat. Cases were also reported in other states of the country, e.g., Mumbai, Kolkata, and Delhi, etc.

Epidemiological Factors

Agent Factor

Pestis is a Gram-negative, nonmotile, coccobacillus, occur in abundance in blood, liver, spleen and other organs of the infected man. In case of pneumonic plague, the bacilli appear in sputum of the patient. The coccobacilli produce exotoxins and endotoxins and spreads over the patient's bloodstream. The bacilli can live and multiply in soil under favourable conditions.

Host Factor

Age and sex : All ages and both sexes can get the disease.

Migration of people : The mobility from one place to another, has the possibility to spread the infection.

Other associated activities, e.g., outdoor movement and activities, e.g., hunting, cultivation harvesting and construction have the opportunities to harbour due to flea man contact.

Environmental Factor

The occurance of disease is associated with climatic changes, which usually appears in September till May. It does not appear in very hot season. In Southern India there is no specific time period of plague, the disease is found active throughout the year due to favourable climatic conditions, for breeding of the field rodents.

Source of Infection

Wild rodents, e.g., field mice, shunks and gabrils are the main reservoir of plague infections. They are found in cultivating fields, deserts, mountains and forests in tropical regions. In India Tatera Indica is the main reservior and not the domestic rat (rattus rattus). The disease is spread by wild rodents and not domestic. These rodents carry the flea which carry *Y. Pestis.*

Vectors of Plague

Rat flea present on wild animals are the carrier of infection. The most common vector for spread of disease is *X. cheopis* and others also transmit *e.g., X. astia, X. brasiliansis* and *P. irritans.* Both the sexes bite and transmit the infection.

Rodents of Plague

Rodents play an important role in spread of infection. Around 200 species of rodents are found to be associated in causation of disease. These rodents may be classified as :

Wild rodents : Main reservoir of plague. The common rodents in India are *Tatera indica, Bandicota bengalensis varius, B.B. Kok. B. indica, M. meltada, M. gleadowi* and *M. booduga.* Though *Tatera indica* is the main source of infection in India.

Commonest rodents : These rodents live close to man, these may be domestic and semi-domestic. Domestic which live in houses like rattus rattus, rattus norvegicus and musculus. The semi-domestic live in the fields or houses, *e.g., R. norvegicus* in sewer drains and the fields.

Mode of Transmission

The spread of infection is very slow from burrow to burrow and field to field taking months to cover vast fields. In this process they infect the house rodents and fleas are present on the household rats from field rodents. The household rodents (rat) die and flea leave the dead body of rat and seek food from man and spread the infection in man by biting.

In case of pneumonic plague the infection is spread through respiratory tract by droplet infection from case.

Types of Plague

Bubonic Plague

The most common disease in man. The rat flea bite the lower exterimities of the man and infect the organisms into the body. They enter the bloodstream and reach the lymphatic system and patient complains of headache, high temperature with chills and rigors, involvements of lymph glands causing infection. The patient has enlarged lymph nodes of axilla, neck and groin, etc. It does not spread by direct man to man contact.

Pneumonic Plague

Pneumonic plague spreads from man to man, by direct droplet infection and is highly infectious. It usually occurs with complication of bubonic plague, when the bacilli enter the lungs and plague bacilli are present in the septum. The incidence is usually below 1 per cent.

Septicaemic Plague

The septicaemic plague is complication of bubonic infection. The infection spreads in the blood and causes septicaemia. Primary septicaemia is rare which occurs from laboratory infection mainly to health personnel.

Prevention and Control of Plague

Protection of Cases

Early diagnosis and treatment of cases : Plague can be diagnosed by blood culture and the clinical manifestations and treatment must be started without waiting for confirmation of the diagnosis. Plague may have 50 per cent mortality, unless promptly treated. Streptomycin (30 mg per kg body weight daily in divided doses for 7–10 days) is the drug of choice. Tetracycline orally (30–40 mg per kg of body weight daily) is another drug and can also be given in combination. Sulphonamide may be given in case above medicines are not available.

Notification : The rodent cases can be notified to the nearest health centre and it has to be notified to International Health Regulation.

Isolation : Bubonic patient does not require any isolation except pneumonic cases. The patient must be isolated and precautions must be taken to prevent the spread of disease.

Confirmation of cases : Streptomycin and tetracycline four time a day is the most effective treatment for plague.

Septron may also be recommended if tetracycline is not available.

Protection from rodents : The rodent growth must be controlled at houses. The rodents can be controlled by improving housing conditions, general cleanliness and raising the standard of living. All possible care must be taken to inhibit the rodents by various household measures, *e.g.*, closing the rat burrows.

Control of fleas : The rat flea (the vector of disease) must be controlled by killing or destroying by using insecticides, *e.g.*, DDT and HCH and malathion. The care must be taken that all the eatable and foodstuffs are covered properly and protected from insecticides, because they are highly poisonous to man. The complete spray must be done especially on the walls and rat burrow.

Surveillance : Surveillance should be carried out in the areas of suspected cases and previous history of cases. The protective measures must be taken in suspected areas.

Immunizations

Plague vaccine is a killed vaccine developed in 1897 by Haffikine, is very effective preventive measure. For its valuable use it must be given in two doses at least a week before the expected outbreak.

Dose

The vaccine is given 0.5 to 1.0 mL at 7 to 15 days interval subcutaneously, single dose does not give any protection against plague. Immunity starts after 5 to 7 days and remains for 6 months. The booster dose can be given in case the infection continue in the area.

Chemoprophylaxis

Tetracycline 500 mg every 6 hourly for 5 days is an effective drug as preventive measure for the people exposed to infection. These can be given to health personnels, laboratory workers, all plague contacts, family members of the patients and others.

Health Education

It is essential to educate the public regarding prevention and control of plague by all above measures.

- Reporting of dead rats and suspected cases for early diagnosis, treatment and preventing the spread.
- Vaccination of people living in suspected areas.
- Environmental and housing cleanliness.
- Regular spray of insecticides to keep the house free from rodents and parasites.
- Use of chemoprophylaxis for those exposed to plague bacilli or flae.

Quarantine

The travellers leaving the epidemic areas of pulmonary plague must be isolated for six days (incubation period) before leaving for other place. The suspected people can be vaccinated against plague.

International Health Regulations

The disease is internationally notifiable. All preventive measures are required to be reported and control its spread to other countries by quarantine, vaccination, keeping the aircraft and ships free from rodents.

•••

Surface Diseases

27

INTRODUCTION

Surface diseases include scabies, leprosy, sexually transmitted diseases (STD), Acquired Immuno-deficiency Syndrome (AIDS), tetanus, reproductive tract infection (RTI), and yellow fever.

SCABIES (ITCH DISEASE)

Definition

Scabies is a skin infection caused by *Sarcoptes scabiei* var hominis a mite (*Acarus*) specific for humans. The infection is caused by the burrowing action of a female parasite resulting in irritation and vesicle or pustule formation.

History

The moslem physician Aveuzoar described the itch mite (*Acarus scabiei*) in the twelfth century, several centuries later (1687) Bonomo described the parasite and Wichmann wrote a monograph on the disease (1786). Herba demonstrated the aetiological relationship between *Sarcoptes scabiei* and scabies.

Epidemiological

The infection is universal and can occur at any age, sex and colour. All persons are susceptible, though it is more common among children. The scabies occurs most commonly where cleanliness is lacking, though it can be found in the homes of well to do people. The disease is spread by direct personal contact with infected person or through indirect contact, with soiled bed linen, clothing and other contaminated objects. Though indirect cause is not very common.

Infectious Agent

The *Acarus* or *Sarcoptes scabiei* is responsible for

lesions of scabies. The parasites both male and female, live in the skin, but the female burrows into the superficial layer of the skin to deposit her eggs. The female can be seen with the naked eyes, but the male, being half her size is not readily detected. The parasites are relatively short-lived, the male dies after mating, and female dies after laying the eggs.

Incubation Period

Incubation period is 1 or two days to 2 weeks.

Clinical Manifestation

The commonest symptom is itching and this may be unbearable at times, particularly at night. The itching is probably thought to be due to movements of the mites, which are more active at night. In the early manifestation there may be few or many burrowing mites but itching will be absent or slight. On careful observation/inspection of affected area with hand lens will reveal burrows, but typical lesions and scratch marks will not be present. After a month of mite activity itching occurs, followed by scratching and its marks. Within few hours of symptoms tissues surrounding the burrows become inflamed and itching begins. The symptoms are relatively few. The systemic manifestations are absent except when secondary infection results, which might involve large areas and cause fever, headache and malaise.

Types of Lesions

Burrows

The tell tale lesion is the burrow, but it is often difficult to find. It is most commonly noted on the web between the fingers. Other frequent

344

locations are natural folds of the skin or pressure areas, such as those about the wrist, elbow, waist, buttocks, axilla or groins. Lesions are often noted about the genitalia in adults. In addition to these areas, lesions are frequently found on the face, scalp, palms and soles. Lesions may occur on any part of the body of infants and small children below 5 years. In women the nipples are commonly affected area and in male the penis in frequently involved (Fig. 27.1).

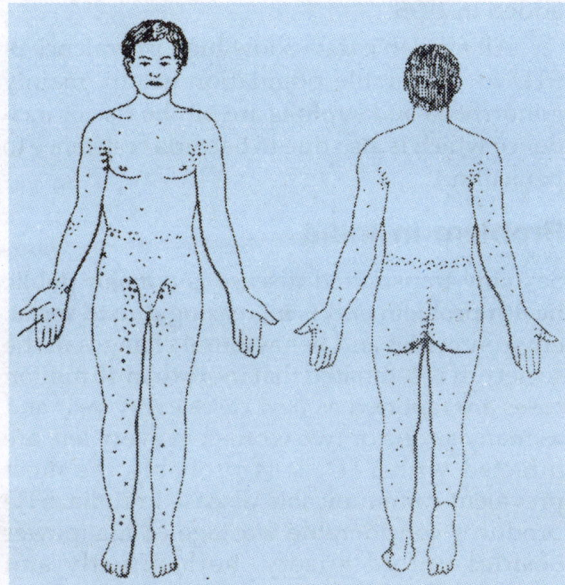

Fig. 27.1 : Common areas of scabies

Papules and Papulovesicles

Scratching may cause modification of lesions, especially when secondary infection occurs. Inflammation may result in pustules and crust formation.

Complications

Long-standing scabies often result in furmentosis, impetigo, paronychia and pyoderma especially in children. Secondary infection with *streptococcus aureus* and *Streptococcus pyogens* is common.

Treatment

Sulphur in varying strength in an ointment base is reliable treatment. The strength of the ointment depends on skin tolerance of the patient and his age. Three per cent ointment is usually prescribed for infants and children, and 5 per cent is used for older children and adults. Two applications of sulphur ointment should be rubbed on skin. Bath is advised before and after completion of treatment. Too free use of sulphur may cause sulphur dermititis. Hence several nonsulphur preparations can be used for treatment.

Treatment of scabies by benzyle benzoate is very effective measure, provided it is applied for prescribed time. The patient is advised to take bath, apply benzyle benzoate (25% in water) to the entire body below the neck, special care to most affected parts. The medication allowed to dry, and the second application is made within 24 hours and at 48 hours a bath is taken, clothes and bedding should be thoroughly washed and sterilised under the sunlight.

Tetmosol (Tetraethylthiuram monosulphide) combined with soap in 20 per cent dilution, may be applied or affected people may be advised to bathe five or six times with tetmosol soap cake, gives eighty per cent cure.

Other ointments *e.g.*, cyclophan ointment applied two times a day for two days give rapid and complete nonpainful cure. There is no reaction, odour or stain on the clothes.

Benzene flexachloride prepared as an emulsion and called Jacutin is cheap, odourless, and very effective as single application.

Effective innovations in treating scabies with 1 per cent gamma benzene hexachloride, it is also known as hexchloracyclohexane is applied for 24 hours.

Nursing Management

Barrier Nursing

Patients under treatment may be cared for aseptic protective measures. The aetiological agent is found in the skin lesions and gowns and gloves must be used while applying the medication. If the patient has secondary infection, *e.g.*, staphylococcal diseases, additional protection may be taken. Clothings and linen used prior to and during treatment should be rolled with the contaminated side innermost and place directly in laundry or drycleaning. Mites may remain in such items and result in reinfection.

Application of specific medication should be followed by bath with soap and warm water. Patient may have skin lesions, and ulcerations from scratching. Treatment for such infection and application of dressings to some lesions may be necessary. Itching may be intense and medication usually relieves it. Use of restrain for the hands especially for children and diversional therapy to distract attention from itching is needed.

The specific therapy is usually followed by soap and water bath and it is important to observe the condition after application and second application may be indicated accordingly. To prevent reinfections, the patient must change the clothes and bedlinen, etc.

Prevention and Control

Personal Hygiene

Proper cleanliness and body care with frequent change of clothes, beddings, are effective control measures. Avoid using clothes, towel, bed of infected person. Children who are infected should not be allowed to attend the school untill disinfected. It is advised for most effective prevention and control. Mass therapy should be used by medicine application to the entire family of the patient and to all the school/class children, if infection appears to large number of children. The people should be given health education on its prevention and control measures.

SEXUALLY TRANSMITTED DISEASES (STD)

Sexually transmitted disease which was named as 'venereal disease' earlier is a group of diseases transmitted by sexual contact and caused by bacterial, viral, protozoan and fungal agents.

Major diseases under sexually transmitted diseases are :
- Venereal syphilis
- Gonorrhoea
- Chancroid
- Lymphogranuloma venereum
- Donovanosis.

Syphilis and gonorrhoea are the most common diseases among all. Syphilis is responsible for many neonatal deaths, mental diseases, blindness and cardiovascular diseases. Gonorrhoea is also considered a dangerous disease for women.

Worldwide Distribution of the Disease

Sexually transmitted disease (STD) is an internationally widespread disease and major public health problem in world with estimation that 333 million new cases of STD had been added in 1995.

All available data show high prevalence of STD in vulnerable population group, mainly gonorrhoea and syphilis are on the rise of incidence which is also due to bacteria resistance to penicillin.

Problem in India

Sexually transmitted disease is a major public health problem and is increasing due to social, environmental and behavioural changes in the society. It is estimated that more than 40 million cases are reported as new cases every year and as many as one or two women in every ten, are infected with STD. It is probably the most prevalent communicable disease in India. STD produces considerable wastage of manpower besides untold misery, both directly and indirectly through their complications.

Syphilis

Syphilis is endemic in large cities, industrial areas, ports and subhimalayan regions. Serological survey is the best source of information on prevalence of syphilis. The survey done in antenatal clinics in Maharashtra and Kerala has shown 2.4 per cent VDRL positive in Maharashtra and 1.4 per cent VDRL positive in Kerala, which is quite high.

Gonorrhoea

Inadequate information is available for gonorrhoea, whereas the prevalence is probably higher than syphilis. About 80 per cent of infected women are asymptomatic carriers.

Chancroid

This also shows high prevalence of the disease.

Lymphogranuloma Venereum (LGV)

This is more prevalent in southern parts of the country, with high incidence in Tamil Nadu, Andhra Pradesh, Maharashtra and Karnataka.

Donovanosis

In 1966, the disease was found in 6.1 per cent males and 6.9 per cent females in the V.D. clinics. It is mainly found in Tamil Nadu, Andhra Pradesh, Maharashtra, Orissa and Karnataka.

Epidemiological Aspects

Agent Factor

A number of agents are responsible in causation of disease:

BACTERIAL	
Syphilis	— *Treponema pallidum* (bacteria)
Gonorrhoea	— *Neisseria gonorrhoea* (bacteria)
Chancroid	— *Haemophilus ducreyi* (bacteria)
Lymphogranuloma venereum	— *Clamydia trachomatis*
Donovanosis	— *Calymmatobacterium* (granuloma inguinale)
Genital herpes	— *Herpes simplex virus*
Genital and anal parts	— *Human papilloma virus*
AIDS	— *Human immunovirus*
Vaginits	— *Candida albicans* and *trichomonas*.

Host Factor

Age

Incidence is high between 15 to 29 years of age, but the highest incidence is seen between 20 to 25 years of age.

Sex

The morbidity rate is higher in men than women, but more severe in women due to pelvic inflammatory diseases.

Marital Status

High incidence is noticed among single, divorced and separated people than married couple.

Socioeconomic Status

The disease has high morbidity among low socioeconomic group than the higher socioeconomic group.

Environmental Factors

The disease is caused by direct sexual contact, therefore, various demographic and social factors are involved in causing the infection.

Social Factors

STD is not merely a medical disease, the social factors are also responsible to spread the infection. These factors may be:

Prostitution

This is a major factor. The prostitutes act as reservoir of infection. Due to rise in industrialisation and urbanisation, the demand of prostitutes has increased. In developed countries, these prostitutes have been replaced as "good time girls".

Broken Homes

The women from broken homes are usually taken for this profession. The homes break due to divorce, separation or death of husband, which leads to unhappy atmosphere or economic constraints, and force women to do such activities.

Easy Money

Due to poverty and lack of employment opportunities, the girls get into prostitution for earning easy money.

Sexual Disharmony

Unhappy married couples, separated or divorced are often involved in prostitutions and greater risk of STD.

Industrialisation and Urbanisation

Increased urbanisation has raised the people's social and geographical mobility and increase in spread of STD cases.

International Travels

They move from one country to another with

infection, thus these travellers export the infection or import the infection of STD.

Social Stigma

This is not socially accepted disease. Therefore, people do not disclose it to medical people and undergo self-treatment and these lead to further spread of infection. Therefore, many hidden and undiagnosed cases are existing in the community.

Alcoholism

Alcoholics have more tendency to go to prostitutes and prostitutes also encourage intake of alcohol.

Preventive Measures

Case Finding

The case detection is an essential component to prevent the spread of infection by screening, case tracing and cluster testing. Easy treatment can cure transmission of infection.

Screening

Control of STD is not possible without screening the cases. Case finding is based on the assumption that at least one other case must be hidden, undiagnosed in the community with the open case. Screening of general public is not possible, hence screening of special groups, *e.g.*, prostitutes, antenatal mothers, blood donors, industrial workers, army, police must be done.

Contact Tracing

The patients are interviewed for their sexual contacts by trained staff. The contact individuals are advised to attend STD clinic for examination and treatment, if needed.

Cluster Testing

The patients are asked to name all those people who had come in contact or have sexual relationships. These people are screened to detect the positive cases.

Treatment

The main aim of the treatment is to turn infectious people into noninfectious, quickly and economically, before they discontinue the treatment.

Syphilis : The treatment for syphilis is a single dose of benezathine penicillin 2.4 million units intramuscular (I.M.).

600,000 (lakh) units of procaine penicillin I.M. × 8 days.

Chronic syphilis requires large dose of benezathine penicillin 7.2 million units total.

2.4 million units weekly for three weeks

Or procaine penicillin 6,00,000 units daily × 15 days.

For pregnant women, same dose depends upon the trimester of pregnancy.

Congenital syphilis : Aqueous crystalline penicillin G 50,000 units/kg/daily in divided doses for ten days.

Or procaine penicillin G 50,000 units/kg body weight daily for 10 days.

If they are sensitive to penicillin then tetracycline or erythromycin 500 mg × 4 times a day for 15 to 20 days can be given.

Gonorrhoea : A single large dosage of penicillin given with procaine penicillin and probenacid is an effective treatment against gonococcal bacilli. Many other drugs like tetracycline, rifampicin, erythromycin and kanamycin are also very effective against infection.

Lymphogranuloma venereum : This can be treated initially by sulphonamide 2 g followed by 0.5 g four times a day for six days. Streptomycin can also be given intramuscularly. If it is not effective, then tetracycline 1 g every 6 hourly/day × 7 days may be given.

Granuloma : Streptomycin 3 g I.M. daily for 10 days or tetracycline 2 g divided doses daily for 10 days.

Contact treatment : All contacts must be diagnosed and treated adequately. The patients may dropout before complete treatment, thus they must be followed-up for complete treatment with recommended requirements for treating STDs.

Follow-up

Syphillis : The syphillis patient with more than one year disease must get venerological examination done for at least 24 months. All detected cases must be regularly visited for complete treatment of the cases.

Gonorrhoea : It has been recommended that every patient with gonorrhoea should be given a further clinical and pathological examination after 7 to 14 days of treatment. Woman must have at least two negative cervical smears and cultures. Women who still show positive culture have to be treated with another antibiotic other than penicillin.

Health Education

Health education is an important component in control of STD to provide general awareness on various sexually transmitted diseases. Health education can be reinforced on prevention and control of infection by safer sex, early diagnosis and the complete treatment and cure is definite for the disease. The special emphasis should be given to teenagers and homosexuals through pamphlets, handbooks and other mass communications.

Sex Education

This is a part of general health education. It should be given to children growing as adolescents by their parents, teachers, in a friendly and honest way.

Personal Protection

Use of condom gives personal protection to the individual. There is minimized risk of spreading the disease. STD is a social as well as medical problem. There must be social rehabilitation along with the treatment. That is :

- Prostitutes must be rehabilitated by education, awareness and making safer sex for people.
- Provision of adequate entertainment facilities for community.
- Raising the standard of living.
- Eliminating the prostitute-encouraging situations.
- Premarital and marital counselling.

STD Clinics

The initial step to control STD is the establishment of STD clinics where all consultation, investigation and treatment, contact tracing and all relevent services are available. Ideally, these services should be free of cost, easily available and accessible to the patients. There must be separate arrangement for female patients. Since the patients desire anonymity and confidentiality, the STD clinics should maintain it. Because of social stigma and shyness in disease, the patient seeks alternative source of medical care or self-medication.

Laboratory Services

Adequate laboratory facilities and trained staff are required for proper diagnosis and treatment of the cases and contacts. Exudates drawn from lesions of the primary and secondary stages may reveal pathogenic treponemes under the dark field microscope. Serological tests for syphilis are VDRL, and slide test, etc. may indicate the presence of infection.

Primary Health Care

The integration of STD control activities has been emphasized into primary health care by including primary health centre (PHC) workers, *e.g.*, village health guides and trained *dais* to provide effective treatment and prevention and control measures. Primary health centre, which is based on principles of community participation, equitable distribution, intersectorial approach and appropriate technology can be best applied in control of STD in the community.

National Notification

It will help to trace out and treat all the contacts of the disease. Population based sample survey may also be useful to identify the carriers, though these surveys are very expensive and are not feasible.

Social Measure

Sexually transmitted disease (STD) is a social problem, hence it is important to imply "social therapy," which would prevent condition like promiscuity. Various social measures, *e.g.*, rehabilitation of prostitutes, provision of recreation therapy, decent living condition, marriage counselling, sex education. Prohibition of sale of stimulating literature, etc.

The control of STD is difficult due to close association with the problem of sex, prostitution and morality. The attitude of people towards venereal diseases ranges from shame and disgrace, in which signs and symptoms are hidden.

In India, STDs are most prevalent in the northern trade routes from Kashmir to Assam and in large cities, syphilis and gonorrhoea are most prevalent and greatest cripplers among the five major diseases.

Syphilis

Syphilis is spirochete caused by cork screw like organism called *Treponema pallidum*, which does not survive outside human body for a longer period. The agent can be destroyed by weak antiseptic, soap and water, by temperature as low as 123°F, by drying and sunlight.

Most cases are contacted through sexual contacts, except congenital syphilis.

Incubation Period

Ten to hundred days, usually 60 days. The disease is clinically menifested by appearance of primary sore that develops at the place of entry of organism. The sore may be usually seen on the penis, labia, cervix, lips, anus or any other moist area. The sore is neither painful nor tender. The patient also develops lymph adenopathy, that is painless and consistent. The organism enters the bloodstream within 6 to 12 weeks of infection. A generalised macule, papule and pustule rash appears on all parts of the body including palms and soles. Patches may also be seen on the mucous membrane of the mouth and throat.

Congenital Syphilis

Syphilis is one of the important causes of abortions and stillbirths. If the baby is born alive, he may or may not exhibit the signs of syphilis. Syphilitic lesions of newborn are usually severe, extensive and highly infectious.

Congenital syphilis can be prevented by VDRL test for every pregnant woman to identify the infection. If test is done in early pregnancy, it must be repeated in late pregnancy too. The cases must be treated to prevent congenital syphilis.

Gonorrhoea

Gonorrhoea is an acute inflammation of genitourinary, anorectal, oesopharyngeal mucous membranous or of conjunctiva causing a purulent discharge due to infection by *Neisseria gonorrhoea*. The infection may spread or be carried by the parts of body such as synovial membrane and fibrous tissue of joints, tendon, the iris and very rare to the endopericardium, pleura and meninges.

Gonorrhoea is a disease usually acquired by contamination by indirect contact. Incubation period is about three days. The first symptoms are redness, burning and tenderness of affected areas, the latent usual complaint of pain while urinating, gonorrhoea is diagnosed by the study of stained smear showing group negative diplococci inside leucocytes.

Treatment consists of cleanliness and medical aid. A person is reinfected as soon as he is exposed to the disease.

The community health nurse should have knowledge about the disease, its prevention and control.

Case Finding

The contacts of all types of cases must be identified by skillful interviewing and teaching the patients at the time of diagnosis.

The nurse tells the importance of diagnosis, treatment and need for control of spread of disease. The nurse may have to visit the home, in case patient is unable to reveal the fact about the ailment. Home visiting nurse must do screening for his wife and children to prevent the spread of infection.

Important and essential case finding method is to make sure that every pregnant woman has blood test for syphilis. Some countries do the test for the couple before they are married.

Case Finding and Follow-up

Home visiting to contact patients who fail to follow thorough treatments is necessary. The home visiting must be carefully planned, the records reviewed to ascertain diagnosis and treatment received and number of contacts examined. Visits may be restricted to infectious cases.

Follow-up of infectious as well as prenatal syphilis is as important as other parts of community health programme. All pregnant women who are diagnosed as having syphilis in any stage of the disease must be visited as often as necessary to ensure adequate treatment and prevent congenital syphilis.

No child will have congenital syphilis, if the mother has received proper prenatal care, which includes proper diagnosis and treatment.

Chancroid (Soft Sore)

Chancroid is a venereal disease characterized by the formation of one or more painful ulcerations at the site of inocculation, with secondary involvement and suppuration of the lymph glands. It is prevalent in areas in which hygienic conditions are poor. The disease is caused by *Haemophilus ducreyi*, transmitted by sexual intercourse, but rarely spreads by extragenital route. It may also spread from the original lesion to other parts of the body.

Incubation period is few hours to few days usually 2 to 7 days.

Signs and Symptoms

The macule or pustule appears at the site of inocculation, usually above the glands of the male and external genitalia in female. The pustule soon ruptures and is followed by formation of soft, painful ragged ulcer surrounded by inflammatory thickening and covered by a dirty looking grey exudate. There may be multiple ulcers. Few days later the regional lymph glands begin to swell and are called buboes, which eventually suppurate. In female the disease spreads to the deep glands surrounding the rectum.

Local medication is not necessary, though saline irrigations are usually advised for cleanliness and hot fomentation is also advisable. Streptomycin and chloramphenicol are the principal drugs of choice.

Granuloma Inguinale (Donovanosis)

It is a chronic, destructive lesion of the groins and anogenital region occurring among young women. It is common in tropics and southern United States. The disease is caused by *Calymatobacterium granulomatis* spread by sexual intercourse and other close contacts.

Incubation period is not known. Lesions develop slowly and persist for a long-time, resisting treatment. These lesions have undermined edges and are surrounded by an overgrowth of granulation tissue. These lesions have grey material that exudes a foul-smelling discharge, contracting scars cause considerable deformity and lymphatic obstruction, which may result in elephantiasis.

Treatment of the disease has been accomplished by streptomycin, chloramphenicol and tetracycline, thorough washing of genitals with soap and water, immediately after sexual intercourse, will help to reduce the possibility of infection.

Maintain the cleanliness by warm saline irrigation.

Lymphogranuloma Venereum

It is an infectious disease that is systemic in nature. It produces specific involvement of lymph nodes, channels of genitalia and rectum, with acute inflammation which extends to lymphatics and tissues of surrounding areas leading lymphoedema, ulceration and disfigurement of genitals.

The disease is caused by psittacosis lymphogranuloma group which is classified between viruses and *Rickettsia* spread by sexual contacts.

Incubation period is 3 to 20 days. Initial lesion may be found at the site of infection, *e.g.*, in male, it is on penis, in female at the cervix. The lesion may be papular, vesicular and ulcerative. There may be slight fever, primary lesion may be absent or may go unnoticed. Multiple small abesses may become hard, painful and reddened. These nodes eventually breakdown and discharge for weeks or months.

Rest is advised during acute stage. Sulphonamide and tetracycline are helpful in the treatment of lymphogranuloma. Incision and drainage is considered unnecessary.

NATIONAL STD CONTROL PROGRAMME

The programme for STD control started in 1949 as a pilot project for control of venereal diseases. In 1955, the Planning Commission recommended the establishment of at least one V.D. clinic in every district and one headquarter clinic and laboratory in every state.

A central V.D. organisation was set-up in the Directorate General of Health Services in 1957 for implementing and coordinating the programme in the country. A free supply of penicillin and VDRL antigen were made available to the VD clinics.

1981-82, the strategy of the programme has been focussed on training, teaching and research in various aspects of STD. New training centres were opened in Madras, New Delhi to provide inservice training to medical and paramedical personnel in venereology. Regional training centres were started in Calcutta and Nagpur. A Regional Reference Laboratory has been functioning at the office of serologist and the chemical examiner to the Government. With the appearance of AIDS, a new dimension has been added to the STD problem in the country. So far, 27 surveillance centres, four reference centres have been established to screen suspected cases.

Under the STD Control Programme in National AIDS Control Programme (NACP II)—504-STD clinics covering all states in the country have been strengthened with equipment and action has been initiated to strengthen 86 more STDs clinics. A massive training programme on syndromic management of STDs have been conducted for all medical officers in the Districts and primary health centres (PHCs) for effective treatment of STD cases based on syndromic approach.

Survey conducted in 257 STD clinics in 27 states reveal that functioning of STD clinics need improvement for maintaining privacy/confidentiality while examining the patients, training of medical and paramedical personnel in management of RTI/STIs, provision of counselling services, availability of condoms and strengthening of laboratory services.

In view of the high incidence of STD in the country, a modest beginning was made at the national level by the Central Government to control the diseases.

Budget Allocation

The allocated funds were gainfully utilized for the establishment of more STD clinics in the States and Union Territories. Second VDRL antigen production unit was set-up at Kolkata.

Training

For proper diagnosis, treatment and patient care, it was highly desirable for adequate number of medical officers and paramedical staffs to be given intensive training and teaching at the two centres. In order to make STD clinics work efficiently, it was desired :

To emphasise upon State Governments that more medical officers and paramedical staff be deputed to undergo training.

The period of three months of training be treated as on deputation.

Need for more STD Clinics

There are 586 districts in the country and still less STD clinics exist.

Health Education Programme

Health education constitutes a very important aspect of STD control programme. More of health education materials, *e.g.*, pamphlets, posters and booklets are being prepared for people's awareness about prevention and control of disease.

LEPROSY

Leprosy is the oldest disease known to mankind. It is a chronic intracellular infectious disease of the skin, the peripheral nervous system and mucous membrane caused by *Mycobacterium leprae*. It also affects the muscles, eyes, bones, testes and internal organs. The disease is not hereditary. Since leprosy bacillus affects the peripheral nerves, patients loss sensation in their hands, feet and eyes. They are unable to feel pain when hurt and hence accidently injure themselves, often very seriously. Therefore, early treatment is essential to prevent deformity.

History

Greek records of post Hippocratic period contain description of a disease which are compatible with present day Lepromatous leprosy. At the time of Galen this was a well known entity as *Elephantiasis graecorum*. Confusion of leprosy with other skin disorders especially psoriasis appeared in some medical literature as late as nineteenth century.

Leprosy has been derived from the Greek word *Leper* meaning scaly. In India leprosy is well known as *Kustha Roga*, which is considered as punishment or curse of God. During middle ages leprosy was widespread in almost all over the world, but it declined slowly in European countries due to improvement in living standards and quality of life.

1873 Hansen of Norway discovered microleprae. For many years there was no effective treatment for leprosy. The only way to handle the patient was to isolate them in special institutions. The introduction of sulphone drug in 1943, has been remarkable treatment of leprosy and domiciliary treatment. Government of India launched campaign against leprosy known as National Leprosy Control Programme (NLCP) in 1955.

1960 : Shepherd discovered that *M. Leprae* could multiply to limited extent when injected into foot pads of mice.

1971 : Kirchheimev in USA reported that armadillos (American ant eater) developed disseminated leprosy when injected *M. Leprae* experimentally.

1980 : A change in the strategy of leprosy control from DDS monotherapy to multidrug therapy (MDT) for more effective treatment.

1983 : National Leprosy Control Programme was redesignated as National Leprosy Eradication Programme (NLEP) with the goal to control the disease by multidrug therapy (MDT).

Worldwide Problem

Leprosy is a major disabling condition in the world with an estimated load of 1.3 million patients. Over 82 per cent of all registered cases in the world are accountable only in five countries, *i.e.*, India, Nigeria, Myanmar, Brazil and Indonesia. One-fourth of estimated cases and 60 per cent of registered cases in the world are in India (Fig. 27.2).

The global statistics on leprosy shows that number of patients registered for treatment in the world had fallen below one million. Almost all registered cases now have access to multidrug therapy, which have led to improved case detection and reduce prevalence rate. Annual detection rate is still high in some countries, *e.g.*, Africa, America, South-East Asia, Eastern Mediterranean, Western Pacific, etc.

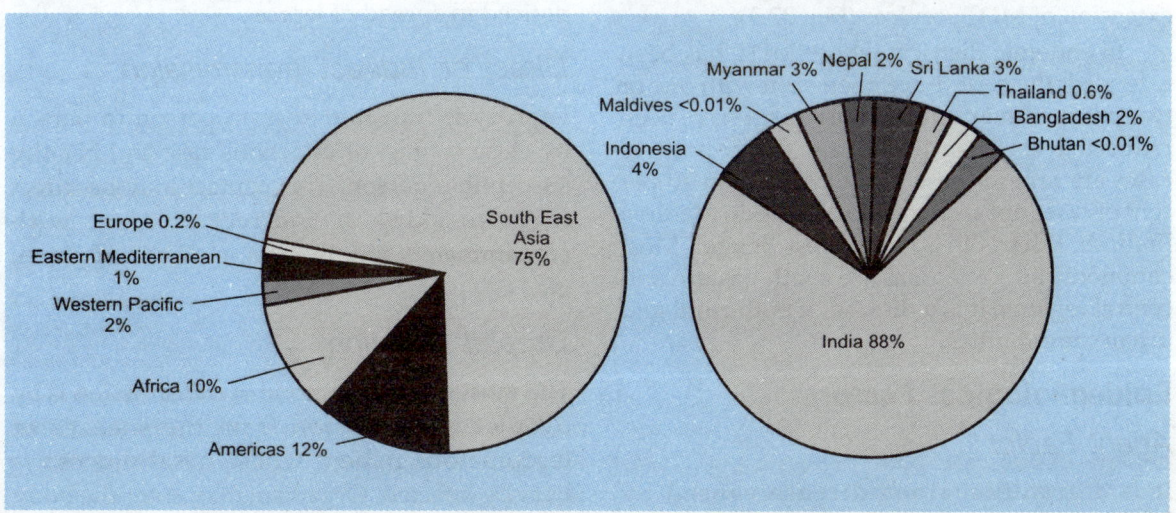

Fig. 27.2 : Distribution of registered cases of leprosy, 2000

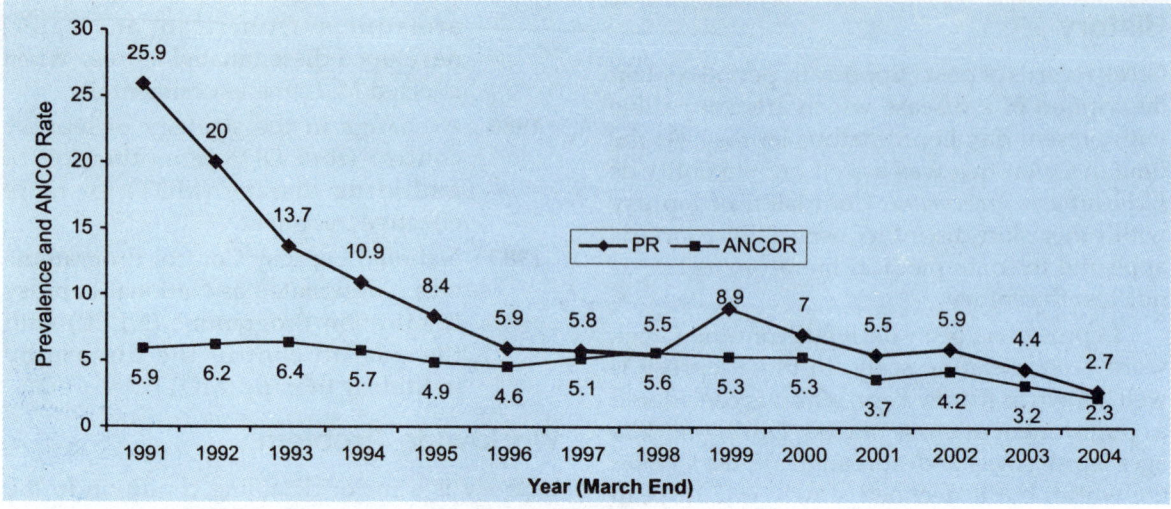

Fig. 27.3 : Trend of leprosy prevalence and annual new case detection rates/10,000 population

In 1996 more than 90 per cent of registered cases have been treated by MDT and 8 million patients have been cured through this treatment. The number of treatment failure and relapses are very low and no drug resistance has been reported.

Problem in India

Leprosy is still a major public health problem in India. One-fourth of estimated cases and 60 per cent of registered cases in the world are in India. The prevalence rate of leprosy in India is 6.7/ 10,000 population, in 201 districts and 15 per cent of the cases are below 15 years of age. Every year 4 million new cases are detected with the extension of MDT services (Fig. 27.3).

In endemic districts where MDT has been extended, the cases have been seen with one or two patches and multibacillary cases have been reduced to less than 10 per cent, smear positive cases are rare in these areas. More than 70 per cent of cases are seen in Uttar Pradesh, Madhya Pradesh, Bihar, Orrisa and West Bengal. Most commonly affected areas are south-eastern and central regions. It is a disease of both rural and urban communities.

Epidemiological Factors

Agent Factor

It is a granulomatous disease caused by *Mycobacterium Leprae*, an acid and alcohol fast

bacillus that has a very slow multiplication time of 12 to 14 days. The bacilli remain dormant in various sites and cause relapse. The bacterial load is highest in the lepromatous cases. The *M. Leprae* can grow in mice and armadillo, but not in artificial media. Local multiplication of the organism in the foot pads of mice is most useful technique for demonstrating the identity and variability of *M. Leprae* and the existence of drug resistant strains for the screening of drugs and for studying vaccine.

Mode of Transmission

The following modes of transmission have been noticed in spread of leprosy.

Direct or Indirect Transmission

Leprosy is transmitted from person to person by close contact of infectious case and healthy susceptible person. This contact may be direct (skin to skin) or indirect (contact with contaminated soil, fomites, clothes and linen, etc.).

Droplet Infection

The most important mode of transmission is by droplet transmission from the sneezes of lepromatous patient whose nasal mucosa is heavily infected. Organism may enter the body through the nasal mucosa or by maculation.

Other Modes of Transmission

Bacilli may also be transmitted through breast milk of lepromatous mothers or insects by maculation through the skin.

Source of Infection

Leprosy cases are the important sources of spread of infection in the community; the current view is that all patients with *'active leprosy'* should be considered infectious. Man is the only source and host of infection.

Host Factor

Age

The higher incidence of leprosy is seen during 10 to 20 years of age, even though the cases have been seen among infants, children and late in age. A high prevalence among children indicates active spread of disease.

Sex

Prevalence of leprosy appears higher in males than females, due to greater mobility. Though sex difference is not found among children below 15 years, whereas it is found among adults.

Immunity

Majority of cases develop lesions and heal spontaneously, indicate the immunity developed through these lesions. Subclinical cases are more common to contribute for active immunity. A certain degree of immunity is also developed through other related mycobacterial infections.

Mobility of People

Leprosy was considered as rural disease. Due to movement of people from rural to urban areas, leprosy is also creating a serious problem in urban community.

Environmental Factors

The poor environmental factors contribute towards spread of leprosy. The presence of infectious cases, the humidity favours the survival of bacilli in the environment. *M. leprae* can survive in dry nasal secretions for at least 9 days and moist soil at room temperature for 46 days. Overcrowding and poor ventilation are the favourable conditions for spread of disease.

Social Factors

Social factors include close contact with the affected cases. There are numerous factors which favour the spread of leprosy among people, *e.g.*, poverty and poverty related factors (overcrowding, poor housing conditions, illiteracy, ignorance, and lack of hygiene). The leprosy is more of a social problem along with medical problem due to guilt, fear, and social stigma about deformity and uncurability.

In spite of scientific information available about leprosy, people have misconception about the disease. This has forced patients to hide their early lesions and thereby delay in treatment, resulting in deformities and delay in cure. Early detection leads to speedy recovery and complete cure.

Incubation Period

It has long incubation period of 3 to 5 years. The tuberculoid leprosy is having shorter incubation period than lepromatous cases.

Classification of Leprosy

Leprosy is manifested in two forms, *Lepromatous* and *Tuberculoid Leprosy*, the two ends of spectrum of disease. Between these two poles occur the borderline and indeterminate type, depending upon the response to infection.

Indeterminate Type

The early infection usually transient and self-healing is indeterminate. This denotes those early cases who develop one or two hyperpigmented macules and definite sensory impairment. These lesions are bacteriologically negative (Fig. 27.4).

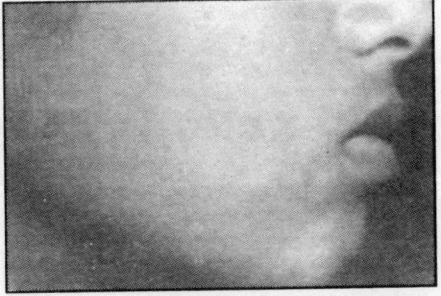

Fig. 27.4 : Indeterminate type leprosy

Tuberculoid Type

There is marked response with vigorous cell mediated immunity around nerves, sweat glands and hair follicles. Organisms are scanty and found mainly in vicinity of terminal nerve endings in the dermis (Fig. 27.5).

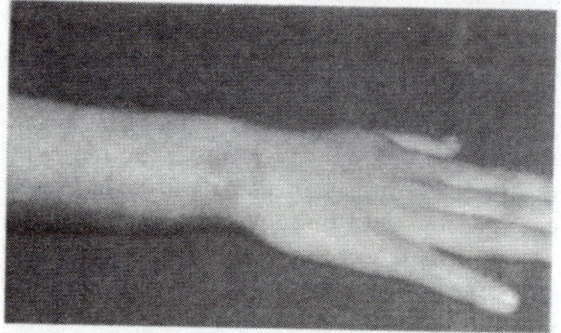

Fig. 27.5 : Tuberculoid type of leprosy

This type denotes four or more lesions which may be flat or raised, hypopigmented or erythematous. These lesions are bacteriologically negative. They tend to heal spontaneously, often without residual disability.

Borderline Type

There are four or more lesions which may be flat or raised well or ill defined, hypopigmented or erythematous with sensory impairment (Fig. 27.6).

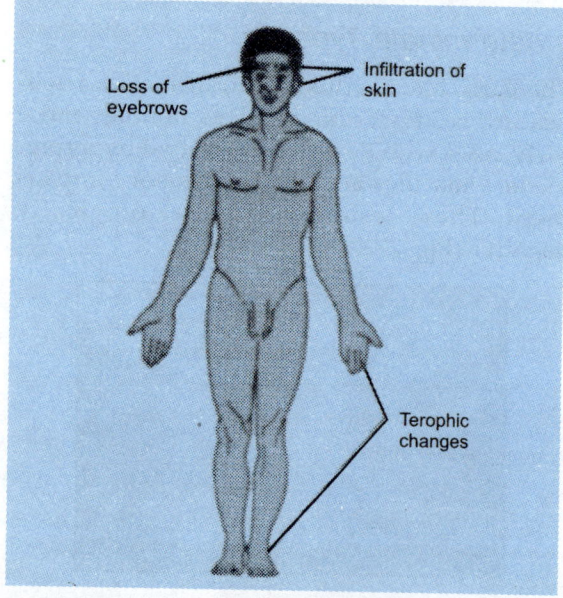

Fig. 27.6 : Boderline type leprosy

They are bacteriologically positive. If untreated they progress to *Lepromatous Leprosy*.

Lepromatous Type

The infective form of disease in which lesions are numerous, flat or raised, shiny, smooth and symmetrically distributed. Sensation is not impaired. They are often inconspicuous except to the trained eyes. As the disease advances the macule lesion become infilterated and succulent, nodular lesions appear especially on the ear pinna, faces and eyebrows.

Pure Neurotic Type Leprosy

These cases show nerve involvement but do not have any lesion in the skin. Clinical evidence of nerve damage appears late in lepromatous leprosy. Anaesthesia and anhidrosis are first detected in the dorsal aspect of the forearms and lower legs later it spreads over the trunk and face. Muscular weakness results from bacillary infiltration as well as from nerve damage.

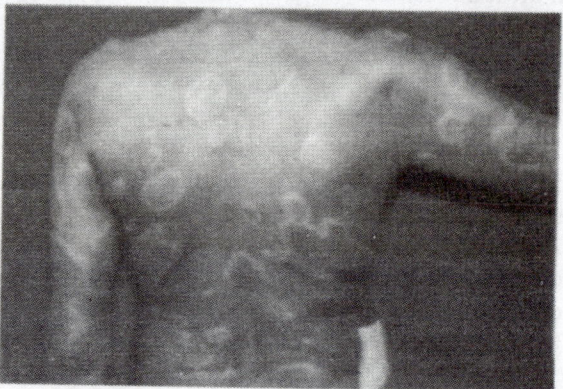

Fig. 27.7 : Neurotic type leprosy

Clinical Manifestation

Leprosy, a chronic bacterial disease with long incubation period between 9 months to 20 years after infection can affect all age groups.

The signs / symptoms may vary between PB to MB depending upon the degree of patient's immunity to *M.leprae*, the causative agent. Nevertheless, 95 per cent of the people in our community are immune to leprosy. Since the leprosy bacilli affect the peripheral nerves and if not properly cared, the patients lose sensation by and large in their hands, feet and eyes and injuries to these insensitive parts may lead to disfigurement, which is main consequence of disease that generates fear and stigma. The early detection and prompt treatment of leprosy with prescribed MDT not only cures leprosy but also interrupts its transmission to others.

Leprosy is clinically characterised by :

- Appearance of hypopigmented and erythematous patches or macules.
- Persistent area of impaired sensation or numbness in the affected areas.
- Presence of thickened nerves.
- Nasal or skin smear shows the presence of acid-fast bacilli.

The disease may also appear acutely with neuritis, iritis and erythema nodosum leprosum.

In advanced cases there is presence of nodules or lump in the skin of face or external ear, loss of fingers or toes, nasal depression, foot drop, ulceration on elbow and toes and other deformities.

Diagnosis

The leprosy patients can be confirmed by physical examination, clinical examination, skin smear, nasal smear, histamine and immunological tests, etc.

Physical Examination

Thorough physical examination of the skin, for thickening and tenderness especially the commonly involved sites, *e.g.*, periphery and cutaneous nerves like ulnar nerve near median epicondyle, greater auricular, lateral popliteal and dorsal branch of the radial.

Examine for loss of sensation of heat, cold, pain, touch at the skin patches. Paresis or paralysis of muscles of hands and feet leading to disability or other deformity.

Clinical Examination

Clinical examination is an effective method of diagnosing leprosy case by taking complete personal history, family history, past history of illness, present complaints and patient's contact with leprosy cases. This history will make the basis for diagnosis of patient.

Skin Smear

Lepromatous and borderline leprosy is diagnosed by presence of *M. leprae* in material obtained by a slit skin smear. The smears are made from skin lesions, ear lobes and dorsum of the ring or middle finger sites on which bacilli multiply readily and persist.

Nasal Smear

Nasal mucus may also contain the organisms in the lepromatous leprosy, which is good indication of infectivity. Nasal smear can be best prepared from early morning mucus material. The patient blows his nose on the clean dry sheet of plastic and smear should be made straightway and fixed, untreated patients will show higher percentage of bacilli.

Bacterial Index

WHO has graded the presence of bacilli :

- No bacilli found in 100 fields—Negative
- One or less bacilli found in each field—One plus (+)
- Bacilli found in all fields—Two plus (++)
- Main bacilli found in all fields—Three plus (+++).

Histamine Test

The test is done by giving histamine phosphate 0.1 mL of 1:1000 solution intradermally into hypopigmented patches. In the normal person, it gives rise to a wheel surrounded by erythematous flare within few minutes (Lewis triple response). In cases of leprosy where nerve supply is destroyed, flare response is lost. Histamine test is usually done when difficult to diagnose, *e.g.*, indeterminate leprosy.

Biopsy

Biopsy is necessary when physical examination does not yield any diagnostic result. It also gives information about the bacterial content of the skin.

Immunological Test

Lepromin test : Lepromin is a suspension of dead *M. Leprae*. The test is performed like tuberculin test, but observed after 4 weeks. The result indicates the degree of cellular hypersensitivity in a patient. Positive reactions are obtained in tuberculoid leprosy, negative responses in lepromatous leprosy and borderline leprosy. This is not confirmatory indication of leprosy, because positive results are also found in normal people and healthy individuals.

Lepra reaction : Any determinate form of leprosy may undergo an acute exacerbation or reaction which is caused by an episode of acute allergic inflammations. In lepromatous disease the reaction lepra, reaction type 2, is due to immune complex mediated vasculitis. In borderline and tuberculoid disease the reaction, lepra reaction type I is due to a sudden increase in cellular hypersensitivity. Borderline reactions are often associated with upgrading or down-grading.

Preventive Measures of Leprosy

Leprosy is a medical as well social problem, because it causes social stigma to leperosy patients. The following elements are considered for its prevention and control measures :

Objectives

- To interrupt the mode of transmission of bacilli
- Early diagnosis, treatment and rehabilitation
- Limitation of deformity or disability.

Early Diagnosis

Leprosy is symptomless initially. Since the incubation period is 3 to 5 years, patient does not know that he has the disease. Even if the patient knows about disease, they do not disclose because of social stigma. Therefore, it is necessary to detect the cases at the early stage with community participation. The health workers need to be trained to make tentative diagnosis of leper patients. Screening of all susceptible individuals in the endemic areas should be done.

The case information should be collected from all sources. Examination of all contacts should be done by survey method. In hyper-endemic area, house to house survey is recommended.

Active and Passive Case Finding

Total population survey to be done for all endemic areas. The survey should be time bound and target oriented and the progress should be monitored at periodic intervals. Contact survey should be undertaken annually. Every effort should be made to examine the contacts every year, highest priority should be accorded to contacts of multibacillary patients because of their greater potential for disease transmission.

Passive Case Finding

Passive case finding mainly depends upon the voluntary reporting, which should be encouraged by intensive health education, to promote the awareness of the disease. Referrals and notifications from the medical institutions within district should also be encouraged by wide dissemination of information regarding salient features of Leprosy Control Programme.

Chemotherapy

Leprosy control is based on effective multidrug therapy since early 1980s. Multidrug therapy has revolutionized the treatment of leprosy. It is a combination of three drugs—rifampicin, clofazimine and dapsone. MDT is supplied by WHO free of cost for treatment of all leprosy cases. Drug is now available free of charge at all primary health centres. Treatment duration varies according to type of disease.

Multibacillary Leprosy (MB)

MB blister packs for 12 months.

Paucibacillary Leprosy (PB)

PB blister packs for six months.

Single Skin Lesions (SSL)

ROM for single dose.

Objectives of Chemotherapy

- To interrupt the channel of transmission of infection in the community, by treating the patient with MDT.
- Early diagnosis and treatment of leprosy patients. Rehabilitation and prevention from deformity and disability.

Multidrug Therapy

It is a combination of rifampicin, dapsone, ethionamide, clofazimine and protionamide which has a bactericidal effect.

Rifampicin : It is now an essential drug in the chemotherapy of leprosy. It is given in combination with other antileprosy drugs, because if given alone may cause resistance to infection.

The single dose of 1500 mg or 600 mg for 3 to 4 days kills 99 per cent of leprosy organism. It is expensive but safe and effective drug. Few side effects, *e.g.*, abdomen pain, anorexia, nausea may be reported. Drug is given under supervision for one hour after administration of drug. Prolonged treatment can be hepatotoxic.

Dapsone (DDS) : It is used worldwide for control of leprosy for last 30 years. It is cheap, safe and easily available.

It is important drug of MDT. The dose of administration is 1 to 2 mg/kg body weight. The common side effects may be haemolytic anaemia, hepatitis, neuropathy, psychosis, agranulocytosis, methaemoglobinaemia. Since dapsone is a haemolytic drug, haemoglobin level must be checked, that it is not less than 60 per cent. DDS syndrome though rare but may cause fever, lymph glands enlargement, hepatitis, dermatitis and maculo papular rashes.

Clofazimine : The dose of clofazimine is 50 mg daily or 100 mg three times in a week (total 6 mg/kg/wk for children). It is an expensive and not very effective like dapsone, but has added advantage in suppressing and preventing reactions. It is used as third drug of MDT. In some cases it may cause dark red skin colour, mucous membrane, urine and sweat, which are temporary changes, not serious and disappear after drug is stopped.

Ethionamide and protionamide : They are bactericidal drugs, more expensive with more toxic effect. WHO has recommended as third drug in case clofazimine is not suitable.

Others : Current MDT has been very effective for prevention and control of leprosy. still other new drugs like quinolines, minocycline, ansamycin, clarithromycin are under trial.

WHO's Recommended Regimens

WHO has recommended the following MDT combination for success of leprosy control:

Rifampicin : 600 mg once a month, under supervision.

Dapsone : 100 mg daily, self-administration without supervision.

Clofazimine : 300 mg once a month with supervision.

50 mg daily self administration.

In case clofazimine is unsuitable, it is replaced by ethionamide or protionamide 250 to 375 mg self administration daily.

Paucibacillary Leprosy

This leprosy is smear negative leprosy which includes tuberculoid, borderline and pure neurotic type of leprosy.

The recommended regimen for paucibacillary cases are :

Rifampicin : 600 mg once a month for 6 months.

Dapsone : 100 mg (1-2 mg/kg/day) for 6 months.

Treatment should continue till clinical symptoms disappear.

Duration of MDT

The duration of treatment depends upon severity of disease. The WHO has recommended the combined therapy for multibacillary leprosy for at least 2 years and continue till smear is negative and for paucibacillary till 6 months and till clinical symptoms subside.

RECOMMENDED REGIMEN OF MDT IN INDIA

Based on WHO regimen for MDT a working group of leprosy has suggested following regimen in India:

Multibacillary Leprosy

For active cases, where all are smear-positive cases.

Dapsone : 100 mg daily.

Rifampicin : 600 mg daily for 2 weeks and then once a month.

Clofazimine : 100 mg, alternate day or 50 mg daily, for 2 years.

Paucibacillary : For active cases but smear is negative.

Dapsone : 100 mg daily.

Rifampicin : 600 mg once a month, supervised for 6 months.

Later dapsone may be continued till symptoms disappear.

The Indian regimen shows some deviation from WHO's recommended regimen.

Surveillance

Clinical and bacteriological surveillance of cases is essential for long-term success of leprosy treatment and early detection of complication or relapse, etc.

Multibacillary Cases

These cases should be examined once a year both clinically and bacteriologically for at least 5 years after treatment.

Paucibacillary Cases

It is recommended that paucibacillary cases should be examined clinically at least once a year for at least 2 years after completion of MDT.

A complete surveillance is when a patient has completed the period of surveillance as per recommended time for paucibacillary and multibacillary and show no sign of relapse.

Immunization

There is no specific vaccine against leprosy. It has been noticed that BCG gives considerable protection against clinical leprosy. BCG vaccine has demonstrated significant level of protection in some of the places, whereas very less protection in other areas. In view of variable protective effect of BCG vaccine against leprosy several other alternative vaccine preparations are under trial. Maximum work has been done on vaccines but no final results are yet attained.

Chemoprophylaxis

Chemoprophylaxis for leprosy is dapsone given for at least three years. Acedapsone (a long acting repository sulphone) was found to be as effective as dapsone. A short course of acedapsone was tried with three injections at the interval of 3 weeks for 210 days and was found effective for 78 per cent protection against leprosy.

Rehabilitation and Disability Limitation of Leprosy Patient

Leprosy is one of the most foremost cause of deformity formation and crippling, which can be prevented by utmost care.

Rehabilitation is *"The physical, mental, social, economical restoration, as far as possible, of all treated patients to normal activity, so that they may be able to resume their place in the home, society and industry"*. It may appear simple but they require systematic and planned medical, surgical, social, educational and vocational training of the leper cases to the highest possible levels of functioning abilities. It requires coordination of health, education and social welfare departments.

Sociotherapy

Leprosy is a social problem, hence chemotherapy alone will not solve the whole problem of the disease and disability. The socioeconomic problems must be identified and solved, which includes social support and assistance, *e.g.,* provision of food, clothings, medical care, job placement, abolishing social evil of beggery. These cases can be referred to social health agencies, voluntary agencies, *e.g.,* Rotary Club, Leprosy Associations, etc., for better living.

Domiciliary Treatment

Leprosy is a chronic disease, hence treatment of the patient at their homes is the only effective way of benefitting the patients. It is also important to take care of hands, feet, eyes and physiotherapy.

Follow-up

The treatment being a long-term therapy, there are chances of discontinuing the treatment (dropouts), and cases may relapse. Therefore, it is necessary to make necessary arrangements for the follow-up of the patient by regular home visits to find out the way for regular treatment and its effectiveness.

Selective Isolation

Hospitalisation of only those patients who are infectious, show acute reactions, complications and require surgical interventions. It has been recommended to make the patients non-infectious by DDS and no need to isolate the patients.

Prevention of Contact

All leprous patients can not be isolated, therefore, it is essential to take preventive measures, to prevent the direct contact of the patient with the susceptible people at home, especially children.

Health Education

Leprosy is psychosocial disease due to misconceptions of mode of transmission. Even the cured people with no disability find it difficult to settle down in life. Health education is an essential component to change the attitude of the people, patient and their families towards leprosy. The patient and his family should be educated about importance of regular treatment, contact examination and self care to prevent disability. Leprosy cannot be controlled unless community involvement, hence people must be educated at mass level about causes of leprosy, mode of transmission, regular treatment, and it is essential to say that leprosy is not a hereditary disease, it is preventable and curable with appropriate treatment. The patient needs social support and sympathy and he should not be disregarded or disrespected or condemned but needs love and affection. Change the superstitions about disease which causes wrong belief and social stigma among leper patients.

Programme Management and Evaluation

Programme planning is essential component for effective leprosy control, this ensures adequate resources (men, money and material), infrastructure regarding supply of drugs, specially trained health personnel and financial resources, etc.

Leprosy control programme in action must be evaluated to assess the effectiveness, efficiency and impact of services provided in terms of reduced leprosy cases in country. These can be measured statistically by using two types of indicators:

- *Operational indicators* to monitor the activities of ongoing functioning in the community which includes case detection, treatment, relapse and disabilities, etc. If there is high prevalence rate of cases, relapses and disabilities, it indicates ineffective health services due to any cause, *e.g.*, facilities inadequacy or lack of awareness among people.
- *Epidemiological indicators* : To find the root cause of achievements or failures of health care is provided by measuring the incidence rates and prevalence rates. The reduced incidence and prevalence rates indicate the effectiveness of control programme.

ANTILEPROSY ACTIVITIES IN INDIA

Antileprosy work has been in action since long, but actual work on leprosy has been recognised since 1874, when Leprosy Mission was founded by **Baily** at Chamba, in the Himachal Pradesh, at present the headquarter is in Purvilla (West Bengal). Since then many organisations have taken up the task for care of lepers, some of these are Hind Kushth Nivaran Sangh, Gandhi Memorial Leprosy Foundation, German Leprosy Relief Association, Damien Foundation, Danish Seva Child Fund, and many other non-government organisations are actively participating and taking care of leprosy patients for rehabilitation, mass education, etc.

International Assistance

There is considerable assistance from international agencies, *e.g.*, SIDA, DANIDA, WHO, UNICEF, Damien Foundation, etc. for antileprosy activities. World Bank supported N.L.E.P. project completed in 2002 and the WHO is providing MDT drugs free of cost worth Rs. 48.00 crores, with objectives to :

- Achieve elimination of leprosy.
- To integrate leprosy services in 27 low endemic areas.
- To provide integrated services at 8 high endemic states *e.g.*, U.P., Bihar, Orissa, M.P., West Bengal, Uttranchal, Chattisgarh and Jharkhand.

The World Health Assembly in 1991 took a major initiative towards global elimination of leprosy, an age old public health problem with devastating effects on its sufferers. The WHO's leadership, strong commitment of endemic countries and active support of NGOs/VOs as well as donor agencies have jointly helped in reducing the global leprosy cases along with proper IEC in the difficult and inaccessible rural/tribal areas as well as slums in urban areas, respectively. A total of 1440 SAPEL/LEC projects have been decentralized along with guidelines to states/Union Territories for implementation during the period 2001–2004 (3 years).

NATIONAL LEPROSY CONTROL PROGRAMME

The Government of India launched the National Leprosy Control Programme in 1954-55. The strategy is based on early detection of cases and sustained regular treatment with dapsone monotherapy.

Objectives

The main objectives are as follows :
- To ensure infectious patients, non-infectious
- To delimit the deformity and disability
- To prevent borderline patients from progressing towards severity of illness
- To control the chain of transmission of disease in community.

Strategy

National Leprosy Control Programme moved ahead initially at a slow pace and gained its momentum during Fourth Five-Year Plan after it was made centrally sponsored programme.

Multidrug Therapy

WHO convened a study group on chemotherapy of leprosy for control programme at Geneva in 1981. The study group recommended the use of MDT based on microbiological principles for the treatment of all multibacillary patients.

In 1980 Government of India declared to eradicate leprosy and constituted a work committee under the chairmanship of Dr. M.S. Swaminathan to suggest strategies for eradication of leprosy by 2000 A.D. The committee had made several recommendations and in persuation of recommendation, the Government is committed to eradicate leprosy by 2000 A.D. The leprosy control programme has been renamed as National Leprosy Eradication Programme (NLEP) and is now included in the 20-point programme to eradicate the disease through reduction of spread of infection in the community and reducing source of infection, breaking the chain of disease transmission.

Objectives

Other recommendations given are :
- Intensive case detection in high endemic areas to identify all hidden cases
- Multidrug therapy in all hyperendemic areas of the country
- Health education campaign to remove social stigma
- Rehabilitation of patients within the community
- Strengthening of voluntary organisations participating in the programme.

NATIONAL LEPROSY ERADICATION PROGRAMME

The Government of India launched National Leprosy Eradication Programme in 1982-83, with an aim to achieve elimination of leprosy by 2000 A.D. and reducing the prevalence by less than 1/10,000 of population strategies. The adopted strategies under the programme involves:
- Provision of domiciliary multidrug therapy, coverage of 201 districts with prevalence of 5 or more leprosy cases for 1000 population by specially trained staff in leprosy
- Provision of MDT services through Mobile Leprosy Treatment Unit (MLTU) with the help of health care centres in 77 endemic districts and 176 low endemic districts
- Health education activities in community
- Appropriate rehabilitation of the cases.

Strategy

The revised strategy is based on early detection of the cases through population survey, school survey, contact examination in the endemic areas. More emphasis should be given on multidrug therapy, health education, referral and rehabilitation activities. The WHO's regimen have been adapted for effective operational and administrative actions.

N.L.E.P. provides Mobile Leprosy Treatment Units (MLTU) and Primary Health Care Units (PHCU) in endemic areas. It also provides free domiciliary treatment of leprosy cases and contacts in endemic districts.

During 2000–2001 a total of 5.59 lakh new cases were detected out of which 58661 (10.5%) were single lesion. Among new cases, children were 18.5 per cent, and 99.5 per cent known cases are put on MDT treatment at present.

Infrastructure

In endemic rural areas, the services are carried out through Leprosy Control Units (LCU), whereas in urban areas they are called as Urban Leprosy Centres (ULC). Temporary hospitalisation wards have 20-bed capacity, at least one in each endemic district to render hospital services to acute patients and complicated cases under the programme—Leprosy Training Centres were set-up to provide training to various categories of health workers in leprosy. By the year 1994, there were 781 Leprosy Control Units, 906 Urban Leprosy Centres, 6097 Survey, Education and Treatment (SET) Centres, 49 Leprosy Training Centres, 291 Temporary Hospitalisation Wards, 285 District Leprosy Units, 75 Reconstructive Surgery Units, 13 Rehabilitation Units, 40 Sample Survey Units.

Targets and Achievements

Presently more than 50 per cent people are getting MDT in the country. MDT is well accepted by the patient, tolerance is good and side effects are minimal. The prevalence rate has come down to 90 per cent in 55 districts, which have completed MDT for 5 years.

ACQUIRED IMMUNO DEFICIENCY SYNDROME (AIDS)

AIDS (Slim disease) is a dreadful, fatal disease caused by retrovirus (HIV), a human immuno deficiency virus which suppresses the body's immune system, resulting that the individual becomes susceptible to various infections in the body. AIDS is the last stage of HIV infections.

Worldwide Distribution and Prevalence

AIDS is a major global problem infecting millions of people including men, women and children in developing and developed countries, including all continents on the earth. Though it was first discovered or identified in 1981, in USA, during 1981 to 85 scientists discovered the virus, modes of transmission, clinical manifestation and large number of infected people all over the world. By late 1992, a total of 6,11,589 cases were reported from all over the world. These cases represent only a tip of the iceberg. There will be many more unrecognised, undiagnosed and unreported cases and infected persons represented by the large hidden part of the iceberg.

The report states the actual cumulative number of cases is much higher than the actual number because of under reporting, under recognition and undiagnosis due to various sociocultural reasons. The number is estimated 2,500,000 (25 lakh) having 2 million adults and 5 lakh children. The total cases reported in 1992 in various continents were as follow :

USA	—	39.5%
Africa	—	34.5%
Europe	—	13.0%
America	—	12.0%
Asia and other	—	0.5%

It was estimated by WHO in 1992, that there were 10 to 12 million people infected with HIV. 16,000 new cases are added every year and 2.3 million people died of AIDS in 1997. They are asymptomatic and transmit the infection to others. Infected women had already given birth to 1 million HIV infected children.

There were 3.1 million new cases in 1996, out of which 1.5 million including 3.5 lakh children died of HIV / AIDS associated illnesses. At present 29.5 million men, women and children are estimated to be HIV / AIDS positive cases.

In the year 1999 more than 34 million people had been estimated with HIV/AIDS. There had been more than 5 million new cases and 2.5 million deaths during 1999.

Although the vast majority of cases have been reported from USA and other developed countries. But the number of AIDS deaths in industrialized countries have recently been falling due to combined antiretroviral therapies introduced during past few years. AIDS incidence has increased to more than 95 per cent in developing countries where the vast majority of HIV infected cases live.

Seventy-five to eighty per cent of this infection in adults is transmitted through sexual contacts, (homosexual, heterosexuals), 30 per cent is from mother to child, 5 to 10 per cent from infected needles.

WHO estimates that, with HIV, more than 1 million adults would get AIDS every year. 15 million children will become orphans. Most of these cases would be in developing countries, *i.e.*, Africa and Asia.

Prevalence in South-East Asia Region

There is an increasing prevalence of HIV infection in South-East Asia Region. The first case was detected in 1985 in male commercial sex worker of Thailand and later in 1986, in most other countries. Since then the incidence is rising rapidly.

Seroprevalence survey carried out in different countries of this region confirm the alarming increase in HIV infection rates in selected high-risk groups like commercial sex workers, I.V. drug users, haemophiliacs and thalasemics.

WHO estimates about 5 million HIV infected people in the region, which comprise 15 per cent of world's population. Beside the prevalance of disease in high-risk group, its alarming increase in rate in general poulation as well. India, Myanmar and Thailand have reported majority of HIV/AIDS cases. The overall HIV infection rate estimated to the region as of March 2001 (Table 27.1) was more than 362/per lakh population, 1345/lakh in Thailand and 760/lakh in Myanmar and 380/lakh in India being the leading contributors. The significant level of HIV/AIDS in these three countries mean that they are now at an advanced stage of the epidemic. The general trend in the rigion shows a pattern of dramatic increase. In june 1996 and 1997, a 150 per cent increase in number of AIDS cases were reported and these are only reported ones. Recent data show that more than 90 per cent of cases are in the age group 15 to 49 years and around 5 per cent children. Mode of transmission in majority of cases are due to sexual contacts (85%) followed by I.V. drug abusers (7%) and transplacental (5%) from mother to foetus.

Table 27.1 : AIDS and HIV infections in the SEA Region, countrywise, March 2001

Country	Reported AIDS cases	Estimated HIV infections	Rate per 100,000 population
Bangladesh	17	13,000	16
Bhutan	1	<100	<16
DPR Korea	0	<100	<1
India	12,239	3,860,000	380
Indonesia	411	52,000	12
Maldives	5	<100	<25
Myanmar	3,817	510,000	760
Nepal	383	33,000	66
Sri Lanka	117	7,300	32
Thailand	156,309	740,000	1,345
South-East Asia Region	173,299	Approx. 6,000,000	>362

The decline in HIV incidence due to 100 per cent condom use programme has received worldwide attention. Even the STD rates are at lower rate than before. Needle exchange programme and community based treatment approach for I.V. drug abusers in Nepal and Myanmar have been effective to change their behaviours and reduce HIV infection.

Prevalence and Epidemiology of AIDS in India

In India, the HIV/AIDS epidemic is now more than a decade old. Within this short period, it has emerged as one of the most serious public health problems in the country. HIV/AIDS, therefore, must be seen as national calamity and can only be fought unitedly by forging co-ordination between people, government organisations and private organisations.

The first case of AIDS in India was, detected in May, 1986 in Chennai. Since then there has been a consistent increase in the number of cases and HIV infection has been reported from almost all States and Union Territories of the country. But the epidemic is still in its early phase except in some of the states like Manipur, Maharashtra and Tamil Nadu.

Most of the cases are among high-risk groups, *i.e.*, female commercial workers, I.V. drug users, haemophiliac and 90 per cent of these cases are below 50 years of age.

The epidemic shifts from high-risk group (sex workers, drug users) to bridge population (clients to sex workers), STD patients and drug users, sex partners, etc.) and then to general population. The trend indicates that HIV infection is spreading in two ways—from urban to rural and from high-risk groups to general population. Data from antenatal clinics indicate rising HIV prevalence among women, which countribute higher incidence in children.

In India about 3.7 million people were showing HIV positive in the year 1999 and prevalence increased to 3.9 million by 2000. Zero surveillance screening for HIV states that 2.6 per cent were zero positive. The cumulative number of AIDS in the country has increased to 12389 females. In the month of June 2000, there were 150 new cases of AIDS detected (Fig. 27.8).

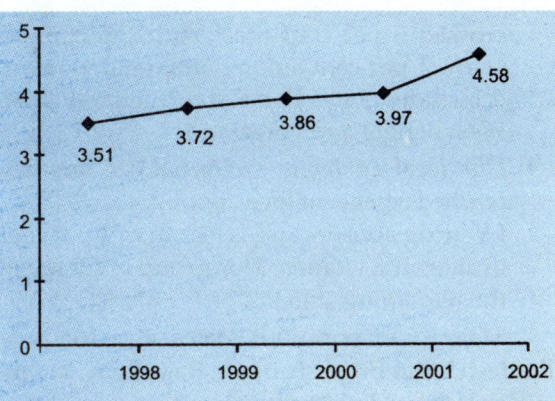

Fig. 27.8 : Magnitude of infection (in million)

The epidemic is increasing across the southern and western states of India and concatenation concentration of HIV through I.V. drug users in the North and East region. In other parts of the country the overall level of HIV are still low.

HIV infection has increased sharply among commercial sex workers and has reached at 60 per cent level in numbar. The incidence is high among STD clinic patients and is increasing in low-risk population (2% among antenatal women attending AN clinics). HIV is spreading rapidly in Manipur and reporting high level of HIV positive cases. Epidemic continues to shift among women and young people, with 21.4 per cent of all HIV cases to be estimated in women with increasing vertical transmission causing paediatric HIV.

Great awareness of HIV has triggered a mixed reponse from community. HIV/AIDS patients are accepted in the society. Home based care is not yet developed in many parts of the country. Mumbai and Imphal report high hospital bed occupancy rate from HIV patients.

The existing sentinel surveillance data for HIV prevalence can be categorised as :

• *Generalised epidemic :* The HIV has crossed 5 per cent in high-risk group, is 1 per cent women and spreading from urban to rural population. These states are Karnataka, Tamil Nadu, Maharashtra, Andhra Pradesh and Manipur.

• *Concentrated epidemic :* The HIV is still concentrated in high-risk groups and has crossed 5 per cent mark, but infection is below 1 per cent among antenatal women. It includes states like Kerala, Gujarat, Goa, West Bengal and Nagaland.

- *Low level epidemic* : When HIV has not reached 5 per cent level among sex workers, I.V. drug abusers and is less than 1 per cent in antenatal women. This group involves all the remaining states.

Majority of populous states, *e.g.*, Madhya Pradesh, Uttar Pradesh, Bihar, Rajasthan, etc. are still in low level of endemic.

Modes of Transmission

Epidemiological studies done throughout the world have documented three modes of transmission.

Sexual Transmission

This refers to transmission through sexual activity, that is genital and/or oral sex. This is the most frequent mode of transmission. The virus can be transmitted from any infected person to his/her sexual partner (man to woman, woman to man and man to man), but less likely from women to women. Anal intercourse has high incidence of disease transmission than vaginal because of more chance of tissue injuries leading to exposure to infection. Women of 15 to 45 years are more exposed to infection.

Blood Transfusion

This refers to transfusion through the infected blood or blood products. That means, this may occur through blood or plasma transfusion when the donor is an infected person and use of blood contaminated needles, syringes or other skin piercing instruments.

It has been seen that the recipient of a single unit of HIV infected blood has hundred per cent possibility of acquiring the infection. In Manipur, the incidence of HIV infection is high among the I.V. drug abusers. Often they exchange the needles and syringes. This can even happen in hospitals and health clinics, if the syringes and needles are not properly sterilized. Thus, HIV

infection may be passed on unknowingly from an infected person to a healthy person.

Perinatal Transmission

This refers to transmission of infection from mother to foetus before, during and shortly after birth. The risk of HIV from mother to child transmission is believed to be 25 to 30 per cent in the uterus and during delivery. It is believed that during the postnatal period, transmission of HIV infection from mother to child occurs through breast milk, but the possibility is low.

Studies indicate that more and more women attending antenatal clinics are testing HIV +ve, thereby increasing the risk of perinatal transmission. Seventy-five per cent infection occurs from sexual route (both homo- and hetrosexual) 8 per cent through blood transfusion and 90 per cent of the cases are occurring in sexually active and socially productive age group. One in every fourth case reported is a woman.

About half the cases occur within 6 months of age and die within 5 years. This is going to nullify the child survival programme of Government of India. The perinatal risk is 30 per cent and there is additional 10 per cent risk of transmission by breastfeeding. In some areas (slum Mumbai) HIV prevalence among ANC attenders is as high as 6 per cent, ANC mothers in metropolitan cities have stabilized in concentrated epidemic. Infection among STD clinic attendents in Mumbai has increased from 23 per cent to 36 per cent in one year. Women were infected by their spouse, who got infection from commercial sex workers or high-risk groups. HIV transmission from pregnant women to newborn has caused the leading problem of paediatric AIDS.

National Aids Control Organisation (NACO) has initiated the programme for prevention of paediatric AIDS through AZT prophylaxis on pilot basis from 1998–99.

HIV is not spread through

- Shaking hands, embracing, contact with objects in phone booth, public transport, door locks, money (coins and notes)

- Shared use of china bone crockery, towels, beddings, linen, toilet articles
- Eating and drinking from communal dishes
- Caressing, petting, kissing
- Masturbation
- Coughing, sneezing, tears
- Normal use of public toilets, swimming pools, community showers
- Medical treatment in hospitals, by doctors and in dental clinics and in all therapy situations where normal rules of hygiene are observed
- Massage, physical therapy, cosmetics (cosmetic treatment), hair dressers, acupuncture, piercing of ears and other comparable treatments, as long as normal standards of hygiene and sterilization are maintained
- Donating blood
- Scratches and bites by pets and insects
- Caring for AIDS victim or HIV positive patients.

Epidemiological Aspect of HIV Infection

Agents

The human immunodeficiency virus was first named in 1986. It is a protein capsule containing two short strands of genetic material—RNA and DNA. It is called retrovirus.

The virus can remain dormant for many years in the host and start destructing the T_4 lymphocytes slowly and lowering the immune system of the body. It can also pass the brain cells and destroy them too. The virus can be killed by heat. It is readily made inactive by acetone and ethanol.

Source of Infection

The virus is found in large quantity in blood, semen and CSF of infected person. It remains in the body lifelong. Less concentration of virus is found in tears, saliva and breast milk, urine, cervical and vaginal secretions. It mainly spreads the infection through blood, semen and placental fluid (Fig. 27.9).

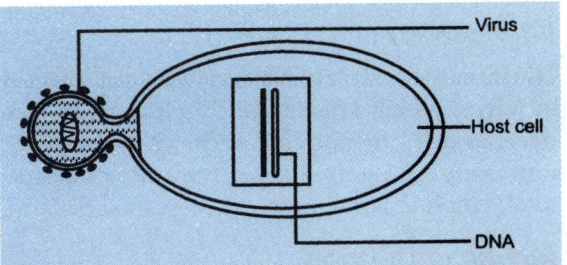

Fig. 27.9 : A virus must attach itself to another cell and use its equipment to reproduce more viruses

Since HIV infected person remains symptomless for many years, hence he can spread the infection to many people.

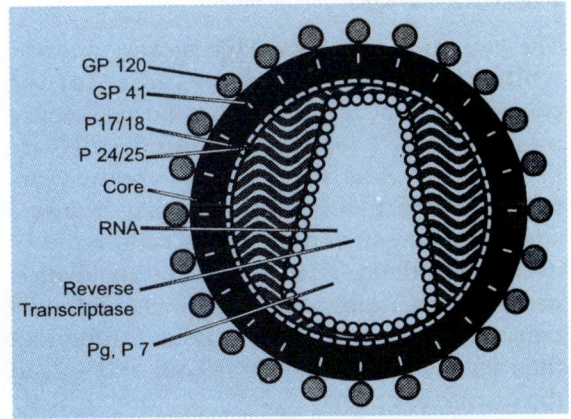

Fig. 27.10 : The human immunodeficiency virus (HIV) consists of genetic information surrounded by a protein layer

Host Factor

Age

Most cases are found among sexually active age group between 20 to 45 years.

Sex

The incidence is higher among homosexual, bisexual men and prostitutes, multiple sex partners, high-risk groups :

- Homosexuals and bisexuals
- Heterosexual partner
- Intravenous drug abusers
- Reciepient of blood and blood product
- Haemophiliac and clients of STD.

Immunology

The immune system of the body gets suppressed by virus, which affects the T helper cells. The decreased 'T' helper cells reduces the cellular immunity and patients get lymphopenia and total lymphocyte count may be less than 500 μm.

Incubation Period

There is no exact evidence of incubation period. It may vary from few months to several years. The virus may remain silent for many years. It is estimated that 75 per cent of HIV infected persons develop AIDS within 10 years. It may be as long as 20 years.

Pathogenesis

The causative organism HIV attacks specific white blood cells that are essential for the coordination of the body's immune defence mechanisms. These white blood cells are destroyed by virus, though it takes many years for the destruction because the virus remains silent for longer period in the cells without destructing them. That is how the incubation period of this disease is very long. Infected persons are likely to be infectious throughout their life due to immune deficiency and spread the disease to others.

Clinical Manifestations

The clinical manifestations of infection with HIV are exceedingly complex. They include all those opportunistic diseases as well as those caused by HIV itself.

HIV infection may be classified into four stages.
- Acute phase
- Asymptomatic stage
- Generalised lymphadenopathy
- AIDS related complex and AIDS.

Acute Phase

Acute HIV disease may occur as early as a week after infection which usually develops 6 to 12 weeks after infection, but may take longer time. Several studies have shown that acute phase starts with fever, lymphadenopathy, night sweats, skin rash, headache and cough.

Persistant Generalised Lymphadenopathy (PGL)

PGL is characterised by enlarged lymph nodes greater that 1 cm involving two or more extra inguinal sites and resting for at least three months, in the absence of any current illness or the use of drugs known to cause lymphadenopathy. The state may progress during the course of disease. Persons with PGL are generally otherwise healthy.

AIDS-related Complex (ARC)

The symptoms generally considered of ARC are weight loss, malaria, fatigue, lethargy, anorexia, abdominal discomfort, fever, night sweat, headache, lymphadenopathy, spleenomegaly, neurological changes leading to loss of memory and peripheral neuropathy.

Many patients develop mucocutaneous lesions, including in particular zoster, seborrhoeic dermatitis, recurrent and persistent orolabial and genital lesions due to herpes virus and leukoplakia.

AIDS

The period between HIV infection and appearance of AIDS symptoms may vary from 6 months to seven years or more. This unrecognised period may be asymptomatic during which an infected person can infect many other people, which interrupts with due control of diseases.

AIDS represents the severe end stage of HIV infection, characterised by bodily infections and tumours, like Kaposi sarcoma which occurs in the presence of cellular immunodeficiency caused by HIV.

Neurological Manifestations

Neurological abnormalities are seen in AIDS patients, *e.g.*, peripheral neuropathy and memory loss. This may be initial manifestation of HIV infection and is atypical. The commonest neurological disorder is subacute encephalopathy characterised by progressive behaviour changes associated with dementia. AIDS encephalopathy or AIDS dementia occurs in one-third of AIDS patients. Common early signs include tremor, slowness and aphasia. The course is usually progressive towards severe dementia. Mutism, incontinence, loss of vision and paraplegia may develop in terminal stage.

Central nervous system involves meningitis, cerebral toxoplasmosis, lymphoma of brain, papova virus, herpes virus, encephalitis, infection with cytomegalovirus, tuberculoid and candidial infection and abscess.

NATIONAL AIDS CONTROL PROGRAMME

Realising the gravity of epidemiological situation of HIV infection, Government of India launched a National AIDS Control Programme (NACP) in 1987. A comprehensive five-year strategic plan was launched during the 8th Plan period with assistance from World Bank.

Objectives

Since AIDS has no cure, the main objectives of the programme is to slow down the spread of HIV/AIDS infection through creation of awareness and aiming at behavioural changes. The main objectives of the programme are:

Strengthening the Programme Management Capacity at National and State Level

A National AIDS Committee, NACO (National AIDS Control Organisation), has been created and is in operation. At the State and Union Territory level, an AIDS Cell has been created in each State/Union Territory. Twenty-three States have been registered for implementation of the programme.

Surveillance and Clinical Management

A surveillance system has been set-up and is functioning in almost all the States and UTs. There are 131 blood testing centres and 9 reference centres. One hundred and eighty sentinel sites have been established to monitor the trend of HIV in various groups of population.

The training of doctors is an ongoing process and trainers are conducting training programme in clinical management including diagnosis of AIDS cases. All States and Union Territories have been provided with funds for management of AIDS patients with opportunistic infections. For protection of health care providers in government hospitals and health centres, there is provision of AZT prophylactically.

Ensuring Blood Safety

The main goal of securing a safe blood supply is being tackled through six major strategies :

- Mandatory licensing of all blood banks.
- Establishment of 154 Zonal Blood Testing Centres (ZBTCs) where HIV testing facilities are available which could be availed by all the blood banks linked with ZBTC.
- Establishment of 40 component separation facilities for reducing the wasteful use of blood, in all 815 blood banks have been modernised in public and voluntary sectors.
- Training of blood bank staff, and
- Promotion of voluntary blood donation.

National blood transfusion councils at national level and state blood transfusion councils at the State/Union Territory level have been constituted. Professional blood donation has been abolished from the country.

CONTROL OF SEXUALLY TRANSMITTED DISEASES (STD)

Importance of STD control measures is one of the main strategies in prevention and control of HIV/AIDS. Steps have been taken to strengthen existing STD control programme through provision of essential equipment to 504 STD clinics, financial assistance for STD drugs and other consumable, and also for the training of the staff. Greater emphasis is placed on strategies to prevent STD through interaction of STD patients, through IEC for HIV prevention. STD services are being made available through integrating STD case management at the first level of health care.

Condom Programme

The Drugs and Costmetic Act, 1940 has been revised to ensure good quality of condoms marketed, meet the international standards.

Information Education and Communication (IEC)

Public Awareness and Community Support

National Aids Control Organisation (NACO) has initiated the programme at national level to spread the awareness about HIV/AIDS through T.V., radio, print material and folk theatres. Efforts are being made to mobilize community support for mass awareness, NGO mobilization, inter-sectorial collaboration and pilot intervention with vulnerable groups of population.

Training and Counselling

National Counselling Training Programme has been launched to train at grass root level counsellors. National AIDS helpline has been set-up with a toll free number 1097 for telephonic counselling which maintains the confidentiality and privacy of the caller.

School AIDs Education Programme has been started to provide lifestyle education and information on HIV/AIDS to students and youths.

Local Surveillance Resources

Awareness

Nurses need to be aware of the National AIDS Prevention and Control Programme in order to :

- Plan relevant health care interventions at the local level.
- Refer suspected cases of HIV infected and AIDS cases to appropriate support services, *e.g.*, testing centres, surveillance centres, referral centres and counselling centres.
- Influence developing priorities of the programme.

Surveillance Resources

Identify the nearest centre to your community/ place of work where you may have to refer your clients for screening, confirmation of diagnosis or for blood testing, etc. Try to obtain the following information on these centres, so that you can develop a working relationship with the centres and help clients utilize their services effectively.

- Location accessibility
- Working schedule
- Policies, any formal procedure to avail the services/referral system
- Kind and nature of services rendered
- *Feedback and follow-up.* Also try to find out the counselling and clinical care facilities available in your area and obtain similar information on these facilities.

Main Components of The National AIDS Control Programme

National AIDS Control Programme (1999–2004) was initiated from 1st April, 1999 for a period of Five years (1999–2004). The programme has two key objectives :

- To reduce the spread of HIV infection; and
- To strengthen the capacity of Central/State governments to respond to HIV/AIDS on a long-term basis.

During 2003–2004, the programme on the prevention and control of HIV/AIDS had been repositioned into a more so address the emerging profile of the epidemic.

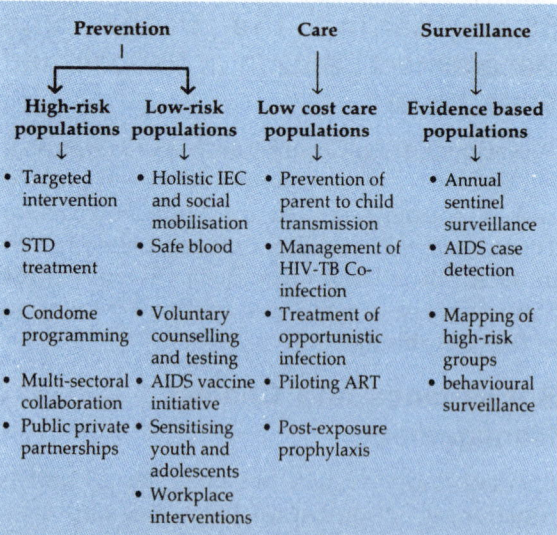

Prevention of HIV Infection in the Community

HIV Transmission

HIV is transmitted through specific individual behaviours and through readily identifiable practices in health care settings, *e.g.*, infection control technique, intravenous infusion and transfusion. Further, HIV transmission requires the active participation of two persons; the chain of transmission can be broken by the individual behaviour of either the infected or the non-infected person or even both.

Elements of Prevention and Control of HIV/AIDS

Primary Element

Primary element of prevention is changing or modifying behaviour through information, education and counselling of people in large and high-risk groups.

Secondary Element

Secondary element of preventing HIV transmission is accessibility of health and social services which include treatment programmes for intravenous drug users, long-term counselling services to infected persons to support responsible behaviour and prevent HIV transmission to others, family welfare services, including supply of good quality condoms and voluntary HIV testing services.

Tertiary Essential Component

Tertiary essential component of preventing HIV transmission is a supportive social environment, so that HIV infected people are accepted and cared by the community.

Nurse's Role in Prevention and Control of AIDS

Nurse's role can be identified based on the background information discussed above and it includes :

- Providing information and education on prevention and control of HIV infection/AIDS to health workers, people at large and high-risk groups in particular.
- Informing people about health and social services available and making referrals.
- Participation in counselling of vulnerable groups and infected persons to motivate a behavioural change.

- Mobilizing community support to find a solution to the problem of rejected HIV-infected/AIDS cases, orphan and terminal cases.

Achievements

Intensive awareness through printed materials and electronic media in urban and rural areas resulted in awareness about the disease, both in the high-risk groups and general population. Awareness level is 60 to 65 per cent in urban and 35 to 45 per cent in rural areas. The highest awareness level is in Tamil Nadu, where it is 95 per cent in urban areas and 75 per cent in rural areas.

Awareness programmes through school and college education has been taken up on the large scale in 18 states.

To ensure blood safety to the population, 815 blood banks in government and voluntary sectors have been modernised and 40 blood component separation facilities have been taken up throughout the country.

For control of STD, which has a direct correlation with HIV/AIDS, 504 STD clinics in district hospitals have been taken up for modernisation. Syndromic management of STD cases has been introduced and doctors are being trained for STD managements.

Indian Medical Association has so far trained more than 20,000 general medical practitioners with support from NACO. Five regional STD centres were upgraded to conduct training, research supervision and monitoring.

TETANUS

Tetanus is an acute infectious disease caused by *Clostridium tetani* clinically characterised by painful muscular contractions of body and neck followed by spasm of muscles especially of spine, chest and abdomen.

Tetanus (Lockjaw/*Dhanushban*)

The organism enters through a break in the skin and the toxin travels and binds the central nervous system tissues causing toxic painful muscular contractions of the body and neck, rigidity, intermittent toxic spasm of cervical muscles, trunk and extremities. The mortality rate is high due to this disease, varying from 40 to 80 per cent.

Worldwide Distribution of the Disease

Tetanus occurs throughout the world and found in most of the countries and most common during summer and among unimmunized or poorly immunized people. It is also an important cause of neonatal deaths in most developing countries, due to poor maternal health services. Contamination of the umbilical cord is the source of infection in the newborn infants. In the older children, the risk is greatest from a deep punctured wound or from an injury associated with tissue necrosis, conditions that favour toxin elaboration.

In spite of highly effective vaccine available, half a million people still die due to this disease every year, mostly in developing countries.

Tetanus is an endemic disease. It tends to occur in areas with poor environmental conditions.

In some countries, the annual incidence rate was 60 per 1000. But in 1994 the number of deaths has fallen down in South-East Asia Region of Bangladesh, India and Indonesia. This is mainly due to effective immunization coverage of antenatal mother and children below 5 years (Fig. 27.11).

Prevalence in India

Tetanus is an important endemic disease in India. It has high incidence and prevalence rate. It was earlier known as *Dhanushban* (like Bow) and was considered to be due to bad wind disease. Tetanus is one of the leading causes of high infant mortality and morbidity ratio, due to poor hand washing practices during delivery by traditional birth attendants. Birth customs are important factors affecting the incidence of disease, especially in rural population.

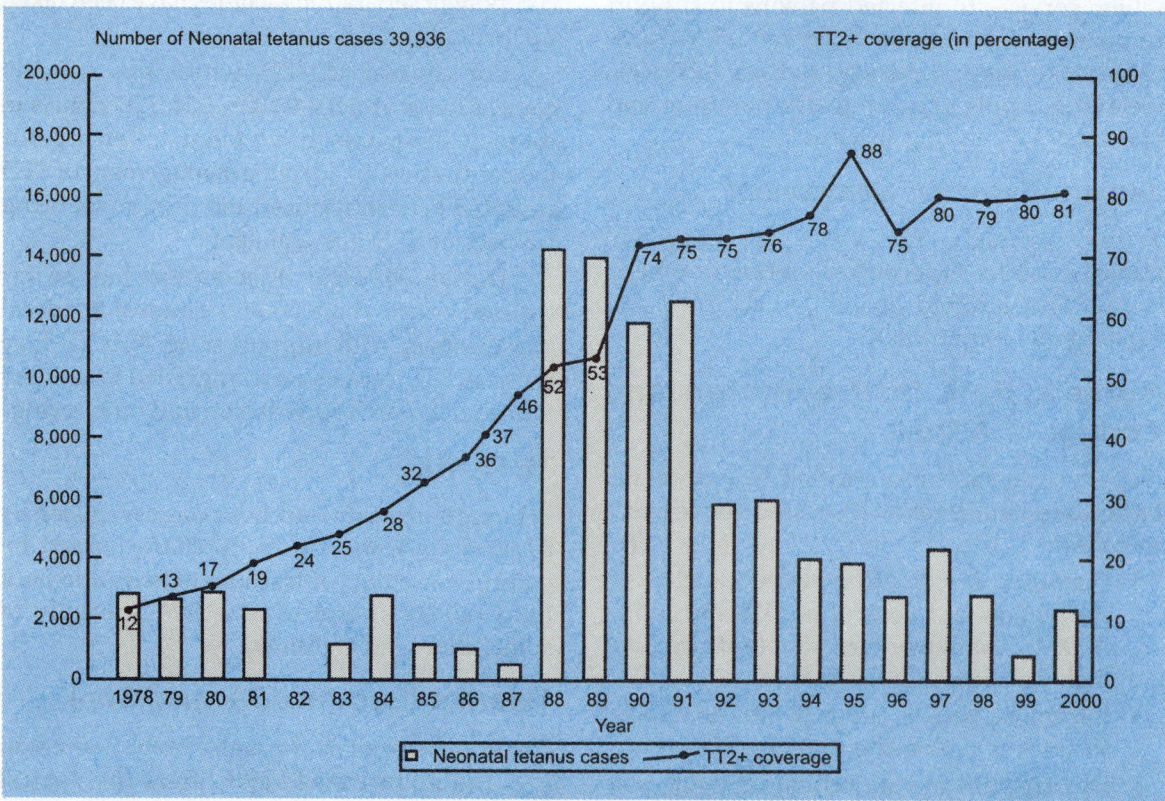

Fig. 27.11 : Trends in reported neonatal tetanus cases and TT2 of Immunization coverage of pregnant women in the SEA Region, 1978 to 2000

The exact cases are not reported about the disease, but available figures show the decline of cases from 26, 232 (1994) to 5,668 (1995). The preventing measures in the high-risk areas like Uttar Pradesh, M.P., Rajasthan, Orissa, Bihar and Assam are being conducted to reduce the number of cases.

In India the goal is set to reduce the neonatal tetanus below one case per thousand of live birth, by 100 per cent immunization coverage to all antenatal mothers with two doses or a booster dose of tetanus toxoid vaccine and proportion of safe deliveries by trained staff.

Epidemiological Factors

Agents

Clostridium tetani is an anaerobic, spore forming, motile Gram-positive bacillus. The spores are highly resistant to many injurious agents and processes including boiling, phenol, cresol and autoclaving. Spores can be destroyed by steam under pressure at 120°C for 20 minutes or by gamma radiation. *C. tetani* survive in soil for years and may be found in house dust, soil and fresh water, etc. They produce two toxins tetanospasmin and tetanolysin. Tetanospasmin is a neurotoxin responsible for clinical manifestation.

Mode of Transmission

The organisms are found in soil, animal dung (horse, cow, sheep, cattle), manure and street dust. Hot climate with fertile soil is favourable environment for the organisms. The organisms are spread through direct or indirect contamination of an obvious or unrecognised wound puncture, scratches, burns, crushed injuries and umbilicus of the newborn are favourable portions of entry.

Host Factor

Age

Infection is more common between 5 years to 40 years of age, due to exposure to high-risk of injuries.

In many developing countries, *Tetanus neonatorum* is a serious problem due to lack of immunization status during antenatal period and poor natal care by untrained *Dais* and customs of applying cow dung on the umbilical cord and cutting the cord with unclean blade or knife, etc.

Sex

The infection is found higher in male than female. Males appear to be more sensitive to exotoxin than females. It is also higher in females in the age group of 15 to 45 years (Reproductive age) due to child bearing factors, like septic abortions and unsafe deliveries.

Population at Risk

All unimmunized people are susceptible and there is no lifelong immunity after one attack. Maternal transfer of immunity to an infant is of short duration. Hence, patients who recover from illness must be immunized to prevent the recurrence of disease.

Environmental Factor

The bacilli are found in soil. The hot climate with fertile soil is a favourable environment for the organisms. The spores of tetanus bacilli survive in soil, street dust, house dust, operation theater, horse and cow dung for very long period. The bacilli produce an exotoxin which is most powerful poison. It acts on skeletal muscles, spinal cord, brain and sympathetic nervous system.

Rural/Urban Areas

The incidence of infection is higher in rural than urban areas because occupation also plays an important role. Agricultural workers are at special risk because of their contact with soil.

Social Factors

Many social factors are involved in causation of disease unhygienic way of cleaning the wound. Most of the deliveries in rural areas are conducted by untrained *Dais* who do not maintain hygiene and a septic technique and use unsterile scissors, knife or blade to cut the umbilical cord. Lack of maternal and child health services and health education are important factors in high incidence of the disease. Most of the cases are due to injury. Infection occurs by contamination of wound with tetanus spores.

Incubation Period

Usually 3 days to 21 days. It may even be shortened till one day or as long as many years.

Clinical Manifestations

The first symptoms are stiffness in the neck, the jaw muscles, the abdomen or the limbs. This stiffness or spasm either rapidly or gradually increases until the jaws are locked (trismus) and cannot be opened. The lips protrude and the corners of the mouth are drawn out of shape, giving rise to the appearance of a sardonic grin (risus sardonicus). This effect is heightened by a simultaneous elevation of the eyebrows and wrinkling of the forehead. The head retracts. The eyes remain partially closed. Gradually other muscles of the body become spastic, and the slightest stimulation of the patient causes frightful convulsions, the back becoming bowed, and the stiffened patient resting on his head and heels (opisthotonos). Even between convulsions the patient is never completely relaxed, the muscles remaining always somewhat spastic, and during convulsions the pain is almost beyond endurance. Profuse sweating is common, and low grade fever the rule, but prior to exitus a terminal temperature of 112º F has been noted. Diffculty in swallowing or breathing is common. The colour is often cyanotic, due to spasm of the larynx and the collection of secretions in the hypopharynx. Voluntary movements are impossible during convulsions, and often in between. The jaws remain clenched at all times. The spasms of tetanus vary from a few seconds to several minutes in duration. They may be precipitated by any form of sensory stimulation, such as a gust of air, turning on the light, walking across the room, slightly jarring the bed, touching the patient, a loud noise. Their number varies from a few to an almost continuous seizure during the twenty-four hours period. Approximately 10 per cent of all cases start as localized tetanus with pain or stiffness around wound of origin, and local spastic rigidity, abdominal muscular stiffness and

trismus appearing later. Occasionally trismus may appear very late.

Types of Tetanus

Tetanus Neonatorum

High infant mortality rate, especially, in rural areas is due to neonatal tetanus. The common cause is the infection of the umbilical cord after birth, due to malpractice of cow dung application on the stump in rural areas.

Traumatic

Injury is the common and major cause of tetanus. Most of the cases of tetanus are due to infected wound.

Otogenic

Ear may be a rare but is the portal of entry of infection. Infected matchstick, pencil or beads may introduce the infection.

Idiopathic

In these cases, the patient has no history of illness. The infection may be introduced either by inhaling or through the alimentary canal.

Prevention and Control of Tetanus

Immunization

Tetanus toxoid is very effective (active immunization) preventive measure against tetanus. It is one of the immunizations taken up by WHO in its expanded programme of immunization and universal immunization programme. The vaccine for use in childhood is usually combined, *i.e.*, DPT. Every effort must be made to ensure that all children get proper course of these vaccines.

The primary course of immunization consists of 3 doses of 0.5 mL of tetanus toxoid at the interval of 4 to 6 weeks, booster at the age of 18 months, second booster at 5 to 6 years, last booster at 10 years and 16 years will give life-long immunity in case of injury.

Rarely, there is reaction to vaccine among children. Local reaction may cause excessive pain, redness, swelling over the injection site persisting for 3 to 4 days.

Passive Immunization

Antitetanus Toxoid (ATS)

ATS is an agent for immediate protection against tetanus. This gives a temporary protection for a wounded patient, therefore, it is not commonly advised. This is a foreign protein. It rapidly eliminates from the body and does not even protect till incubation period (1-3 day).

Human Immunoglobulin

Human immunoglobulin is the best tetanus prophylaxis for all ages. The dosage is 250 to 500 International Units. It is given intra-muscularly and does not produce any serum sickness or anaphylatic shock. It gives passive immunity for longer period of 30 days or more. But this is very expensive, therefore, may not be commonly taken.

Active and Passive Immunization Combined Therapy

Active and passive are commonly used together by giving ATS in one arm and T.T. in another arm and repeating it after 6 weeks and 6 to 12 months.

Prevention of Tetanus after Injury Care of Wound

The wound should be protected from dust and proper cleaning must be done to prevent the entry of bacilli. The patient may be given T.T., 0.5 mL and repeat the dose after 6 weeks and 6 to 12 months. ATS may also be given for immediate protection of the wound.

Prevention of Tetanus Neonatorum

It is an important cause of high infant mortality rate. This can be prevented by giving complete doses of tetanus toxoid vaccines to antenatal mother by administering doses at least at the

16-20 weeks	Ist dose
20-24 weeks	IInd dose
36-38 weeks	IIIrd dose

Two doses are also recommended at the 5th and 7th month of pregnancy. If mother delivers within one year of previous pregnancy, she needs to have only one T.T. dose for second pregnancy. The delivery must be conducted by trained *Dais* and in hygienic condition.

REPRODUCTIVE TRACT INFECTION (RTI)/SEXUALLY TRANSMITTED INFECTION (STI)

RTIs include a variety of bacterial, viral and protozoal infections of the lower and upper reproductive tract of both sexes. Many RTIs are sexually transmitted. RTIs pose threat to women's lives and well-being throughout the world. RTI includes sexually transmitted infections (STIs): related to procedures such as unsafe deliveries and abortions or intrauterine devices (IUD) insertions: and infection due to overgrowth of organism normally found in the genital tract. Men also experience RTIs, particularly STIs, but the prevalence and the consequences for women are much more severe. A high incidence of infertility, tubal pregnancy and poor reproductive outcome is an indirect reflection of high prevalence of RTI/STI in India.

Vaginal discharge is amongst the first 25 common reasons to consult a doctor, 405 gynaecological OPD attendance is because of RTI and 15 per cent of Gynaecological admissions are due to pelvic inflammatory disease (PID).

Three out of four women affected with RTI are below the age of 25 years. The incidence decreases with increasing age.

CAUSES OF RTI

Infections caused by overgrowth of organism normally found in the genital tract is known as endogenous infections. These infections are associated with inadequate personal, sexual and menstrual hygiene.

Sexually transmitted diseases (STDs) are a specific group of communicable diseases that are transmitted through unsafe Sexual contact.

Infections due to inadequate medical procedures, such as, unsafe abortion, unsafe delivery or unhygienic IUD insertion.

Factors Influencing Prevalence of RTI/STI in Developing Countries

RTIs/STIs are widespread due to biomedical, behavioural and societal factors. Most of these societies are in transition, young population is moving about with increasing urbanisation and less restraints. There is low level of education, health information is lacking, local customs and tradition also encourage infection, menstrual hygiene is poor, because daily bath is not taken and under clothing are not changed regularly, financial and social status of women is low, thus they suffer in silence. On the other hand, having multiple sex partner for male is common.

Mode of Transmission

RTIs/STIs are infectious diseases which can be transmitted from an infected person to a healthy person through unprotected sex and in case of RTI also through improper aseptic precaution during gynaecological procedures, such as unsafe abortion, unsafe deliveries by untrained persons menifestations.

Clinical of RTIs/STIs

Screening and diagnosis of RTI/STI is based on identifying groups of easily recognised signs and symptoms (syndromes).

Symptoms of RTIs/STIs can appear anywhere from 2 to 3 days up to several months and even years after having sex with an infected partner. Some men and women with RTI/STI may be asymptomatic or have minimal discomfort and so do not seek health care. The common signs and symptoms of RTI/STI are as follows :

- Vaginal discharge in women which looks and smells differently from the usual discharge.
- Urethral discharge in men is often associated with ulcers in the external genitalia.
- Genital ulcers in both men and women. (An ulcer is a break in the continuity of skin or mucous membrane which occurs in the external genital due to RTI STI).
- Lower abdominal pain in women can be pelvic inflammatory disease (PID) which is infection of the female genital tract, PID occurs as a result of ascending RTI/STI. The seriousness of PID lies in the fact that the condition can lead to fatal illness.
- Scrotal swelling occurs when the testis is infected. This is a very painful condition. If

early effective treatment is not given, the inflammatory process will resolve and healing occurs with fibrous scaring and destruction of testicular tissues. This will render the men subfertile.

- Inguinal bubo in both men and women is a painful swelling of the lymph nodes in the inguinal region resulting from any kind of acute infection of skin on the pubic area, genitals, buttocks, anus, thighs, legs, feet and toes. These are common symptoms of RTI/ STI which is often associated with genital ulcers.
- Neonatal conjunctivitis is an acute infection of the eyes in a baby less than one month of age. Such condition occurs in a newborn baby where the mother is infected with RTI/ STI.

Complications of RTI/STI

Apart from individual suffering the main significance of RTI/STI lies in complications and long-term sequel from these infections such as :

- Infertility—inability to conceive
- Ectopic pregnancy, *i.e.*, pregnancy occurring outside normal uterine cavity
- Lower abdominal pain in women can be because of infection of the female genital tract
- Irregular menstruation
- Cancer of the anus and genitals
- Abortion and stillbirth
- Infections in newborn
- Increased risk of transmission of HIV infection.

Management of RTI/STI and other Complications

Comprehensive case management of RTI/STI is the cornerstone of control programme. Prompt and effective case detection and treatment result in immediate health benefits for individual patients.

In order to manage patients with any kind of illness, the health worker needs to know what symptoms and signs they have. To find out their symptoms, history is taken and signs are discovered on examination. This will help the health worker to decide to treat the patient appropriately or refer the patient to the primary health centre or children health centres as the case may be.

Prevention of RTI/STI

A comprehensive RTI/STI control programme requires three levels of action :
- Primary prevention
- Secondary prevention
- Tertiary prevention.

Primary Prevention

Avoiding acquisition of infection through infected sexual partner. Strategy of primary prevention includes education and counselling about safe sex practices and sexual hygiene and promotion of condom use. Use of condom prevents transmission of RTI/STI. Improving access to safe delivery and safe abortion services.

Secondary Prevention (Identification and Treatment)

Secondary prevention aims at early detection and treatment of RTI/STI, so that spread of infection to others is curtailed. Strategy for secondary prevention is continued education of health workers for prompt diagnosis and treatment, strengthening the existing referral system, education and counselling to promote health seeking behaviour in community by reducing the number of sexual partners, ideally sticking to one regular sexual partner avoiding sex with a person who has many sex partners and practising safe sex by correct use of condoms and also seek prompt treatment and counselling for RTI/STI. Use of most appropriate antibiotics, practising proper asepsis during reproductive interventions and treatment and education of sex partners. Presence of RTI/STI increases the risk of HIV/AIDS transmission by at least 5 to 10 times.

Tertiary Prevention

Tertiary prevention envisages controlling complications of RTI, for example, preventing lower genital tract infection from ascending to the upper genital tract leading to tubal damage.

Prompt diagnosis and treatment of RTI/STI during pregnancy prevents foetal wastage (abortion and stillbirth). Strategies for tertiary prevention includes actively screening for presence of infection in high-risk group and appropriate treatment.

Adolescents and young adults are especially vulnerable to RTIs/STIs. Targeting the younger generation with information regarding the correct practices and providing them knowledge about the causation, prevention and treatment of RTIs is essential for a successful prevention of RTI/STI.

The role of men in the prevention and control of RTIs/STIs among women is significant as men act as a source of spread of infection to their sexual counterpart. Hence they must take precautionary measures for prevention of RTI, by having safe sex, use of condom and sex hygiene, etc.

YELLOW FEVER

Yellow fever is a zoonotic disease caused by a filterable arbovirus, affects mainly monkeys and other vertebrates and is transmitted to man by a vector *Aedes Aegyp'ti*, a semi-domestic mosquito clinically characterised by viral haemorrhagic with severe involvement of liver and kidneys. Severe cases develop jaundice and internal haemorrhage with symptoms of brown vomiting, malena and epistaxis, albuminuria or anuria, shock, stupor and coma. The symptoms are fatal, hence the patient dies within five to ten days of illness.

Worldwide Problem

The major epidemic of yellow fever has been documented in twentieth century. Attempts were made towards eradication, but it failed due to epidemic in South America in 1928. Although,
- Incidence of yellow fever is increasing like other mosquito borne diseases mainly in Africa and America.
- Countries of South America have been reported free of disease. In some of the countries yellow fever remains endemic throughout.
- Rural population are at greater risk, with more cases occurring among young adult

males who work in the forests. Recently yellow fever epidemic in Africa shows the higher incidence rate among children. The largest number of cases during last 40 years was reported during 1980 to 1990 and was followed by epidemic of yellow fever in Kenya in 1992. Outbreak in Peru in 1995 was reported with 440 cases in first six months of the year.

WHO estimates around two lakh cases and 20,000 deaths due to the yellow fever disease every year.

The highest incidence has been recorded in America. Most of the cases are reported from Bolivia, Brazil, Colombia and Peru. There is no evidence of any case of yellow fever in Asia.

Epidemiological Factors

Agent

Causative organism : It is a filterable virus belonging to a group of B arbovirus named as *Flavivirus fibricus*, is a member of Togavirus family. It is recognized in two forms–*classic yellow fever* transmitted from man to man by a vector *aedes aegyp'ti* (Fig. 27.12) a semi-domestic mosquito. *Jungle yellow fever or sylvatic yellow fever* occurring among wild animals and is transmitted to man by several genus of mosquito vectors.

Reservoir of infection : Monkeys and culicine mosquito are mainly the reservoir of infections in forest area; whereas infected man is the reservoir of infection clinically or for subclinical period.

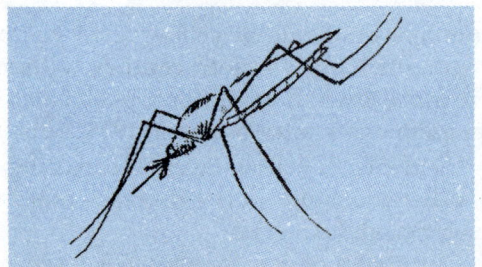

Fig. 27.12 : Vector Aedes Aegyp'ti causing Yellow Fever

Mode of transmission : The virus of yellow fever is transmitted to man by the bite of an infected mosquito. The cycle of transmission being Man—Mosquito—Man. Studies have shown that laboratory workers may get infection by inhalation of aerosols containing virus but that is very rare transmission.

Host Factor

Age and Sex

All ages and both the sexes are susceptible to infection. The adult male may be the victim of jungle yellow fever.

Immunity : Attack of yellow fever is more often on male than female, due to his nature of work which brings him closer to the natural habitat of the vector. It gives lifelong immunity, second attack is rarely seen. Children born to immune mothers are immune up to 4 to 6 months of the age.

Occupation

People working in the forest are more susceptible to the disease.

Environment and Climate

Yellow fever virus can multiply in the mosquito under favourable temperature of 25 °C and mosquito can survive for longer period under 60 per cent of humidity. Hence the disease will show higher prevalence under such climatic conditions.

Social Factor

Various social factors contribute to the increasing number of cases of yellow fever. These factors may be urbanization, mobility of the people and increasing population.

Mode of Transmission

Man to Man Transmission

The *Aedes Aegyp'ti* is transmitted form infected cases to susceptible host in the urban areas. The case is usually infected from the forest areas and has brought the disease to the urban area. The disease may also be spread by infected monkeys entering the residential areas of the city, is bitten by mosquito and spreads the infection which is very rare.

Monkey to Man

It is transmission of yellow fever from monkey to the mosquito of Genus *Haemogogus*. Transmission from monkey to man is accidental and is the result of human penetration.

Incubation Period

Incubation period of the disease is 3 to 6 days.

Clinical Manifestation

Yellow fever may be mild or severe, the onset is abrupt with hyperpyrexia to 104°F with bradycardia, myalgia, headache, dizziness, nausea, vomiting, etc., jaundice and haemorrhage may appear after two days of fever. There may be bleeding from gastrointestinal tract called as *"black vomit"*. Haemorrhage from other orifices of the body may appear. Urine output decreases.

The patient becomes weak, hypotensive, collapse, weak pulse and may die.

Diagnosis

May be done by serological tests and isolating virus from blood and determining the specific antibody titer.

Treatment

There is no specific treatment for yellow fever. Symptomatic therapy of analgesic, antipyretic and blood transfusion, electrolyte balance may be given to patient.

Control of Jungle Yellow Fever

Yellow fever is preventable by vaccination and destruction of *Aedes aegyp'ti* and breeding places. Jungle yellow fever continues to be a major public health problem and is an intolerable disease. The virus survives in animal kingdom and mosquito control is difficult. Vaccination is the only preventive measure for yellow fever.

Urban Yellow Fever Vaccination

Immunization to population at risk is the most effective preventive measure for yellow fever. Internally approved vaccine 0.5 mL of 17 D is a live attenuate and freeze dried vaccine. It should be stored between the temperature +5 to – 3 °C.

Preferably below 0°C, the reconstituted vaccine should be kept in ice, away from sunlight and discarded within half an hour, if not in use.

The vaccine dose of 0.5 mL is given subcutaneously to all the age groups. WHO recommends revaccination after 10 years of the first dose.

Contraindication

The immunization should be avoided during pregnancy and children below one year of age, if there is no risk of exposure to infection.

Side Effects

The post-vaccine reaction may be seen as headache, malaise, mild fever may occur in 2 to 5 per cent of vaccinees.

Vector Control Measures

The yellow fever can be prevented through vector control measures to reduce or stop the transmission quickly.

These measures have been proved very effective in America in control of spread of the disease. The mosquitoes can be controlled by anti-adult and antilarval measures by eliminating the breeding places, health education and community participation. Personal protection from mosquito bite by use of repellents, mosquito nets, mosquito coils and other measures.

Surveillance

Surveillance should be done in the endemic areas for early detection of virus present in the human host, based on WHO's, index known as *Aedes aegyp'ti Index*.

Reporting of all cases required by all countries and the vaccination should be given to all above six months of age.

Nursing Management

The patient's room should be well secured. Isolation and disinfection are necessary. Rooms may be sprayed with insecticides having residual effects. The patient should be provided complete bed rest and quiet environment.

Continuous monitoring of the patient is necessary. Bedrails and restrains must be provided to prevent from injury to delirium patients. Special personal care of patient with fever must be taken. Oral fluid should be encouraged, if there is no vomiting. Constant observation on total blood loss and its replacement. Progress depends upon the severity of the disease. Mild cases may recover within a week, whereas severe cases may terminate fatally in three to four days. If patient recovers, convalescence is generally prolonged.

INTERNATIONAL HEALTH REGULATIONS

Though yellow fever does not exist in India, but climatic conditions are favourable in most parts of the country and these conditions would permit the development of yellow fever. The virus of yellow fever could enter in India through infected travellers (Cases and Carriers) and through infected mosquitoes. Hence WHO has listed the measures for its control.

Vaccination

The Indian population is not vaccinated against yellow fever and a valid certificate is required for vaccination against yellow fever from travellers coming from infected areas. Vaccination against yellow fever is valid for 10 years and needs to revaccinate, if required. The certificate must be valid and duly certified by Ministry of Health, Government of India.

Travellers

All the travellers passing through endemic areas must possess a valid certificate of vaccination. If they do not get the vaccination then they are kept in quarantine for 6 days (as incubation period).

Mosquito Protection

Effective preventive measures are taken to keep the airports, seaports and dockyards free from mosquito breeding. The specific measures are used to disinfect the ships and aircrafts coming from the endemic areas.

●●●

28

Emerging and Re-emerging Infectious Diseases

INTRODUCTION

Emerging and re-emerging diseases are defined as those for which the incidence in humans has either increased or threatens to increase in the near future. This includes newly appearing infectious diseases and those spreading to new geographical areas. Also includes the diseases where the infectious agent has developed resistance to antimicrobials used in case management. Re-emerging infectious diseases are those that reappear after a significant decline in their incidence during last two decades.

Emerging-infectious diseases are newly identified and previously unknown infections which cause public health problems either locally or internationally. Recent emerging diseases include highly fatal respiratory diseases caused by a virus called *Sin Nombre*, a variant of Creutzfeldt-Jakob disease, a disease of central nervous system, HIV infection which causes AIDS and ebola haemorrhagic fever and haemol uraemia syndrome (HUS). Other newly detected infectious diseases of global concern include, a new form of cholera, a haemolytic uraemia syndrome. Hepatitis C, B, E, etc.

Re-emerging infectious diseases are those reappearing infectious diseases, which were known but had formerly fallen to a level so low that they were no longer considered a public health problem. Re-emerging infectious diseases often reappear in epidemic proportions. Tuberculosis is increasing worldwide due to its close association with HIV infections. Cholera has been reintroduced in countries where it had previously disappeared and can spread further because their water and sanitation system have deteriorated. Dengue has started to occur in urban areas where mosquito control has broken down. Other major diseases such as malaria, plague, yellow fever, meningococcal meningitis, diphtheria have re-appeared as public health threat in many countries after many years of decline.

Infectious diseases are still the major health problem of the majority of people all over the world. In the developing countries the principal causes of death are infectious and parasitic diseases that drain the capacities of humans to work and to learn. Thus, conquering of these diseases is necessary for economic self-sufficiency and national development. In the industrialized countries, the mortality from infectious diseases has declined dramatically but these diseases represent the most frequent problems requiring professional attention accounting for a large portion of the loss of health care.

Although many infectious diseases have been conquered, new and emerging problems have been created.

On the other hand, the advancement in modern medicine have led to the development of more antimicrobial drugs and the ability to cultivate viruses in tissues culture, as well as an increase knowledge about immunity.

Epidemiology is the science concerned with the study of the history and occurance of disease, along with those factors that may directly or indirectly favour the development of a disease. A chain of events is necessary, continue spread of infectious disease beginning with causative agent which may be bacteria, viral, rickettsial, protozoal, fungal or helminthic, infection by each type of organism gives rise to specific reactions in the infected organism.

NEW EMERGING AND RE-EMERGING INFECTIOUS DISEASES

In global eradication of smallpox in 1977 and the discovery of antibiotics and vaccines led to an optimism and a sense of complacency that infectious diseases could be eliminated as public health problems. Today, infectious diseases are the leading cause of death worldwide and at least 17 million people die from these diseases each year. The South-East Asian region accounts for almost 41 per cent (7 million) of these deaths.

Emerging and re-emerging infectious diseases have become a major global health problem which are highly complex and challenging. Majority of the diseases are responsible for high mortality and morbidity with widespread epidemics in the world and cause a lot of misery to mankind, disturb economic development. Diseases like malaria and tuberculosis are re-emerging with a greater force. Plague, diphtheria, dengue, meningococcal meningitis, yellow fever and cholera are also reappearing in some parts of the world. HIV/AIDS, hepatitis C and ebola haemorrhagic fever are the new diseases identified.

Global Health Problem

Emerging and re-emerging infectious diseases have become the major global health problem which are highly complex and challenging. Majority of the diseases are responsible for high mortality and morbidity with widespread epidemics in the world and cause a lot of misery to mankind and disturb international trade and economic development. Diseases like malaria and tuberculosis are re-emerging with a greater force. Plague, diphtheria, dengue, meningococcal meningitis, yellow fever, and cholera are also re-appearing in some parts of the world : HIV/AIDS, hepatitis-C and ebola type haemorrhagic fever are the new diseases identified.

In India as there is greater emergence and re-emergence of many infectious diseases in comparison to the other developing countries which have created serious health problems and a great challenge to India. The diseases are also responsible for highest number of deaths and illnesses causing invasive disruption of national economy. Recently India has experienced outbreak of epidemics of plague and dengue which had not only taken precious lives but also created panic, fear and sufferings amongst the people. Illiteracy, ignorance, low socioeconomic status and high population growth, unplanned urbanization are some of the factors responsible for the present situation. Spread of infectious diseases in India is directly linked to low environmental sanitation as large number of people are living in unhealthy environments due to lack of basic amenities of life. The infectious diseases can easily be prevented by creating public awareness leading to active community participation and timely response by the community at local level.

Causes of Emergence and Re-emergence of Infectious Diseases

Several factors contribute to emergence and re-emergence of infectious diseases but most of them can be linked with the growth of population unplanned and underplanned urbanization, rapid and intense international travel, overcrowding in cities with poor sanitation, changes in handling and processing of large quantities of food and increased exposure of humans to disease vectors and reservoirs in nature. Other factors include a deteriorating public health infrastructure which is unable to cope up with population demands and the emergence of resistance to antibiotics due to their increased misuse.

People in India tend to self-medication and start using drugs/antibiotics indiscriminately. They take these medicines when not required and where these are required they sometimes do not adhere to full course of the treatment. It results in drug resistance of many bacteria/micro-organisms.

Emerging and re-emerging infections reflect the constant struggle of micro-organisms to survive. One of the ways micro-organisms have found for surviving is to overcome the barriers which normally protect humans from infections. This may follow deforestation which forces forest animals to come close to man in search of food and failure to control mosquitoes and other carriers of diseases to humans. Breakdown in water and sanitation systems, failure to detect diseases early and failure of immunisation programmes and high-risk human behaviour are some of the other reasons for the spread of infectious diseases.

Major Emerging and Re-emerging Infectious Diseases

Emergence of HIV / AIDS infections (the deadly disease) is a serious public health problem of the world. It has infected millions of women, men and children in developed as well as developing countries. About 8000 cases of AIDS are detected worldwide every day and the number of cases is on rise in the third world. The root cause of the spread of AIDS in the third world is economic as well as social. WHO estimates that in December 1996, 21.8 million adults and more than 83 million children were living with HIV / AIDS worldwide. Since the beginning of the epidemic, WHO has predicted that by the beginning of the next century 30 to 40 million people will be affected.

Entering Diseases

Tuberculosis (TB) still kills adults more than any other disease. Since 80 per cent of these deaths is among the most productive age group (15–59 years), it has a serious impact on socioeconomic development. It was estimated that 3.5 million new cases would have occurred in the South-East Asian region during 1995, which represented about 40 per cent of the global burden of the disease. An estimated 1.2 million people must have died from TB in the region in 1995, which was also nearly 40 per cent of the global TB deaths. TB / HIV coinfection is expected to increase dramatically to nearly to a level of one-in-five of all TB cases in the South-East Asian region in comming future. Emergence of drug-resistance tuberculosis in the region is now a serious concern.

Strong and sustainable National Tuberculosis Control Programmes (NTBCPs) need to be established to achieve the global targets of 85 per cent cure rate and 70 per cent case finding by the year 2020. Countries in the region have made considerable progress since 1993 in implementing the DOTS strategy. All countries in the region (except DPR Korea—no information available) have adopted DOTS and are implementing the strategy in at least the demonstration areas. The most successful is the Bangladesh tuberculosis programme, which presently covers 58 million population and is further expanding with assistance from NGOs such as BRAC. Damion Foundation and other NGOs engaged in leprosy elimination activities.

All countries have manuals / guidelines for TB control based on DOTS and have prepared 5-year plans for their National Tuberculosis Programmes (NTPs). The challenge in the Region is to expand the DOTS coverage as soon as possible. However, the expansion should not compromise the quality of programme delivery, which should be closely monitored through supervision / support visits and reporting on case finding / treatment outcomes.

It is anticipated that in the next two years, the DOTS coverage in the region will increase from the present level of less than 10 per cent to approximately 20 per cent of the population. By the end of 1999 all countries in the region, except India and Indonesia, will achieve countrywide DOTS coverage and by the year 2001, India and Indonesia will achieve 50 to 60 percent coverage (Fig. 28.1).

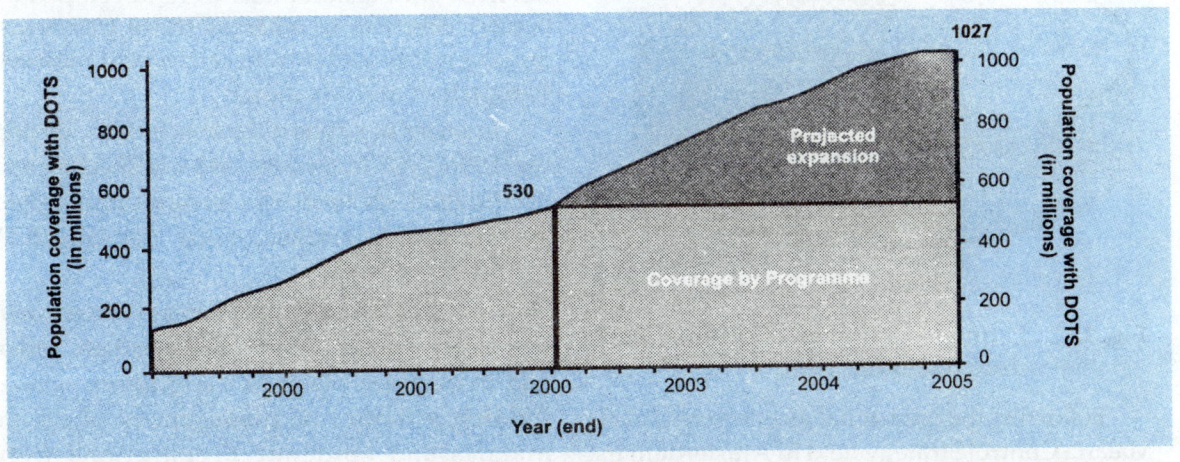

Fig. 28.1 : DOTS Coverage

Two main obstacles are slowing the implementation of DOTS in the region. First, there is lack of strong political commitment for controlling tuberculosis. Despite recent increases in the staff and national budgets for tuberculosis in many countries, there is still a severe lack of human and financial resources for rapid action. Second, there is lack of commitment of health services for implementing the DOTS strategy. This is often gauged by the limited support provided for new and demanding activities for tuberculosis control, such as training, supervision and regular monitoring.

Malaria is another ancient scourge that still dominates the disease pattern in the region. It is estimated that 1.2 billion people in the region live in malarial areas. The number of malaria cases in 1995 in the region was estimated at 23.6 million with almost 40,000 deaths. An alarming feature is the increase in the proportion of *P. falciparum* cases. The development of resistance of the parasite to the commonly available antimalarial drugs is emerging as a serious problem in many countries. Development of resistance of the mosquito vectors to insecticides is another problem hampering the control programmes (Fig. 28.2).

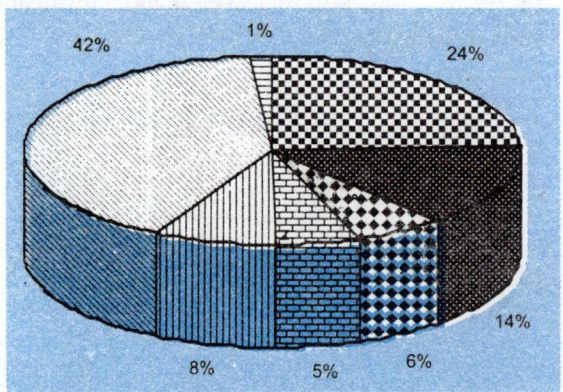

Fig. 28.2 : Estimated number of antimalarial drug resistance 1995

Following the ministerial meeting on Global Malaria Control Strategy held in Amsterdam in October 1992. WHO/SEARO organized a

Regional Working Group Meeting on Malaria in March 1993 to review the situation and to adopt the global strategy (Fig. 28.3).

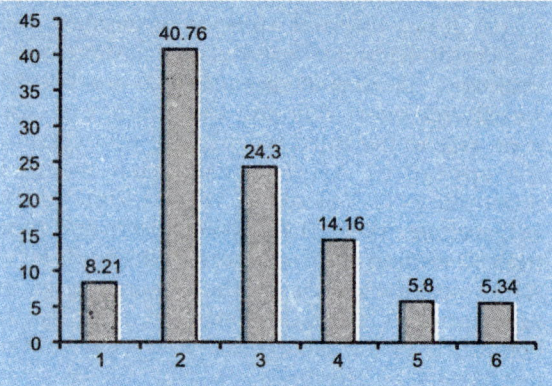

Fig. 28.3 : Estimated turberculosis cases by WHO Region, 1998

In March 1995, an Intercountry Consultative meeting organized by WHO/SEARO considered multidrug-resistant malaria in border areas as a priority problem for the region, in the light of its global malaria control strategy, WHO/SEARO initiated a regional collaborative programme on drug resistant malaria and control of malaria in border areas. Series of meetings to review the situation in the border districts which had identified malaria and kala-azar as common border health problems between Bangladesh, Bhutan, India and Nepal were organized during 1995-96, by WHO/SEARO. Joint action plans were developed by border districts to address these problems. Similar collaboration was carried out between Bangladesh and Myanmar.

In order to support these activities, during the 1996-1997 biennium, WHO/SEARO had established an umbrella programme called Technical Co-operation among countries ICP, TCC 031.

Learning from country experiences with epidemics during 1994-95 in Rajasthan, India, and in northern plains of Bangladesh, several training activities on management of severe malaria and epidemic preparations were undertaken, with assistance from SEARO and

Headquarter. These training activities were conducted during 1995-1996 in Bangladesh, Bhutan, India, Myanmar and Nepal.

Dengue/Dengue Haemorrhagic Fever (DHF) is a leading cause of hospitalisation and death among children in many countries of the region. It was estimated that there were 400,000 cases and 8,000 deaths from DHF in the region in 1995. During 1996, an increasing trend in morbidity associated with dengue and DHF had been observed in India, Indonesia and Sri Lanka. In an outbreak in Delhi alone, during August-November (1996), about 10,000 cases and 400 deaths were reported (Table 28.1).

In October 1995, a Regional Consultative Meeting on Prevention and Control of Dengue/ DHF was organized at WHO/SEARO. This meeting reviewed the present situation and developed a revised strategy and plan of action for prevention and control of this disease at the national and regional levels. Development of a training module for case management of dengue/DHF/DSS was in process.

WHO provided technical support to the countries of the region in containment of dengue outbreaks. A special consultative meeting on Management of Dengue Epidemic was conducted in November 1996 at WHO/SEARO.

Tetravalent live attenuated dengue vaccine has been developed by Mahidol University in Thailand, with support from WHO and clinical trials of this vaccine in children are underway. This is the first time a developing country has successfully carried out the development of a vaccine for human use.

Hepatitis B is a growing problem in the region. It is estimated that there are more than 80 million carriers (more than 5 per cent of the total population) in the region. These carriers will help to spread this disease in the general population and infected mothers will pass on

Table 28.1 : Cases registered and deaths due to Dangue/DHF during 1998 to March 2004

S. No.	States	1998		1999		2000		2001		2002		2003		2004 (up to March)	
		C	D	C	D	C	D	C	D	C	D	C	D	C	D
1	Andhra Pradesh	0	0	0	0	5	0	1	0	61	3	95	5	1	0
2	Bihar	0	0	0	0	0	0	0	0	1	0	0	0	0	0
3	Chandigarh	0	0	0	0	0	0	0	0	15	0	0	0	0	0
4	Delhi	333	5	168	2	180	2	322	3	45	2	2882	35	4	0
5	Goa	0	0	0	0	0	0	1	0	0	0	14	2	0	0
6	Gujarat	0	0	92	0	29	0	69	0	40	0	249	9	0	0
7	Haryana	14	0	3	0	2	0	260	5	3	0	95	6	0	0
8	Karnataka	115	3	39	0	196	0	220	0	428	1	1296	7	4	0
9	Kerala	6	0	0	0	0	0	41	0	219	2	3546	68	113	2
10	Maharashtra	193	5	59	12	66	3	54	2	370	18	772	45	0	0
11	Orissa	11	0	0	0	0	0	0	0	0	0	0	0	0	0
12	Punjab	0	0	419	1	91	1	49	0	27	2	848	13	0	0
13	Rajasthan	2	0	1	0	0	0	1452	35	325	5	685	11	21	0
14	Tamil Nadu	33	5	135	2	81	1	816	8	392	0	1600	8	60	0
15	Uttar Pradesh	0	0	28	0	0	0	21	0	0	0	738	8	0	0
	Total	707	18	944	17	650	7	3306	53	1926	33	12750	217	203	2

C = Case   D = Death

the disease to their babies. The majority of those infected are likely to die of liver cancer and cirrhosis (Fig. 28.4).

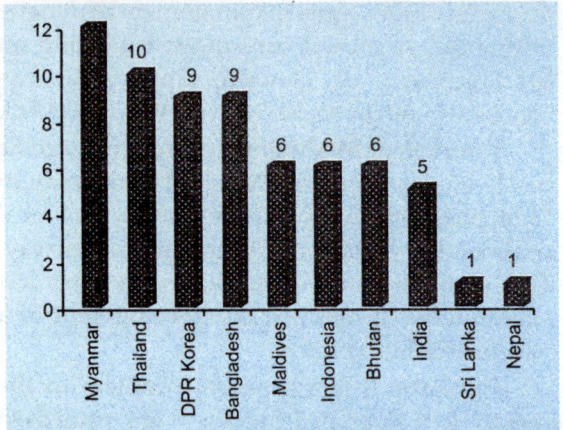

Fig. 28.4 : Hepatitis B Prevalence rate in SEAR Region by 2000

WHO supported establishment of hepatitis B control programmes in countries of the region. During 1992 to 1994 Indonesia, Maldives and Thailand introduced hepatitis B vaccine within the framework of EPI. Sri Lanka introduced vaccination for medical personnel in 1995. Sero-epidemiological studies were carried out in Bhutan and Bangladesh. Commencing in 1996. Bhutan introduced hepatitis B vaccine within the framework of EPI. A demonstration project on hepatitis B immunization was started in New Delhi in October 1996. Hepatitis B vaccine had been produced in DPR Korea and Indonesia. Large-scale production started in Myanmar in 1997. WHO supported the mandatory screening of blood and blood products, both technically and financially and the same is now being carried out in all countries of the region except Bangladesh and Nepal.

Hepatitis C virus (HCV) infection is prevalent in the countries of the region. In India, antibody to HCV has been found in 2 per cent voluntary blood donors, while in Indonesia, Myanmar and Thailand the figures are 2.5 per cent, 3.9 per cent and 1.4 per cent respectiveiy. The testing of blood from patients with hepatocellular carcinoma showed that 42 per

cent of these samples in India, 29 per cent in Indonesia, 35 per cent in Myanmar and 8.4 per cent in Thailand had markers of HCV infection. Mandatory screening of blood and blood products for the presence of HCV markers has been established in Thailand, but only limited numbers of blood and blood products are screened for HCV markers in India, Indonesia and Sri Lanka.

WHO supported the seroepidemiological studies of hepatitis C infection in countries of the region.

Hepatitis E virus (HEV) infection is very common in the region. During 1995 to 1996 water-borne outbreaks of HEV were reported in Bangladesh, India, Indonesia, Myanmar and Nepal. This infection caused high mortality in pregnant women.

WHO provided the necessary diagnostic reagents to these countries.

Meningococcal meningitis had been reported in almost all countries of the region. With an estimated 20,000 cases and 5,000 deaths in 1995, this disease had the potential to develop into explosive outbreaks if not diagnosed and treated early enough. The disease can also cause very high death rates as levelled by the epidemic currently prevailing in Africa.

WHO provided information to member countries regarding the African situation and suggested special steps towards the vaccination and active surveillance of pilgrims to and from Mecca. WHO also provided diagnostic kits to Bangladesh, Bhutan, Maldives, Myanmar and Nepal.

Japanese encephalitis (JE) is another emerging public health problem, particularly in India, Nepal, Sri Lanka and Thailand. It was estimated that 20,000 cases and 4,000 deaths occurred in the region in 1995. This disease is particularly dangerous as a majority of patients who recover, suffer from varying degrees of brain damage. The disability requires lifelong care, either in institutions or at home, thereby adding considerably to the health care costs of the country. The human immunization strategy to control JE is used in Thailand, India and Sri Lanka. In 1995, Thailand introduced a mass vaccination campaign in 30 per cent of the provinces. Starting from 1996, it is expected that this campaign will cover all rural areas in Thailand.

WHO provided technincal information to endemic countries and helped in the procurement of JE vaccine.

Rabies continues to be a major public health problem in some countries of the region. It is estimated that about 30,000 people in India, 2,000 people in Bangladesh and about 400 people each in Bhutan, Indonesia, Nepal, Sri Lanka and Thailand died of rabies every year.

WHO technically facilitated large-scale dog vaccination programme and improved human post-exposure treatment in Indonesia, Sri Lanka and Thailand. Support was also provided to India, Indonesia and Thailand in the development and production of cell culture vaccine.

Antimicrobial Resistance

There has been unrestricted, improper and indiscriminated use of chemotherapeutic agents in countries of our region in the recent years. This has resulted in the emergence of resistant organisms which are spreading rapidly. Today drug-resistant salmonellosis, shigellosis and gonococcal, staphylococcal, streptococcal and pneumococcal diseases have been detected in countries of the region.

These organisms are posing serious threat to the treatment of infectious diseases which are expensive to treat and the cost burden can hardly be afforded by developing countries. Moreover, the laboratory systems for detecting resistance are inadequately controlled and monitored, resulting in delays in effective response to emerging problems. A co-ordinated multidisciplinary approach is required to tackle this problem as a strategic priority.

In order to address the issue of laboratory based surveillance, WHO, in 1995-96, supported the setting up of a Gonococcal Antimicrobial Sensitivity Programme (GASP) in the region. This involved the establishment of a network of laboratories to the quality of data generated.

WHO also prepared a manual on standard operational procedure for isolation, identification and antimicrobial susceptibility in *Neisseria gonorrhoeae* which will be disseminated to the concerned laboratories of the region. Dissemination of these manuals will always keep information updated.

RE-EMERGING DISEASES

The sudden re-appearance of human plague in India, in 1994, after a period of 27 years caused global concern. It created a sense of panic, both within and outside the country and led to the imposition of unwarranted trade and travel restrictions by several countries. There is a need to be vigilant since the natural foci of infectious plague exist in India, Indonesia, Myanmar and possibly Nepal.

During 1995-1996, WHO trained nationals from India. Indonesia, Myanmar, Nepal, Sri Lanka and Thailand in laboratory diagnosis and surveillance of plague. As a result of this training, India is producing diagnostic reagents for plague at the Haffkine Institute, Mumbai.

Kala-azar almost disappeared from the South-East Asian region during the early 1960s due to insecticide spraying under the Malaria Control Programme (MCP). Subsequently, as the MCP entered the maintenance phase, insecticide spraying was withdrawn and kala-azar vectors started breeding profusely. Kala-azar continues to be a health problem of importance in primarily the rural areas of India, Bangladesh and Nepal, where approximately 110 million people are at risk. It was estimated that 100,000 cases and 5,000 deaths occurred in these three countries in 1995.

In 1993, WHO/SEARO conducted a consultative meeting on visceral leishmaniasis control to review the situation and to formulate country objectives for the control of the disease. Subsequently, WHO assisted the endemic countries in the formulation of control strategies and supported national training courses on case management, laboratory diagnosis and vector control. As a result of the implementation of this strategy, India reported a decline of incidence and deaths during 1994-1995. Some progress has also been made in Bangladesh and Nepal through the integration of vector control programmes.

In August 1995, during the border meeting involving districts from Bangladesh, Bhutan, India and Nepal, malaria and kala-azar were identified as common health problems. The meeting, which was organized by WHO/SEARO developed a district joint action plan to address kala-azar problems in border areas between Bangladesh, India and Nepal. WHO supported the countries in evaluating their collaborative activities.

Potential Emerging Diseases

In addition to the current infectious disease problems in SEAR, there are potential problems associated with an increase in the number of drug-resistant bacterial and parasitic diseases and emergence of new viral infections. The potential emerging infections in SEAR are hanta-virus, yellow fever and Ebola like haemorrhagic fever and E. coli 0157.

Hantavirus infection causing haemorrhagic fever with renal syndrome (kidney disease) has been reported only from Myanmar and Sri Lanka. Antibody studies in India, Indonesia and Thailand, however, suggest that there is wide circulation of this virus, which poses a potential threat to the countries.

Yellow fever has never been reported from this region. However, the recent epidemic in Kenya poses a threat as the mosquito vector (Aedes aegyp'ti) is widely prevalent in the region and yet the people have no immunity against the disease. If yellow fever virus is introduced in this region, there will be large epidemics with very high death rates (50–80%). Thus, there is need for extra vigilance to protect the region against yellow fever.

Though Ebola haemorrhagic fever has not occurred in the region, antibodies to Ebola related filoviruses have been detected in a species of monkeys in Indonesia. E. coli 0157 causes diarrhoea which has a wide range presentation from the mild without blood to stools that are virtually all blood. Very often, it causes fatal haemolytic uraemic syndrome (HUS). There have been reports of several serious outbreaks in USA, Japan, South Africa and Australia. In each outbreak, many people were affected with high complication and fatality rates. The disease has potential of emerging into the region.

Bovine spongiform encephalopathy (BSE) which possibly links with a form of brain disease in humans—a new variant of Creutzfeldt-Jakob Disease (CJD)—has not been reported in South-East Asia. However, India and Thailand have reported sporadic cases of CJD.

WHO provided technical information and recommendations regarding the prevention and control of these potential, emerging infectious diseases.

Causes of Emerging Diseases

There is no single factor responsible for the emergence of these diseases but rather the inter-action of multifactors. Poverty is on the increase and millions of people, by virtue of their living conditions, are exposed daily to the hazards of infectious diseases. Environmental degradation is another factor that contributes to the increasing disease burden.

Rapid population growth combined with uncontrolled urbanization means that millions of city dweller are forced to live in overcrowded and unhygienic conditions lacking clean water and adequate sanitation. These conditions provide ample breeding grounds for infectious diseases.

Migration and displacement of people due to wars, civil strike and natural disasters like floods and earthquakes, also provide fertile breeding grounds for these diseases. The rapid increase in international travel and growing trade and tourism have implications for the spread of infectious diseases from one country to another.

Also, mutation results in new strains of infectious agents and antimicrobial resistance. These, together with vector resistance to insecticides, are also important factors in the emergence of new diseases.

But, perhaps one of the most important factors contributing to the emergence of infectious diseases is the low priority and support given to public health services in many countries.

Economic Impact of New Emerging and Re-emerging Diseases

The economic impact of these diseases can be enormous. For example, during the plague outbreak in 1994, India is estimated to have suffered loses in trade, employment and tourism amounting to over US $ 1.5 billion. Similarly, as a result of the cholera epidemic in 1991, Peru lost an estimated US $ 770 million. More recently, the mad-cow disease in UK has resulted in a loss of billions of pounds sterling following the ban imposed by the European Community on the import of British beef. In Thailand, a well-documented study estimates that health care costs of an AIDS patient varies from US $ 1,500 to 5,000.

Priority Areas for Action and Future Plans

WHO has identified three priority areas for national and international action during the next five years.

The first priority is to achieve the eradication or elimination of diseases such as poliomyelitis, dracunculiasis, leprosy and measles which does not require large expenditure. If the necessary resources are not mobilized, however, there is every likelihood of these diseases will return with a vengeance, negating previous efforts.

The second priority is the prevention and control of diseases which are major public health problems in the region such as tuberculosis, malaria, viral hepatitis, dengue/dangue haemorrhagic fever, Japanese encephalitis, meningococcal meningitis, HIV/AIDS, acute respiratory infections and diarrhoeal diseases, through the establishment of appropriate national and regional surveillance mechanisms.

The third priority is to take short-term and long-term action to combat newly emerging diseases. Since speedy response is needed to effectively contain outbreaks, rapid response mechanisms need to be built into the surveillance system.

The following are priority activities for the coming few years towards the prevention and control of emerging and re-emerging of communicable diseases :

- Strengthening epidemiological surveillance
- Strengthening laboratory capabilities and services
- Establishment of rapid response team
- Monitoring antimicrobial resistance
- Establishment of international disease surveillance networking
- Advocacy and mobilization of international support.

●●●

UNIT VII

HEALTH INFORMATION AND STATISTICS

- **Vital Health Statistics**

Vital Health Statistics

29

INTRODUCTION

Vital health statistics is an essential part of health information system. A health information system may be defined as :

"A mechanism for the collection, processing, analysing and transmission of information required for organizing and operating health services and also for research and training".

"Statistics is a science of collection of numerical data and the technique of analysing the data and draw conclusions from such data". Vital health statistics are the statistics related to births, deaths, sickness that occur in a community. Vital health statistics indicate the health status of a community and provide guidelines necessary for planning and health administration.

The vital health statistics is useful in determining the target health programmes. The main objective of vital health statistics is to provide adequate, factual, reliable, complete, timely and updated information.

Definition

Vital health statistics has been defined as *"The facts, systematically collected and compiled in numerical form, related to, or derived from records of vital events".*

These vital events are births, deaths, marriages, illnesses of a particular community. These vital events serve as "Yard Sticks" that measure the health status of a population.

Use of Vital Health Statistics

The vital health statistics are the most essential components in planning and organizing the health services of a particular community. Therefore, the accurate and complete statistics will be useful in various aspects.

- To measure the health status in a country, to identify the health needs of various population groups, so that the health care can be utilized with maximum efforts.
- To plan and organise the health services and for proper utilization of the resources (men, money and materials) available.
- To evaluate the utilisation of health services about its progress, success or failure of health programme and services being provided.
- For comparison of health status at local, national and international levels.
- To assess whether health services are achieving their objectives in terms of its effectiveness and efficiency.
- To conduct the research studies in community health problems and its management.

Components for Vital Health Statistics

- Demographical aspects and vital events in relation to population factors, *e.g.,* deaths, births, marriages and illnesses, etc.
- Environmental health statistics in relation to water, air, noise and other factors.
- Health resources and utilization of resources in hospitals and related health agenices, *e.g.,* facilities, beds and health manpower.
- Utilization of health services, *e.g.,* bed occupancy, admissions and discharge.
- Financial utilization (cost-effectiveness) related to health. This shows the balance between expenditure and output in terms of improvement in healthy status of people.

Sources of Health Information

Different vital statistics at various time periods are as given below :

Census

The census is an important source of health statistics. It is taken in almost all over the world at regular interval of every ten years. In census every member of the population is contacted in a given time to collect the essential information. It needs sufficient preparation and time for many years to collect, analyse and report the data.

Census is defined as *"the total process of collecting, compiling and publishing demographic, economic and social data pertaining at a specified time or time to all persons in a country or territory"*.

The first census was taken in 1881 in India and were repeated every ten years interval. The last census was held in 2001. Census is usually conducted at the end of first quarter of the year (March-April) because most people are usually found at home, during this period.

Census helps to provide demographic information like total population, according to :

- Age and sex distribution
- Social and economical characteristics of the people
- Working and living conditions
- Any other information.

Population information helps to plan the health service planning according to age, income and living conditions, etc., with census data, it is not possible to obtain the qualified health, demographic and socioeconomic indicators.

Registration of Vital Events

It is the second important source of health statistics. If registration of vital events is complete and accurate, it can serve as a reliable source of health information. Therefore, more importance has been given to vital events in almost all the countries.

Vital events are defined as the *"legal registration, statistical recording and reporting of the occurrence of collection, compiling, presentation, analysis and distribution of statistics pertaining to vital events, i.e., live births, deaths, foetal deaths, marriages, divorces, adoptions and legal separations"*.

Government of India passed the Birth and Death Registration Act in 1873, but the act provided only voluntary registration, hence the registration system was inaccurate, incomplete, unreliable. This was because of ignorance, illiteracy, lack of concern and poor motivation.

There was no uniformity and standard system of collecting the information. Large number of deaths and births were not registered. The registration varied from 30 to 90 per cent in different states. Therefore, registration was of little value.

The Central Births and Deaths Registration Act 1969

To improve the registration system, Government of India amended Central Birth and Death Registration Act which came into force on first April 1970. This Act limited the time for registration of birth within 14 days and death within 7 days. In case of failure, a fine of Rs 50 may be imposed. According to the Act it is compulsory to register these vital events. The registration is done by *village chowkidars, Anganwari workers*, health workers, heads of the hospitals, nursing homes and municipal corporation in the cities. The Act made the beginning of new events of history of health statistics registration.

Lay Reporting

Some countries have adopted lay reporting, due to slow development of registration system. Lay reporting is defined as *"the collection of information, its use and its transmission to other levels of health system by nonprofessional health workers"*.

In this, primary health workers are employed to collect and record data in his or her defined area. They also give sufficient information of places where registration of vital events are not practiced.

Sample Registration Survey

It is a dual record system. One system consists of continuous counting of births, deaths and another system consists of every six months survey by an investigator. Hence the information becomes more reliable by compiling both the informations. Sample registration survey was initiated in 1960 in India, to provide more reliable source of statistics. Sample registration survey (SRS) now covers the entire country. It is a major source of information for births, deaths and age-specific fertility and mortality rates, infant and adult mortality have become available.

Notification of Diseases

Notification means reporting of the specific communicable and noncommunicable disease, as and when they are identified, the notification of diseases was limited to few diseases, but the number of diseases have increased. Though notification of diseases vary from country to country, mainly six diseases have been listed by WHO for notification, *e.g.*, cholera, plague, yellow fever, polio, influenza, rabies to national and international health agencies. The basic purpose of notification is to prevent and control various diseases. The notification is often done to village health guide and multipurpose health workers.

Notification gives an important morbidity data and gives valuable information about disease frequency, incidence and prevalence of disease. We can also assess the geographical distribution of diseases and their rise and fall.

Even though it is an important source of data, still it has limitations because it covers only the morbidity data of public, and may not have complete data. Some diseases may go unnoticed due to lack of investigation facilities. In spite of limitations, it still provides valuable information about occurrence of diseases. It provides early warning about epidemic of disease and helps in planning and implementing the programme for control. Noncommunicable diseases, *e.g.*, cancer, cardiovascular disease, diabetes, accidents and mental illness also help to know the incidence and prevalence of the diseases.

Institutional Records

Hospitals, dispensaries, primary health centres (PHCs), secondary centres (SCs) prepare monthly annual reports. These records also give valuable and a wide variety of information, mainly regarding morbidity data. Hospital records give a basic information about prevalence of illness in the public. These can be collected from various sources. They are good source of health statistics.

The main drawback of these records are :

- They provide the limited information of only those cases which come to the health agencies. Mild cases may not seek the treatment.
- Even admission policy may vary from institution to institution, leaving a wider scope of limitation of available information.

Hence, these records are considered as the poor guide for estimation of diseases but still they supplement lot of information about health problems and activities. These hospital records provide important information regarding age and sex distribution of disease, geographical distribution, socioeconomical and biological factors, cost of care and bed occupancy rate, etc. These medical records again help in effective utilization of resources and planning the health activities according to health needs.

Disease Registers

The specific disease registers are maintained by various hospitals and health centres, which provide the useful data on morbidity, mortality, the treatment given and progress made. These registers are valuable to know about specific morbidity and mortality rate. They are also essential for continuous treatment and follow-up of the patients. These registers are maintained only for certain diseases like cardiovascular disease, cancer, congenital defects, diabetes and communicable diseases like tuberculosis, rabies, malaria, leprosy and STD, etc. These are the permanent records which are prepared monthly and annual compiling of data.

Health Record Linkage

These records are collecting and compiling all the records of a person, which gives the overall picture of one's health; the data like disease, marriage, birth, death and absenteeism from workplace are compiled to bring conclusion to the health status of course. Due to limited use, these records are listed in selected areas like longitudinal studies, chronic illness and congenital diseases.

Epidemiological Surveillance

These surveys help in collecting certain information about community from time to time. They are important source of information regarding incidence and prevalence of various communicable and noncommunicable diseases. In many countries including India where many diseases are endemic (e.g., malaria, leprosy, filaria and T.B.), special control/eradication programmes have been set. These surveillances provide adequate data regarding occurrence of new cases and effect of prevention control measures.

Health Service Records

Information can also be collected from government hospitals, primary health centres, private hospitals, general clinics and specialised clinics. All these informations are helpful in assessing the various aspects of health situation of the countries.

Population Survey

Varieties of surveys conducted by different agencies at different time periods of the year, supplement the additional information regarding population in general, which may give data regarding health services or health problems. These surveys can be cross-sectional or longitudinal.

Health Manpower Statistics

Though not very important, but still some information can be estimated by calculating the nurse-population or doctor-patient ratio. Number of various health professionals available for providing health services to the people.

Environmental Health Data

Information regarding air, water, soil, noise pollution and pollution from harmful industrial and household wastes. It helps to identify the potential health problems and precautionary action may prevent various diseases, due to pollution.

Method of Data Collection

The data obtained from various sources is classified, analysed and tested for accurate statistical method and for easily understanding the health statistics. There are various methods of collecting the statistical data.

Questionnaire

One of the most commonly used methods of data collection is questionnaire. It is a tool in which the questions are formed in predetermined fashion, which are to be filled up by the respondents. Questionnaire can either be administered in person or sent by post.

Advantages

- Less expensive
- Easy to administer
- Less time consuming because many questions can be administered at a time and many people can administer questionnaires at a time.

Disadvantages

- Only literate people can fill questions
- Respondents may interpret the questions in different manner and may reply differently
- Mailed questions may be difficult to understand and clear their doubts.

The questionnaire can be structured in which limited answers are set and unstructured in which different views are received from the respondents.

Interviewing

Very common method of data collection. Interview is direct conversation between interviewer and interviewee. In interview, the interviewer asks the set questions to the interviewee and gets the responses which are recorded simultaneously.

Advantages

- Face to face interaction may help the interviewer to clear any doubt.
- Interviewer can get correct response from respondent.
- Can also be used for illiterate people.

Disadvantages

- Time consuming and not possible to get large information at a time by interviewing
- Interviewee may not give correct answer to the direct interviewer due to lack of confidentiality
- Needs experienced person to conduct the interview
- Interviewee may not feel comfortable to answer in front of the interviewer.

Observation

It is an effective tool in community health, because many things can be interpreted by observational skills, while talking, which may not be interpreted by observer, *e.g.*, housing condition, breastfeeding practices and child care, etc. Observer must develop the skill of accurate and correct observation and timely recording. If good observation is made it gives an effective information regarding health, which can be supplemented to the interview or questionnaires.

Surveillance

The surveillance is supervision and close observation especially for the suspected persons. Epidemiological surveillance is the common observation of the factors that determine the occurrence and distribution of disease and other conditions regarding diseases. Surveillance is the means of collecting the factual information which is not otherwise available from other sources. When health professional wants to know or search for some measures, they need to collect a lot of information, which can be done on a sample of population, which in turn is the representative of the whole population.

Surveillance system is usually done to study the occurrence of the endemic diseases, e.g., plague, cholera, typhoid, etc.

Health Survey

The term health survey, is used to survey the health status, *e.g.*, morbidity pattern, mortality and nutritional status. The health survey conducted are mainly :

- Evaluating the health status of the people, by knowing health problems and aid in planning the health services.

- Factors affecting the health and illness in a particular area.
- Utilization of health services by the people cost-effectiveness of the health services and evaluating the health needs being met and helps in replanning of programmes.

Survey can be crosssectional or longitudinal.

- In crosssectional survey the sample population is surveyed for the required data at one time. It provides information regarding incidence and prevalence of disease.
- In longitudinal survey the population is followed up for a fixed period of longer duration. It provides the information regarding history of diseases and factors affecting health and illness.

Levels of Health Surveillance

Individual Surveillance

The surveillance of an individual who may be infected and as long as, he is the source of infection to others, *e.g.*, cholera, typhoid and their cases and carriers.

Local Population Surveillance

It includes active and passive survey for prevention and control of disease.

(*a*) Active surveillance.

(*b*) Passive surveillance.

National Surveillance

It is done countrywide in cases of disease eradication like leprosy, polio, guinea worm infestation, etc.

International Surveillance

International surveillance for those diseases which spread internationally like influenza, yellow fever. These surveillances are usually taken up by WHO, the information and notification conveyed to all countries of the world for timely action.

Disease Surveillance

Epidemiological surveillance is a process of watchfulness over health events which may occur in a population. It has been defined as *"the ongoing and systematic collection, analysis, and interpretation of health data in the process of describing and monitoring health event with the objective of supporting the planning, implementation and evaluation of public health interventions"*. All countries of the region have developed surveillance systems for specific diseases, such as the EPI-target diseases, malaria, leprosy, tuberculosis and HIV / AIDS. However, only a few countries have disease surveillance data for other communicable diseases.

Countries with well-established surveillance systems, such as Sri Lanka and Thailand, publish comprehensive weekly surveillance reports on all nationally reportable diseases. In 1997, Nepal established an early warning reporting system for important epidemic prone diseases, and India publishes a monthly newsletter on communicable diseases. However, disease surveillance and early warning systems in countries of the region need further improvement.

To improve national capacity in epidemiology and disease surveillance, three-month Field Epidemiology Training Programmes (FETPs) for medical officers and senior public health staff have been organized annually since 1996 at the WHO collaborating centre for epidemiology and training (the National Institute of Communicable Diseases) in New Delhi, India. Outbreak investigation training has been organized at the WHO collaborating centre (Naval Medical Research Unit, No. 2) in Jakarta, Indonesia.

In addition to training efforts, other activities include the development of case definitions for eleven important communicable diseases with epidemic potential. This effort was undertaken through an intercountry consultation held in Sri Lanka in 1997. WHO has also provided technical support for the development of an ASEAN plan of action for strengthening disease surveillance and co-ordination for the control of communicable diseases among ASEAN countries which have common borders and close communication.

All countries of the South-East Asian region are encouraged to develop early warning systems and rapid response mechanisms which will enable them to respond early and effectively to potential disease outbreaks. Unfortunately, several countries in the region do not yet have effective surveillance systems. That these are urgently required is continually reinforced in the discussions about the bacterial, viral and parasitic diseases of public health importance in the region today.

Statistical Data

The word **'Statistics'** has been derived from the Latin word *'status'* meaning **"a political state"**. Initially, statistics was simply the collection of numerical data on different aspects of the life of the people useful to the state. Subquantly, its scope broadened to include collection of numerical data in tabular and graphical form. By the end of nineteenth century, statistics began to concern itself not only with the collection and presentation of data but also with the interpretation and drawing of inferences (conclusions) from data.

Statistics play an important role in everyday life and has proved to be of utmost use in every field of scientific enquiry. The word 'statistics' is used both in its singular as well as plural senses. In singular sense, statistics is a science which concerns itself with the collection, presentation and drawing of conclusions from numerical data. In its plural sense, statistics means numerical facts or observations collected with a definite object in view, *e.g.*, statistics of the population of a country; total number of males and females, total income and expenditure of an individual, etc.

The statistical data must be arranged and compiled in a systematic and organised way for comprehensive understanding of the compiled information. The data can be presented by various methods like tabular form, graphical presentation, pictorial diagrams and charts.

Characteristics of Statistics

- Statistics are expressed quantitatively and not qualitatively.
- Statistics are a sum total of observations. A single observation does not form statistics.
- Statistics are collected with a definite purpose.

- Statistics in an experiment are comparable and can be classified in different groups.

(Comparable means an experiment is repeated and data collected each time as comparable).

TYPES OF DATA

Statistical data are of two types. When an investigator collects data himself with definite plan or design in his mind it is called primary data. This data is therefore, highly reliable and relevant. However, it is not always possible for an investigator to collect primary data due to lack of time, money and resources. Many times, he uses the data collected by someone else, may be in the form of published reports, or official statistics collected by the government, etc. Since the same data can serve various purposes, it is therefore, possible that the data collected by an individual is used by another for his own investigation. Such data that is collected by someone else in another context and used by investigator for his experiment, is called as secondary data. Secondary data should be used with great care since they are collected with a purpose different from that of investigator and may lose some details and may not be fully relevant to the investigations.

Presentation of Data

As soon as collection of data is over, the investigator has to find ways to condense them in a tabular form in order to study their salient features. Such an arrangement of data is called as presentation of data.

Suppose weight of 10 school children ranges like: 30 kg, 35 kg, 25 kg, 25 kg, 40 kg, 42 kg, 42 kg, 38 kg, 41 kg, 41 kg.

The data in this form is called as raw or ungrouped data. If we want to assess the nutrition status of 10 children. The data in raw form does not give us a clear picture of the group. If we arrange them in ascending or descending order, it gives us a slightly better picture. In ascending order. the data looks as follows :

25, 25, 30, 35, 38, 40, 41, 41, 42, 42 kg.

The data arranged in this fashion is called array data. Presentation of data in this form is quite a tedious and time consuming job particularly when the number of observations

are large. To make it easily understandable and clear, we can tabulate data in the form given below :

Table 29.1 : Frequency distribution of ungrouped data

25	—	2
30	—	1
35	—	1
38	—	1
40	—	1
41	—	2
42	—	2
		10

The quantity that we measure from observation to observation is called as variate and arranged groups of observations securing particular number is the frequency of variate. Table 29.1 shows the frequency-distribution of ungrouped data.

Arranging data in ascending or descending order is tedious work and does not tell much except the minimum and maximum of data. Therefore, to bring out certain salient features of the data, we further simplify the presentation of data and condense them into classes or groups. Presenting data in this form enables us to receive certain salient features at a glance. However, in this kind of presentation of data we have one shortcoming. Each frequency for a particular data is supposed to be at its mid-point.

Table 29.2 : Frequency distribution of grouped data

25–30	—	3
31–35	—	1
36–40	—	2
41–45	—	4
		10

This is called as frequency distribution table (Table 29.2) for grouped data or simply frequency table. This is better way of presentation of data as compared to the earlier ones. Since simply by looking at it, we draw the conclusion that most of the students obtained weight in the range 41 to 45. In other words, the group of students is an average of 41 to 45 kg. The above table shows the number of more students having body weight between lower limit and upper limit of various class intervals. The lower limit between 25 to 30 kg and upper limit between 41 to 45 kg.

Points to Keep in Mind

1. The classes should be nonoverlapping.
2. There should be no gaps between classes.
3. As far as possible, open ended classes should be of same size.
4. Limits of each class should be so chosen that there is no ambiguity as to which class a particular item of the data belongs to.

Steps in Forming Classes

1. Determine the minimum and maximum values of variable occurring in the data, *e.g.*,

   Wt : Minimum = 25 kg

   Maximum = 42 kg

2. Decide the number of classes to be formed. There is no special rule to decide this, but we usually keep the number of classes in the range of 5 to 15.

3. Decide "maximum value – minimum value", by the number of classes to be formed to determine the class interval. Such a quotient gives us approximate size of a class, and we choose a convenient number around the quotient = 20

   $45–25 = 20 ÷ 4 = 5$. Four classes at intervals of 5.

   The difference between maximum and minimum value is called range.

4. Include the minimum and maximum occurring in the data. *e.g.*, 25–30 and 40–45.

5. Take each item from raw data, one at a time and put a *tally mark* (|) against the class to which the item belongs (See Table 29.3). Record the tally marks of five into bunches of five, the fifth one crossing diagonally the other four. For example, 25 – 30 = |||| = 5

6. By counting, it determines the total number of tally marks in each class, which gives us the frequency of the class. The total of all frequencies and title of a frequency distribution table may be properly given so that, it conveys exactly what the table is about.

For example, Frequency distribution table showing weight in kg of school children.

The total frequencies of a particular class and of all classes prior to that particular class is called Cumulative frequency (CF) of that class – for calculating Cumulative frequencies, the classes should be written in ascending order. Table 29.3 showing the manner in which Cumulative frequencies are distributed over various classes is called a **Cumulative frequency** (CF) (Table 29.3).

Graphical Representation of Statistical Data

After collecting statistical data, they must be arranged purposefully in graphical form in order to bring out the important points clearly. Therefore, the way in which data is presented is very important. The data represented in graph make it more comprehensive and easy to understand.

Purpose

The data represented in graphical and tabular forms gives a better perspective by representing pictorally, since pictures or graphs, if drawn attractively, are eye-catching and make unwieldy data easily understandable, and more comprehensive. Graphs are good visual aids.

Types

Some of these graphic aids given overleaf can be used to present the data.

Tables : Easiest and most commonly used method of presentation.

Table 29.3 : Showing frequency and Cumulative frequency

Grouping	Frequency	Tally Mark	Cumulative Frequencies
25-30	4	||||	4
31-35	8	||||| |||	4 + 8 = 12
36-40	9	||||| ||||	4 + 8 + 9 = 21
41-50	13	||||| ||||| |||	4 + 8 + 9 + 13 = 34
	34	34	CF = 34

Charts : The useful variety of charts can be used for comparing, contrasting and presenting data.

Diagrams and pictures : Attractive, comprehensive and simple to be understood at a glance and also a common man can understand things.

Graphs : Useful method to show the progress of a particular event over a period of time.

Special curves : Shows the rise and fall of data.

Tabulation

Tabulation is the first step before analysing, interpreting the information. There are certain principles to be kept in mind before preparing tables.

1. There must be a heading of the table in brief descriptive way.
2. It should indicate the sample size of the information.
3. It Should not be too long to read.
4. Table enumerate the factual data.
5. Explanation must be there for each table at the bottom of the tables.

An example of a simple table is given below :

Table 29.4 : Trend of Population in India

Year	Population
1991	
1992	
1993	

Charts

Charts depict the pictorial and written information in an effective manner. It shows between two or more aspects.

The chart may be prepared according to information to be presented. The useful variety of charts can be used for comparing, contrasting and presenting data. Charts can present any information other than graphical presentation in an easy understanding way. Charts are "the visual symbol summarizing or comparing or contrasting or performing other helpful services in explaining subject motto".

Diagrams and Pictures

The diagrams and pictures look attractive and are simple to be understood at a glance and thus a common man can understand things.

Graphs

These are the visual acts based on the use of visual symbolic and visual abstract than words, numbers and formulae.

Graphs are useful methods of presenting simple statistical data. They are useful methods to show the progress of a particular event over a period of time. The special curves show the rise and fall of the data.

Maps

Maps are the accurate and measurable representative diagram of the geographical area drawn. These maps can be used for community exploration.

Types of Charts and Graphs

The data can be presented on the charts or in the graphical presentations, for the chart visibility of the statistical data, graphical presentation is functional form of art as much as modern painting.

Curve or Line Chart (Graph)

It is most widely used method of presenting statistics graphically. This type of chart is simple to construct. The plotted points of data are connected by a solid or symbol line. Fluctuation of this line shows the variation in trend, the distance of the plotted form, the baseline of the graph indicates the quantity. For example, the occurrence of any illness may show rise and fall of prevalence during particular year of time on the lines (Fig. 29.1).

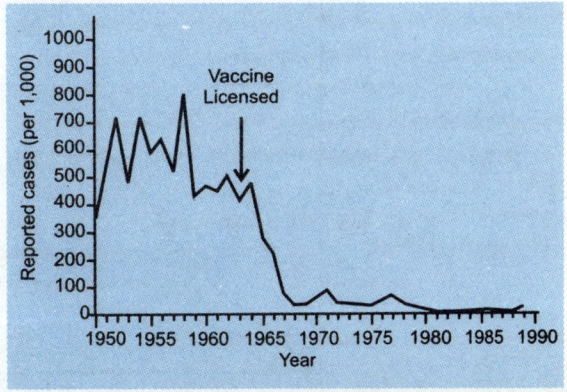

Fig. 29.1 : Measles (Rubeola) by year of report, 1950-1989

Multiple Curve

Multiple curve charts compare two or more related trends. If too many curves appear on one chart, the plotting becomes indistinguishable. Therefore, two or more separate graphs should be made for better comprehension (Fig. 29.2).

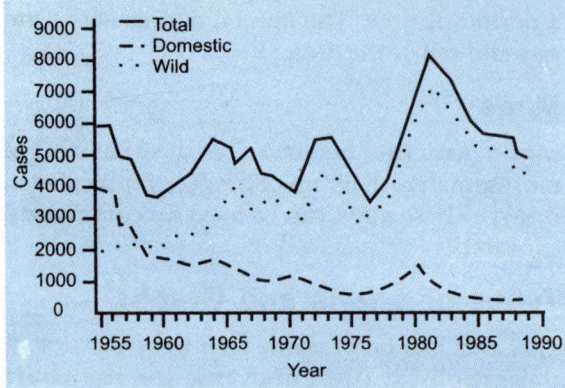

Fig. 29.2 : Rabies, wild and domestic animals by year of report, 1955-1989

Cumulative Curve

Cumulative curve is used when the primary interest is in the cumulated picture of an extended period of time. This cumulation of data tends to smooth the fluctuation of the curve (Fig. 29.3).

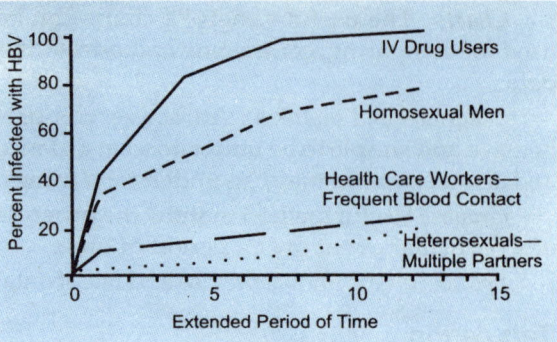

Fig. 29.3 : Cumulative incidence of hepatitis B virus infection by duration of high-risk behaviour

Simple Surface Chart

Simple surface chart depicts the single trend. Its layout and plotting are similar to those of line chart; shading, cross-hatching, photographs or illustrations are used to fill in the area below trend line (Fig. 29.4).

Bar Charts

They are also called as column charts, primary purpose is to depict numerical values of a given item over a period of time. These values either absolute or per cent are represented by the height of the column. The layout of the column chart

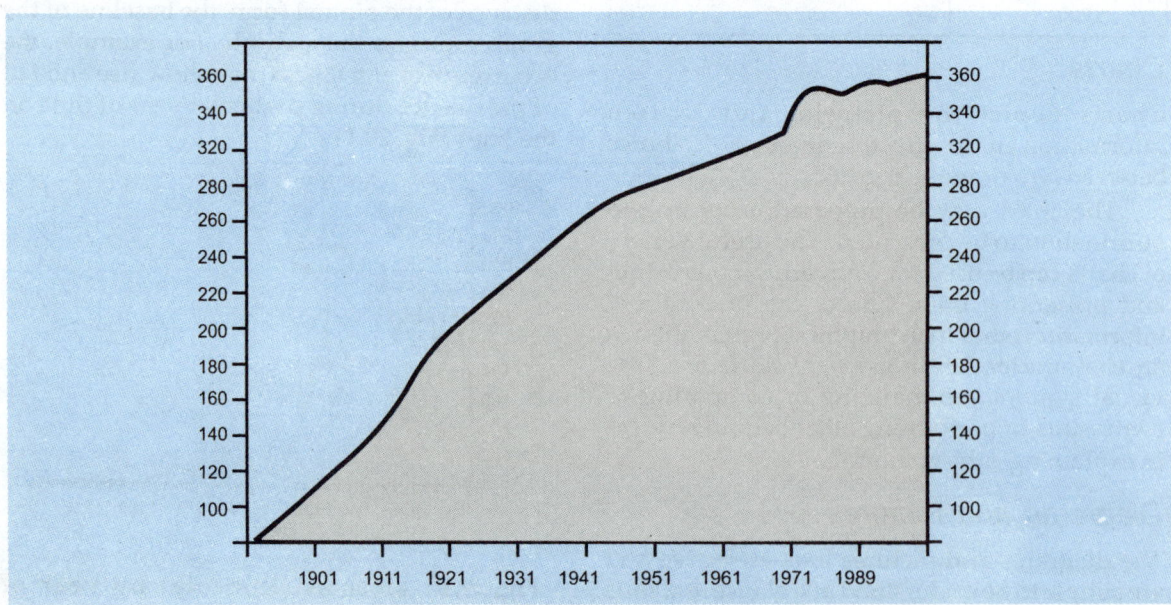

Fig. 29.4 : Population trend in India

requires special care as to spacing and widthwise, *e.g.*, grouped bars, subdivided and deviation bars.

Bar charts are simplest form of graph comparing different items as of the specific data. The bars originating at the right of the common baseline are measured by a few vertical scale lines or ticks. Bar charts are the popular media of presenting statistical data because they are easy to prepare and enable values to be compared visually. The following are some examples of bar charts :

Simple Chart

Bar may be vertical or horizontal. The bars are usually separated by appropriate spaces with an eye to neatness and clear presentation. A suitable scale must be choosen to present the length of the bars (Fig. 29.5).

Multiple Bar Chart (Graph)

When it is necessary to confirm number of items in two respect, two or more bars can be grouped together.

For Example

Trends in life-expectancy in SEAR by country 1950–2000 (Fig. 29.6).

Component Bar Chart

The bar may be divided into two or more parts, each part representing a certain item and proportional to the magnitude of that particular item. It gives a general picture of the composition of each bar. The fewer the segments, the easier the chart will be to read (Fig. 29.7).

Deviation Columns

Deviation columns provide a method for plotting positive and negative data over a period

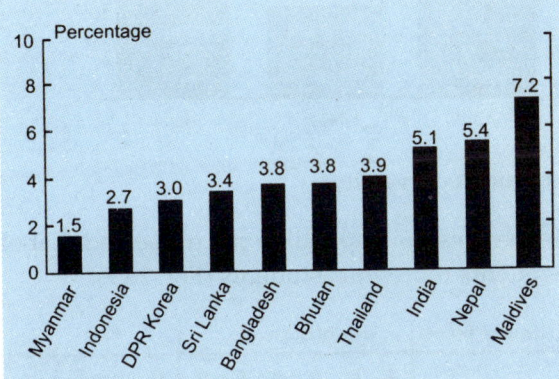

Fig. 29.5 : Total health expenditure (THE) as percentage of GDP in the SEA region, by country, 1998

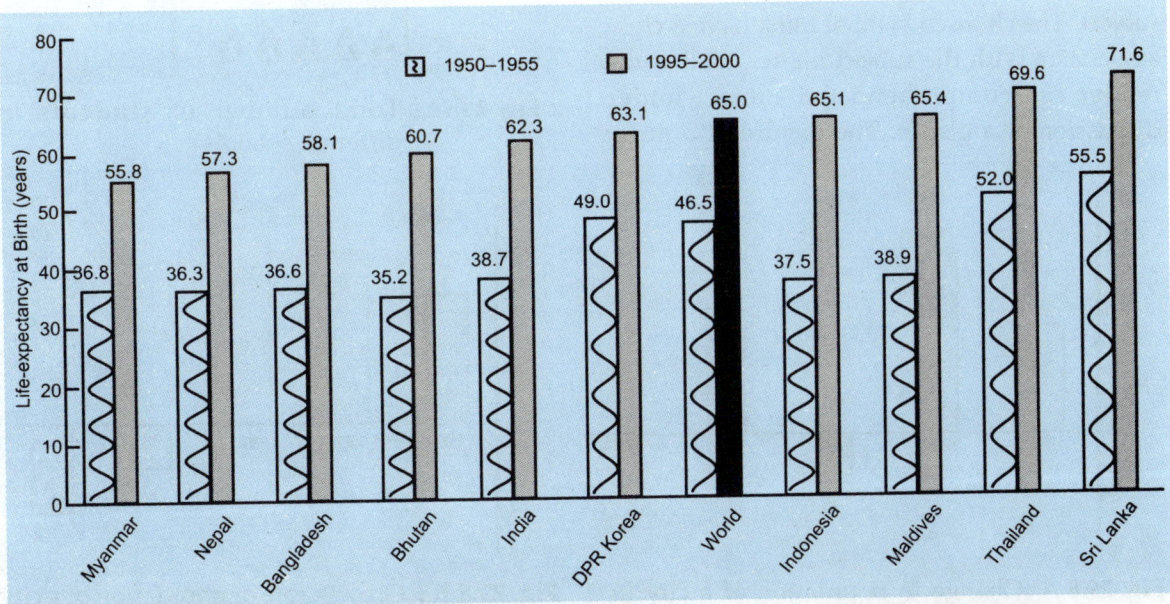

Fig. 29.6 : Trends in life-expectancy in the SEA region, by country, 1950–2000

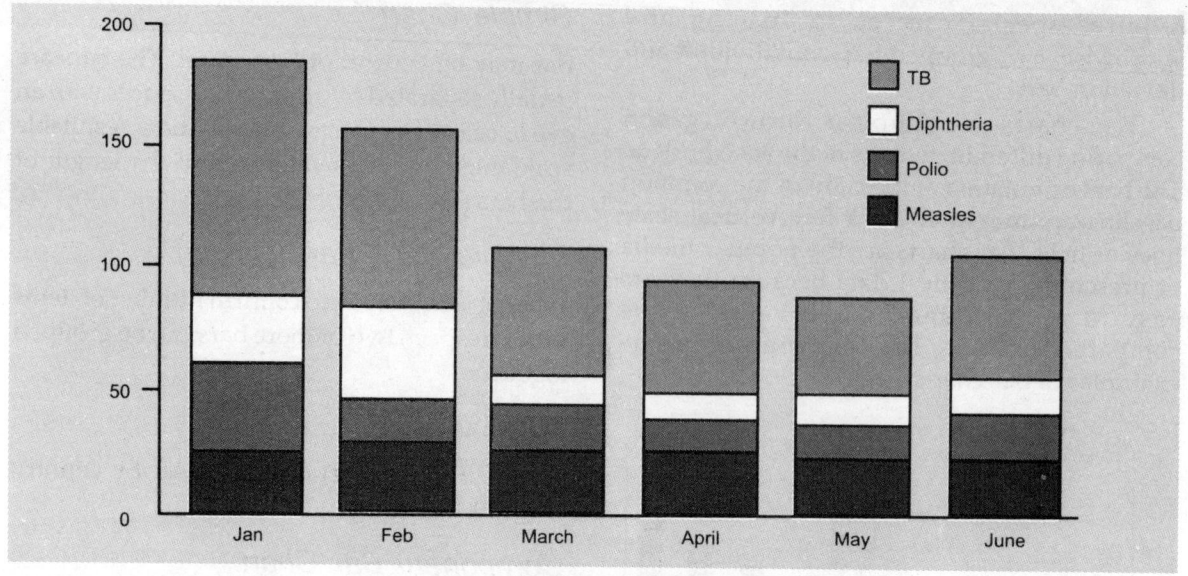

Fig. 29.7 : No. of children infected in a city

of time. This is increase and decrease, losses and gains elevations from requirement of norms (Fig. 29.8).

Pictogram

Illustrate statistical data by means of pictorial symbol. Pictograms are the popular method of presenting data for layman. It can add great interest to what might otherwise be a dull subject. The choosen symbol must have a close association with the subject matter, so that the reader can comprehend the subject under discussion at a glance. The picture of a nurse

represents the population per nurse and that of students represents students (Fig. 29.9).

Name of School	No. of Students	Key
A	🧍 🧍 🧍 🧍 🧍 🧍	🧍 = 100 Students
B	🧍 🧍 🧍 🧍	
C	🧍 🧍	
D	🧍 🧍 🧍 🧍 🧍	

Fig. 29.9 : Total number of students in different schools

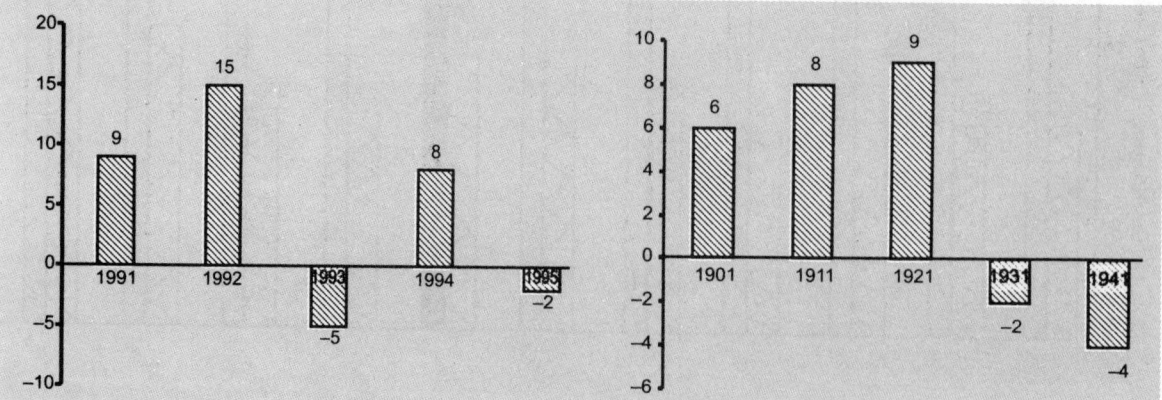

Fig. 29.8 A : Change in population of a city in Europe

Fig. 29.8 B : Growth rate of population of a city in an European country

Pie Graph

The circle is divided into different segments to show the frequency of information out of hundred. The whole pie graph as '100' is divided into percentage to show the different statistical information number of segments percentage. The area of each segment depends upon the angle. Instead of comparing the length of a bar, the areas of segments of a circle are compared. It is often necessary to indicate the percentage in the segments, because it is not very easy to compare the area of segments sometimes.

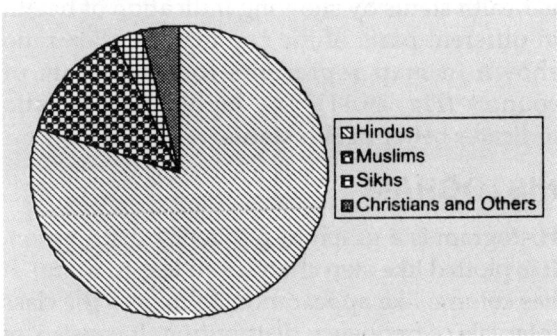

Fig. 29.10 : Composition of Indian population

Statistical Maps

The statistical data is represented on geographical map, showing the incidences, prevalences of any disease or the progress made

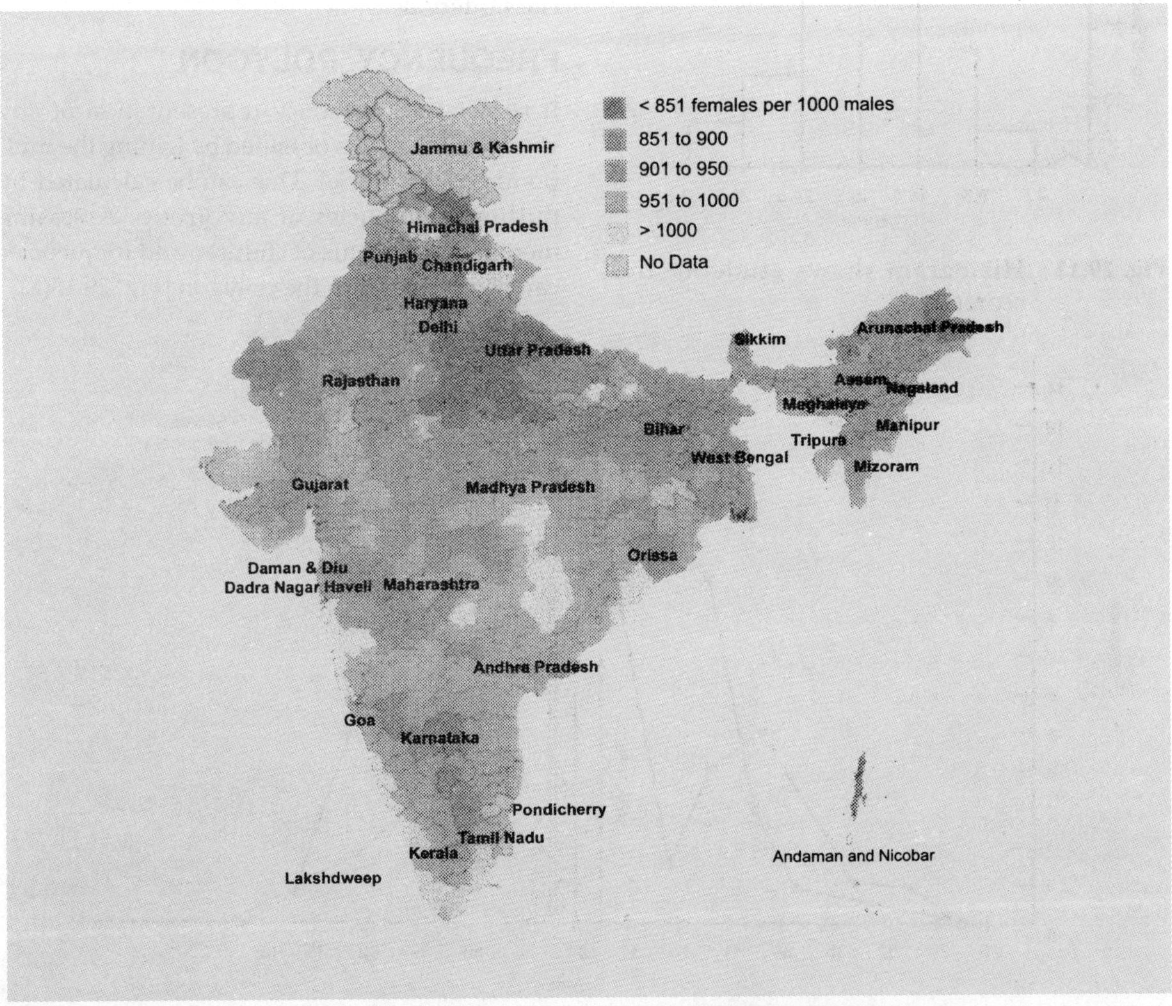

Fig. 29.11 : Map showing statewise sex ratio

in health status by showing indication of health in different parts of the country, *e.g.*, Sex ratio shown in map represents for each state of country (Fig. 29.11). The higher female ratio indicates better health status.

HISTOGRAM

Histogram is a graph of frequency distribution. It is plotted like step chart (from less to more). It has column like appearance, delineates the class intervals of frequency distribution. It consists of series of blocks. These intervals are given along the horizontal axis and the frequencies along the vertical axis, and construct the rectangles with class intervals as bases and respective frequencies as heights. The determination of scale depends upon our convenience and type of data.

Since the scale in 'X'-axis starts at 4.5 a (kink break) is indicated near the origin to signify that the graph is drawn to scale beginning at '4.5' and not at the origin, the same technique can be employed on 'Y'-axis, if necessary (Fig. 29.12).

In above case, the class intervals are continuous. In any case where class intervals are not continuous it is necessary to convert the given class interval into continuous intervals and then draw the histogram with reference to continuous class intervals.

FREQUENCY POLYGON

It shows the frequency representation of any statistical data. It is obtained by joining the midpoints of the blocks. This can be calculated by putting frequencies of any group. Assessing mental health status of children and frequencies can be presented in the polygon [Fig. 29.13(a)] .

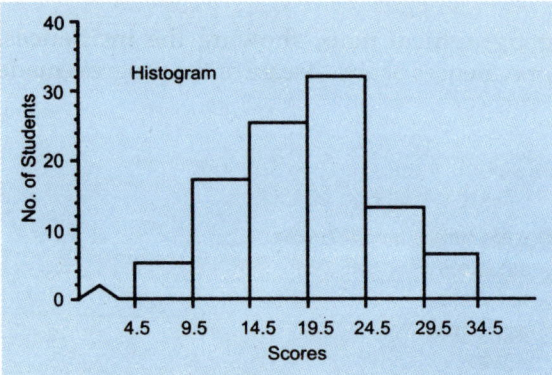

Fig. 29.12 : Histogram shows students and scores

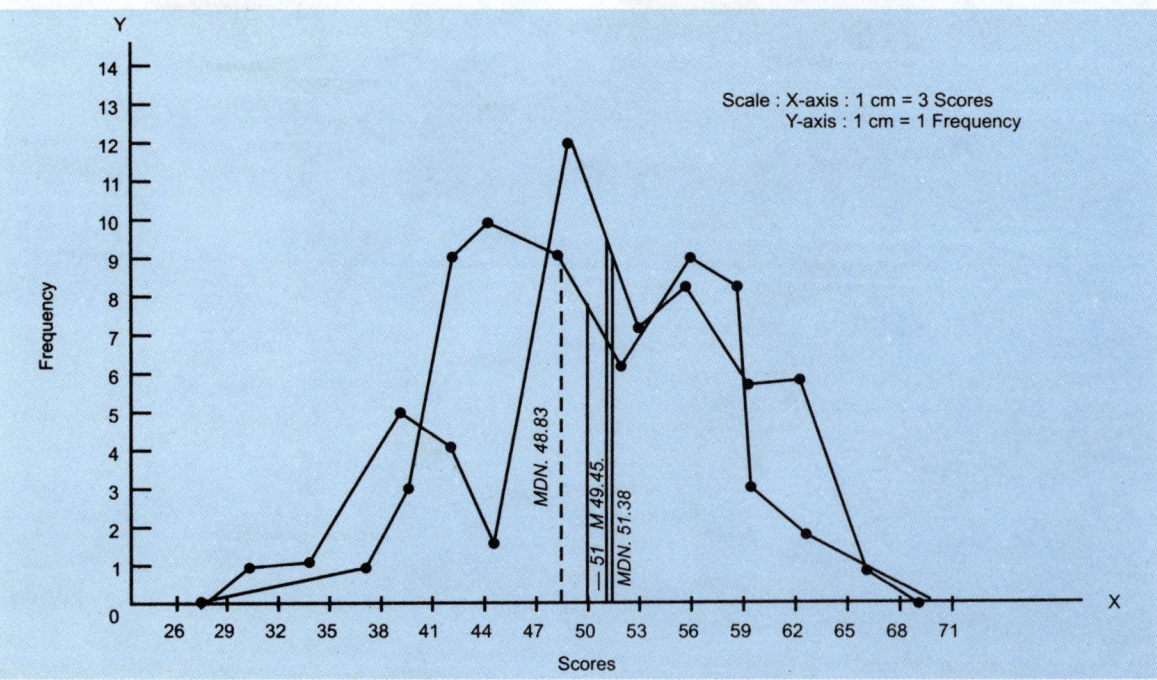

Fig. 29.13(a) : Frequency polygon representing mental health status scores of 60 childrens each in the age group of 7 and 8 years

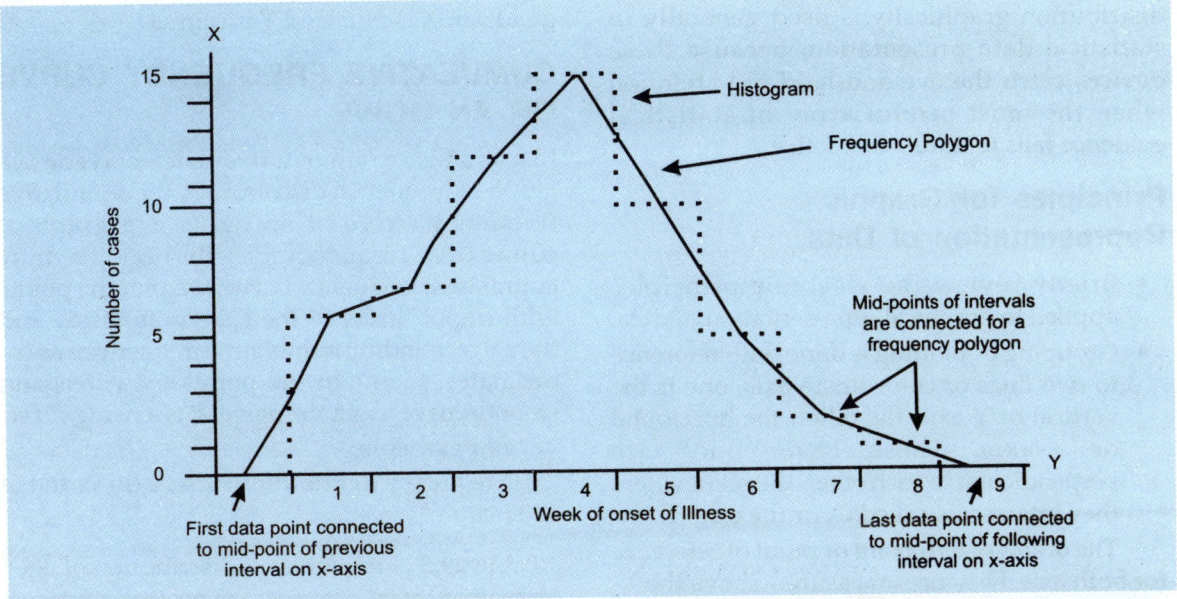

Fig. 29.13 (b) : Histogram and polygon showing week of onset of Illness

A frequency polygon is *drawn by joining the middle points of the upper sides (tops) of the adjacent rectangles of a histogram by means of line segments* (Fig. 29.13(b)]. To compare the polygon, the end points obtained above are joined, the mid-points of the immediately lower or higher imagined class intervals of zero frequency. This ensures the total area of a frequency polygon is the same as that of the corresponding histogram. A frequency polygon can also be drawn independently by plotting the class intervals along the X-axis and the frequencies along the Y-axis and then joining the plotted points by segment lines.

Construction of Frequency Polygon

Labelling the Points on the Baseline

To label the scores on the X-axis, the scores can be labelled from below the last score and above the higher score, and vertical axis has been moved in the convenience.

Plotting Mid-points

Frequencies of each interval are plotted above the mid-points of the interval on the Y-axis in Fig. 29.12.

Drawing the Frequency Polygon When all the Points have been Located in the Diagram

They are joined by a series of short lined to form the frequency polygon to complete the polygon one additional interval at the lower and one additional interval at the higher ·of the distribution are added on the X scale. The frequency on each of these intervals remains zero, therefore, by adding these frequencies to the scale it remains the same. To begin the polygon one-half interval below the first, and end it half interval above the last interval on the X-axis.

Dimensions of Frequency Polygon

To balance the polygon and symmetry, the unit distance must be selected carefully, to represent the intervals on the X-axis and frequencies on the Y-axis. Too long unit tends to stretch out the polygon, while too short X units crowd the separate points. On the other hand, too long by unit (frequencies) elaborate the changes from intervals and too short 'Y' makes the polygon too flat. A good rule is to select X and Y units which will make the similar height and width (X + Y) or height should be graphical representation of the frequency distribution.

The method of representing a frequency distribution graphically is used generally in statistical data presentation, because these devices catch the eye and hold the attention when the most careful array of statistical evidence fails to attract the notice.

Principles for Graphic Representation of Data

- Briefly review the algebraic principles applied to graphical representation of data.
- Grouping or plotting is done with reference to two lines or co-ordinate axis, one is the vertical or Y axis, the other, the horizontal or X-axis. These basic lines are perpendicular to each other, the point where they intersect is called O, or the origin.

The origin is zero point or point of reference for both axis. Distances measured above the X-axis to the right of O are called positive and distances measured along the X-axis to the left of O are called negative. Similarly, distance measured on the Y-axis above O is positive distance and below O negative. In the four quadrants, the upper right division or first quadrant both X and Y measures are (++). In the upper left division or second quadrant by X is minus and Y is plus (– +). In the lower left quadrant or third quadrant both X and Y are negative (– –), while in the lower right or fourth quadrant X is plus and Y is minus (+ –).

CUMULATIVE FREQUENCY CURVE OR AN OGIVE

Just as a histogram or a frequency polygon is a graph of frequency distribution, the cumulative frequency curve or an ogive is a graph of cumulative frequency distribution. To draw cumulative frequency curve, we plot the points with upper limits of the classes abscissae and the corresponding cumulative frequencies as co-ordinates, then join the points by a freehand smooth curve to get the ogive. It is a rising curve.

For example,

Frequency distribution of Age (in years) of 100 people.

Table 29.5 : Frequency of distribution of age

Age	People
0 – 10	7
11 – 20	10
21 – 30	23
31 – 40	51
41 – 50	6
51 – 60	3
Total	100

Table 29.6 : Showing cumulative frequency

Distribution	C.F.
10	7
20	17 (10 + 7)
30	40 (23 + 17)
40	91 (51 + 40)
50	97 (6 + 91)
60	100 (3 + 97)

- The upper limits of the classes are 10, 20, 30, 40, 50, 60.
- The upper limits of classes are responding the X-axis.
- The cumulative frequencies of respective classes are representing along the Y-axis.
- The points so plotted are joined by a free-hand curve to obtain a cumulative frequency curve.

While drawing a cumulative frequency curve or an ogive, we assume that there are class intervals before the given class intervals with zero frequency.

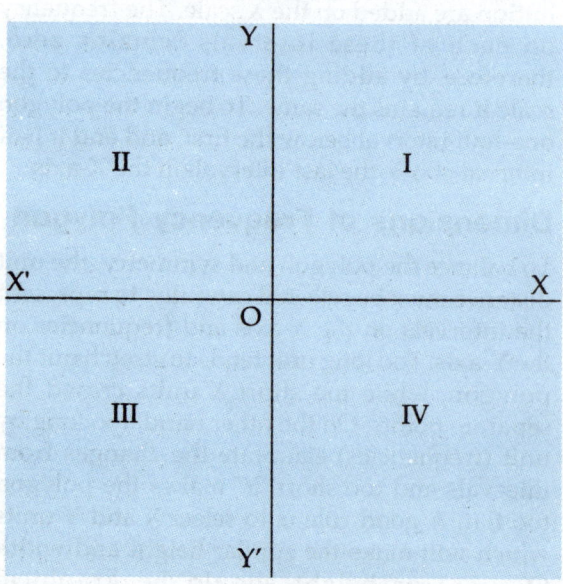

Fig. 29.14

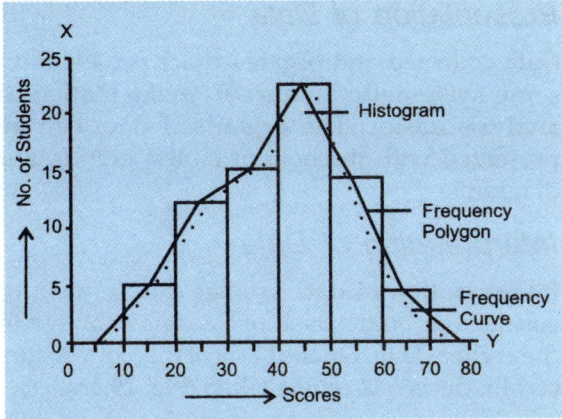

Fig. 29.15 : Histogram, frequency polygon and frequency curve

Measurement may be of several kinds and may be taken to various degrees of precision. When people or objects have been ranked or arranged in an ordinal series with respect to some factors, it is termed as simplest type of measurement. These factors may be according to salaries, positions, e.g., school children according to marks in an examination. Measurement of individual performance by means of tests is usually expressed as a score. These scores may be with reference to amount of workdone in a given time and mental tests scores, physical trait scores or time taken to complete a given task. When the scores are expressed in equal units these are called as interval scale. Continuous and discrete series while measuring physical and mental traits most of the variables fall into continuous series, that means these are capable of any degree of subdivision. The series which shows real gap between two intervals is called discrete series. The average number of children of a community is said to be 2.57 at an average.

Test Scores in Continuous Series

The score of continuous series are said to be distance with continum, rather than discrete points. The exact mid-point of 130.5 – 131.5 = 131.

Other score may be interpreted likewise. The score of '10' may include 9.5, 10 and 10.5, etc. The statistical measuring of a score is an interval which extends along some dimension from 5 unit or below to 5 unit and above the face value of the score.

As per second method, the score of 130 means it is less than 130 and not 131, that means any fractional value greater than 130 but less than 131 which may be 130.3, 130.5 130.8, etc. The mid-point is 130.5. Both the ways of calculating scores are valued and valid. If the height of 10 people is recorded as 170 inches that means the height varies from 169.8, 170.3, 170.5 or 170.7, etc. and not between 170–171.

When to Use the Frequency Polygon and When to Use Histogram

The frequency polygon is less precise than the histogram in that it does not represent accurately, i.e., in terms of area, the frequency upon each interval. In comparing two or more graphs plotted on the same axis, however the frequency polygon is likely to be more useful, as the vertical and horizontal lines in the histograms will often coincide.

Methods of Computing Statistical Data

Health information can be collected at any setting, at any level of precision desired within the constraints of available resources. This data can be cross-sectional, longitudinal, descriptive or analytic or both. Surveys carried out by either single or repeat visits provide direct estimates of vital events. Follow-up surveys on the same households within short intervals (e.g., 6 months) provide more accurate estimates of vital health statistics but may be too expensive for monitoring purposes.

Data is first obtained which is subsequently classified, analysed and tested for accuracy by statistical methods. The data that is obtained directly from an individual is called primary data for example the census 1991, data collecting from people is primary data. The data collected from outside source is called secondary data. Primary data gives precise required information, which secondary data may not give.

Types of Data Analysis

Descriptive Methods

• Collection and classification of data

- Presenting them in tabular and diagrammatic forms
- Calculating summary indices to measure certain characteristics of data.

Quantitative Data

In quantitative data, the variables are measured in numerical terms, *e.g.*, taking temperature, height and weight measurement of an individual, etc. Their values can be expressed numerically.

Qualitative

Sometimes it is not possible to measure variables numerically, for example attitudes of people, intelligence of individual and aptitude, etc. can not be measured numerically like height and weight. Therefore, we may rank them according to quality of their attributes. There may be comparison ranking. The ranks may be used as numerical measurements for purposes of statistical analysis. Empirical and quantitative analysis are mostly used in technical problems and physical sciences. The empirical methodology consists of making observations and collecting information, analysing the information and drawing conclusions and retesting these conclusions by further observations and laws are made.

Empirical Methods and Quantification

Empirical methods are based on experience. A scientific method of investigation is associated with empirical method. An empirical investigation is an investigation where facts are collected through observation.

Steps of Data Analysis

Collection of Data

This is the first step in the statistical study and is foundation of statistical analysis. Therefore, data should be gathered with maximum care by the investigator and obtained from reliable sources.

Organisation of Data

The information collected by investigator needs to be organised by editing, classifying and tabulating.

Presentation of Data

Data collected and organised are presented in some systematic manner to make statistical analysis easier. The organised data can be presented with the help of tables, graphs and diagrams.

Interpretation of Data

Interpretation of data implies the drawing of conclusions on the basis of the data analysed in the earlier stage. On the basis of this conclusion, certain decisions can be taken (Fig. 29.16).

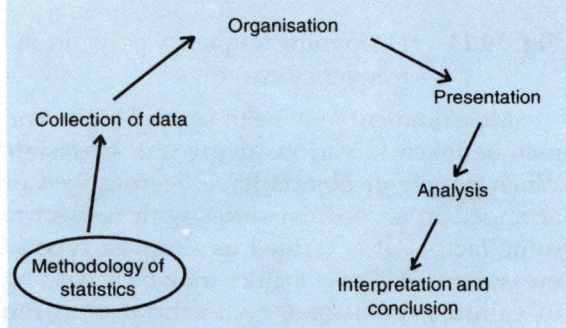

Fig. 29.16 : Steps of data analysis and interpretation

MEASUREMENT OF CENTRAL TENDENCY

Measurement of central tendency refers to central position with reference to graph's performance. It is an average and represents all the scores obtained from the group. It not only gives the concise description of the performance of the group but also enables to compare two or more groups in terms of mean or average.

One of the most important objects of statistical analysis is to get one single value that describes the characteristics of the entire mass of unwieldy data. Such a value is called the central value or an average. The word average is very commonly used in day-to-day conversation. For example, if we talk about average boy in the class or average height or life of an Indian, average income, etc. When we say he is an average student in the class that means he is neither very good nor very bad, just a mediocre type of student. However, in statistics, average has different meaning. It may be defined as that value of a distribution which is considered as the most representative or typical value for a group of numbers.

Such a value is of great significance because it depicts the characteristics of the whole group. Since an average represents the entire data, its value lies somewhere in between the two extremes, *e.g.*, the largest and the smallest items. For this reason, an average is frequently referred to as a measure of central tendency.

Object of Averaging

There are two main objects of the study of averages :

To Get One Single Value

It describes the characteristics of the entire group.

Measures of central value by condensing the mass of data in one single value, enable us to get a bird's eye-view of the entire data. Hence, one value can represent thousands, lakhs and even millions of value. For example, it is impossible to remember incidence and prevalence of disease in thousands or millions, but if the average figure is taken it is easy to remember. We take one single value that represents the entire population. Such a figure will throw light on the intensity of disease in a defined population.

To Facilitate Comparison

Measures of central value by reducing the mass of data in one single figure, enable comparisons to be made. Comparisons can be made either at a point of time or over a period of time, for example, the percentage results of the students of different colleges in a certain examination; if we want to compare the health status of two countries and we can take the average of diseases, deaths, births and socioeconomic conditions. Such comparisons are of immense help in planning and organising suitable health policies to improve the health status.

TYPES OF AVERAGE

The following are the types of average :
  (*a*) Arithmetic mean,
  (*b*) Median,
  (*c*) Mode,
  (*d*) Geometric mean, etc
  (*e*) Hormonic mean.

Arithmetic Mean

The most popular and widely used measure for representing the entire data by one value is said to be an average and statistically called arithmetic mean. Its value is obtained by adding together all the items and by dividing this total by number of items.

Calculation of Arithmetic Mean

The process of computing mean in case of individual observation : (1) add together various values of the variable, *e.g.*, weight of 10 children and divide the total by number of students :

For example, 16, 15, 10, 10, 18, 18, 17, 12 11, 14

$$= \frac{141 \text{ kg}}{10} = 14.1 \text{ kg}$$

Hence, the average weight of
10 children = 14.1 kg

The statistics does not allow the term 'average' because it has too loose a connotation. It has different meanings, *e.g.*, average person, average salary, or height, etc. It can refer to either mean, median, mode, geometric mean, hormonic mean or any other average.

Computation of Mean, Median and Mode

Mean is the most common measure of Central tendancy, represented by $\bar{X}$. To find out the mean, all the individual observations are added together, and then divided by the number of total observations. The process of adding together is called as summation and is denoted by the sign Σ or S. The individual sign is denoted by η and mean is indicated as $\bar{X}$.

For example, the incidence of malaria in seven months is 20, 30, 40, 35, 25, 30, 35 then mean of these seven months incidence of malaria is 20 + 30 + 40 + 35 + 25 + 30 + 35/7 = 215/7 = 30.7

Mean is easy to calculate and to understand. It gives a comprehensive figure about any big figures. Mean is considered to be the most useful in statistical average; even though it may sometimes be unduly influenced by abnormal values in distributions.

The formula is represented as :

$$\overline{X} = \frac{\Sigma X}{n} = \otimes$$

$\overline{X}$ = represents mean

Σ = A sign (The capital greek letter sigma) that stands for addition of all values

n = number of values

X = denotes measure of a variable, i.e., scores

If X = represents the weight of (5) infants = 9 kg, 10 kg, 11 kg, 8 kg, 6 kg

∴ Total weight of 5 infants

ΣX = 9 + 10 + 11 + 8 + 6 = 44 kg

n = 5

$$\overline{X} = \frac{\Sigma X}{n}$$

Mean of weight of 5 infants = $\frac{44}{5}$ = 8.8 kg

Hence, the average weight of 5 infants is 8.8 kg.

Median

It is the middle value in a series that is arranged from smallest to largest.

For example, the median of 5 infants weight :

6 kg + 8 kg + 9 kg + 10 kg + 11 kg
= 9 kg

Hence, the median of weight of 5 infants is 9 kg in which two scores are above and two scores below :

To obtain median, the data is first arranged in an ascending or descending order and then the value of middle figure is obtained, which is called median.

Another example: The number of fever cases every month.

20	15
15	20
30	25
40	30 **Median**
25	35
35	40
45	45

If the number of values or items is even, the practice is to take the average of two middle values. For example, if there are eight values instead of seven, the median is worked out by taking average of two middle values.

In case of even numbers of values, the middle two scores are divided by 2 to take the median.

For example : 6 + 8 + 9 + 10 + 11 + 12

Median = $\frac{9 + 10}{2}$ = $\frac{19}{2}$ = 9.5 kg

Hence, the median of above value is 9.5

Mode

It is the number most frequently observed during the observation; as per following values:

2 4 3 6 7 6 6 6 3 4 4 7 7

frequency of	2	=	1	
	4	=	3	
	3	=	2	
	6	=	4	**Mode**
	7	=	3	

Out of mean, median and mode, central tendency mean is generally preferred to other average, because of its greatest stability and arithmetic mean is also needed for computing standard deviation and test, etc.

Median is computed when exact mid-point or 50 per cent value of distribution is desired. Mode gives a quick or approximate measure of central tendency and especially when most typical value is needed.

Procedure for Computation of Mean and Median

Based on following data, you need to find the mean by using formula :

Mean $\overline{X}$ = $\frac{\Sigma fx}{n}$

$\overline{X}$ = Mean

fx = frequency multiplied by mid-point

Σfx = sum total of frequencies multiplied by mid-point (the value is now frequent)

n = sum of frequencies

Total no. of score = 50; Class interval = 4

Class interval	f (Frequency)	Mid-point (X)	fx
90 – 94	1	92	92 = 92
85 – 89	3	87	87 × 3 = 261
80 – 84	4	82	82 × 4 = 328
75 – 79	5	77	77 × 5 = 385
70 – 74	6	72	72 × 6 = 432
65 – 69	8	67	67 × 8 = 536
60 – 64	10	62	62 × 10 = 620
55 – 59	6	57	57 × 6 = 342
50 – 54	6	52	52 × 6 = 312
45 – 49	2	47	47 × 2 = 94
40 – 44	4	42	42 × 4 = 168
35 – 39	3	37	37 × 3 = 111
30 – 34	2	32	32 × 2 = 64
	n = 60		Σfx = 3745

$$\text{Mean} = \overline{X} = \frac{\Sigma fx}{n} \text{ or } \overline{X} = \frac{3745}{60} = 62.416$$

Median

Procedure for computing median. Median is the 50 per cent point in the distribution. Therefore, we take $\frac{N}{2}$ scores to find median in above table

$N = 60$, $\frac{N}{2} = \frac{60}{2} = 30$, the median is that point in the distribution which has 30 scores on each side.

- Start with small score distribution (30 – 34) and add up frequencies till you locate the score where median lies and till that class interval of 60 – 64, $f = 10$.
- Next interval is 65 – 69, $f = 8$, where you need formula to calculate median is given below :

$$\text{Median (Me)} = I + \left(\frac{\frac{N}{2} - f}{f_m} \right) i$$

I = Exact lower limit of the class interval upon which median lies. In the table the class interval in which median lies is 60 – 64, therefore, lower limit is 59.5.

$\frac{N}{2}$ = Half of the total number of scores $\frac{60}{2} = 30$.

f = Sum of the scores on all intervals below I, i.e., below 59.5 the number of score is 23.

f_m = Frequency (Number of scores) within the interval upon which median falls. Here the f on which median fall is 10.

i = Length of class-interval, which is 5 as given in table above.

$$\text{Hence, Median} = I + \left(\frac{N/2 - f}{f_m} \right) i$$

$$= 59.5 + \frac{\frac{60}{2} - 23}{10} \times 5$$

$$= 59.5 + \frac{30 - 23}{10} \times 5$$

$$59.5 + \frac{7}{10} \times 5 = 59.5 + 3.5 = 63$$

Median = 63.

Mode

The third type of 'Central value' or centre of the distribution is the value of greatest frequency or more precisely of greatest frequency density. In graphical representation, its value is on the 'X'-axis and highest frequency point is as shown below :

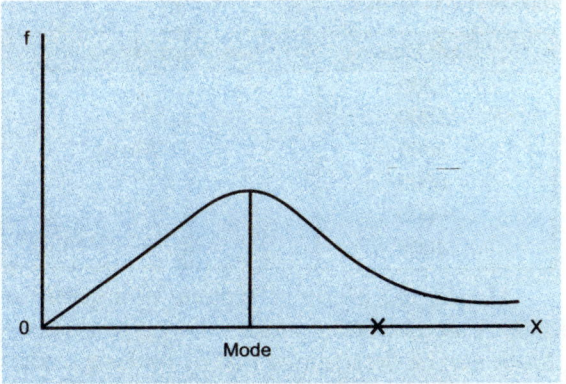

Mode is said to be the value which occurs most frequently. It is the value which has the greatest frequency density in its immediate neighbourhood. Mode is also called the most typical value of a distribution.

The value of the variable at which the curve reaches the maximum is called the mode. It is the value around which the items tend to be most heavily concentrated.

Calculation of Mode

To determine mode, count the number of times of various values repeated themselves and the value which occurs the maximum number of times is the modal value. The more often the modal value appears relatively the more valuable the measure is as an average to represent data.

There are many situations in which arithmetic mean and median fail to reveal the true characteristics of data. For example, when we say about most common height, most common weight or income, we keep in mind mode and not arithmetic mean or median. The mean does not always provide an accurate reflection of data due to presence of extreme items. Median may also prove unrepresentative of the data for an uneven distribution of the series. The short-comings of both mean and median may be overcome by mode which refers to the value which occurs most frequently in a distribution. Moreover, mode is the easiest to compute since it is the value corresponding to the highest frequency.

The mode can be calculated by counting the maximum number of an item, *e.g.*,

Total Income	(in Rupees)	
1000	3	
5000	4	
3000	7	**Mode**
6000	6	
10000	5	
4000	4	

Hence, the mode of income of a group is 3000. Calculation of mode—Discrete series—Mode can be determined just by looking to that value of the variable around which the items are most heavily concentrated.

Height in inches	No. of People	
58	4	
60	6	
62	20	
63	25	
64	60	
66	65	**Mode**
68	20	
70	1	

The mode of height in inches is 66 in which most number of people are lying.

Calculation of Mode

Continuous series : By preparing grouping table and analysis table or by inspection, ascertain the modal class.

- Determine the value of mode by applying the following formula-I.

$$M_1 = L_1 + \left(\frac{\Delta_1}{\Delta_1 + \Delta_2}\right) \times i$$

L_1 = lower limit of modal class.

Δ_1 = difference between modal class and pre-modal class.

Δ_2 = difference between modal class and post-modal class.

i = Size of class-interval of modal class.

Formula II

$$M_0 = L_1 + \frac{f_1 - f_0}{2 f_1 - f_0 - f_2} \times i$$

L_1 = lower limit of modal class

f_1 = frequency of modal class

f_0 = frequency of class preceding the modal class

f_2 = frequency of the class succeeding the modal class.

While applying this formula, the class interval should be informed throughout. If they are unequal they should first be made equal so that frequencies are equally distributed throughout the class otherwise mode may not be accurate.

Formula III : Mode = 3 Median – 2 Mean.

Graphic Representation of Mode

In a frequency distribution, the value of mode can also be determined graphically. The steps in calculation are :

- Draw a histogram of the given data.
- Draw two lines diagonally in the inside of the modal class bar, starting from each upper corner of the bar to the upper corner of the adjacent bar.
- Draw perpendicular line from the intersection of the two diagonal lines to the 'X'-axis (horizontal line which gives us the modal value).

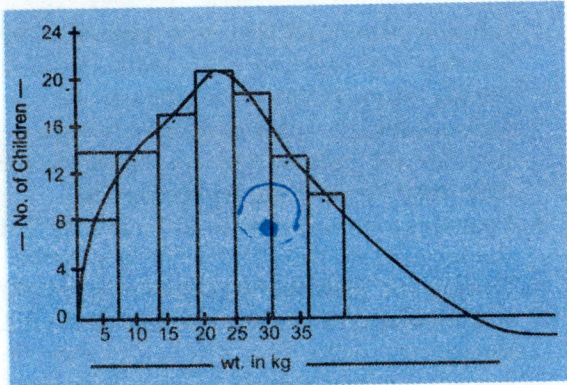

Fig. 29.16 : Graphic representation of Mode

Relationship between Mean, Median and Mode

A distribution in which the value of Mean, Median and Mode coincide is known as a symmetrical distribution, and when they do not coincide is known as asymmetrical or skewed. In moderately skewed or asymmetrical distribution, an important relationship exists among mean, median and mode (Fig. 29.17). The distance between mean and median is about one-third the distance between mean and the mode.

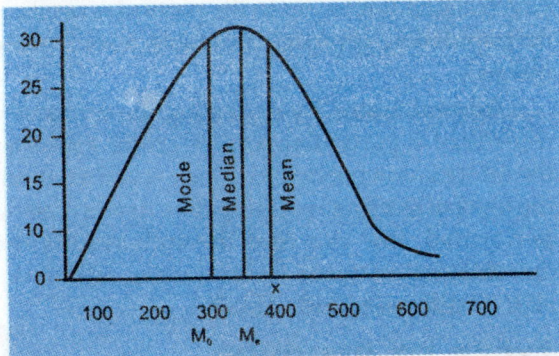

Fig. 29.17 : Frequency polygon showing relationship between mean, median and mode

Standards of Accuracy in Computation

Sometimes, by discarding decimals, throws away legitimate data. More often, however, he tends to retain too many decimals, a practice which may give a false appearance of great precision not always justified by the original material.

Some of the generally accepted principles which apply to statistical calculation are :

- **Rounded number :** The numbers are usually rounded in calculations for accuracy demanded by figures. Convenient rules for rounding numbers to two decimals are as follows : When the third decimal is less than 5 drop it; when greater than five increase the preceding figure by 1. When exactly five compute the fourth decimal and correct back to the second place, when exactly 5 followed by zeros, drop it and make no corrections.

A mean of 52.6872 is reported as 52.69

Median of 12.3842 = 12.38

Plotting of two frequency distributions of scores on the same axis when sample differ in size.

In order to provide a more detailed comparison of the two types of frequency graphs, the distribution is plotted on the same co-ordinate axis as a frequency polygon and as a histogram. The increased number of cases and the more symmetrical arrangement of scores in the distribution make these figures more regular in appearance. These polygons provide an immediate comparison of the relationship between two groups.

RECORDS, REPORTS, REGISTERS

Health records are the means of providing information about health of an individual, family or community. These may be regarding socioeconomic, psychological and environmental conditions. Records are practical and indispensible aid to health personnel for giving best possible proper care to individual or family. Records are the effective means of communication between family and health workers. Information noted during observation on records, may be studied by other health professionals for further action. CHN, before she goes to the family will read the record and get knowledge about family members and their health, and he / she will not be treated as stranger because by this time they are successful to create good personal rapport.

Effective record must include health situations and home conditions affecting the individual and family.

Each record must show the essential aspects of health care, so that next health personnel should come to know what is done and what has to be done. Records not only ensure effective services, but also save the time, effort and money.

PURPOSES OF MAINTAINING RECORDS

- Helps in determining the work done.
- Helps in collection of statistics of the community.
- Helps in assessing the health statistics of the people.
- Determines the evaluation of health care.
- Helps as a tool for educating the people.
- Essential legal documents.
- Determines continuity of the care.

Principles of Maintaining Records

- Flexibility should be there in maintaining records.
- Written clearly, legibly. Illegible records are waste of time, effort and money.
- Records serve as legal documents, and should contain facts based on observation, communication and action.
- Records should be brief, clear, complete and accurate.
- Records must be written with ink, avoid overwriting of records and signature for the accountability of work recorded.
- Meaningful and understandable records will be used for references by other people.
- Should be carefully handled because they are valuable documents filed in systematic organised way.

Functions of Record System

The well maintained records and reports system serves several functions.

- Provides a service accounting system that documents what exactly has been done. Information on records must be eventful about precise care given and the level of

nursing personnel that was required. The number and types of visits paid. The data on the records must be answerable for accountability. Information necessary to identify the patient and his eligibility for care must be accurate and complete.

- Provides a control system and assumes that the services are provided according to plan. During the process of goal setting certain specific outcomes have been identified, with measurable indication. The information on records must be secured to correct any error or omission or misdirection of efforts. The record system must supply the basic data required for making these estimations.
- Record system provides a rich source of information for planning and evaluating the nursing service provided.

Identification of population characteristics may determine the health needs of specific group of people, e.g., if the community has more number of infants, hence the care can be planned on care of infants on immunization, nutrition and assessment of growth and development.

By reviewing records and reports, community health nurse has a basis for deciding the extent to which action is relevant to the particular needs of the population, approach is suitable, resources are utilized.

Administrator, by reviewing the composite records of a particular service group provides the information needed to decide whether or not the level of staffing is appropriate to work being performed. She can find through results the documentation needs for proposing additional staff or different kind of staff.

TYPES OF RECORDS

Cumulation or Continuing Records

These are the continuation of all records of an individual's lifetime, having one basic record for health.

The antenatal mother record will continue throughout pregnancy, childbirth, infant, toddler and pre-school and record is handed over to the school administration. This helps the community health nurse to know previous health conditions and problems which help in dealing with present problems.

These records save time and are economical and help to evaluate the progress over a long period.

System of using one record for home and clinic services in which home visits are recorded in red and clinic visits in blue ink helps co-ordinate the services and saves the time of all the personnel concerned.

Family Records

Family is the basic unit of health services. Hence the central record unit should also have a family record.

Family folder which contains all the individual records of one family has all the identifying data plus observations about general, social and environmental factors that affect health in family. There may also be a summary of health status of the family, with space of periodical evaluation. Record outlines are usually printed. Nurse should see that the family folder or records are complete and accurately filled.

Salient Features of Record Keeping

- Records are usually started when individual seeks medical care at home or centre. The nurse at centre should be comfortably seated in a quiet private room to maintain the confidentiality.
- Do not force the person on economic and social informations unless he/she is willing to tell the fact.
- Explain the reason for recording and ensure for confidentiality of information.
- Ask questions in a friendly way, but in definite and direct manner.
- Write brief notes of all informations.
  - (a) Reason of visit
  - (b) Observations made
  - (c) What has been done
  - (d) Plan for next visit
  - (e) Attitude of the care-seeker
  - (f) Referral, if any.
- Record should have chronological progress, e.g., height and weight of child shows

progress. Antenatal mother progressing with good health, etc.

REPORTS

The data collected (authentic) for records are periodically synthesized into reports, which serve as a check in progress, as a guide for future action and as a basis for reporting for agency or programme as a whole. These reports contain statistical and narrative contents. They may be required on daily, weekly, monthly, quarterly or yearly basis.

1. The quarterly reports can be integrated into yearly reports.
2. Sufficiently long for some trend in, or result forms provide service to the people and is sufficient.
3. Sufficiently short to permit quick rectification of misdirected activities.

Reports are the forms of analysis of some aspects of a service. Reports summarise the services of the nurse or the agency. Usually, reports are written daily, weekly, monthly and annually.

Daily Reports

These are the day-to-day activities of the agency. These are the daily summarising of the work done.

Weekly

The daily reports are completed at the end of every week to assess the activities performed and helps for future planning.

Monthly

Monthly reports provide an opportunity to present the problems for administrative consideration.

Annual Reports

Every year compilation of reports help in preparing the overall health activities, achievements, vital events, utilization of resources and helps for further planning for health care and resources.

Purpose

Reports are written to :
- Interpret the health service rendered over a specific period of time.

- Determine the progress made in achieving the goals.
- Study the health condition and health status.
- As a guide for further planning and organising health programmes.
- Helps in interpretation of service to public and other related agencies.

Principle of Report Writing

- Based on factual data and not opinion.
- Based on reporter's observation, conversation and action.
- Short, concise, clear and comprehensive.
- Clearly understood by others, only standard abbreviations must be written.
- Confidentiality must be maintained.

Statistical Content of Reports

The nursing actions or efforts can be shown statistically to show the progress or organisation of work for its usefulness. The statistical data are more useful if they contain an element of comparison, *e.g.*, if community health nurse shows the number of home visiting done during current year, may not solve any purpose, instead she may show the comparison on home visiting done in the current year and the previous year will show the progress in work. The immunization covered for number of children within periods of time.

Trends of average time spent on various programmes, *e.g.*, home care and nursing care in the clinics will show the utilisation of time in different activities performed.

Narrative Report

This report explains the progress and problems faced during care. It should be closely related to statistical statements. It provides opportunity to relate and explain statistical report finding, regarding problems encountered and suggest remedies, *e.g.*, if more time is spent on travelling by nursing care personnel then geographically may be divided according to convenience of staff to work efficiently.

The narrative report provide opportunity in identification of community leaders, which may help in health programme.

This report is also useful for administration, since this report narrates about problems and accomplishments and often indicates that staff education or consultative or administration's support may be needed to improve the field situations. This may also clarify nurse's own understanding of the situation.

Annual Report

The community health nurse, who is writing an annual report should not only consider as means of information, but also means of communicating to them about the significance of what has been done. Annual report should identify service problems with which nurse must deal.

Principles of preparing annual report :

1. Develop an outline of content and general method of presentation.
2. Collect information and material of the whole year and put the whole information at the end to write the report.
3. Organise the report to locate the essential information.
4. Choose the style that will suit the audience. The administrator will be reviewing many such reports. Hence a clear and readily located summary must be highlighted.
5. Emphasise other agencies, divisions or persons who have helped the programme.

Criteria for Record System

Record system should possess sufficient uniformity to provide for easy recording, tabulation, collation and to permit interunit and interservice comparisons.

Record system should require the minimal amount of time that is consistent with the records purpose. It is quite possible to reduce record time, at the expense of reducing efficiency and effectiveness of the service, *e.g.*, community health nurse must not waste her time in neatly recording system and pay attention to quality and quantity.

Records should be made easily available for users. The individual service records, family records, and school records should be available for effective use in planning and providing care to the person.

Record System Should Require Reasonable Storage Space

Each agency must have a period of record retaining, so as to have sufficient space for new records. A short period saves the space, but it may create problem in certain situations. In some agencies the retaining period is 5 to 10 years.

Record system should be susceptible to co-ordinate those parameters considered important for planning and evaluation.

The records of the type of needs of community is important to identify the health situation, whether it is in the centre, schools, or any other place.

Record System Should Provide Confidentiality of Record Content

Assurance of privacy is one of the big problems in developing community co-ordinated health care information systems. In the use of data processing system in hospitals, special keys are issued to those who are entitled to use. In certain circumstances, data has to be disclosed, where family consent has to be taken. Community health nurse needs to be responsible for careful observation of agency policies regarding release of information and when necessary, working out special methods for storing and handling sensitive information.

Computer

The electronic data processing and other automated systems are assuming an increasingly important role in other managements and the management of health services. Properly used data processing reduces clerical work for professionals to make information avaiable in a short time, and to provide large number of relationships or corrections that could not be readily secured through other methods of data handling. In short time it is possible to secure it in minutes. Detailed information related to the health care provided to an individual or family for various health problems.

Nurses must find out what computer can do for them, what combination of information they may get with respect to nursing input, what material on population may be useful in planning the nursing programme. Community health nurse can find the data processing system a new and powerful resource for care.

Records Must be Used

Records must be used for planning and evaluating the health care service to the community. The analyzing of record data and studying the implications for one's own work will place the individual nurse in the total picture of the health efforts of which she is such an important part.

Computer provides several advantages over paper based record system. Information can be stored in smaller areas, search and analytic tasks can be performed and information can be obtained more efficiently. But if used improperly, can magnify weakness in an organisation. It can be applied in three catagories :

1. Clinical system
2. Management information system
3. Educational system.

Advantages

- Physician can enter diagnosis and clinical notes directly into computer and nurses can not change the treatment.
- Computer analyses data and facilitate communication about patient's health care providence.
- Patient monitoring system, record patient responses and can alert nurses to changes.
- Computer can record patient's progress on paper or on the monitor, sound an alarm and often transmit information from patient's bedside. Through computer monitoring, nurses can respond quickly to changes in patient's conditions.
- Computer has many applications in management information system. They can be used for patient classification system, supplies and material management, staff scheduling, policy and procedures changes and announcements, patient charges, budget information and management, personnel records, statistical reports, administration reports and memos.
- *Education system :* Computer assisted instructions allow students to proceed at

their own speed, provides immediate feedback and allows dissemination of information to remote areas.

Registers

The registers usually provide only an indication of the total volume of service and of the types of cases seen. It gives no idea of the quality of services or the results achieved. However, untill individual records and fitting system are developed, registers must be continued. It is necessary to keep each register up-to-date and accurate. A good record system provides all the information available from the usual clinic register, adds more useful information. Once established, a good record system consumes little time in its maintenance.

EXERCISES

1. What do you understand by vital health statistics? List the sources of vital health statistics. Discuss any two of the sources of valid health statistics.
2. Define health information system. Describe the uses of health information system.
3. Define statistics. Discuss methods of statistical presentation of data.
4. Discuss the purposes and significance uses of records and reports on community health nursing. Describe the types of records maintained for quality care.
5. Write short notes on:
   (a) Census
   (b) Tabulation of data
   (c) Uses of graphical presentation
   (d) Use of computer for records

●●●

Sample Questions

QUESTION BANK

1. (a) Enumerate the causes of diarrhoea.
   (b) How would you identify mild moderate and severe diarrhoea ?
   (c) Describe the oral rehydration therapy as a lifesaving remedy for diarrhoea.

2. (a) Describe the modes of transmission of diarrhoea.
   (b) Discuss briefly the National Diarrhoea Disease Control Programme.
   (c) Role of nurse in prevention of diarrhoea.

3. A five year old child comes to clinic with acute respiratory infection, as a community health nurse what health education would you provide for care of the child and its prevention and control?

4. (a) List the early signs of pneumonia.
   (b) Describe the nursing and medical management of pneumonia.
   (c) What are complications of pneumonia ?

5. (a) Discuss the acute respiratory infection control programme.
   (b) Explain the responsibilities of community health nurse, for prevention and control of ARI.

6. (a) Describe the causation of meningitis and the transmission of disease.
   (b) How would you manage the case with meningococcal meningitis ?
   (c) Describe its prevention and control.

7. (a) Enumerate the clinical manifestation of dengue fever.
   (b) What is the nursing intervention for a case of dengue fever ?
   (c) List the complications of dengue fever and its management.

   (d) Role of nurse in prevention of dengue fever.

8. (a) Describe the epidemiological factors in causation of T.B.
   (b) Discuss the Revised National Tuberculosis Control Programme and Dot therapy in T.B.
   (c) Role of nurse in BCG vaccination.

9. (a) Discuss the levels of prevention of disease in case of T.B.
   (b) Explain the responsibilities of community health nurse in prevention of T.B.
   (c) Plan health education session for group of T.B. patients on prevention and spread of infection.
   (d) Describe the agent factor, mode of transmission and reservior of infection of T.B.
   (e) Plan health education and home care for chronic T.B. patients.

10. (a) Describe the transmission of measles among children.
    (b) How would you identify the child in the measles ?
    (c) Explain the steps to prevent the spread of measles.

11. (a) Few cases of measles have been identified in a community. Discuss the steps to be followed for its prevention and control.
    (b) How would you plan for immunization of children against measles ?

12. (a) Explain the epidemiological trial of tetanus.
    (b) Describe the immediate measures you would adopt in case of injury to a child.

(c) Role of nurse while immunizing community against tetanus.

13. (a) Describe the clinical manifestation of tetanus.

(b) Explain the prevention and control measures of tetanus.

(c) Prevention of neonatorum tetanus.

14. (a) What is neonatorum tetanus ?

(b) How would you prevent neonatorum tetanus ?

(c) Describe its management.

15. (a) Describe the causative organisms and mode of transmission of rabies.

(b) Discuss the steps you would follow in case of dog bite.

(c) Role of nurse in prevention of dog bite.

(d) What is agent, host and environment in rabies ?

(e) Describe the prevention and control rabies.

16. (a) 'Hepatitis B' is one of the major public health problem. Justify it.

(b) As a community health nurse what steps would you adopt for its prevention and control of hepatitis in your community?

17. As community health nurse, you find the tuberculosis incidence rising in your area.

(a) Describe the steps to be followed for its prevention and control.

(b) How would you provide specific protection to children below one year ?

18. (a) Explain the distribution of T.B. in India.

(b) Describe reasons for its rising problem.

(c) Discuss the steps undertaken by the Govt. of India for effective prevention and control.

19. (a) Describe the clinical manifestation of T.B.

(b) Explain the multidrug therapy as an effective management for treatment and prevention and spread of T.B.

(c) Role of nurse in prevention and control of T.B.

20. (a) Explain the epidemiological factors and causation of chickenpox.

(b) As a community health nurse, what preventive measures would you adopt in control of chickenpox.

21. (a) Describe the mode of transmission of chickenpox.

(b) Explain the role of nurse in prevention and control of chickenpox.

22. (a) Enumerate the epidemiological triad in causation of malaria.

(b) Describe the modified plan of operation for malaria.

(c) Explain the role of nurse in prevention of malaria.

23. A case of fever comes to you in the health centre. As a community health nurse, how would you diagnose the cause and what steps would you follow for treatment and prevention and spread of disease?

24. You find number of fever cases in the community. Describe the steps you would follow to identify the cases as malaria. What preventive and control measures you will adopt?

25. (a) Describe the mode of transmission of poliomyelitis.

(b) List the clinical manifestation of poliomyelitis.

(c) Explain the role of nurse in early diagnosis and treatment of poliomyelitis.

26. (a) Explain the epidemiological factors of polio-myelitis.

(b) What steps would you follow in prevention and control of poliomyelitis ?

27. (a) What do you understand by epidemic of plague ?

(b) Describe the reservoir of infection and causative organism of disease.

(c) Describe the role of nurse in preventing the spread of infection.

28. (a) Explain the agent, host and environmental factors in causation of hepatitis B.

(b) Describe the high-risk groups.

(c) Enumerate the significant control measures for hepatitis B in a community.

29. (a) Describe the distribution of disease in India.

(b) Why it is considered as a major health problem?

(c) Discuss briefly about the National Filaria Control Programme.

30. (a) Discuss the causation, organism and mode of transmission of filaria.

(b) Describe the preventive and control measures for filaria.

31. (a) "Diarrhoea is one of the major killer disease among children". Give reason.

(b) Describe the steps undertaken by Govt. for its control measures.

(c) Describe the role of nurse in prevention of diarrhoea.

32. (a) Explain the clinical manifestation of diarrhoea.

(b) As a community health nurse how you prevent dehydration among children with diarrhoea?

(c) List the complications of dehydration.

33. (a) Define community health and community health nursing.

(b) Explain the principles of community health nurse.

(c) Discuss the role of community health nurse.

34. (a) Discuss the levels of prevention of disease with relation to tuberculosis.

(b) Explain the concept of epidemiological triad.

(c) Discuss the epidemiological factor in causation of malaria.

35. (a) List the food and water-borne diseases.

(b) Discuss role of nurse in prevention and control of any one of the water-borne disease.

(c) Define mental health.

(d) List the characteristics of mentally healthy person.

(e) How would you promote the mental health of a sick persons?

36. Define vital health statistics. Explain the different types of vital health statistics record to be collected in India.

37. (a) Discuss the important vital health statistic for collecting health information.

(b) How these informations are tabulated and why?

38. (a) Discuss the methods of compiling and presenting different vital health statistics.

(b) What is the significance of these informations?

39. List the major STD problems in India and its distribution.

40. Describe the social causes for STD as a community health nurse, how would you plan to prevent the STD?

41. Describe the epidemiological factors causing STD.

42. Discuss briefly the National STD Control Programme.

43. Discuss about the increasing number of AIDS cases.

44. Describe the National AIDS control programme.

45. (a) Discuss the epidemiological triad for AIDS.

(b) Why AIDS has very long incubation period?

(c) Describe the role of nurse in prevention of AIDS.

46. (a) Describe three levels of prevention of disease in AIDS.

(b) Functions of community health nurse in controlling spread of AIDS.

47. (a) Explain the multifactorial causation of diabetes.

(b) Describe the role of nurse in three levels of prevention of disease.

48. (a) Explain agent, host and environment of diabetes mellitus.

(b) Describe the objectives of giving nursing care to diabetic patient.

(c) What health education would you give to patients with diabetes mellitus?

49. (a) Describe the aetiological factors in causation of cardiovascular diseases.

    (b) What are the preventive measures of cardiovascular diseases ?

    (c) Explain the role of nurse in giving care to patient with cardiovascular disease.

50. (a) Discuss the three levels of prevention of disease in cardiovascular diseases.

    (b) Explain the national cardiovascular diseases.

51. Cancer has become a major public health problem in India :

    (a) Describe the causes of cancer.

    (b) Explain the clinical features of cancer.

    (c) Discuss the National Cancer Control Programme in India.

52. As a community health nurse, how would you help the community in early diagnosis and treatment of cancer?

53. Describe briefly the National Cancer Control Programme.

54. (a) Describe the three levels of prevention of disease in case of cancer.

    (b) Explain the nurse's responsibility in prevention of cancer.

55. (a) Explain the concept of health and disease.

    (b) Describe the dimensions of health.

    (c) Role of nurse in maintaining health and preventing diseases.

56. Explain the factors affecting health with examples.

57. Discuss the levels of prevention of diseases. Illustrate your answer with examples.

58. Describe the epidemiological triad in causation of disease with examples.

59. (a) Describe the different modes of transmission of diseases.

    (b) As a community health nurse, what measures would you adopt to prevent and control the diseases?

60. (a) Define immunity and immunization.

    (b) List the types of immunization.

    (c) As a community health nurse, what immunization schedule would you follow for 0-1 year old child.

61. (a) Explain immunization process.

    (b) How would you organize the immunization session ?

62. Write short notes on the following :

    (a) Food poisoning and its prevention.

    (b) Information Education Communication in diarrhoea.

    (c) Causes of diarrhoea.

    (d) Health education on diarrhoea.

    (e) ORT.

63. Write short notes on the following :

    (a) Prevention and control of cholera.

    (b) Prepare a health education session for a group of mothers for prevention and control of diarrhoea.

    (c) Plan a health education session for group of mothers on prevention of worm infestation among children.

    (d) BCG Vaccination.

    (e) DOT therapy.

64. Write short notes on the following :

    (a) Role of nurse in control of T.B.

    (b) Domicillary T.B. care.

    (c) National T.B. Control Programme.

    (d) Clinical manifestation of T.B.

    (e) National T.B. Control Programme.

65. Write short notes on the following :

    (a) Nursing care to a child with mumps.

    (b) Care of child with measles.

    (c) Nursing intervention for child with chickenpox.

    (d) Prevention of influenza.

    (e) Triple vaccine.

66. Write short notes on the following :

    (a) Wound care in case of dog bite.

    (b) Vaccination against rabies.

    (c) Direct observed therapy for T.B.

    (d) Multidrug therapy.

    (e) BCG vaccination.

67. Write short notes on the following :

    (a) Health education to T.B. patient.

    (b) Prevention and control measures of T.B.

    (c) Agents and host environment factors in T.B.

    (d) Pulse Polio Programme.

    (e) Immunization against poliomyelitis.

68. Write short notes on the following :
    (a) Presumptive and radical treatment for malaria.
    (b) National malaria control programme.
    (c) Role of nurse in prevention of malaria.
    (d) Types of plague.
    (e) Vector of plague.
    (f) Medical management of plague.

69. Write short notes on the following :
    (a) Syphilis and its prevention.
    (b) Congenital syphilis.
    (c) Diarrhoea as a public health problem.
    (d) AIDs is a major, public health problem.
    (e) Role of NACO.
    (f) Mode of transmission of AIDS.

70. Write short notes on the following :
    (a) Prevention and control of accidents.
    (b) Cardiovascular accident.
    (c) Lung cancer.
    (d) Breast cancer.
    (e) Cancer of cervix.

MULTIPLE CHOICE QUESTIONS

1. The sore throat and moist lesion in patients mouth indicate that the patient has probably contacted syphilis patient in the following manner :
   (a) By kissing an infected sex partner
   (b) By sexual contact with infected friend
   (c) By having it since birth
   (d) From public toilet, etc.

2. Which of the following age group has the greatest prevalence of AIDS ?
   (a) Below 24 years
   (b) Between 20 to 40 years
   (c) Above 40 years
   (d) At birth

3. All of the following diseases are entirely preventable except :
   (a) Mumps
   (b) Measles
   (c) Diphtheria
   (d) Influenza

4. If complicating pregnancy, which of the following diseases may result in serious teratogenic defects in offspring?
   (a) Rubella
   (b) Rubeola
   (c) Variola
   (d) Varicella

5. If complicating pregnancy, which of the following diseases are believed to result in abortion or congenital defect in children?
   (a) Mumps
   (b) Influenza
   (c) German measles
   (d) All of the above

6. The first census of India during the British period was held during the tenure of :
   (a) Lord Mayo
   (b) Lord Ripon
   (c) Lord Mountbatton
   (d) Lord Irwin

7. As a CHN, you are expected to motivate the people's behaviour towards healthy habits. Most effective health education approach will be :
   (a) Service approach
   (b) Health education
   (c) Legislative
   (d) All of the above

8. The health education to a group of alcoholic people should be able to :
   (a) Change their behaviour
   (b) Teach the bad effects of alcoholism
   (c) Inform about the constituents of alcohol
   (d) Discuss and create awareness among them about family crisis

9. To prevent cardiovascular accidents among the community people you need to advice on :
   (a) Prevent hypertension
   (b) Regular check-up for high B.P.
   (c) Prevent other associated problems
   (d) All of the above

10. The most important aspect of previous history of patients with CVA will include :
    (a) Cancer
    (b) Hypertension
    (c) Congenital anomaly
    (d) Paralysis

11. The life-expectancy at birth in India is :
    (a) 50 years for males and 60 years for females
    (b) 57 years for males and 59 for females
    (c) 60 years for males and 61 years for females
    (d) 58 years for both males and females

12. All of the following are negative indicator except :
    (a) Death rate
    (b) Infant mortality rate
    (c) Perinatal mortality rate
    (d) Life-expectancy at birth

13. Society may be defined as :
    (a) Social relationship between families
    (b) System of social relationship between individuals
    (c) Relationship between individual and people
    (d) Relationship between individual, family and people

14. When a group of 6 to 8 qualified experts discuss a topic in front of audience is said to be :
    (a) Panel discussion
    (b) Group discussion
    (c) Seminar
    (d) Workshop

15. The most common cause of blindness is :
    (a) Trachoma
    (b) Glaucoma
    (c) Cataract
    (d) Vitamin A deficiency

16. The measurement of obesity can be done by the method called :
    (a) Height weight chart
    (b) Skin fold thickness
    (c) Body weight / age
    (d) Basal calorie consumption

17. The major cause of accidents is :
    (a) Unsafe facilities
    (b) Unsafe security
    (c) Negligence
    (d) None of the above

18. Pap smear among women is done to detect:
    (a) Cancer of cervix
    (b) Cancer of lungs
    (c) Breast cancer
    (d) Any cancer in the body

19. Pap smear examination to detect cancer of cervix is :
    (a) Primary level prevention
    (b) Secondary level prevention
    (c) Tertiary level prevention
    (d) All of the above

20. The major cause of MMR in India is :
    (a) Anaemia
    (b) Haemorrhage
    (c) Toxaemia of pregnancy
    (d) Abortion

21. MMR vaccine is given appropriately at the age of :
    (a) 9 to 12 months
    (b) 0 to 40 days
    (c) 1½ to 2½ months
    (d) At any age

22. Universal programme for immunization includes all except :
    (a) BCG
    (b) DPT
    (c) Typhoid
    (d) Measles

23. Numerator for neonatal mortality rate is calculated by newborn death within :
    (a) 24 hours
    (b) one week
    (c) 28 days
    (d) one year

24. Maternal mortality rate is measured as per :
    (a) 100 deliveries
    (b) 1000 deliveries
    (c) 1000 pregnancies
    (d) 1000 live births

25. The major cause of infant mortality rate in India is :
    (a) Acute respiratory infection
    (b) Prematurity
    (c) Diarrhoea
    (d) Congenital anomalies

26. As a community health nurse, a 4 years old child comes to you with complaint of ARI. You will advice :
    (a) Syrup ampicilin 125 mg four times daily
    (b) Paediatric septran 3 tab., twice daily
    (c) Syrup amoxycilin 125 mg thrice daily
    (d) Paediatric septran 2 tab. twice daily

27. One of the following is not a risk factor for cancer of breast :
    (a) Early menarche
    (b) Early menopause
    (c) (Oral contraceptive) High fat diet
    (d) Late first pregnancy

28. The earliest clinical sign of vitamin A deficiency is :
    (a) Bitot spot
    (b) Keratomalacia
    (c) Conjunctival xerosis
    (d) Nyctalopia

29. According to W.H.O., blindness is defined as "visual acquity is less than" :
    (a) 6/6
    (b) 6/60
    (c) 1/60
    (d) 18/60

30. The MMR in India according to 2001 is :
    (a) 4/1000
    (b) 2/1000
    (c) 3/1000
    (d) 5/1000

31. The major cause of IMR in India is :
    (a) Malnutrition
    (b) Infection
    (c) Congenital anomaly
    (d) All of the above

32. The cases of measles is most commonly found in :
    (a) Summer season
    (b) Winter season
    (c) Rainy season
    (d) Spring season

33. Tetanus spores can be killed by :
    (a) Phenol
    (b) Autoclaving for 10 minutes
    (c) Ultraviolet rays
    (d) All of the above

34. As a community health nurse, which preventive measures you will adopt for prevention of rabies ?
    (a) Restraint of dogs in public places
    (b) Licencing of all domestic dogs
    (c) Vaccination of dogs
    (d) All of the above

35. The most common mode of transmission of Leprosy is :
    (a) Vectors
    (b) Fomites
    (c) Droplet
    (d) Direct skin contact

36. As a community health nurse, the most effective means of filaria control measure to be advised, will be :
    (a) Personal protection
    (b) Hetrazan mass treatment
    (c) Adequate sewage
    (d) Insecticidal measures against culex mosquito

37. Malaria prophylaxis to the people living in endemic areas should be given for :
    (a) 1 day
    (b) 1 week
    (c) 3 weeks
    (d) 4 weeks

38. Typhoid bacilli survive longest in :
    (a) Ice cream
    (b) Water
    (c) Soil irrigated with sewage
    (d) Sweets

39. The type of plasmodium not found in India is :
    (a) P. ovale
    (b) P. falciparum
    (c) P. vivex
    (d) P. malariae

40. Primaquine is given in *P. falciparum* cases to prevent :

(a) Recurrence

(b) Treatment

(c) Transmission to others

(d) Susceptibility

41. After leaving malaria endemic area, the people getting chroloquine, prophylaxis should be stopped :

(a) Immediately

(b) 2 days

(c) 2 weeks

(d) 6 weeks

42. Reservoir of infection in plague is spread mainly by :

(a) Domestic rats

(b) Rat flaes

(c) Wild rodents

(d) All of the above

43. Infectious hepatitis virus is found in :

(a) Urine of infected person

(b) Faeces of infected person

(c) Nasopharynx of infected person

(d) None of the above

44. Chickenpox is more severe in case of :

(a) All ages

(b) Adults

(c) Young children

(d) Infants

45. Incidence of a disease is defined as :

(a) Number of old cases present during a specific period in a given period

(b) Number of cases existing in a given population at a given time

(c) Number of cases existing in a given period

(d) Number of new cases occurring in a specific period

46. All of the following are quarantinable diseases except :

(a) Malaria

(b) Cholera

(c) Plague

(d) Yellow fever

47. Disinfectant is an agent which :

(a) Destroys disease producing micro-organism, but not necessary the spores

(b) Prevents the growth of micro-organisms

(c) Destroys disease producing micro-organisms including spores

(d) All of the above

48. Which one of the following immuno-globulin can cross human placenta ?

(a) IgM

(b) IgG

(c) IgA

(d) IgE

49. Which of the following chemical is most powerful disinfectant ?

(a) Dettol

(b) Phenol

(c) Lysol

(d) $KMnO_4$

50. Epidemiology is defined as :

(a) Study of distribution and determinants of disease prevalence in man

(b) Study of determinants of disease prevalence in man

(c) Study of epidemics

(d) Study of distribution of disease in man

51. Which one of the following is not a live attenuated vaccine ?

(a) Hepatitis B

(b) Measles

(c) Chickenpox

(d) OPV

52. The following are internationally quarantinable diseases :

(a) Yellow fever

(b) Cholera

(c) Plague

(d) All of the above

53. Health surveillance is said to be :

(a) Collection of relevant data

(b) Interpretation of data

(c) Collection and interpretation of data

(d) Monitoring the programme

54. As per time distribution of epidemic disease occurring every three year is called as :
    (a) Annual trend
    (b) Cyclical trend
    (c) Rendemic trend
    (d) Secular trend

55. Quarantine against a particular disease is done for a period of :
    (a) Maximum incubation period
    (b) Minimum incubation period
    (c) Serial interval
    (d) Period of infectivity

56. The following is the milk-borne disease :
    (a) Leptospirosis
    (b) Brucellosis
    (c) Q fever
    (d) All of the above

57. Dry heat is not used for sterilisation of :
    (a) Liver
    (b) Glassware
    (c) Paraffin oil
    (d) Telcom powder

58. The best method for sterilization of disposable items are by :
    (a) Dry heat
    (b) Gases
    (c) Steam
    (d) Chemical agent

59. In Chickenpox isolation of a case is recommended till :
    (a) Fever persists
    (b) Lesions have crusted
    (c) Crusts have fallen
    (d) Skin is clear

60. A child comes to health centre with Chickenpox, you as a community health nurse would advice for :
    (a) Vitamin suppliment
    (b) Antibiotic
    (c) Watch for pneumonia
    (d) All of the above

61. One year old unimmunized child exposed to measles case two days before he comes to in health centre, as a CHN you would advice for :
    (a) Immunoglobulin
    (b) Measles vaccine
    (c) Prophylaxis vitamin supplement
    (d) None of the above

62. The process of restriction of movement of persons who have come in contact of diseased person is called as :
    (a) Active surveillance
    (b) Quarantine
    (c) Isolation
    (d) Passive surveillance

63. The Polio vaccine should be preserved at :
    (a) 2 to 8°C
    (b) −2 to −8°C
    (c) 0 to 4°C
    (d) Below 0°C

64. Direct transmission includes all except :
    (a) Fomites
    (b) Droplet
    (c) By bite
    (d) Contact with soil

65. Blood transfusion does not transmit :
    (a) AIDS
    (b) Syphilis
    (c) Malignancy
    (d) Hepatitis B

66. The chickenpox rashes can be described as following, except :
    (a) Scabs are noninfectious
    (b) Centrifugal
    (c) Pleomorphic
    (d) All of the above

67. B.C.G vaccine once constituted should be used within :
    (a) 24 hours
    (b) 12 hours
    (c) 6 hours
    (d) 3 hours

68. Congenital anomalies in newborn is seen in pregnant women who gets infected with :
    (a) Rubella
    (b) Rubeola
    (c) Herpes
    (d) Toxoplasma

69. Lowest incidence rate of trachoma is found in :
    (a) Delhi
    (b) Punjab
    (c) Orissa
    (d) Tamil Nadu
70. The most common agent for causation of diarrhoea among children is :
    (a) Adenovirus
    (b) Ribovirus
    (c) Rotavirus
    (d) None of above
71. Oral rehydration solution contains all except :
    (a) Calcium lactate
    (b) Sodium chloride
    (c) Bicarbonate
    (d) Glucose
72. The best treatment of diarrhoea among children is :
    (a) I.V. fluids
    (b) ORS
    (c) Antibiotic
    (d) Antidiarrhoeal drugs
73. The best method to prevent pulmonary tuberculosis is :
    (a) Case isolation
    (b) B.C.G vaccination
    (c) Treatment of cases
    (d) Chemoprophylaxis
74. Dengue is spread by :
    (a) Anopheles
    (b) Culex
    (c) Droplet nuclei
    (d) Aedes
75. Tuberculin test is observed after :
    (a) 24 hours
    (b) 48 hours
    (c) 72 hours
    (d) 96 hours
76. For effective treatment of tuberculosis, the combination of antitubercle drugs are :
    (a) INH + ethambutol
    (b) INH + PAS
    (c) INH + streptomycin
    (d) INH + thiacetazone

77. A child comes to you with complain of diarrhoea and mild dehydration. You as a community health nurse will advice :
    (a) 600 mL ORS per day
    (b) 600 mL of Ringers lactate
    (c) 600 mL of sugar-salt solution
    (d) 600 mL of N/2 saline orally
78. Glucose is added to antidiarrhoeal solution because :
    (a) It tastes sweet
    (b) Increases absorption of amino acid
    (c) Increases absorption of sodium
    (d) All of the above
79. Salk vaccine for poliomyelitis is a :
    (a) Live attenuated vaccine
    (b) Killed vaccine
    (c) Immunoglobulin
    (d) Toxoid
80. All the following are live vaccine except :
    (a) BCG
    (b) DPT
    (c) Sabin
    (d) 17 D vaccine
81. Effective prophylactic measure for cholera is :
    (a) Water purification
    (b) Early case detection
    (c) Chemoprophylaxis
    (d) Surveillance
82. The freshly prepared ORS (oral rehydration solution) should be used within :
    (a) 12 hours
    (b) 24 hours
    (c) 36 hours
    (d) 48 hours
83. Transplacental immunity is seen in all except :
    (a) Diphtheria
    (b) Polio
    (c) Pertussis
    (d) Measles
84. The following vaccine should not be given, if child has convulsion :
    (a) OVP
    (b) DPT
    (c) BCG
    (d) Tetanus toxoid

85. Which of the following is not incubatory carrier :
    (a) Measles
    (b) Typhoid
    (c) Cholera
    (d) Tetanus

86. Most common causes of malnutrition in diarrhoea is due to :
    (a) Malabsorption
    (b) Anorexia
    (c) Restricted food intake
    (d) Hypersecretion

87. If child comes to health clinic with diarrhoea, the antibiotics can be given only in case of :
    (a) Shigella infection
    (b) Salmonella type
    (c) Enterotoxigenic
    (d) S. typhi

88. A mother brings her child with diarrhoea to the clinic, as a community health nurse you will advice her to give :
    (a) Substitute animal milk by soya mix
    (b) Half diluted animal milk
    (c) No milk or any other feed except ORS
    (d) Milk combined with cereals

89. When a child comes for immunization to the health centre, you as a community health nurse will not give it, if child has :
    (a) Diarrhoea
    (b) Cough and cold
    (c) Mild fever
    (d) None of the above

90. The reservoir of infection is only human host in case of :
    (a) Rabies
    (b) Poliomyelitis
    (c) Measles
    (d) Influenza

91. If a group of children comes with complaint of vomiting after meals at noon, the causative organism for food poisoning will be :
    (a) Staphylococcus
    (b) Salmonella
    (c) Botulism
    (d) Virus

92. The following diseases can be eradicated except :
    (a) Malaria
    (b) Measles
    (c) Polio
    (d) Tuberculosis

93. After reconstitution of measles vaccine it should be used within :
    (a) One hour
    (b) 2 hours
    (c) 3 hours
    (d) 4 hours

94. The permanent carrier in typhoid is considered who excretes bacilli for more than:
    (a) 3 months
    (b) 6 months
    (c) One year
    (d) Two years

95. The best control method you would like to adopt is :
    (a) Early diagnosis and treatment
    (b) Chemoprophylaxis
    (c) Vaccination
    (d) Health education

96. Healthy carriers are present in all the following except :
    (a) Cholera
    (b) Typhoid
    (c) Pertussis
    (d) Diphtheria

97. During cholera outbreak, the best emergency sanitatory measures to be adopted will be :
    (a) Chemoprophylaxis
    (b) Mass vaccination
    (c) Disinfection of stool
    (d) Provision of chlorinated water

98. The effective preventive measures for AIDS is use of condom, which provides protection against :
    (a) Inhibition of sperm action
    (b) Spermicidal action
    (c) Agglutination of spermatozoa
    (d) All of the above

99. A female multipurpose worker should be able to identify all except :
   (a) Anaemia
   (b) Hydramnios
   (c) Malpresentation
   (d) Renal disease

100. To prevent vitamin A deficiency, you will advice mother to give the child :
   (a) Banana
   (b) Eggs
   (c) Milk
   (d) Green leafy vegetables

101. Vitamin A supplementation given to children from the age of 1 to 6 years should be every :
   (a) Monthly
   (b) 6 months
   (c) 9 months
   (d) Yearly

102. The complete biological food is said to be :
   (a) Milk
   (b) Wheat
   (c) Rice
   (d) All of the above

103. The health education to prevent malnutrition among children will include :
   (a) Nutritional education
   (b) Supplementary feeding
   (c) Comprehensive child care
   (d) Nutritional rehabilitation

104. Which of the following is associated with air pollution :
   (a) Lung cancer
   (b) Emphysema
   (c) Bronchial asthma
   (d) All of the above

105. The most leading source of air pollution is :
   (a) Power plants
   (b) Transportation
   (c) Industries
   (d) Space heating

106. The causative organism of filaria is :
   (a) W. bancrofti
   (b) Plasmodium
   (c) Female anopheles
   (d) Bacilli

107. Causative agent of malaria is :
   (a) Plasmodium
   (b) B. malayi
   (c) Female anopheles
   (d) Virus

108. The mode of transmission of disease by flies is :
   (a) Defecation
   (b) Mechanical transmission
   (c) Vomit drop
   (d) Chemical transmission

109. Sample registration system (SRS) was started to collect information regarding :
   (a) Population mobility
   (b) Birth and death rate in states and country
   (c) Morbidity rate of different diseases
   (d) Death rate of rural areas

110. The death is to be registered in India within :
   (a) 7 days
   (b) 15 days
   (c) 21 days
   (d) one month

111. The birth is to be registered in India within :
   (a) 7 days
   (b) 15 days
   (c) 25 days
   (d) 30 days

112. Sample registration system survey is done after every :
   (a) 6 months
   (b) Year
   (c) Two years
   (d) Three years

113. Census are taken every :
   (a) Yearly
   (b) 2 yearly
   (c) 5 yearly
   (d) 10 yearly

114. The following are the most effective bicommunication except :
   (a) Symposium
   (b) Lecture
   (c) Group discussion.
   (d) Panel discussion.

115. Community participation means :
    (a) Provision of manpower and logistics support by community
    (b) Involvement of community in planning and evaluation
    (c) Use of health services by the community
    (d) All of the above

116. Primary health care includes all except :
    (a) Low cost
    (b) Equitable distribution
    (c) Community participation
    (d) Latest technology

117. The primary health centres staffing includes that the best method of teaching urban-slum about ORS will be :
    (a) Demonstration
    (b) Role play
    (c) Lecture
    (d) Discussion

118. The Govt. of India has announced National Health Policy in the year :
    (a) 1978
    (b) 1981
    (c) 1982
    (d) 1990

119. National Health policy of India is based on :
    (a) Primary health care
    (b) Basic health care
    (c) Health for all
    (d) a and c

120. The population covered by one subcentre as per National Health Policy is :
    (a) 1000
    (b) 3000
    (c) 5000
    (d) 10,000

121. Each primary health centre is expected to cover a population around :
    (a) 30,000
    (b) 40,000
    (c) 50,000
    (d) 1 lakh

122. National Tuberculosis Control Programme is implemented through :
    (a) Primary health centre
    (b) District T.B. hospital
    (c) Urban health centre
    (d) All of the above

123. The female multipurpose worker does not do :
    (a) Birth and death registration
    (b) Distribution of condom
    (c) Malaria surveillance
    (d) Supervision of health volunteers

124. Most effective way to teach student is by :
    (a) Lecture
    (b) Film show
    (c) Demonstration
    (d) Exhibition

125. A positive case of tuberculosis comes to the health centre, you as a community health nurse will advice :
    (a) Mantoux test
    (b) B.C.G vaccination
    (c) DOT therapy
    (d) X-ray chest

126. Mantoux test is done in tuberculosis :
    (a) To diagnose the case
    (b) To treat the case
    (c) To prevent the disease
    (d) All of the above

127. Mode of transmission of pneumonic plague is :
    (a) Indirect transmission
    (b) Direct transmission
    (c) Arthropodes transmission
    (d) Vector borne disease

128. Rat flea is responsible in causation of :
    (a) Plague
    (b) Rabies
    (c) Yellow fever
    (d) Dengue fever

ANSWERS

1. (b)	2. (b)	3. (d)	4. (a)	5. (c)	6. (b)
7. (b)	8. (a)	9. (d)	10. (b)	11. (c)	12. (d)
13. (c)	14. (a)	15. (a)	16. (b)	17. (c)	18. (a)
19. (a)	20. (b)	21. (a)	22. (c)	23. (c)	24. (b)
25. (c)	26. (b)	27. (b)	28. (c)	29. (c)	30. (a)
31. (a)	32. (d)	33. (c)	34. (d)	35. (c)	36. (a)
37. (d)	38. (c)	39. (c)	40. (b)	41. (a)	42. (c)
43. (b)	44. (b)	45. (d)	46. (a)	47. (a)	48. (b)
49. (c)	50. (a)	51. (a)	52. (d)	53. (c)	54. (b)
55. (a)	56. (d)	57. (a)	58. (a)	59. (b)	60. (c)
61. (a)	62. (b)	63. (b)	64. (d)	65. (c)	66. (b)
67. (d)	68. (b)	69. (b)	70. (c)	71. (a)	72. (b)
73. (c)	74. (d)	75. (c)	76. (d)	77. (a)	78. (c)
79. (a)	80. (b)	81. (a)	82. (b)	83. (?)	84. (b)
85. (d)	86. (c)	87. (a)	88. (b)	89. (d)	90. (c)
91. (a)	92. (d)	93. (a)	94. (c)	95. (a)	96. (c)
97. (d)	98. (a)	99. (d)	100. (d)	101. (b)	102. (a)
103. (c)	104. (c)	105. (b)	106. (a)	107. (a)	108. (b)
109. (b)	110. (a)	111. (b)	112. (a)	113. (d)	114. (b)
115. (b)	116. (d)	117. (a)	118. (c)	119. (d)	120. (b)
121. (b)	122. (a)	123. (a)	124. (c)	125. (a)	126. (b)
127. (a)	128. (b)				

Previous Years University Papers

QUESTION PAPER-1
B.Sc.–April 2000
(Epidemiology and Preventive Medicine)
Time Allowed : 3 Hours   Max. Marks : 75

Instructions: *Attempt any five questions only.*
Each question carry equal marks.

1. (a) Define the term immunity.
   (b) Explain in brief the different types of immunity.
   (c) Describe the hazards of immunization. (2+5+8 = 15)

2. (a) Describe the determinants of health.
   (b) List down the major health problems of India.
   (c) Explain the changing concept of health. (5+5+5=15)

3. You are deputed as a community health nurse in a cyclone hit area where water is highly polluted.
   (a) List down the expected diseases to be reported from this area.
   (b) Describe in brief the sources of water pollution.
   (c) Explain your role in prevention of diseases reported from this area. (5+5+5=15)

4. (a) Explain the term disease prevention.
   (b) List down the level of disease prevention.
   (c) Describe in detail the primary level of disease prevention. (2+5+8=15)

5. (a) Explain the ecological triads in causations of measles.
   (b) List down the signs and symptoms of measles.
   (c) Describe in brief the preventive and control measures that you would suggest to prevent further spread of this disease. (5+5+5=15)

6. Write short notes on any *three* of the following :
   (a) The uses of Epidemiology.
   (b) Noise pollution.
   (c) Anti-rodent measures.
   (d) The disease cycle.

QUESTION PAPER-2
B.Sc. (Hons.) – April 2001
(Epidemiology and Preventive Medicine)
Time Allowed : 3 Hours   Max Marks : 75

Instructions : *Attempt any five questions only.*
Each question carry equal marks.

1. (a) Explain the concept of "Epidemiological Triad" in causation of a communicable disease.
   (b) Describe the agent, host and environmental factors in causation of tuberculosis. (5+10)

2. (a) Define epidemiology.
   (b) Describe how the knowledge of epidemiology is useful in prevention and control of diseases.
   (c) Explain the role of a nurse in application of epidemiology. (2+10+3)

3. (a) Briefly explain the different levels of prevention of disease.
   (b) Describe the levels of prevention of disease in poliomyelitis among children. (5+10)

4. (a) Explain the concept of health and disease.
   (b) Enumerate the factors affecting health of an individuals.
   (c) Describe the role of nurse in promotion of health of a given community. (4+7+4)

5. (a) List the major environmental pollutants causing health problems among the individuals.
   (b) Describe the various health hazards due to air pollution.
   (c) Briefly explain the measures adopted or can be adopted to prevent air-borne diseases. (3+5+7)

6. Write short notes on any *three* of the following:
   (a) Nurses responsibility in prevention of cardiovascular diseases.
   (b) Methods of sewage disposal.
   (c) Quarantine and incubation period.
   (d) UNICEF and its role in health sector.
   (e) Health indicators.

QUESTION PAPER-3
B.Sc. 2002
(Epidemiology and Preventive Medicine)
Time Allowed: 3 Hours   Max Marks : 75

Instructions : Attempt any five questions only.
Each question carry equal marks.

1. (a) Define immunity and immunization.
   (b) Briefly, explain the different types of immunity.
   (c) What immunization would you advice to mothers of 0 to 1 year old children?
   (2+7+6=15)

2. (a) List the major public health problems in India.
   (b) Describe the population as a problem in India and its impact on health and disease.
   (c) Explain the role of nurse in educating the public about existing population as a problem.
   (2½+7½+5=15)

3. (a) Explain the concept of disease.
   (b) Discuss the epidemiological triad in causation of disease in relation to AIDS occurrence in the community. (3+12=15)
   OR
   (a) Discuss the epidemiological triad in causation of tetanus in the community.
   (b) Explain the primary prevention of tetanus.
   (10+5=15)

4. Discuss briefly the mortality and morbidity indicators which are significant for measurement of health status of a country of community.
   (15)

5 (a) State the effect of Poor Sanitation on health of a man.
   (b) Describe the different methods of solid waste disposal.
   (c) Explain the modern methods of sewage treatment.
   (4+6+5=15)

6. Write short notes on any *three* :
   (a) Descriptive epidemiology.
   (b) Spectrum of health.
   (c) World health organisation and its role in prevention of epidemic diseases.
   (d) Preventive measures for diabetes mellitus.
   (e) Societal health problems.
   (f) Chinese system of medicine.
   (5×3=15)

QUESTION PAPER-4
B.Sc. 2003
(Epidemiology and Preventive Medicine)
Time Allowed: 3 hours   Max Marks : 75

Instructions : Attempt any five questions only.
Each question carry equal marks.

1. (a) Explain the concept of health and positive health.
   (b) "Health is multidimensional." Justify the statement with examples.
   (c) Briefly, describe the determinants of health.
   (2+6+7)

2. (a) Discuss the modes of transmission of tuberculosis.
   (b) Enumerate the role of Nurse in prevention and control of tuberculosis in a community.
   (7+8)
   OR
   (a) Explain the natural history of disease in causation of measles.
   (b) What preventive measure would you follow to control the spread of measles in the community?
   (8+7)

3. (a) Explain the concept of safe and wholesome water.
   (b) Identify the sources of water pollution and list the water-borne diseases.
   (c) State the role of nurse in prevention of water-borne diseases.
   (4+6+5)

4. (a) Define epidemiology and list its uses.
   (b) As a community health nurse, how the study of epidemiology will help you in preventing communicable and non-communicable diseases?
   (5+10)

5. Discuss the levels of prevention of communicable diseases with examples, and nurse's responsibility at each level of prevention of disease.
   (15)

6. Write briefly on any *three* of the following :
   (a) Objectives of Pulse Polio Programme.
   (b) Prevention and control of xerophthalmia in children.
   (c) UNICEF and its role in child health.
   (d) Indian systems of Medicine.
   (e) Changing concepts of Public Health.
   (f) Rural environment as health hazard.
   (g) Multifactorial causation of diseases.
   (5×3=15)

QUESTION PAPER-5

B.Sc. Nursing – April 2004
(Epidemiology and Preventive Medicine)

Time Allowed : 3 Hours   Max Marks : 75

Instructions : Attempt any five questions only.
Each question carry equal marks.

1. (a) Describe the sources of air pollution.
   (b) Briefly explain the impact of air pollution on health of people.
   (c) Identify the preventive measures to control air pollution.   (5+5+5=15)
2. (a) List the helminthic infestations and its causes, which commonly occur among children.
   (b) What health education would you give to prevent helminthic infestations to school children?   (5+10)
3. Explain any *two* of the following :
   (i) Descriptive epidemiology in study of disease.
   (ii) Web of causation of disease.
   (iii) Epidemiological triad in disease causation.
   (iv) Prevention and control of occupational diseases.   (7½+7½)
4. (a) Discuss the modes of transmission of filaria.
   (b) Enumerate the role of nurse in prevention and control of filaria in a community.   (5+10)
5. (a) Explain the risk factors in causation of cardiovascular diseases.
   (b) Describe the role of nurse in prevention and control of cardiovascular diseases.   (5+10)
6. Write short notes on any *three* :
   (i) Morbidity indicators.
   (ii) F.A.O.
   (iii) Immunity and types of Immunity.
   (iv) Healthy carrier.
   (v) E.S.I.
   (vi) Health problems due to industrialization and urbanisation.   (5+5+5)

QUESTION PAPER-1

B.Sc. Nursing – April 2000
(Community Health Nursing)

Time Allowed : 3 Hours   Max Marks : 75

Instructions : Attempt any five questions only.
Each question carry equal marks.

1. (a) Define community identification.
   (b) What is the importance of community identification in community health nursing ?
   (c) Explain with example the categories of factual information that you would like to collect.   (2, 4, 9)
2. (a) What is meant by "couple protection rate"?
   (b) Write the objectives of family welfare programme "to achieve NRR-1 by the year 2000 AD."
   (c) Discuss the roles and functions of community health nurse in family welfare programme.   (2, 4, 9)
3. (a) Explain the concept of ecosystem and ecology.
   (b) Discuss ecological factors affecting health of the urban and rural community.   (5, 10)
4. Plan nursing interventions for any *three* of the following situations:
   (a) An *anganwadi* worker reports a large number of cases with history of fever with chills and rigor.
   (b) An adolescent school girl wants to have guidance on menstrual hygiene.
   (c) School teacher reports that many primary school children are having dental problem.
   (d) A mother reports that her nine years old son is having worm infestation.   (5×3)
5. (a) Define "primary health care".
   (b) Describe the Government's policy of primary health care at village level.   (3, 12)
6. Write short notes on any *three* of the following :
   (a) Panchayati Raj.
   (b) Mass Media for effective communication.
   (c) Minimum needs programme.
   (d) Family as a unit of health and disease.
   (e) Occupational hazards.   (5+5+5)

QUESTION PAPER-2
B.Sc Nursing – April 2001
(Community Health Nursing)
Time Allowed: 3 Hours   Max Marks : 75

Instructions : Attempt any five questions only.
Each question carry equal marks.

1. As a community health nurse you are assigned a community of urban slum of 3000 population for providing comprehensive health care services. Describe the steps you will take to provide comprehensive health care services to this community.   (15)

2. (a) Explain the concept and scope of family planning.
   (b) Discuss the impact of population explosion on health and development.
   (c) Explain the impact of family planning on the health of women and children.
                                                    (5+5+5)

3. (a) Explain the concept of health education.
   (b) Discuss its importance in community health nursing practice.
   (c) As a community health nurse how would you organise mass health education programme for community under your care ?   (5+5+5)

4. Discuss briefly :
   (a) National Tuberculosis Control Programme in India.
   (b) Roles and responsibilities of community health nurse in prevention and control of tuberculosis.   (9+6)

5. (a) List the objectives of appointing Kartar Singh Committee.
   (b) Discuss the recommendations given by this committee.   (5+10)

6. Write short notes on any *three* of the following :
   (a) National strategy for health for all 2000 AD.
   (b) Community involvement.
   (c) Functions of voluntary health agencies.
   (d) Health threat and foreseable crisis situations in the family.
   (e) Records and reports.
   (f) Presumptive treatment of malaria.
                                                    (5×3=15)

QUESTION PAPER-3
B.Sc Nursing – April 2000
(Community Health Nursing)
Time Allowed: 3 Hours   Max Marks : 75

Instructions : Attempt any five questions only.
Each question carry equal marks.

1. (a) Define community health nursing.
   (b) What do you understand by community "Health and Nursing needs" assessment ?
   (c) Discuss the methods of assessment of health and nursing needs.   (2+8+5=15)

2. (a) List down the common occupational health hazards among textile industrial workers.
   (b) Describe the measures you would take to prevent and control these hazards.
                                                    (6+9=15)

3. (a) What is "couple protection rate"?
   (b) List the scope of family planning services.
   (c) Enumerate the goals of National Family Welfare Programme.
   (d) As a community health nurse what methods would you suggest for spacing ?   (2+3+4+6=15)

4. (a) What do you understand by maternal mortality rate?
   (b) Explain the causes of high maternal mortality rate in India.
   (c) What is your role as a community health nurse in bringing down the maternal mortality ?   (3+6+6=15)

5. (a) Explain the concept of ecology.
   (b) Discuss ecological factors affecting health of the urban community.
                                                    (5+10=15)

6. (a) Define disaster and disaster nursing.
   (b) List the objectives of disaster nursing.
   (c) Describe in brief the role of community health nurse in disaster nursing services.
                                                    (4+4+7=15)

7. Write short notes on any *three* of the following :
   (a) Principles of health education.
   (b) WHO.
   (c) Ways and means of community participation.
   (d) ICDS programme.
   (e) National health Policy.   5×3=15

QUESTION PAPER-4
B.Sc. Nursing – April 2003
(Community Health Nursing)

Time Allowed: 3 Hours   Max Marks : 75

Instructions : Attempt any five questions onlty.
  Each question carry equal marks.

1. "Community identification is the initial step of providing comprehensive health care to community"
   (a) Describe the factors you would like to study to identify health needs of community.
   (b) State the sources and methods of community identification.   (10+5=15)

2. "Vector-borne diseases are major health problems in India."
   (a) List the common vector-borne diseases.
   (b) Discuss the National Control Programme on any one of the vector-borne diseases.   (3+12)

3. (a) Explain the concept of family health care.
   (b) Describe the importance of identifying health risk factors in providing family health care.
   (c) Briefly state the steps of providing family health care with examples.   (2+5+8)

4. (a) List the important sources of vital health statistics.
   (b) Describe any two of the significant sources of collecting health information.
   (c) Identify the role of nurse in gathering relevant health information.   (5+6+4)

5. (a) Enumerate the health indicators which reflect the health status of mothers and children.
   (b) Briefly discuss the components of RCH (Reproductive and child health) Programme initiated by Government of India, to reduce maternal and child mortality.
   (c) List the functions of community health nurse in RCH programme.   (3+8+4)

6. "Nutritional problems are the major health hazards among children."
   (a) List the nutritional problems in children.
   (b) As a community health nurse, what health education would you plan for children with P.C.M.? (Protein calorie-malnutrition)   (4+11)

7. Write briefly notes on the following :
   (a) Primary health care at grass roots level.
   (b) Community health team functioning.
   (c) Records and Reports in Community health.   (5×3=15)

QUESTION PAPER-5
B.Sc. Nursing – April 2004
(Community Health Nursing)

Time Allowed: 3 Hours   Max Marks : 75

Instructions : Attempt any five questions only.
  Each question carry equal marks.

1. (a) Define comprehensive family health care.
   (b) Discuss in brief the importance of family centered care.
   (c) Explain the steps of family health nursing process.   (2+5+8=15)

2. Your are working in a rural health agency. You are required to visit the following families under your care. Plan nursing intervention for *three* of the following families :
   (a) Where antenatal mother is anaemic and her two year-old child is having diarrhoea.
   (b) Where 7-year-old child is suffering from measles.
   (c) Where 10-year old child is bitten by a dog..
   (d) Where 2 year old child is having upper respiratory-tract infection.   (5×3=15)

3. (a) Define ecology.   (2+7+6=15)
   (b) Explain ecosystem. List the factors affecting ecosystem.
   (c) Discuss any *one* of the factors and it's impact on health of the community.

4. (a) Define primary health care.(2+6+7=15)
   (b) Describe briefly the principles of primary health care.
   (c) Health education is one of the important elements of primary health care. Justify.

5. Discuss ways and means of improving nutritional status of school children through actions of community health nursing personnel in low income level urban community.   (15)

6. Write short notes on any *three* of the following:
   (a) Records and reports in community health agency and it's importance.
   (b) Community identification.
   (c) Fertility and factors influencing change in fertility.
   (d) Maternal mortality rate.
   (e) High health risk family.   (5×3=15)

●●●

APPENDICES

APPENDICES

Information on Health Indicators

Indicator		Latest available data	Year	Source	Remarks
Population with adequate excreta	Total	36.0	1998–99	4	
disposal facilities available (%)	Urban	80.7	1998–99	4	
	Rural	18.9	1998–99	4	
(Population with toilet/latrine facility)					
Health Resources					
Facilities					
Number of hospital beds		665,639	1998	5	As of 1/1/1998
Population per hospital bed		1,451	1998	5	For hospitals only
Hospital beds per 10,000 population		6.9	1998	5	
Number of health centres :					
(a) Subcentres		137,006	1998	5	
(b) Primary health centres		23,179	1998	5	
(c) Community health centres		2,913	1998	5	
Human resources					
Number of physicians		503,900	1998	5	Registered
Population per physician		1,916	1998	5	Computed value
Physicians per 10,000 population		5.2	1998	5	
General nurse midwives		607,376	1997	5	Registered
Auxiliary nurse midwives / health workers		301,691	1997	5	
Budgetary resources					
Total Expenditure on Health as % of Gross Domestic Product (GDP)		5.1	1998	6	
Public Expenditure on Health as % of Total Expenditure on Health		18.0	1998	6	
Private Expenditure on Health as % of Total Expenditure on Health		82.0	1998	6	
Public Expenditure on Health as % of General Government Expenditure		5.6	1998	6	

Indicator	Latest available data	Year	Source	Remarks
Social Security Expenditure on Health as % of Public Expenditure on Health	...	1998	6	
Tax funded Health Expenditure as % of Public Expenditure on Health	96.4	1998	6	
External Resources for Health as % of Public Expenditure on Health	3.6	1998	6	
Private Insurance for Health Risks as % of Private Expenditure on Health	...	1998	6	
Out-of-Pocket Spending on Health as % of Private Expenditure on Health	97.3	1998	6	
Per capita Total Expenditure on Health at official Exchange rate (Exchange Rate per US$)	22	1998	6	
Per capita Public Expenditure on Health at official Exchange rate (Exchange Rate per US$)	4	1998	6	
Per capita Total Expenditure on Health in international dollars (int'l $)	110	1998	6	
Per capita Public Expenditure on Health in international dollars (int'l $)	20	1998	6	
Health Services				
Pregnant women attended by trained personnel during pregnancy (%) Total	65.1	1995–96	4	
Urban	85.6	1995–96	4	
Rural	59.3	1995–96	4	
Deliveries attended by trained personnel (%) Total	42.3	1995–96	4	
Urban	73.5	1995–96	4	
Rural	33.5	1995–96	4	
Women of childbearing age using family planning (%)	48.2	1998–99	4	
Eligible population (i.e., infants reaching their first birthday) that has been fully immunized according to national immunization policies	34.5 / 49.0	1998–99 / 2001	4 / 7	As of Oct 2001
Infants reaching their first birthday who have been fully immunized against diphtheria, tetanus, and whooping cough (%)	52.1	1998–99	4	
Infants reaching their first birthday who have been fully immunized against measles (%)	41.7	1998–99	4	
Infants reaching their first birthday who have been fully immunized against poliomyelitis (%)	69.1	1998–99	4	

Indicator		Latest available data	Year	Source	Remarks
Women who have been immunized with tetanus toxoid (TT) during pregnancy (%)		66.8	1995–96	4	
Health Status					
Life expectancy at birth (Years):	Male	62.4	1996–2001	5	Projected values
	Female	63.4	1996–2001	5	
Infant mortality rate (per 1000 live births)		68	1994–98	4	
Under-five mortality rate (per 1000 live births)		95	1994–98	4	
Maternal mortality ratio (per 100,000 live births)		407	1998	8	

Sources : 1. India, *Census of India 2001 : Provisional Population totals*, March 2001.

2. India, *Sample Registration System, Statistical Report 1998*, October 2000.

3. India, *Sample Registration System, SRS Bulletin*, April 2001.

4. India, *National Family Health Survey (NFHS–2), 1998–99*, October 2000.

5. India, *Health Information of India 1997 and 1998*, July 2000.

6. Adapted from "WHO Geneva, *The World Health Report 2001 : Mental Health, New Understanding, New Hope*", October 2001.

7. India, Press Briefing by the Minister of Health, 23 October 2001.

8. India, *Sample Registration System, SRS Bulletin*, April 2000.

Self Breast Examination for Early Detection of Breast Cancer

Observe for symmetry, Lump Nipple retraction for failure of nipple erection.

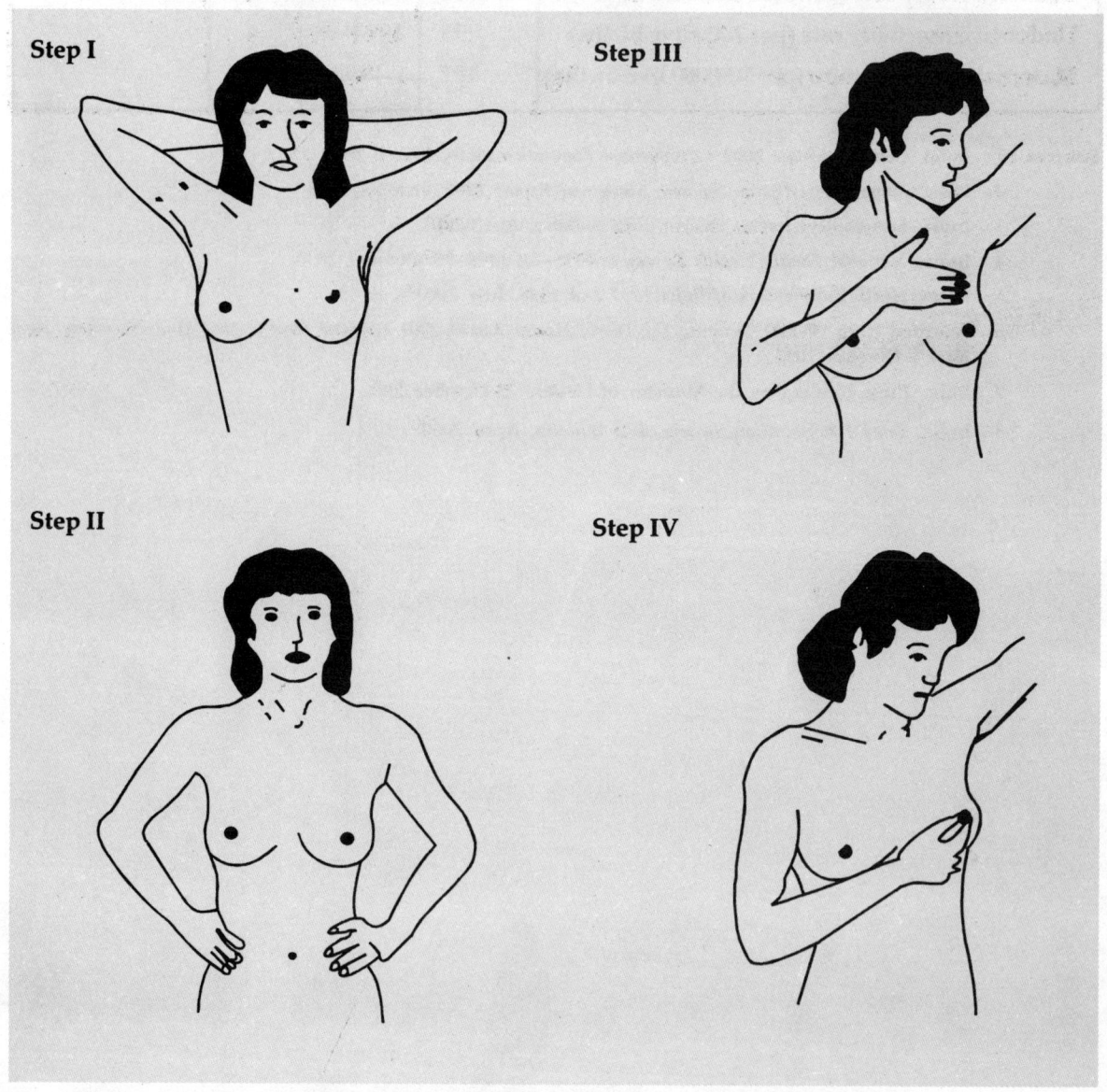

Step I

Step II

Step III

Step IV

Step V

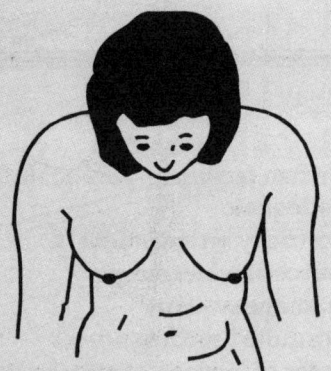

Step VIII

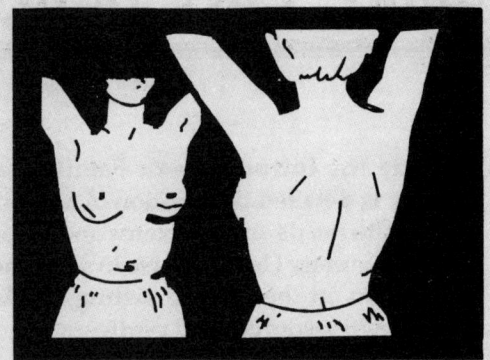

Step VI

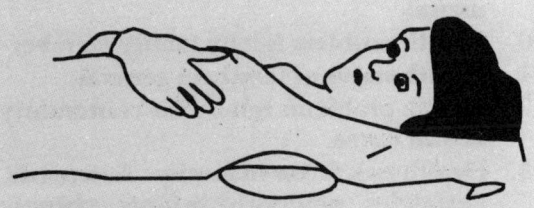

Step IX

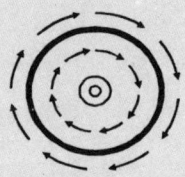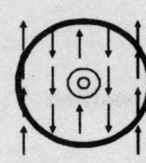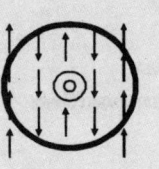

Step VII

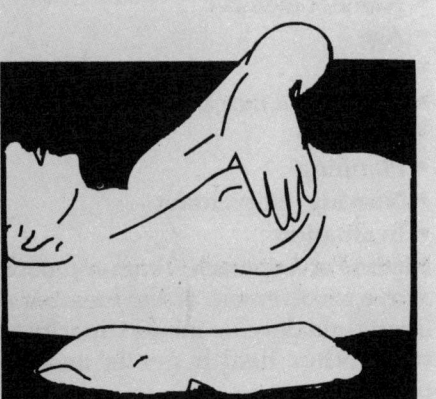

Step X

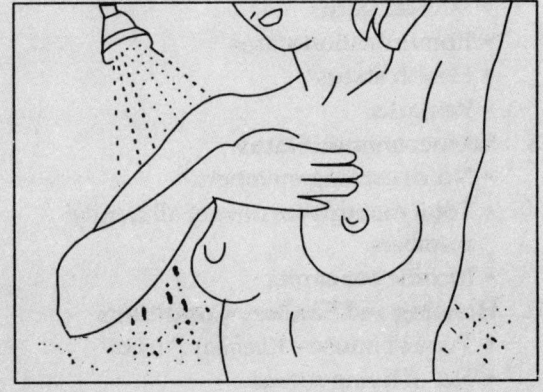

Family Care Study

1. **Guide for Introduction** : Family Care Study is detailed description of a family, its health needs and problems and Heofts of Community Health Nurse to solve their problems in their home settings within their own resources and participation.

2. **Identification Data**
   - Name of the head of the family
   - Address

3. **Family Characteristics**
   - Type of family
   - Size of family
   - Religion
   - Caste
   - Chief diet

4. **Family Composition**
   - S. No.
   - Name
   - Age
   - Sex
   - Relationship with head of the family
   - Education occupation
   - Marital status
   - Immunization status
   - Health status
   - Remarks

5. **Socioeconomic Status**
   - No. of earning members
   - Total monthly income of all family members.
   - Income per capita

6. **Housing and Sanitary Conditions**
   - Type of house – *Kuchha / Puckka*
   - No. of living rooms
   - Living space per head – Adequate / Inadequate
   - Ventilation of rooms – Satisfactory / Unsatisfactory

   - Kitchen facilities – Adequate / Inadequate
   - Electricity arrangement
   - Source of water supply
   - Drainage system
   - Mosquito breeding areas
   - Types of latrines – Sanitary / Manual
   - Method of waste disposal –Satisfactory / Unsatisfactory.

7. **Knowledge about health and diseases**

8. **Personal habits** : Smoking, alcoholism

9. **Nutritional status of the family (one day menu)**

10. **Health problem felt by family member**

11. **Health status of family in general**

12. **Health problems felt by the community health nurse**

13. **Health risk factor in family** : Antenatals, geriatrics, newborn, infants, chronic illness etc.

14. **Family Care Plan**
    - S. No.
    - Name of member
    - Age
    - Sex
    - Health risk factor
    - Objective
    - Planning
    - Nursing intervention
    - Evaluation

15. **Method of Approach** : Team approach with active involvement of the member of the family and develop family capacity to deal with other health needs and health problems.

16. **Family Visit** : Nurse may plan 5 to 10 visits for giving care to a family based on health risk situation, high-risk, moderate or low risk. She needs to plan for the care based on priority needs of family members and

divide the objectives for consecutive visits till she terminates the care.

- *Plan for frequency and number of visits :* Depends upon the overall objectives and needs of family once or twice a week, etc.
- *Date and time of visits :* To plan with the family, because it should be suitable to family members and nurse.
- *Setting of objectives and plan for care :* Nurse sets the overall objectives and then plans the daily objectives. Plan for care to be given including health education.
- *Observations during visit :* It is one of the essential skill of nurse, she must observe carefully the family actions and living conditions during family visit.
- *Care given and discussion :* Nurse gives the care as for plan. But care remains flexible in case of priority needs at home. For example, if she plans to give health education to infant for immunization and she finds child with severe diarrhoea, her plan may change from giving health education on immunization to demonstration of ORS (Oral Rehydration Solution) to give the child and referrals for advise, etc. Nurse discusses the care with family members. It must be based on felt needs of the family as well. All family members are considered during care, which is based on priority needs.

- *Health education :* The complete health care involves need based health education to infants, elders, mothers and fathers, etc.
- *Recording of subsequent visit :* Docomentation of planning and accountability giving care is essential to ensure the work done and avoid repetition. It also helps to get cumulative health status of family.
- *Termination of visit :* The visit must be terminated by proper information to family members and they must be guided to whom to approach in need.

17. **Summary and Conclusion :** Total visits, overall planning, implementary paid and evaluation of nursing intervention must be summarised by indicating the effects of visit and impact on health status of family.

Community Health Nursing Exercise

Objectives

1. To apply statistical methods to selected health data.
2. To appreciate implication of the data for the community and for the public health nurse.

Trends in community population : Complete the table below, providing population, birth rates, and death rates for the years selected.

	1981	1991	2001	After 2004
Population of community (local)				
Birth rate				
National				
State				
Local				
Death rate				
National				
State				
Local				

HOME VISIT RECORD

Objective : To accumulate a concise record of family nursing experience.

While working with the family, keep a record of your findings and your service. Include visits to the home, consultations, referrals, and other activities undertaken on behalf of the family in relation to its needs. Your record should indicate both your planning for and evaluation of each.

Date	Record of Service

Signature

Identification of Families Coping Behaviours/Functional Abilities

Family assessments helps to identify the family at different levels according to their characteristics and coping behaviours and functional abilities which provides data for planning, organising, implementing and evaluating nursing intervention. Family functioning can be improved by effective nursing action for effecture changes in behaviour by regular family visits and working with them.

The family can be divided into 'V' levels (Tapia's classification)

1. **Level I :**

   Chaotic family : This type of family is :
   - Disorganized, difficulty in meeting needs
   - Distrust of others, roles are confused
   - Parents assume inappropriate adult roles
   - Hostility and resistance towards others of help
   - Children may take up adult roles
   - Child abuse and neglect or removal from home.

2. **Level II :** Intermediate family :
   - Less disorganized, better able to meet its roles than chaotic family
   - Roles are confused but family willing to use available services and make changes
   - Children are neglected but remain in the home.

3. **Level III :** Normal family with conflicts and problems :
   - Basic needs are met.
   - Higher degree of trust among family members
   - *Parents maturity level varies :* One more mature than the other
   - Confusion among children about appropriate roles
   - Family recognizes its problems
   - Utilise the resources available
   - Tries to make necessary behaviour and attitudinal changes.

4. **Level IV :** *Family with solutions :*
   - Normal, stable, healthy and happy family with fewer problems and conflicts
   - Basic needs are met :
   - When they arise
   - Parental roles are clear
   - Children have appropriate role models to support their growth and development.

5. **Level V :** Ideal, Independent Family ;
   - Able to fulfil the functions and roles
   - Resolve problems as they arise
   - Seek help in crisis situation.

Identification of Risk Factors in Families

Assessment of family will identify actual or potential risk factors. These factors can be categorised :

1. **Developmental factors :** These relate to events that occur as the result of normal growth of the individual family members. These are present throughout :
   - Infancy
   - Toddlerhood
   - School age
   - Adolescence
   - Adulthood
   - Marriage
   - Childbirth
   - Menopause
   - Retirement
   - Death

2. **Environmental factors :** These are related to the surroundings which have a bad effect on the health. For example :
   - Factors outside the house
     Collection of refuse, breeding of disease carrying insects
     Stray dogs, open drains, unhygienic eating places, unprotected electrical installations
   - Factors inside the homes
     Open fires for heating and cooking, sharp instruments
     Overcrowding
     Use of unsafe water for drinking
     Unsanitary disposal of water, wastes and solids.
   - Factors at workplace
     Accidents related to agricultural tools
     Machines, poisonous insects, snakes and scorpions, etc.
     Use of pesticides, dyes, stone crushing and plants and pollens, etc.

3. **Hereditary factors :** These are the factors that places an individual at risk because of family history. For example :
   - Cardiovascular diseases
   - Diabetes
   - Haemophilia.

4. **Situational factors :** Factors that may appear unexpectedly and unpredictable with no time for preparation. For example :
   - Acute illness, chronic illness or disabilities

- Accidents
- Assaults
- Rape
- Murder
- Flood
- Earthquake
- Death, etc.

5. **Lifestyle factors :** Factors related to lifestyle behaviours, *i.e.*, the way of living, habits, customs, attitudes, nutritional and health practices. For example :
   - Alcohol and drug abuse
   - Smoking
   - Lack of regular exercise and rest
   - Juvenile delinquency
   - Depression
   - Parental discord, etc.
   - Single parent family
   - Large family with limited physical facilities.

6. **Socioeconomic factors :** Factors related to the availability and utilization of financial resources. For example :
   - Poverty
   - Ignorance or lack of knowledge
   - Illiteracy
   - Indifferent attitude
   - Nonutilization or underutilization of facilities
   - Nonaccessibility
   - Nonacceptance, and
   - Nonperception, etc.

Role of Nurse : Identification of risk factors will help community health nurse to identify those factors which affect the health of every individual during developmental stage. So that she can identify those factors, try to overcome for better health care plan.

Perineal Care

INTRODUCTION

Perineal hygiene involves cleaning the external genitalia and surrounding area. The perineal area is conductive to the growth of pathogenic organism because it is warm, moist and is not well ventilated. Since there are many orifices situated in this area, the pathogenic organisms can enter into the body. Thorough cleanliness is essential to prevent infection, bad odour and provide a sense of well-being.

Definition

An antiseptic irrigation or sponging of the vulva and perineum given after voiding or defecation in a specified period following delivery or an operation on the birth canal, perineum, urinary meatus or anus is termed perineal care.

Indications

Special attention to the perineal area is essential when:
(a) The patients is having inability
(b) The patients genitourinary tract infection
(c) Incontinence of urine and stool
(d) Excessive vaginal discharge
(e) Indwelling catheter
(f) Postnatal mothers
(g) Before and after surgery on the genitourinary system
(h) Injury, ulcer or surgery on the perineal area or rectum
(i) After abortion
(j) Gynaecological problems

Purposes for Perineal Care to Post-Natal Mothers

1. To inspect the colour, odour, amount of lochia and condition of perineum
2. To clean the skin and mucous membrane under aseptic conditions
3. To discourage the growth of bacteria by application of antiseptics
4. To relieve inflammation and congestion
5. To relieve pain
6. To stimulate circulation
7. To prevent infection and promote healing
8. To enhance comfort.

Principles

1. Always select a safe place which is little at higher site.
2. Create clean field before placing the bag.
3. Keep the bag on clean field facing outer pocket outside.
4. Wash hands and take out all needed equipment and supplies at a time and close the bag.
5. Ensure privacy during the procedure.
6. Maintain maximum asepsis.
7. Strength of the solutions : Dettol 1:60, Savlon 1:100 to 120.
8. Temperature of solutions should not be more than 105° F.
9. Avoid friction over the stitches.
10. Do not contaminate dressing set and arms.
11. Used pad or cloth should be collected in a paper bag or leaf and should be burnt or discarded properly after the procedure.
12. Do not put used swabs in the bedpan.
13. Clean and boil contaminated instruments and equipment before returning them into the nurse's bag .

NURSE'S RESPONSIBILITY IN THE PERINEAL CARE

A. Preliminary Assessment

1. Assess the condition of the perineal skin— any itching, irritation, ulcers, oedema, drainage, etc.
2. Assess the need and frequency of perineal care.
3. Assess whether the perineal care should be done under aseptic technique or a clean technique.
4. Check the physician's orders for any special instructions.
5. Assess the patient's ability for self care.
6. Assess the patient's mental state to follow instructions.

B. Preparation of the Articles

Articles	Purpose
Handwashing articles	To prevent cross infection
Mackintosh with paper lining	To protect the bed
Drape sheet	To drape the patient
Bedpan (if available)	
A Jug with warm water or antiseptic solution	To clean the perineum
A sterile bowl with 8 to 10 boiled cooled swabs	To clean the perineum
Artery clamp—1	To hold the swabs for
Thumb forceps—1	cleaning
Spoon—1	To measure solution
Antiseptic solution —Dettol or Savlon	To clean the perineum
Spirit, Mercurochrome or	To apply over stitches
Betadine	For protection and to
Pad, Bandage	absorb discharge
Paper bag	
Extra cotton and paper	
Inch tape	

C. Preparation of Patient and Unit

1. Explain the procedure to the patient.
2. Wash hands.
3. Provide privacy by screen on drapes.
4. Remove all articles that may interfere with the procedure.
5. Place mackintosh with paper lining under the buttocks over the bedsheet.
6. Offer the bedpan.
7. Untie the pad if any and observe the discharge, its colour, odour, amount, etc. and discard the pad in the paper bag.
8. Massage the uterus and expel out the clots.

D. Procedure

1. Wash hands with soap and water.
2. Pour water over the perineum.
3. Clean the perineum using boiled cooled swabs.
   (a) Hold the swabs with artery clamp and clean from above downwards towards the anal canal.
   (b) Use one swab for one swabbing.
   (c) Clean the perineum from the midline outward in the following order : The vulva, the labia minora on both sides, labia majora on both sides, clean the perineal region and the anus thoroughly.
4. Give care to stitched area with spirit swab and apply mercurochrome or betadine.
5. Put sterile pad. Do not touch the surface of the pad which will come in contact with the vulva and perineum.
6. Remove the bedpan and mackintosh.
7. Make the mother comfortable.
8. Wash hands and measure the fundal height.
9. Clean all articles, boil the forceps and replace the articles.
10. Remove the screen and tidy up the unit.
11. Either burn the paper bag with pads or discard it in the dustbin.
12. Wash hands.
13. Record the procedure with date and time and observations made.

Surgical Dressing at Home

INTRODUCTION

Home hazards and minor accidents resulting in cuts and minor injuries are very common in community and home situation. It is necessary for the nurse to dress traumatic wounds and lesions particularly in rural areas where other medical services are not available.

Definition

Wound

A wound is a cut or break in the continuity of any tissue.

Surgical Dressing

This procedure applies to dressings that are done at traumatic and other lesions in the home, school, centre or in an industrial health office.

Purposes

(a) To remove and dispose of soiled dressings to prevent spread of infection.
(b) To cleanse area around the wound to prevent further infection and tissue damage.
(c) To apply sterile dressing to prevent other infections and to promote healing.
(d) To absorb inflammatory excedate and to promote drainage.
(e) To convert the contaminated wound into a clean wound.
(f) To prevent haemorrhage.
(g) To prevent skin excoriation.
(h) To apply the medication on the wound.
(i) To restore the function of the part.

Principles of Wound Care

(a) Micro-organisms are present in the environment, on the articles and on the skin. Pathogenic organisms are transmitted from the source to the new host directly or indirectly.

(b) Bacteria travel along with the dust particles.
(c) Cleaning on area where there is less number of organisms, before cleaning an area where there are more organisms, minimize the spread of organisms to the clear area.
(d) A break in the skin and the mucous membrane acts as a portal of entry for the pathogenic organisms.
(e) Respiratory tract harbours micro-organisms that can enter the wound.
(f) Nutrients and oxygen are carried to the wound via bloodstream and are essential for collagen formation.
(g) Moisture facilitates growth and movement of micro-organisms.
(h) Fluid moves downward as a result of gravitational pull.
(i) Fluid moves through materials by capillary action.
(j) Unfamiliar situation produce anxiety.
(k) Systematic ways of working saves time, energy and material.

General Instructions for Dressing

(a) Practice strict aseptic technique.
(b) Wash hands before and after the procedure.
(c) Dressing should not be changed for at least 15 minutes after the room has been swept or cleaned.
(d) Instruments used for one dressisng are not be used for another until they have been resterilized.
(e) Create a clean field round the wounds.
(f) Avoid talking, coughing and sneezing when wound is open.
(g) During the procedure, the nurse works carefully to avoid contaminating the patients skin, clothing and bed linen with soiled instruments and dressing. All the soiled dressings and contaminated instruments

should be carefully collected and disposed safely.

(h) Cleaning the wound should be done from cleanest area to the less clean area.

(i) If dressing are adherent to the wound, wet it with normal saline before it is removed from the wound.

(j) While dressing the wound, keep the wound edges as clear as possible to promote healing.

(k) Before doing the dressing inspect the wound for any complication. If any, do the needful.

(l) Avoid meal timings.

(m) Give analgesics prior to the painful dressings.

NURSE'S RESPONSIBILITY IN THE WOUND DRESSING

Preliminary Assessment

(a) Check the general condition of the patient.

(b) Check the purpose for which the dressing is to be done.

(c) Check the condition of the wound, i.e., the type of wound and dressing to be applied, etc.

(d) Check the physician's order, e.g., type of dressing, the specific instructions, if any, regarding the cleaning solution, application of medicine, etc.

(e) If any previous card is available find out the general condition of the wound and patient from the card.

(f) Check the articles available in the house.

(g) Look for the other members who can follow instructions and look after the client.

Preparation of Articles

Articles	Purpose
1. Hand washing articles.	To prevent cross infection
2. Makintosh with paper linings.	To protect the bed, garments
3. Bowl containing spoon, disecting forcep, artry clamp and swabs. (to be boiled).	To clean the wound
4. Scissors.	To cut dressing material
5. Sterile dressing and cotton swabs.	To clean and dress the wound
6. Sterile swab sticks.	To apply medicine
7. Antiseptic lotion/ ointment/powder	To apply on wound
8. Paper bag	To collect waste
9. Saucepan with lid.	To boil the articles

Preparation of the Patient Working Field and Environment

(a) Knock the door, introduce yourself to the patient and relative. Develop interpersonal relationship and explain the procedure to them to gain confidence.

(b) Keep home visit bag at bedside either on box, extra charpoy, chair or table.

(c) Take out hand washing article from outer pocket and wash hands thoroughly.

(d) Arrange the work area. Keep required articles for boiling and arrange them.

(e) Provide privacy.

(f) Apply restrain (if required) in case of children.

(g) Ask the patient to void prior to dressing.

(h) Shave the area if required.

(i) Place the patient in a comfortable and relaxed position depending on the area to be cleaned.

(j) Give proper support to the body parts of the patient which has to be raised and hold it in a position for a considerable time.

(k) See that the patient's room is in order with no unnecessary articles.

(l) Put off fan and close the doors and windows if draft is present.

(m) Adjust the height of the bed for comfortable working.

(n) Call for assistance, if required.

(o) Protect the bed with makintosh and paper lining.

(p) Expose only the necessary part.

(q) Untie the bandage or adhesive and remove them.

Steps of Procedure

(a) Wash hands thoroughly with soap and water.

(b) Remove bandage and outer dressing and put it in the paper bag. Note the type and amount of drainage present.

(c) Pour small amount of cleansing solution into the bowl.

(d) Clean the wound from the centre to periphery discarding the used swabs after each stroke.

(e) After thorough cleaning of the wound, dry the wound with dry swabs using the same precautions.

(f) Apply medications using swab sticks.

(g) Apply sterile dressing and do the bandaging.

(h) Explain the condition to the patient and the relatives and give advice regarding care, rest, exercise and diet. Urge the person to come to the centre for dressing. See to the comfort of the patient.

(i) Wash hands.

(j) Record the condition of the patient's wound, type and amount of drainage, the care given and medication used with date and time.

After Care of the Patients and the Articles

(a) Help the patient to dress-up and take a comfortable position in the bed. Change the garments and bed linen (if required).

(b) Remove the makintosh with paper lining.

(c) Wrap soiled dressing and burn if possible (or direct the relative to do so).

(d) Wash used instruments, boil with soap and water, rinse and boil.

(e) Wash hands.

(f) Return clean boiled instruments to the home visit bag.

(g) Record the procedure in the card.

Eye Care at Home

INTRODUCTION

Eyes are the one of the vital sense organ of the body. To see this beautiful world we need beautiful eyes. So this has to be taken care from the birth. In newborn a common problem of the eyes is discharges that dry on the lashes as crusts, which can lead to eye infection, if not taken care of.

Definition

Eye care is a procedure of cleaning the eyes by maintaining asepsis.

Purpose

- To clean the eyes
- To protect the eyes
- To prevent infection
- For the sense of well-being
- To promote and maintain the health of the eyes
- For aesthetic sense.

Principles

1. Always keep the bag on a higher place with a paper lining.
2. Wash hands before taking out the articles.
3. All articles needed are taken out at one time, then close the bag.
4. Never mix the bag articles with the home articles.
5. Wash and boil the article before use.
6. Never keep moist article inside the bag.

Eyes

1. Asepsis should be maintained while giving eye care.
2. One swab for one stroke only.
3. Move from less infected to more infected area.

4. Surrounding area should be clean.
5. From inner canthus to outer canthus.
6. Position of the child : Lying on the back and near the nurse.

Preparation of the Articles

1. Place the bag on the higher surface.
2. Take out the hand washing articles.
3. Take out the articles needed for the eye care.

Articles	Purpose
Bowl with boiled cooled Swabs	For eye care
Spoon	To take out the swabs from bowl
Extra cotton	To plug the ears
Paper bag	To put the waste and to squeeze the swabs, into the paper bag.

Preparation of the Patient and the Surrounding Area

- Explain the procedure to patient and relatives.
- Adjust the article nearby.

Procedure

Steps of procedure

- Wash the hands
- Plug the ear
- Take out the swab from the bowl with spoon
- Take the swab from spoon touching only one side of swab, squeeze in the paper bag.
- Clean from the inner canthus to outer canthus with one swab for one stroke and discard the swab in the paper bag.
- Continue cleaning till all discharge is removed from the eyes.

Points to be Kept in Mind

(a) Area of the swab touched by the fingers should not come in contact with the eyes.

(b) Squeeze off the excessive water from the swabs.

(c) No pressure on the eyeball should be given.

(d) Gently wipe the lids from the inner to outer canthus.

(e) One swab for one swabbing.

(f) Separate swab for separate eyes.

After Care

- Make the patient comfortable.
- Boil and dry the articles and place in bag.
- Record due procedure done.

•••

Glossary

Absorption Field : The element of a septic system in which the liquid portion of waste is distributed.

Accreditation : The process by which an agency or organization evaluates and recognizes an institution as meeting certain predetermined standards.

Acculturated : The cultural modification of an individual or group by adapting to or borrowing traits from another culture.

Acid rain : Both wet and dry acidic deposits, which occur both within and downwind of areas that produce emissions containing sulphur dioxide and oxides of nitrogen (also called acid deposition).

Activities of Daily Living (ADLs) : Eating, toileting, dressing, bathing, walking, getting in and out of a bed or chair, and getting outside.

Acute disease : A disease in which the peak severity of symptoms occurs and subsides within three months of onset, usually within days or weeks.

Administration for Children and Families: An parenting division of the DHHS that co-ordinates programmes which promote the economic and social well-being of families, children, individuals, and communities.

Administration on Aging : An operating division of the DHHS designated to carryout the provisions of the Older Americans Act of 1965.

Adolescents and Young Adults : Individuals between the ages of 15 and 24 years.

Adult Day Care Programmes : Daytime care provided to seniors who are unable to be left alone.

Aetiology : The cause of disease (*e.g.*, the aetiology of mumps is the mumps virus).

Affective Disorder: Mental disorder characterized by a disturbance of mood, either depression or elation (mania); for example, bipolar disorder, major depression.

Aftercare : The continuing care provided to the former drug abusers or drug dependent persons.

Age Pyramid : A conceptual model that illustrates the age distribution of a population.

Age-adjusted Rates : Rates used to make comparisons of relative risks across groups and overtime when groups differ by age structure.

Aged : The state of being old.

Agency for Healthcare Research and Quality (AHRQ) : An operating division of DHHS created by superfund legislation to prevent or mitigate adverse health effect and diminished quality of life resulting from exposure to hazardous substances in the environment. It is a part of the Public Health Service.

Agent (pathogenic agent) : The cause of the disease or health problem, the factor that must be present in order for the disease to occur.

Ageing : The physiological changes that occur normally in plants and animals as they grow older.

Aid to the Permanently and Totally Disabled (APTD) : 1962 amendments to the Social Security Act aimed at providing federal funds for social services to the mentally ill.

Aid to Families with Dependent Children (AFDC) : Programme of the Administration for Children and Families that provides cash assistance based on need, income, and resources to single mother and their children who find themselves with minimal resources.

Air Pollution : The contamination of the air by gases, liquids, or solids that interfere with the comfort, safety, or health of living organisms.

Air-borne Disease : A communicable disease that is transmitted through the air (*e.g.*, influenza).

Alcoholics Anonymous (AA) : A fellowship of recovering alcoholics who offer support to anyone who desires to stop drinking.

Alcoholism : A disease characterized by impaired control over drinking, preoccupation with drinking, and continued use of alcohol despite adverse consequences.

Alien : A person born in and owing allegiance to a country other than the one in which he or she lives.

Allied Health Care Professionals : Health care workers who provide services that assist, facilitate, and complement the work of physicians and other health care specialists.

Allopathic Providers : Independent health care providers whose remedies for illnesses produce effects different from those of the disease. These people are doctors of medicine (MDs).

Ambulatory : "Free-standing" health care facilities that provide a wide and rapidly expanding array of services.

American Cancer Society : A voluntary health agency dedicated to fighting cancer and educating the public about cancer.

American Health Security Act of 1993 : The comprehensive health care reform introduced by then President Clinton, but never enacted.

Amotivational Syndrome : A pattern of behaviour characterized by apathy, loss of effectiveness, and a more passive, introverted personality.

Amphetamines : A group of synthetic drugs that act as stimulants.

Anabolic Drugs : Compounds, structurally similar to the male hormone testosterone, that increase protein synthesis.

Analytical Study : A type of epidemiological study aimed at testing hypotheses (*e.g.*, case/control study, cohort study).

Anthroponosis : A disease that infects only humans.

Aquifers : Underground water reservoirs.

Asbestos : A naturally occurring mineral fibre that has been identified as a class A carcinogen by the Environmental Protection Agency.

Aseism : Prejudice and discrimination against the aged.

Assisted-living Residence : "A special combination of housing, personalized supportive services and health care designed to meet the needs—both scheduled and unscheduled—of those who need help with activities of daily living" (see Chapter 9, reference 22).

Attack Rate : A special incidence rate calculated for a particular population for a single disease outbreak and expressed as a per cent.

Automatic (passive) Protection : The modification of a product or the environment in such a way as to reduce unintentional injuries.

Bacteriological Period : The period in public health history from 1875 to 1900 during which the causes of many bacterial diseases were discovered.

Barbiturates : Depressant drugs based on the structure of barbituric acid; for example, phenobarbital.

Behavioural Health Care Services : The managed care term for mental health and substance abuse/dependence care services.

Benzodiazapines : Non-barbiturate depressant drugs; examples : librium, valium.

Binge Drinking : Consuming five or more alcoholic drinks in a row.

Biogenic Pollutants : Air-borne biological organisms or their particles or gases or other toxic materials that can produce illness.

Biological Hazards : Living organism (and viruses), or their products, that increase the risk of disease or death in humans.

Biosphere : The zone of the earth where life is found, including parts of the atmosphere, earth, surface and ground water, the ocean and their sediments.

Bipolar Disorder : An affective mental disorder characterized by distinct periods of elevated mood alternating with periods of depression.

Birth Rate : Number of livebirths per 1000 of estimated midyear population in a given year".

Blood-alcohol Concentration (BAC) : The percentage of concentration of alcohol in blood; a BAC of 0.08 per cent or greater is regarded as the legal level of intoxication in most states.

Body Echo : The offspring of those in the Baby Boom generation.

Body Mass Index (MBI) : The ratio of weight (in kilograms) to height (in meters, squared). To calculate in pounds and inches divide (weight in pounds)/2.20 by [(height in inches)/32.27²].

Bottle Bills : Laws that require consumers to pay refundable deposits on beer and soft drink containers.

Bottom-up Community Organization : Organization efforts that begin with those who live within the community affected.

Brownfields : Abandoned gas stations, industrial plants and commercial work sites most of which are contaminated with hazardous chemicals.

Bureau of Alcohol, Tobacco, and Firearms (ATF) : The Federal Agency in the Department of the Treasury that regulates alcohol and tobacco.

Bureau of Indian Affairs (BIA) : The Original Federal Government Agency charged with the responsibility for the welfare of Native Americans.

Byssionosis : Acute or chronic lung disease caused by the inhalation of cotton, flax, or hemp dusts; those affected include workers in cotton textile plants (sometimes called brown lung disease).

Capitation : See prepaid health care.

Carcinogens : Agents, usually chemicals, that cause cancer.

Care Manager : One who helps identify the health care needs of an individual but does not actually provide the health care services.

Care Provider : One who helps identify the health care needs of an individual and also personally performs the care giving service.

Carrier : A person or animal that harbours a specific communicable disease agent in the absence of discernible clinical disease and serves as a potential source of infection to others.

Carrying Capacity : The amount of resources (air, water, shelter, etc.) of a given environment to support a certain-sized population.

Case Fatality Rate (CFR) : The percentage of cases of a particular disease that result in death.

Case/Control Study (retrospective study) : An epidemiological study that seeks to compare those diagnosed with a disease (cases) with those who do not have the disease (controls) for prior exposure to specific risk factors.

Cases : People afflicted with a disease.

Categorical Programmes : Those programmes available only to people who can be categorized into a specific group based on disease, age, family means, geography, or other variables.

Cause-specific Mortality Rate (CSMR) : An expression of the death rate due to a particular disease; the CSMR is calculated by dividing the number of deaths due to a particular disease by the total population and multiplying by 100,000.

Census : The enumeration of the population of the United States that is conducted every ten years; begun in 1790.

Centre for Mental Health Services (CMHS) : The Federal Agency, housed within the Department of Health and Human Service's Substance Abuse and Mental Health Services Administration, whose mission it is to conduct research on the causes and treatments for mental disorders.

Centers for Disease Control and Prevention (CDCP) : One of the operating divisions of the Public Health Service; charged with the responsibility for surveillance and control of diseases and other health problems.

Cerebrovascular Disease (Stroke) : A disease in which the blood supply to the brain is interrupted.

Certified Safety Professional (CSP) : A health and safety professional, trained in industrial and workplace safety, who has met specific requirements for board certification.

Chain of Infection : A model to conceptualize the transmission of a communicable disease from its source to a susceptible host.

Chemical Hazards : Hazards caused by the mismanagement of chemicals.

Chemical Straitjacket : The concept of a mental patient's behaviour being restrained or subdued by a drug (Chemical) such as Thorazine instead of by a physical straitjacket.

Child Abuse : The intentional physical, emotional, verbal, or sexual mistreatment of a minor.

Child Maltreatment : The act or failure to act by a parent, caretaker, or other person as defined under state law, which results in physical abuse, neglect, medical neglect, sexual abuse, emotional abuse, or an act, or failure to act which presents an imminent risk of serious harm to the child.

Child Neglect : Infectious diseases that normally affect people in their childhood (*e.g.,* measles, mumps, rubella, and pertussis).

Children : Persons between 1 and 14 years of age.

Chiropractor : A nonallopathic, independent health care provider who treats health problems by adjusting the spinal column.

Chloroflurocarbons (CFCs) : A family of chemical agents used in industry for such items as propellants, refrigeration, solvent cleaning, and insulation.

Chlorpromazine : The first and most famous anti psychotic drug introduced in 1954 under the brandname Thorazine.

Chronic Disease : A disease or health condition that lasts longer than three months, sometimes for the remainder of one's life.

Citizen Initiated Community Organization : See bottom-up community organization.

Clean Air Act (CAA) (P.L. 88-206) : A 1963 law that provided the Federal Government with authority to address interstate air pollution problems.

Clean Water Act (CWA) (P.L. 92-500) : A 1972 law that provided the federal government with authority to ensure water quality by controlling water pollution; first known as Federal Water Pollution Control Act Amendments.

Club Drugs : A general term for those illicit drugs, primarily synthetic, that are most commonly encountered at night clubs and "raves". Examples include MDMA, LSD, GHB GBL, PCP, Ketamine, Rohypnol, and methamphetamines.

Coal Workers' Pneumoconiosis (CWP) : Acute and chronic lung disease caused by the inhalation of coal dust (sometimes called black lung disease).

Cosmic Radiation : The radiation which comes from outer space and the sun.

Criteria Pollutants : The most pervasive air pollutants in the United States.

Crude Birth Rate (CBR) : An expression of the number of livebirths per unit of population in a given period of time. For example, the crude birth rate in the United States in 1999 was 14.5 births per 1,000 population.

Crude Death Rate (CDR) : An expression of the total number of deaths (from all causes) per unit of population in a given period of time. For example, the crude death rate in the United States in 1999 was 877.0 per 100,000 population.

Crude Rate : A rate in which the denominator includes the total population.

Cultural Competency : A set of congruent behaviours, attitudes, and policies that come together in a system, agency, or among professionals that enables effective work in cross cultural situations.

Culturally Sensitive : Having respect for cultures other than one's own.

Curriculum : Written plan for instruction.

Cycles per Second (CPS) : A measure of sound frequency.

Death Rate : See mortality rate.

Decibels (DB) : A measure of sound amplitude.

Deductible : The amount of expense that the beneficiary must incur before the insurance company begins to pay for covered services.

Definitive Host : Host in which the parasite attains maturity or passes its sexual stage is primary or definitive host.

Deinstitutionalization : The process of discharging, on a large scale, patients from state mental hospitals to less restrictive community settings.

Demographic : Statistics of human population.

Demography (demographers) : The study of a population and those variables bringing about change in that population.

Department of Health and Human Services (DHHS) : The second largest federal department in the United States government, formed in 1980 and headed by the secretary who is a member of the president's cabinet.

Depressant : A psychoactive drug that slows down the central nervous system.

Descriptive Study : An epidemiological study that describes an epidemic with respect to person, place, and time.

Designer Drugs : Mind-altering drugs, synthesized in clandestine laboratories, that are similar to but structurally different from known controlled substances.

Diagnosis-related Groups (DRGs) : A procedure used to classify the health problems of all medicare patients when they are admitted to a hospital.

Direct Instruction : Pattern of instruction in which subject matter is identified as a separate subject and is allocated a specific amount of teaching time in the school day.

Direct Transmission : The immediate transfer of an infectious agent by direct contact between infected and susceptible individuals.

Disability-adjusted Life-expectancy (DALE) : The number of healthy years of life that can be expected, on average, in a given population.

Disability-adjusted Life Years (DALYs) : A measure for the burden of disease that takes into account premature death and years lived with disability of specified severity and duration. One DALY is one lost year of healthy life.

Disabling Injury : An injury causing any restriction of normal activity beyond the day of the injury's occurrence.

Disease Prevention (DP) : "As the process of reducing risks and alleviating disease to promote, preserve, and store health and minimize suffering and distress" (see Chapter 5, reference 15).

Diseases of Adaptation : Diseases that result from chronic exposure to excess levels of stressors which elicit the General Adaptation Syndrome.

Disinfection : The killing of communicable disease agents outside the host, on counter tops, for example.

Dose Rate : The rate at which a dose of radiation is received.

Drug (Chemical) Dependence : A psychological and sometimes physical state characterized by a craving for a drug.

Drug : A substance other than food or vitamins, that upon entering the body in small amounts, alters one's health or well being.

Drug Abuse Education : Providing information about the dangers of drug abuse, changing attitudes and beliefs about drugs, providing skills necessary to abstain from drugs, and ultimately changing drug abuse behaviour.

Drug Enforcement Administration (DEA) : The Federal Government's lead agency with the primary responsibility for enforcing the Nation's drug laws, including the controlled substances Act of 1970.

Drug Misuse : Inappropriate use of prescription or nonprescription drugs.

Drug Use : A nonevaluative term referring to drug taking behaviour in general; any drug-taking behaviour.

Dumps : Open pits in which solid waste is placed.

Earth Day : Annul public observance for concerns about the environment; the first was held April 22, 1970.

Ecology : Inter-relationship between organisms and their environment.

Elderhostel : Education programmes specifically for seniors, held on college campuses.

Elderly (or elder) : Individuals over 65 years of age.

Elderly Support Ratio : The support ratio that includes only the elderly.

Eligible Couple : Couples who are in the reproductive period, and are capable of producing children.

Employee Assistance Programme (EAP) : That aspect of a workplace drug programme devoted to assisting employees in recovering from their alcohol or other drug problems.

Endemic Disease : A disease that occurs regularly in a population as a matter of course.

Environment : All the external conditions, circumstances and influences surrounding, and affecting the growth and development of an organisms.

Environmental Hazards : Factors or conditions in the environment that increase the risk of disease or death in humans.

Environmental Health : The study and management of environmental conditions that affect the health and well-being of humans.

Environmental Sanitation : The practice of establishing and maintaining healthy or hygienic conditions in the environment.

Environmental Tobacco Smoke (ETS): Tobacco smoke in the ambient air.

Epidemic : An unexpectedly large number of cases of disease in a particular population for a particular time period.

Epidemic Curve : A graphic display of the cases of disease according to the time or date of onset of symptoms.

Epidemiologist : One who practices epidemiology.

Epidemiology : The study of the distribution and determinants of diseases and injuries in human populations.

Equilibrium Phase : Last phase of the population growth S-curve, when the birth and death rates are equal.

Eradication : The complete elimination or uprooting of a disease (*e.g.*, smallpox eradication).

Evaluation : Determining the value or worth of the objective of interest.

Exclusion : A health condition that is written into the health insurance policy indicating what is not covered by the policy.

Exclusive Provider Organization (EPO) : Similar to a preferred provider organization but with fewer providers and stronger financial incentives. See preferred provider organization (PPO).

Experimental Study : An epidemiological study carried out under controlled conditions, usually to determine the effectiveness of a vaccine, therapeutic drug, or surgical technique.

Exponential Phase : Middle phase of the population growth S-curve, when the birth rate is greater than the death rate.

Family and Medical Leave Act : Federal legislation that provides up to a 12-week unpaid leave to men and women after the birth of a child, an adoption, or an event of illness in the immediate family.

Family Planning : The process of determining the preferred number and spacing of children in one's family and choosing the appropriate means to achieve this preference.

Family Violence : The use of physical force by one family member against another, with the intent to hurt, injure, or cause death.

Fatal Injury : An injury that results in one or more deaths.

Fecund : A woman in reproductive period, who has the physiological ability, to produce children when exposed to its risk.

Federal Emergency Response Agency (FEMA) : The nation's official emergency response agency.

Federal Water Pollution Control : Act Amendments, see Clean Water Act.

Fee-for-service Indemnity : A method of paying for health care in which after the care (service) is rendered, a bill (fee) is paid.

Fertility Rate : The number of livebirths per 1,000 women of childbearing age (15-44 years).

Fixed Indemnity : The maximum amount an insure will pay for a certain service.

Foetal Alcohol Syndrome (FAS) : A group of abnormalities that may include growth retardation, abnormal appearance of face and head, and deficits of central nervous system function including mental retardation in babies born to mothers who have consumed heavy amounts of alcohol during their pregnancies.

Foetal Deaths : Deaths in utero with a gestational age of at least 20 weeks.

Food and Drug Administration (FDA) : An operating division of DHHS that regulates all food, over-the-counter and prescription drugs, medical devices, and cosmetics. It is part of the Public Health Service.

Food-borne Disease : A disease transmitted through the contamination of food.

Food-borne Disease Outbreak (FBDO) : The occurrence of two or more cases of a similar illness resulting from the ingestion of food.

Formaldehyde (CH_2O) : A water soluble gas used in aqueous solutions in hundreds of consumer products.

Formative Evaluation : The evaluation that is conducted during the planning and implementing processes to improve or refine the programme.

Freight or Flight Reaction : An alarm reaction that prepares one physiologically for sudden action (heart rate, blood pressure, and respiration increase).

Frequency : The rate of vibrations created by the transmission of energy. In the case of sound, it is measured in cycles per second, hertz, or vibration per second.

Full-service Hospital : Hospital that offer services in all or most of the levels of care defined by the spectrum of health care.

Functional Limitations : Difficulty in performing personal care and home management tasks.

Gag Rule : Regulations that barred physicians and nurses in clinics receiving federal funds from counselling clients about abortions.

Gatekeeper : Those who control, both formally and informally, the political climate of the community.

General Adaptation Syndrome (GAS) : The complex physiological responses resulting from exposure to stressors that can in time result in health deficits.

General Fertility Rate : Number of livebirths per thousand women in the reproductive age (15-45) in a given year.

Geriatrics : The branch of medicine that deals with the structural changes, physiology, diseases, and hygiene of old age.

Gerontology : The study of aging, from the broadest perspective.

Global Warming : The gradual increase in the earth's surface temperature.

Government Hospital : One that is supported and managed by governmental jurisdictions.

Grass-roots Community Organizing : A process that begins with those affected by the problem/concern.

Greenhouse Effect : The tapping of heat in the atmosphere by greenhouse gases.

Greenhouse Gases : Atmospheric gases, principally carbon dioxide, the CFCs, methane, and nitrous oxide, that are transparent to visible light but absorb infrared radiation (heat).

Gross Reproductive Rate (GRP) : Number of girls that would be born to a woman if she experiences the current fertility pattern throughout her reproductive span (15-45) assuming no mortality.

Groundwater : Water located under the surface of the ground.

Group Model HMO : See staff model HMO.

Hallucinogens : Drugs that produce profound distortions of the senses.

Hard-to-reach Population : Those in a target population that are not easily reached by normal programming efforts.

Hazard : An unsafe act or condition.

Hazardous waste : A solid waste or combination of solid wastes which—because of its quantity, concentration, or physical, chemical, or infectious characteristics—may : (A) cause or significantly contribute to an increase in mortality or an increase in serious irreversible, or incapacitating reversible, illness; or (B) pose a substantial present or potential hazard to human health or the environment when improperly treated, stored, transported, or disposed of, or otherwise managed.

Health : A dynamic state or condition which is multidimensional in nature and results from a person's adaptations to his/her environment; it is a resource for living and exists in varying degrees.

Health Care Financing Administration (HCFA) : An operating division of the DHHS that oversees the expenditure of all federal monies appropriated for health care services.

Health Education : "Any combination of planned learning experience based on sound theories that provide individuals, groups, and communities the opportunity to acquire information and the skills to make quality health decisions".

Health Maintenance Organization (HMOS) : Groups that supply prepaid comprehensive health care with an emphasis on prevention.

Health Physicist : A safety professional with responsibility for monitoring radiation within the plant environment, developing instrumentation for the purpose, and developing plans for coping with radiation accidents.

Health Promotion (HP) : "As any planned combination of educational.

Health Promotion Programme (HPP) : A programme aimed at improving the health of the target population through changes in behaviour and lifestyle. Health Resources and Services Administration (HRSA). An operating division of the DHHS established in 1982 to improve the nation's health resources and services and their distribution to underserved populations. It is part of the Public Health Service.

Health Resources Development Period : The period in public health history from 1900 to 1960; a time of great growth in health care facilities.

Health School Environment : "The promotion, maintenance, and utilization of safe and wholesome surroundings, organization of day-by-day experiences and planned learning procedures to influence favourable emotional, physical and social health" (see Chapter 6, reference 25).

Healthy People 2010 : The third set of health goals and objectives for that defines the nation's health agenda and guides its health policy.

Herbicide : A pesticide designed specifically to kill plants.

Herd Immunity : The resistance of a population to the spread of an infectious agent based on the immunity of a high portion of individuals.

Heroin : The most widely abused narcotic drug, a derivative of morphine and a schedule 1 drug.

Home Health Care : Care that is provided in the patient's residence for the purpose of promoting maintaining, or restoring health.

Home Health Care Services : Health care services provided in the patient's place of residence (home or apartment).

Homebound : A person unable to leave home for normal activities such as shopping, meals, or other activities.

Hospital Survey and Construction Act of 1946 (Hill-Burton Act) : Federal legislation that provided substantial funds for hospital construction.

Host : A person or other living animal that affords subsistence or lodgment to a communicable agent under natural conditions.

Hydrologic Cycle : The endless movement of water from the earth's surface to the atmosphere and back to the earth's surface.

Hypercholesterolaemia : High levels of cholesterol in the blood.

Hyperendemic : A persistent intense transmission of infectious disease or agent in a given community.

Hypertension : A chronic condition characterized by a resting blood pressure reading of 140/90 mm of mercury or higher.

Illegal Alien : An individual who entered this country without permission.

Illicit (illegal) Drugs : Drugs that cannot be legally manufactured, distributed, bought, or sold and that lack recognized medical value.

Immigrant : Individuals who migrate to this country from another country for the purpose of seeking permanent residence.

Impairments : Defects in the functioning of one's sense organs or limitations in one's mobility or range of motion.

Implementation : Putting a planned programme into action.

Imunoglobulins : All types of proteins with antibody activity.

Incidence Rate : The number of new cases of a disease in a population-at-risk during a particular period of time, divided by the total number in the same population.

Incineration : The burning of solid wastes.

Incubation Period : The period of time between exposure to an infectious agent and the onset of symptoms.

Independent Practice Association (IPA) Model HMO : An HMO in which individual physicians contract with the HMO to provide care for a certain number of enrollees.

Independent Providers : Health care professionals with the education and legal authority to treat any health problem.

Indian Health Service (IHS) : An operating division of the DHHS whose goal is to raise the health status of the American Indian and Alaska Native to the highest possible level by providing a comprehensive health services delivery system. It is a part of the Public Health Service.

Indirect Transmission : Communicable disease transmission involving an intermediate step; for example, air-borne, vehicle-borne, or vector-borne transmission.

Indoor Air Pollution : The build-up of undesirable gases and particles in the air inside a building.

Industrial Hygienist : A health professional concerned with health hazards in the workplace, including such things as problems with ventilation, noise and lighting; also responsible for measuring air quality and with recommending plans for improving the healthiness of work environments.

Infant Mortality Rate : The number of deaths of children under one year of age per 1,000 live-births.

Infants Death (infant mortality) : Death of a child under one year of age.

Infants Mortality Rate : Number of infants (0-1 yr) in a given year per live births of the year.

Infection : The lodgment and growth of a virus or microorganism in a host organism.

Infectious Disease : See communicable diseases.

Infectivity : The ability of a pathogen to lodge and grow in a host.

Informal Caregiver : One who provides unpaid care or assistance to one who has some physical, mental, emotional, or financial need that limits his or her independence.

Inhalants : Breathable substances that produce mind altering effects; for example, glue.

Injury : Physical harm or damage to the body resulting from an exchange, usually acute, of mechanical, chemical, thermal, or other environmental energy that exceeds the body's tolerance.

Injury Prevention (control) : An organized effort to prevent injuries or to minimize their severity.

Injury Prevention Education : The process of changing people's health-directed behaviour in such a way as to reduce unintentional injuries.

Insecticides : Pesticides designed specifically to kill insects.

Insidious : Slow and secret onset of disease in the body.

Instrumental Activities of Daily Living (IADL): Measure of more complex tasks such as handling personal finances, preparing meals, shopping, doing homework, travelling, using the telephone, and taking needs.

Integrated Instruction : Pattern of instruction in which a certain subject matter is the vehicle used to teach other subjects.

Intensity : Cardiovascular workload measured by heart rate.

Intentional Injury : An injury that is judged to have been purposely inflicted, either by the victim or another.

Intermediate Host : Those hosts in which parasites are in a larval or asexual stage are intermediate hosts.

Intern : A first year resident.

Internal Radiation : Radiation in the human body that occurs as a result of ingesting food or inhaling air.

Intervention : An activity or activities designed to create change in people.

Intimate Partner Violence (IPV) : Rape, physical assault, or stalking perpetrated by current or former dates, spouses, or cohabiting partners, with cohabiting meaning living together at least some of the time as a couple.

Isolation : The separation of infected persons from those who are susceptible.

Joint Commission on Accreditation of Health Care : Organizations (JCAHC). The predominate organization responsible for accrediting health care facilities.

Labor-force Support Ratio : A ratio of the total number of those individuals who are not working (regardless of age) to the number of those who are.

Lag Phase : Initial phase of the population growth S-curve, when growth is slow.

Leachates : Liquids created when water mixes with wastes and removes soluble constituents from them by percolation.

Lead : A naturally occurring mineral element found throughout the environment and is produced in large quantities for industrial products.

Licensed Practical Nurse (LPN) : Those prepared in one-to two-year programmes to provide nontechnical bedside nursing care under the supervision of physicians or registered nurses.

Life-expectancy : The average number of years a person from a specific cohort is projected to live from a given point in time.

Limited (restricted) Care Providers : Health care providers who provide care for a specific part of the body; for example, dentists.

Limited-service Hospitals : Hospital that offer only the specific services needed by the population served.

Litigation : The process of seeking justice for injury through courts.

Long-term Care : Different kinds of help that people with chronic illnesses, disabilities, or other conditions need to deal with the circumstances that limit them physically or mentally.

Low Birth-weight Infant : An infant that weighs less than 2,500 grams, or 5.5 pounds, at birth.

Low Enforcement : The application of federal, state, and local laws to arrest, jail, bring to trial, and sentence those who break drug laws or break laws because of drug use.

Lyme Disease : A systematic bacterial, tick-borne disease with symptoms that include dermatologic, arthritic, neurologic, and cardiac abnormalities.

Mainstream Tobacco Smoke : The smoke of burning tobacco inhaled and exhaled by the smoker.

Major Depression : An affective mental disorder characterized by a dysphonic mood, usually depression, or loss of interest or pleasure in almost all usual activities or pastimes.

Majority : Those with characteristics that are found in the over 50 per cent of a population.

Malignant Neoplasm : Uncontrolled new tissue growth resulting from cells that have lost control over their growth and division mental health care services.

Managed Care : Health plans that integrate the financing and delivery of health care services to covered individual by means of arrangements with selected providers to furnish comprehensive services to members; explicit criteria for the selection of health care providers; significant financial incentives for members to use providers and procedures associated with the plan; and formal programmes for quality assurance and utilization review.

Marijuana : Dried plant parts of Cannabis sativa.

Maternal Morality : The death of a woman while pregnant or within 42 days of termination of pregnancy, irrespective of the duration and the site of the pregnancy, from any cause related to or aggravated by the pregnancy or its management.

Maternal Mortality : Death of women during pregnancy or within 42 day of termination of pregnancy for any maternal cause, but not from accident or incidental cause.

Maternal Mortality Rate : No. of women during reproductive age (15-45) due to maternal cause per 1000 livebirths.

Maternal Mortality Rate : Number of mothers dying per 100,000 livebirths in a given year.

Maternal, Infant and Child Health : The health of women of childbearing age from pre-pregnancy, through pregnancy, labour and delivery, and the postpartum period and the health of the child prior to birth through adolescence.

Meals-on-Wheels Programme : A community supported nutrition programme in which prepared meals are delivered to elders in their homes, usually by volunteers.

Medicaid : A national health insurance programme for the poor.

Medicare : A national health insurance programme for people 65 years of age and older, certain younger disabled people, and people with permanent kidney failure.

Medigap : Private health insurance to supplement medicare benefits—that is, to fill in the gaps of medicare.

Mental Disorder : Deficiency in one's psychological resources for dealing with everyday life, usually characterized by distress or impairment of one or more areas of functioning.

Mental Health : Emotional and social well-being, including one's psychological resources for dealing with the day-to-day problems of life.

Mental Hygiene Movement : A movement by those who believed that mental illness could be cured if identified and treated at an early stage; proponents were Adolph Meyer and Clifford Beers.

Mental Illness : A collective term for all mental disorders.

Metastasis : The spread of a disease, such as cancer, by the transfer of cells by means of the blood or lymphatics.

Methamphetamine : The amphetamine drug most widely abused.

Methcathinone ("cat") : An illicit, synthetic drug, similar to the amphetamines, that first appeared in the United States in 1991.

Migration : Movement of people from one country to another.

Minority Groups : Subgroups of the population that consist of less than 50 per cent of the population.

Minority Health : The morbidity and mortality of American Indians / Alaska Natives, Asian Americans and Pacific Islanders, black Americans, and Americans of Hispanic origin in the United States.

Model for Unintentional Injuries : The public health triangle (host, agent, and environment) modified to indicate energy as the causative agent of injuries.

Modern Era of Public Health : The era of American public health that began in 1850 and continues today.

Modifiable Risk Factor : Factors contributing to the development of a noncommunicable disease that can be altered by modifying one's behaviour or environment; for example, cigarette smoking is a modifiable risk factor for coronary heart disease.

Moral Treatment : Treatment for mental illness in eighteenth and nineteenth centuries, based on belief that mental illness was caused by moral deterioration.

Morbidity Rate : The rate of illness in a population.

Mortality (fatality) Rate : The rate of deaths in a population.

Multicausation Disease Model : A visual representation of the host, together with various internal and external factors that promote and protect against disease.

Municipal Solid Waste : Waste generated by individual households, businesses, and institutions located within municipalities.

Narcotics : Drugs similar to morphine that reduce pain and induce a stuporous state.

Natality (birth) Rate : The rate of births in a population.

National Alliance for the Mentally Ill (NAMI) : A national voluntary health agency that advocates for the mentally ill.

National Ambient Air Quality Standards (NAAQSs) : Standards created by the EPA for allowable concentration levels of outdoor air pollutants.

National Institute for Mental Health (NIMH) : The agency of the National Institutes of Health whose mission is to conduct research on the causes of and treatments for mental disorders.

National Institute for Occupational Safety and Health (NIOSH) : A research body within the centers for Disease Control and Prevention, Department of Health and Human Services, that is responsible for developing and recommending occupational safety and health standards.

National Institute on Drug Abuse (NIDA) : The Federal Government's lead agency for drug abuse research, of the National Institutes of Health.

National Institutes of Health (NIH) : The Federal Government's lead agency for drug abuse research, of the National Institutes of Health and also the research division of the DHHS. It is a part of the Public Health Service.

National Mental Health Association (NMHA) : A national voluntary health association that advocates for mental health and for those with mental illnesses; it has 600 affiliates in 43 states.

Natural Hazards : Conditions of nature that increase the probability of disease, injury or death of humans.

Need Assessment : The process of collecting and analyzing information, to develop an understanding of the issues resources, and constraints of the target population, as related to the development of HP / DP programmes (Chapter 5, reference 20).

Neonatal Death (neonatal mortality) : Deaths occurring during the first 28 days after birth.

Neonatologist : A medical doctor who specializes in the care of newborns from birth to two months of age.

Net Migration : The population gain or loss resulting from migration.

Net Reproductive Rate (NRR) : Number of daughters a newborn girl will bear during her lifetime, assuming a fixed age specific fertility and mortality rate.

Neuroleptic Drug : A drug that reduces nervous activity; another term for antipsychotic drug.

Noise Pollution : Excessive sound.

Nonallopathic Providers : Independent providers who provide nontraditional forms of health care.

Noncommunicable Disease (noninfectious disease) : A disease not caused by a communicable agent, and that thus cannot be transmitted from infected host to susceptible host.

Nontarget Organisms : All other susceptible organisms in the environment, for which a pesticide was not intended.

Notifiable Diseases : Any abnormal condition or disorder, other than one resulting from an occupational injury, caused by an exposure to environmental factors associated with employment.

Occupational Health Nurse (OHN) : A registered nurse whose primary responsibilities include prevention of illness and promotion of health in the workplace.

Occupational Injury : An injury that results from exposure to a single incident in the work environment (*e.g.*, cut, fracture, sprain, amputation).

Occupational Safety and Health Act of 1970 (OSHAct) : Comprehensive federal legislation aimed at assuring safe and healthful working conditions for working men and women.

Occupational Safety and Health Administration (OSHA) : The federal agency located within the Department of Labour and created by the OSHAct that is charged with the responsibility of administering the provisions of the OSHAct.

Odds ratio : A probability statement about the association between a particular disease and a specific risk factor, often the outcome of a retrospective (case/control) study.

Office of National Drug Control Policy (ONDCP) : The headquarters of America's drug control effort, located in the executive branch of the Federal Government, and headed by a director appointed by the President.

Official Health Agency : See governmental health agency.

Old : Those who are 65 years of age and older.

Old Old : Those who are 75 to 84 years of age.

Older Americans Act of 1965 : Federal legislation to improve the lives of elders.

Oldest Old : Those who are 85 years of age and older.

Operationalize (operational definition) : Provide working definitions.

Osteopathic Providers : Independent health care providers whose remedies emphasize the interrelationships of the body's systems in prevention, diagnosis, and treatment.

Outside Community Organization : Organization efforts that begin with individuals from outside the affected community.

Over-the-counter (OTC) Drugs (nonprescription drugs) : Drugs (Except tobacco and alcohol) that can be legally purchased without a physician's prescription; example, aspirin.

Ownership : A feeling that one has a stake in or "owns" the object of interest.

Ozone Layer : Ozone gas (O_3) found in the stratosphere.

Pandemic Disease : An epidemic over a wide geographical area or even worldwide.

Pandemic : An outbreak of disease over a wide geographical area, such as a continent.

Parity : The concept of equality in health care coverage for people with mental illness and those with other medical illnesses or injuries.

Passive Smoking : The inhalation of environmental tobacco smoke by nonsmokers.

Pathogenicity : The capability of a communicable agent to cause disease in a susceptible host.

Per Counselling Programmes : School-based drug education programmes in which students discuss alcohol and other drug-related problems with other students.

Pest : Any organism—multicelled animal or plant, or microbe—that has an adverse effect on human interests.

Pesticides : Synthetic chemicals developed and manufactured for the purpose of killing pests.

Phasing in : Implementation of an intervention with small groups prior to the implementation with the entire target population.

Philanthropic Foundation : An endowed institution that donates money for the good of humankind.

Photochemical Smog : A secondary air pollutant created when primary pollutants react with oxygen and sunlight.

Physical Dependence : Drug dependence in which discontinued use results in the onset of physical illness.

Physician-hospital Organization (PHO) : Various agreements between physicians and hospitals to form units to negotiate with insurers as managed care organizations.

Pilot Test : Presentation of the intervention to just a few individuals, who are either from the intended target population or from a very similar population.

Placebo : A blank treatment (*e.g.*, a sugar pill).

Pneumoconiosis : Fibrotic lung disease caused by the inhalation of dusts, especially mineral dusts.

Point Source Epidemic Curve : An epidemic curve depicting a distribution of cases that can all be traced to a single source of exposure.

Point Source Pollution : Pollution that can be traced to a single identifiable source.

Point-of-service (POS) Option : An option of a health maintenance organization plan that allows enrollees to be at least partially reimbursed for selecting a health care provider outside the plan.

Pollutant Standard Index (PSI) : A scale developed by the EPA which relates air pollutant concentrations to health effects.

Polydrug Use : Concurrent use of multiple drugs.

Population Health : The health status of people who are not organized and have no identity as a group or locality and the actions and conditions to promote, protect and preserve their health.

Population-at-risk : Those in the population who are susceptible to a particular disease or condition.

Postneonatal Deaths (postneonatal mortality) : Deaths that occur between 28 days and 365 days after birth.

Pre-existing Condition : A medical condition that had been diagnosed or treated usually within six months. Before the date a health insurance policy goes into effect.

Preferred Provider Organization (PPO) : An organization that buys fixed-rate (discount) health services from providers and sells them (via premiums) to consumers.

Premature Infant : One born following a gestation period of 38 weeks or less, or one born at a low birth weight.

Prenatal Health Care (prenatal care) : One of the fundamentals of a safe motherhood programme and includes three major components: risk assessment, treatment for medical conditions or risk reductions, and education. Prenatal health care should begin before pregnancy when a couple is considering having a child and continue throughout pregnancy.

Prepaid Health Care : A method of paying for covered health care services on a pre-person premium basis for a specific period of time prior to service being rendered. Also referred to as capitation.

Pre-placement Examination : A physical examination of a newly hired or transferred worker to determine medical suitability for placement in a specific position.

Prevalence Rate : The number of new and old cases of a disease in a population in a given period of time, divided by the total number of that population.

Prevention : The planning for and taking of action to forestall the onset of a disease or other health problem before the occurrence of undesirable health events.

Preventive Care : Care given to healthy people to keep them healthy.

Primary Medical Care : The provision of integrated, accessible health care services by clinicians who are accountable for addressing a large majority of personal health care needs, developing a sustained partnership with patients, and practicing in the context of family and community.

Primary Prevention : Preventive measures that forestall the onset of illness or injury during the prepathogenesis period.

Private (proprietary) Hospitals : For-profit hospitals.

Problem Drinker : One for whom alcohol consumption results in personal, economic, medical, social, or any other type of problem.

Pro-choice : A medical/ethical position that holds that women have a right to reproductive freedom.

Professional Nurse : A registered nurse holding a bachelor of science degree in nursing (BSN).

Programme Planning : A process by which an intervention is planned to help meet the needs of a target population.

Programme Support Center : An operating division of the DHHS established in 1995 to provide cost effective, efficient, and responsive administrative support to the DHHS and other Federal agencies.

Prolife : A medical/ethical position that holds that performing an abortion is an act of murder.

Propagated Epidemic Curve : An epidemic curve depicting a distribution of cases traceable to multiple sources of exposure over time.

Proportionate Mortality Ratio (PMR) : The percentage of overall mortality in a population that can be assigned to a particular cause or disease.

Prospective Pricing System (PPS) : One in which providers are paid predetermined amounts of money per procedure for services provided.

Prospective Study : An epidemiological study that begins in the present and continues into the future for the purpose of observing the development of disease (*e.g.*, cohort study).

Providers : Those individuals educated to provide health services, such as physicians, dentists, nurses, etc.

Psychoactive Drugs : Mind-altering drugs; drugs that affect the central nervous system.

Psychological Dependence : A psychological state characterized by an overwhelming desire to continue use of a drug.

Psychopharmacological Therapy : Treatment for mental illness that involves medications.

Psychotherapy : A treatment methodology based on the Freudian concept of emotional (catharsis) release, sexual conflict resolution, and subconscious drives.

Public Health : The health status of a defined group of people and the governmental actions and conditions to promote, protect and preserve their health.

Public Health Practice : Incorporates interventions aimed at disease prevention and health promotion, specific protection, and case findings.

Public Health Professional : A health care worker who works in a public health organization.

Public Health Service (PHS) : An agency in the Department of Health and Human Services (HHS) that is comprised of eight of the 12 operating divisions of HHS.

Public Hospitals : Hospitals that are supported and managed by governmental jurisdictions.

Public Policy : The guiding principles and courses of action pursued by governments to solve practical problems affecting society.

Quarantine : Limitation of freedom of movement of those who have been exposed to a disease and may be incubating it.

Quasi-governmental Health Organizations : Organizations that have some responsibilities assigned by the government but operate more like voluntary agencies; for example, the American Red Cross.

Radiation : Energy released when an atom is solid or naturally decays from less stable to a more stable form.

Radon : A naturally occurring radioactive gas that cannot be seen, smelled, or tasted.

Rate : The number of events (cases of disease) that occur in a given period of time.

Recycling : The collection and reprocessing of a resource after use so it can be reused for the same or another purpose.

Reform Phase of Public Health : The period of public health from 1900 to 1920, characterized by social movements to improve health conditions in cities and in the workplace.

Refugee : A person who flees one area or country to seek shelter or protection from danger in another.

Registered Nurse (RN) : An associate or baccalaureate degree-prepared nurse who has passed the state licensing examination.

Regulation : The enactment and enforcement of laws to control conduct.

Rehabilitation Centre : A facility in which restorative care is provided following injury, disease, or surgery.

Relative Risk : A statement of the relationship between the risk of acquiring a disease when a specific risk factor is present and the risk of acquiring that same disease when the risk factor is not present.

Rem (roentgen equivalent man) : A measure of the biological damage of radiation to human tissues.

Resident : A physician who is training in a specialty.

Residues and Wastes : Unwanted by-products of human activities.

Resource Conservation and Recovery Act of 1976 (RCRA) : A federal law that sets forth guidelines for the proper handling and disposal of solid and hazardous wastes.

Respite Care : Planned short-term care, usually for the purpose of relieving a full-time informal caregiver.

Restorative Care : Care provided to patients after a successful treatment or when the progress of a incurable disease has been arrested.

Retirement Communities : Residential communities that have been specifically developed for those in their retire.

Retrospective Study : An epidemiological study that looks into the past for clues to explain the present distribution of disease.

Risk Factors : Factors that increase the probability of disease, injury, or death.

Roe vs. Wade : A 1973 Supreme Court decision that made it unconstitutional for state laws to prohibit abortions.

Rohypnol (flunitrazepam) : A depressant in the benzodiazepine group that has achieved notoriety as a date rape drug.

Rollover Protective Structures (ROPSs) : Factory-installed or retrofitted reinforced framework on a cab to protect the operator of in case of a rollover.

Safe Drinking Water Act (SDWA) : A 1974 federal law that instructed the EPA to set maximum contaminant levels for specific pollutants in drinking water.

Safety Engineer : A health and safety professional, sometimes with an engineering background, employed by a company for the purpose of reducing unintentional injuries in the workplace.

Safety Programme : The part of the workplace health and safety programme aimed at reducing unintentional injuries at the job.

Sanitarians : Environmental workers responsible for inspection of restaurants, retail food outlets, public housing, and other facilities to assure compliance with public health codes.

Sanitary Engineer : Environmental worker responsible for management of waste water and solid waste for a community.

Sanitary Landfill : A waste disposal site located on land suited for this purpose and pon which solid waste is spread in thin layers and covered with a fresh layer of soil.

School Health Coordinator : Person who co-ordinates the school health programme for a school district.

School Health Education : "Planned, sequential, K-12 curriculum that addresses the physical, mental, emotional and social dimensions of health. The curriculum is designed to motivate and assist students to maintain and improve their health, prevent disease, and reduce health-related risk behaviours" (Chapter 6, reference 19).

School Health Policies : Written statements that describe the nature and procedures of a school health programme.

School Health Services : Health services provided by school health workers to appraise, protect and promote the health of students and school personnel.

School Health Team : Those individuals who work together to plan and implement the school health programme.

Scope : Part of the curriculum that outlines what will be taught.

Screening : Investigating person's history to identify one's who require care.

Secondary Medical Care : Specialized attention and ongoing management for common and less frequently encountered medical conditions, including support services for people with special challenges due to chronic or long-term conditions.

Secondary Prevention : Preventive measures that lead to early diagnosis and prompt treatment of a disease or injury to limit disability and prevent more severe pathogenesis.

Second-hand Smoke : Environmental tobacco smoke (ETS); tobacco smoke in the ambient air that can be inhaled.

Secured Landfill : A double-lined landfill located above flood plain and away from a fault zone, equipped with monitoring pipes for seepage, used primarily for hazardous waste.

Self-help Support Groups : Groups of concerned citizens who are united by shared interest, concern, or deficit not shared by other members of the community; alcoholics Anonymous, for example.

Self-insured Organization : One that pays the health care costs of its employees with the premiums collected from the employees and the contributions made by the employer.

Senior Centers : Facilities where seniors can congregate for fellowship, meals, education, and recreation.

Septic Tank : A watertight concrete or fibreglass tank that holds sewage; one of two main part of a septic system.

Sequence : Part of the curriculum that states in what order the content will be taught.

Service Demands : Things that those in the target population believe they must have or be able to do in order to solve a problem.

Service Needs : Needs that health professionals believe the target population must have fulfilled in order to resolve a problem.

Sick Building Syndrome : A term to describe a situation in which the air quality in a building produces generalized signs and symptoms of ill health in the building's occupants.

Sidestream Tobacco Smoke : The smoke that comes off the end of burning tobacco products.

Silicosis : Acute or chronic lung disease caused by the inhalation of free crystalline silica; those affected include workers in mines, stone quarries, sand and gravel operations, and abrasive blasting operations.

Sliding Scale Fee : A fee based on ability to pay.

Sludge : A semi-solid mixture of solid waste that includes bacteria, viruses, organic matter, toxic metals, synthetic organic chemicals, and solid chemicals.

Smokeless Tabacco (spit tobacco) : Snuff and chewing tobacco.

Social Security Administration (SSA) : An independent federal agency that administers programmes that provide financial support to special groups of Americans.

Socio-economic Status : A demographic term which takes into consideration the combination of social and economic factors.

Solid Waste : Solid refuse from households, agriculture, and businesses, including garbage, yard waste, paper products, manure, excess stone generated from mining, and building material scraps.

Solid Waste Management : The collection, transportation and disposal of solid waste.

Sound-level Meter : Instrument used to measure sound.

Source Reduction : A waste management approach entailing the reduction or elimination of use of materials that produce an accumulation of solid waste.

Special Supplemental Food Programme for Women, Infants, and Children : See WIC.

Specific Rate : A rate of a specific disease in a population or the rate of events in a specific population (*e.g.,* cause-specific death rate, age-specific death rate).

Spectrum of Health Care Deliver : The array of types of care—from preventive to continuing, or long-term, care. It comprises six levels of care.

Spiritual Era of Public Health : A time during the Middle Age when the causation of communicable disease was linked to spiritual forces.

Staff Model HMO : A health maintenance organization that hires its own staff of health care providers.

Standard of Acceptability : A comparative mandate, value, norm, or group.

Standard Precautions : Disease prevention guidelines for health care workers and other who may come in contact with human body fluids, which involve the use of appropriate barriers to reduce or eliminate exposure to these fluids.

State Children's Health Insurance Programme (SCHIP) : A title insurance programme under the Social Security Act that provides health insurance to uninsured children.

State Implementation Plans (SIPs) : Documents submitted by each state to the EPA outlining their plan for achieving and maintaining air-quality standards.

Stimulant : A drug that increases the activity of the central nervous system; for example, methamphetamine.

Student Assis Programmes (SAPs) : School-based drug education programmes to assist students who have alcohol or other drug problems.

Substance Abuse and Mental Health Services Administration (SAMHSA) : An operating division of the DHHS, whose stated mission is the reduction of the incidence and prevalence of alcohol and other drug abuse and mental disorders, the improvement of treatment outcomes, and the curtailment of the consequences of mental health problems for families and communities. It is part of the Public Health Service.

Sudden Infant Death Syndrome (SIDS) : Sudden unanticipated death of an infant in whom, after examination, there is no recognized cause of death.

Summative Evaluation : The evaluation that determines the impact of a programme on the target population.

Superfund Legislation : See Comprehensive Environmental Response, Compensation, and Liability Act.

Supplemental Security : Programme of the Social Security Administration that provides cash benefits to elderly, blind, and disabled with minimal resources.

Support Ratio : A ratio that compares the number of individuals whom society considers economically productive (the working population) to the number of those it considers economically unproductive (the nonworking or dependent population).

Surface Water : Water that is found on the earth's surface (*e.g.*, oceans, rivers, streams, ponds, lakes, etc.).

Survey of Occupational Injuries and Illnesses (SOII) : An annual survey of injuries and illnesses from a large sample of U.S. employees (approximately 250,000) maintained by the Bureau of Labour Statistics in the Department of Labour.

Synar Amendment : A federal law that requires states to set the minimum legal age for purchasing tobacco products at 18 years and that requires states to enforce this law.

Synesthesia : Impairment of mind (by hallucinogens), characterized by a sensation that senses are mixed (*e.g.*, seeing sounds and hearing images).

Tardive Dyskinesia : Irreversible, involuntary, and abnormal movements of the tongue, mouth, arms and legs which can result from long-term use of certain antipsychotic drugs such as chlorpromazine.

Target Organism (target pest) : The organism for which a pesticide is applied.

Target Population (audience) : Those whom a planned programme is intended to serve.

Technical Nurse : An associate degree-prepared registered nurse.

Terrestrial Radiation : Radiation that comes from radioactive minerals within the earth.

Third-party Payment System : A health insurance term indicating that bills will be paid by the insurer (the government or private insurance company) and not the patient (first party) or the health care provider (the second party).

Thorazine : See chlorpromazine.

Title X : A portion of the Public Health Service Act of 1970, that provides funds for family planning services for low-income people.

Tolerance : Physiological and enzymatic adjustments that occur in response to the chronic presence of drugs, reflected in the need for ever-increasing doses to achieve a previous level of effect.

Unsafe Act : Any behaviour that would increase the probability of an injury occurring.

Unsafe Condition : Any environmental factor or set of factors (physical or social) that would increase the probability of an injury occurring.

Urbanization : The process by which people come together to live in cities.

Utilization Review or Utilization Management : Provided health care is analyzed by someone other than the patient and provider for its appropriateness.

Vector : A living organism, usually an arthropod, that can transmit a communicable disease agent to a susceptible host (e.g., mosquitoes, ticks, lice, fleas).

Vector-borne Disease : A communicable disease transmitted by insects or other arthropods; for example, St. Louis encephalitis.

Vector-borne-disease Outbreak (VBDO) : The occurrence of two or more cases of a vector-borne disease.

Vehical : Inanimate materials or objects, such as clothes, bedding, toys, hypodermic needles; or nonliving biological materials such as food, milk, water, blood, serum or plasma, tissues or organs, that can serve as a source of infection.

Vehicle-borne Disease : A communicable disease transmitted by nonliving objects; for example, typhoid fever can be transmitted by water.

Visitor Services : A community social service involving one individual taking time to visit with another who is unable to leave his/her residence.

Vital Statistics : Statistical summaries of vital records—records of major life events, such as births, deaths, marriages, divorces, and infant deaths.

Volatile Organic Compounds (VOCs) : Compounds that exist as vapours over the normal range of air pressures and temperatures.

Voluntary (independent) Hospital : A nonprofit hospital administered by religious, fraternal, and other charitable community organizations.

Voluntary Health Agency : A nonprofit organization created by concerned citizens to deal with health needs not met by governmental health agencies.

Waste Water : The aqueous mixture that remains after water has been used or contaminated by humans.

Waste-to-energy (WTE) Plants : Incinerators that are able to convert some heat generated from the burning of solid waste into steam and electricity.

Water Pollution : Any physical or chemical change in water that can harm living organisms or make the water unfit for other uses.

Water-borne Disease : A disease that is transmitted through contamination of water.

Water-borne-disease Outbreak (WBDO) : The occurrence of two or more cases of a similar illness resulting from the ingestion of drinking water or after exposure to water used for recreational purposes and epidemiological evidence that implicates water as the probable source of illness.

WIC (also known as the Special Supplemental Food Programme for Women, Infants, and Children) : A federal programme sponsored by the United States Department of Agriculture designed to provide supplemental foods, nutrition and health education, and referrals for health and social services to improve the health of at-risk, economically disadvantaged woman who are pregnant or are caring for infants and children under age of five.

Worker's Compensation Laws : A set of federal laws designed to compensate those workers and their families who suffer injuries, disease, or death from workplace exposure.

World Health Assembly : Body of delegates of the member nations of the World Health Organization.

World Health Organization (WHO) : Most widely recognized international governmental health organization today. Created in 1948 by representatives of United Nations countries.

Years of Potential Life Lost (YPLL) : The number of years lost when death occurs before the age of 65 or 75.

Young Old : Those 65 to 74 years of age.

Youth Gang : A self-formed association of peers, bound together by mutual interests, with identifiable leadership and well-defined lines of authority, who act in concert to achieve a specific purpose and whose acts generally include illegal activity and control over a territory or an enterprise.

Zero Population Growth (ZPG) : A state in which the birth and death rates for a given population are equal.

Zoonosis : A communicable disease transmissible under natural conditions from vertebrate animals to man.

●●●

Index

D